# FIGHTING
# SUDDEN CARDIAC DEATH

◆

# A Worldwide Challenge

*edited by*

**Etienne Aliot, MD, FESC, FACC**
*Chief, Department of Cardiology*
*Central Hospital*
*University of Nancy*
*Nancy, France*

**Jacques Clémenty, MD, FESC**
*Chief, Department of Cardiology*
*Haut-Levêque Hospital*
*University of Bordeaux*
*Bordeaux, France*

**Eric N. Prystowsky, MD, FACC**
*Director, Clinical Electrophysiology Laboratory*
*St. Vincent Hospital*
*Indianapolis, Indiana;*
*Consulting Professor of Medicine*
*Duke University Medical Center*
*Durham, North Carolina*

Futura Publishing Co., Inc.
Armonk, New York

Library of Congress Cataloging-in-Publication Data

Fighting sudden cardiac death : a worldwide challenge / edited by Etienne Aliot,
Jacques Clementy, Eric N. Prystowsky.
    p. ; cm.
  Includes bibliographical references and index.
  ISBN 0-87993-460-3
    1. Cardiac arrest. I. Aliot, Etienne. II. Clementy, Jacques. III. Prystowsky,
Eric N.
[DNLM: 1. Death, Sudden, Cardiac. WG 205 F471 2000]
RC685.C173 F54 2000
616.1'23—dc21

                                            00-037655

*Published by*
Futura Publishing Company
135 Bedford Road
Armonk, New York 10504

LC#: 00-037655
ISBN#: 0-87993-460-3

Every effort has been made to ensure that the information in this book is as up to
date and accurate as possible at the time of publication. However, due to the constant developments in medicine neither the author, nor the editors, nor the publisher can accept any legal or any other responsibility for any errors or omissions
that may occur.

Printed in the United States on acid-free paper.

*This book is dedicated to our patients,
nurses, and to*

*Chris, wife of Etienne Aliot, MD,
and children, Delphine, Sophie, and Romain;
Anne, wife of Jacques Clémenty, MD,
and children, Sebastien and Nicolas;
Bonnie, wife of Eric N. Prystowsky, MD,
and children, David and Daniel.*

# Contributors

**Etienne Aliot, MD**
*Chief, Department of Cardiology, Central Hospital, University of Nancy, Nancy, France*

**Frederic Anselme, MD**
*Cardiology Service, Charles Nicolle Hospital, Rouen, France*

**Charles Antzelevitch, PhD**
*Masonic Medical Research Laboratory, Utica, New York*

**Dominique Babuty, MD, PhD**
*CHU Trousseau, Hôpitaux de Tours, Cardiology B and Laboratoire d'Electrophysiologie Cardiaque, Tours, France*

**Cristina Basso, MD, PhD**
*Institute of Pathological Anatomy, University of Padua Medical School, Padova, Italy*

**Henry Marc Becane, MD**
*Service de Cardiologie, Hôpital Cochin, Université René Descartes and Institut de Myologie Hôpital de la Salpetriere, Paris, France*

**Lance B. Becker, MD**
*Section of Emergency Medicine, Department of Medicine, The University of Chicago, Chicago, Illinois*

**Omer Berenfeld, PhD**
*Department of Pharmacology, SUNY Health Science Center, Syracuse, New York*

**Jean-Jacques Blanc, MD**
*Professor of Cardiology, Head, Department Cardiology, Brest University Hospital, Brest, France*

**Dirk Böcker, MD**
*The Hospital of the Westfälische Wilhelms-University, Department of Cardiology and Angiology and Institute for Arteriosclerosis Research, Münster, Germany*

**Gisele Bonne, PhD**
*Service de Cardiologie, Hôpital Cochin, Université René Descartes and Institut de Myologie Hôpital de la Salpetriere, Paris, France*

**Martin Borggrefe, MD**
*The Hospital of the Westfälische Wilhelms-University, Department of Cardiology and Angiology and Institute for Arteriosclerosis Research, Münster, Germany*

**Leo Bossaert, MD**
*Executive Director European Resuscitation Council, University of Antwerp-Belgium, Antwerp, Belgium*

**Günter Breithardt, MD**
*The Hospital of the Westfälische Wilhelms-University, Department of Cardiology and Angiology and Institute for Arteriosclerosis Research, Münster, Germany*

**Josep Brugada, MD, PhD**
*Arrhythmia Unit, University of Barcelona, Barcelona, Spain*

**Pedro Brugada, MD, PhD**
*Professor of Cardiology, Cardiovascular Research and Teaching Institute Aalst, Cardiovascular Center, OLV Hospital, Aalst Hospital, Belgium*

**Ramon Brugada, MD**
*Cardiology Department, Baylor College of Medicine, Houston, Texas*

**Fiorella Calabrese, MD**
*Institute of Pathological Anatomy, University of Padua Medical School, Padova, Italy*

**Hugh Calkins, MD**
*Associate Professor of Medicine, Director of Electrophysiology, Division of Cardiology, Department of Medicine, The Johns Hopkins University School of Medicine, Baltimore, Maryland*

**A. John Camm, MD**
*Professor of Clinical Cardiology, Cardiological Sciences, St. George's Hospital Medical School, London, United Kingdom*

**Riccardo Cappato, MD**
*Medizinische Abteilung, AK St. Georg, Hamburg, Germany*

**Danielle Casset-Senon, PhD**
*Cardiology B Department and UMR CNRS 6542, Trousseau Hospital, Tours, France*

**Agustin Castellanos, MD**
*Division of Cardiology, University of Miami Medical Center, Miami, Florida*

**Maxime Chalumeau, MD**
*Cardiology Service, Charles Nicolle Hospital, Rouen, France*

**Jean-Christophe Charniot, MD**
*Cardiology B Department and UMR CNRS 6542, Trousseau Hospital Tours, France*

**Nipon Chattipakorn, MD, PhD**
*Cardiac Rhythm Management Lab, Division of Cardiovascular Disease, Department of Medicine, The University of Alabama at Birmingham, Birmingham, Alabama*

**Jay Chen, BSc**
*Department of Pharmacology, SUNY Health Science Center, Syracuse, New York*

**Jacques Clémenty, MD**
*Chief, Department of Cardiology, Haut-Levêque Hospital, University of Bordeaux, Bordeaux, France*

**X. Copie, MD**
*Department of Cardiology, Broussais Hospital, Pierre and Marie Curie University, Paris, France*

**Domenico Corrado, MD**
*Consultant Cardiologist, Institute of Pathological Anatomy, University of Padua, Padova, Italy*

**Pierre Cosnay, MD**
*CHU Trousseau, Hôpitaux de Tours, Cardiology B and Laboratoire d'Electrophysiologie Cardiaque, Tours, France*

**Philippe Coumel, MD**
*Department Head, Professor of Cardiology, Cardiology Department, Lariboisière University Hospital, Paris, France*

**Alain Cribier, MD**
*Cardiology Service, Charles Nicolle Hospital, Rouen, France*

**Lia Crotti, MD**
*Molecular Cardiology Laboratories, Fondazione Salvatore Maugeri IRCCS, Pavia, Italy*

**Michael Davies, MD**
*British Heart Foundation Professor of Cardiovascular Pathology, St. George's Hospital Medical School (University of London), London, United Kingdom*

**C. de Chillou, MD**
*Department of Cardiology, University of Nancy, Nancy, France*

**Michel de Lorgeril, MD**
*The French Centre National de la Recherche Scientifique (CNRS), Département des Sciences de la Vie, Paris, France*

**Jacqueline de Vreede-Swagemakers, MD**
*Department of Cardiology, Academic Hospital Maastricht, Maastricht, The Netherlands*

**S. Digeos-Hasnier, MD**
*Department of Cardiology, Broussais Hospital, Pierre and Marie Curie University, Paris, France*

**Denis Duboc, MD, PhD**
*Service de Cardiologie, Hôpital Cochin, Université René Descartes and Institut de Myologie Hôpital de la Salpetriere, Paris, France*

**Perry M. Elliott, MD**
*Lecturer, Department of Cardiological Sciences, St. George's Hospital Medical School, London, United Kingdom*

**Nabil El-Sherif, MD**
*Cardiology Division, Department of Medicine, State University of New York Health Science Center and Veterans Affairs Medical Center, Brooklyn, New York*

**Fabrice Extramiana, MD**
*Cardiology Department, Lariboisière University Hospital, Paris, France*

**Jean-Paul Fauchier, MD**
*CHU Trousseau, Hôpitaux de Tours, Cardiology B and Laboratoire d'Electrophysiologie Cardiaque, Tours, France*

**Laurent Fauchier, MD**
*CHU Trousseau, Hôpitaux de Tours, Cardiology B and Laboratoire d'Electrophysiologie Cardiaque, Tours, France*

**Guy Fontaine, MD, PhD**
*Hôpital Jean Rostand, Ivry sur Seine, France*

**F. Fontaliran, MD**
*Hôpital Jean Rostand, Ivry sur Seine, France*

**P. Fornes, MD, PhD**
*Service d'anatomopathologie, Hôpital Broussais, Paris, France*

**R. Frank, MD**
*Hôpital Jean Rostand, Ivry sur Seine, France*

**Jean-Marie Freyssinet, PhD**
*Institut d'Hématologie et d'Immunologie, Faculté de Médecine, Université Louis Pasteur, Strasbourg, France*

**Martin Fromer, MD**
*Division of Cardiology, Centre Hospitalier Universitaire Vaudois, Lausanne, Switzerland*

**Anton M. Gorgels, MD**
*Department of Cardiology, Academic Hospital Maastricht, Maastricht, The Netherlands*

**Colette M. Guiraudon, MD**
*Professor of Pathology, University of Western Ontario, London, Ontario, Canada*

**Gerard M. Guiraudon, MD**
*Professor of Surgery, SUNY at Buffalo, New York; Director, Clinical Trials, University of Ottawa Heart Institute, Ottawa, Ontario, Canada*

**L. Guize, MD**
*Department of Cardiology, Broussais Hospital, Pierre and Marie Curie University, Paris, France*

**Susanne Herwig, MD**
*University of Bonn, Department of Cardiology-Medicine, Bonn, Germany*

**Boyu Huang, PhD**
*Cardiology Division, Department of Medicine, State University of New York Health Science Center and Veterans Affairs Medical Center, Brooklyn, New York*

**Bénédicte Hugel, PhD**
*Institut d'Hématologie et d'Immunologie, Faculté de Médecine, Université Louis Pasteur, Strasbourg, France*

**Raymond E. Ideker, MD, PhD**
*Professor of Physiology, Medicine, and Biomedical Engineering, Cardiac Rhythm Management Laboratory, Division of Cardiovascular Disease, Department of Medicine, The University of Alabama at Birmingham, Birmingham, Alabama*

**Alberto Interian, Jr, MD**
*Division of Cardiology, University of Miami Medical Center, Miami, Florida*

**Karl Isaaz, MD**
*Professor of Medicine, Chief, Division of Cardiology, University of Saint-Etienne, Sainte-Etienne, France*

**José Jalife, MD**
*Professor and Chairman, Department of Pharmacology, Professor of Medicine and Pediatrics, SUNY Health Science Center, Syracuse, New York*

**Michiel J. Janse, MD**
*Cardiovascular Research, Academic Medical Center, Meibergdreef, Amsterdam, The Netherlands*

**Luc J.L.M. Jordaens, MD**
*Thoraxcentre, Academic Hospital Rotterdam, Rotterdam, The Netherlands*

**Werner Jung, MD**
*University of Bonn, Department of Cardiology-Medicine, Bonn, Germany*

**Salem Kacet, MD**
*Cardiology Department, Lille University Hospital, Lille, France*

**George J. Klein, MD**
*Professor of Medicine, Chief of Cardiology, London Health Science Center, London, Ontario, Canada*

**Martin Kloosterman, MD**
*Division of Cardiology, University of Miami Medical Center, Miami, Florida*

**Claude Kouakam, MD**
*Cardiology Department, Lille University Hospital, Lille, France*

**Dmitry O. Kozhevnikov, MD**
*Cardiology Division, Department of Medicine, State University of New York Health Science Center and Veterans Affairs Medical Center, Brooklyn, New York*

**Henri E. Kulbertus, MD**
*Centre Hospitalier Universitaire de Liège, Service de Cardiologie, Universitaire du Sart Tilman, Liège, Belgium*

**T. Lavergne, MD**
*Department of Cardiology, Broussais Hospital, Pierre and Marie Curie University, Paris, France*

**Ralph Lazzara, MD**
*Director, Cardiac Arrhythmia Research Institute, University of Oklahoma Health Sciences Center, Cardiovascular Section; Veterans Administration Medical Center, Oklahoma City, Oklahoma*

**Arnaud Lazarus, MD**
*Service de Cardiologie, Hôpital Cochin, Université René Descartes and Institut de Myologie Hôpital de la Salpetriere, Paris, France*

**Antoine Leenhardt, MD**
*Professor of Cardiology, Cardiology Department, Lariboisière University Hospital, Paris, France*

**J.Y. Le Heuzey, MD**
*Department of Cardiology, Broussais Hospital, Pierre and Marie Curie University, Paris, France*

**Guy Lesèche, MD**
*Service de Chirurgie Thoracique et Vasculaire, Hôpital Beaujon, Clichy, France*

**Aimée Lousberg, MD**
*Department of Cardiology, Academic Hospital Maastricht, Maastricht, The Netherlands*

**Jerry C. Luck, MD**
*Section of Cardiology and Cardiovascular Center, Penn State University College of Medicine, Hershey, Pennsylvania*

**Berndt Lüderitz, MD**
*Professor of Medicine, Head, Department of Medicine and Cardiology, University of Bonn, Department of Cardiology-Medicine, Bonn, Germany*

**I. Magnin-Poull, MD**
*Department of Cardiology, University of Nancy, Nancy, France*

**Pierre Maison Blanche, MD**
*Cardiology Department, Lariboisière, University Hospital, Paris, France*

**Marek Malik, MD, PhD**
*Professor of Cardiac Electrophysiology, Department of Cardiological Sciences, St. George's Hospital Medical School, London, United Kingdom*

**Ziad Mallat, MD, PhD**
*INSERM U141, Hôpital Lariboisière, Paris, France*

**Ravi Mandapati, MD**
*Department of Pediatrics (Cardiology), SUNY Health Science Center, Syracuse, New York*

**Moussa Mansour, MD**
*Department of Pharmacology, SUNY Health Science Center, Syracuse, New York*

**Jacques Mansourati, MD**
*Department of Cardiology, Brest University Hospital, Brest, France*

**Christian Marchal, MD**
*Hopitaux de Tours, Tours, France*

**Barry J. Maron, MD**
*Director, Cardiovascular Research, Minneapolis Heart Institute Foundation, Minneapolis, Minnesota*

**William J. McKenna, MD**
*Professor of Cardiac Medicine, Department of Cardiological Sciences, St. George's Hospital Medical School, London, United Kingdom*

**Paul Milliez, MD**
*Cardiology Department, Lariboisière University Hospital, Paris, France*

**Raul M. Mitrani, MD**
*Division of Cardiology, University of Miami Medical Center, Miami, Florida*

**Arthur J. Moss, MD**
*Professor of Medicine (Cardiology), Director, Heart Research Follow-up Program, University of Rochester Medical Center, Rochester, New York*

**Robert J. Myerburg, MD**
*Division of Cardiology, University of Miami Medical Center, Miami, Florida*

**Gerald V. Naccarelli, MD**
*Professor of Medicine, Head, Section of Cardiology, Director, Cardiovascular Center, Penn State University College of Medicine, The Milton S. Hershey Medical Center, Hershey, Pennsylvania*

**Christian Neel, MD**
*Hopitaux de Tours, Tours, France*

**Owen A. Obel, MD**
*Specialist Registrar in Cardiology, Cardiological Sciences, St. George's Hospital Medical School, London, United Kingdom*

**Zine Ounnoughenne, MD**
*Service de Cardiologie, Hôpital Cochin, Université René Descartes and Institut de Myologie Hôpital de la Salpetriere, Paris, France*

**Hemantkumar T. Patel, MD**
*Section of Cardiology and Cardiovascular Center, Penn State University College of Medicine, Hershey, Pennsylvania*

**O. Piot, MD**
*Department of Cardiology, Broussais Hospital, Pierre and Marie Curie University, Paris, France*

**Philippe Poret, MD**
*CHU Trousseau, Hôpitaux de Tours, Cardiology B and Laboratoire d'Electrophysiologie Cardiaque, Tours, France*

**Silvia G. Priori, MD, PhD**
*Molecular Cardiology Laboratories, Fondazione Salvatore Maugeri IRCCS, Pavia, Italy*

**Eric N. Prystowsky, MD**
*Director, Clinical Electrophysiology Laboratory, St. Vincent Hospital, Indianapolis, Indiana; Consulting Professor of Medicine, Duke University Medical Center, Durham, North Carolina*

**Antonio Raviele, MD**
*Chief, Division of Cardiology, Umberto I Hospital, Mestre-Venice, Italy*

**N. Sadoul, MD**
*Department of Cardiology, University of Nancy, Nancy, France*

**Sanjeev Saksena, MD**
*Clinical Professor of Medicine, Robert Wood Johnson School of Medicine; Director, Arrhythmia and Pacemaker Service, Eastern Heart Institute-Atlantic Health System, Millburn, New Jersey*

**Nadir Saoudi, MD**
*Cardiology Service, Charles Nicolle Hospital, Rouen, France*

**Irina Savelieva, MD**
*Department of Cardiological Sciences, St. George's Hospital Medical School, London, United Kingdom*

**Arnaud Savoure, MD**
*Cardiology Service, Charles Nicolle Hospital, Rouen, France*

**Ketty Schwartz, PhD**
*Unité INSERM, Institut de Myologie, Groupe Hospitalier Pitié-Salpêtrière, Paris, France*

**Peter J. Schwartz, MD**
*Professor and Chairman, Department of Cardiology Policlinico S. Matteo IRCCS and University of Pavia, Pavia, Italy*

**Jeffrey Simmons, MD**
*Division of Cardiology, University of Miami Medical Center, Miami, Florida*

**Paul Sorajja, MD**
*Clinical Research Fellow, Department of Cardiological Sciences, St. George's Hospital Medical School, London, United Kingdom*

**Bela Szabo, MD, PhD**
*University of Oklahoma, Veterans Administration Medical Center, Cardiac Arrhythmia Research Institute; Cardiac Arrhythmia Research Institute, Oklahoma City, Oklahoma*

**Alain Tedgui, PhD**
*INSERM U141, Hôpital Lariboisière, Paris, France*

**David Tena-Carbi, MD**
*Cardiology B Department and UMR CNRS 6542, Trousseau Hospital, Tours, France*

**Gaetano Thiene, MD**
*Professor of Cardiovascular Pathology, Department of Pathology, Institute of Pathological Anatomy, University of Padua Medical School, Padova, Italy*

**Jeffrey Towbin, MD**
*Department of Pediatrics, Baylor College of Medicine, Houston, Texas*

**Marialuisa Valente, MD**
*Institute of Pathological Anatomy, Department of Cardiovascular Pathology, University of Padua, Padova, Italy*

**Jean Varin, MD**
*Service de Cardiologie, Hôpital Cochin, Université René Descartes and Institut de Myologie Hôpital de la Salpetriere, Paris, France*

**Elisabeth Villain, MD**
*Service de Cardiologie Pédiatrique, Hôpital Necker Enfants-Malades, Paris, France*

**Hein J.J. Wellens, MD**
*Department of Cardiology, Academic Hospital Maastricht, Maastricht, The Netherlands*

**Thomas Wichter, MD**
*The Hospital of the Westfälische Wilhelms-University, Department of Cardiology and Angiology and Institute for Arteriosclerosis Research, Münster, Germany*

**Deborah L. Wolbrette, MD**
*Section of Cardiology and Cardiovascular Center, Penn State University College of Medicine, Hershey, Pennsylvania*

**Christian Wolpert, MD**
*University of Bonn, Department of Cardiology-Medicine, Bonn, Germany*

**Wojciech Zareba, MD, PhD**
*Associate Professor of Medicine (Cardiology), University of Rochester Medical Center, Rochester, New York*

# *Preface*

Sudden cardiac death (SCD) is a worldwide problem and a leading cause of death in adults in the Western world. It all too often claims the lives of people who were seemingly in good health. The fight against SCD remains a major challenge to cardiologists and electrophysiologists, and will be won through a better understanding of both the pathophysiological mechanisms of SCD as well as identification and appropriate treatment of patients at risk for a primary event. This book analyzes SCD from multiple perspectives, incorporating state-of-the-art knowledge of genetic disorders to randomized clinical trials. Using this knowledge, we hope the reader will gain a more united view of SCD, and a more directed approach to its primary and secondary prevention.

We express our sincere gratitude to the contributors of this book, often pioneers in their specific areas of expertise. We also thank our editor at Futura, Linda Shaw, for her tireless efforts in this project.

We also want to thank the Working Group on Arrhythmias and the Working Group on Cardiac Pacing of the French Society of Cardiology for their contribution to this work.

Etienne Aliot, MD
Jacques Clémenty, MD
Eric N. Prystowsky, MD

# Contents

# I

# *Definition, Epidemiology, and Mechanisms*

# 1

# Definitions and Epidemiology of Sudden Cardiac Death

*Robert J. Myerburg, MD, Raul M. Mitrani, MD, Alberto Interian, Jr, MD, Martin Kloosterman, MD, Jeffrey Simmons, MD, and Agustin Castellanos, MD*

## Introduction

The importance of sudden cardiac death as a public health problem has been recognized for less than 50 years.[1-3] As medical science advanced during the past 2 decades, appreciation of its impact and attention to its prevention became a major focus of scientific and clinical medicine. This attention derived from estimates of the magnitude of the problem,[4,5] in parallel with developments that made intervention and prevention strategies realistic goals for the medical enterprise.[6] In order to achieve these goals, however, it is necessary to recognize ways in which patients at risk can be identified and understand the features of the sudden cardiac death syndrome that are amenable to interventions.

## Definitions

Sudden cardiac death is defined by the following medical terminology: *"Natural death due to cardiac causes, heralded by abrupt loss of consciousness within 1 hour of the onset of acute symptoms; preexisting heart disease may have been known to be present, but the time and mode of death are unexpected."* [7] The key operational term is the unexpectedness of the event, since victims of sudden cardiac death can range from those with minimal or no known previous structural heart disease to those with advanced disease under continuous medical care. In the majority of instances, the terminal event results from an

Dr. Myerburg's research is funded in part by the American Heart Association Chair in Cardiovascular Research at the University of Miami.
From: Aliot E, Clementy J, Prystowsky EN (editors). *Fighting Sudden Cardiac Death: A Worldwide Challenge.* ©Futura Publishing Company, Armonk, NY, 2000.

electrical disturbance of the heart, which creates the inability to maintain organ perfusion. However, the definition of the specific electrical disturbance is important, because it determines both the potential effectiveness of interventions and prognosis.[8] Therefore, the definition should be qualified by the term "due to," which links the event to its mechanism. Moreover, the definition of the term "death" should be distinguished from the term "cardiac arrest" (Figure 1), since the former is literally an irreversible event characterized by the cessation of all biological functions, while cardiac arrest is potentially reversible for some period of time after the event.

The most common mechanism of cardiac arrest is ventricular fibrillation (Figure 2). Various studies of community-based event rates have suggested that ventricular fibrillation is the mechanism of cardiac arrest leading to sudden cardiac death in 65–80% of victims,[7] depending in part on the nature of the underlying disease. The second most common mechanisms of cardiac arrest are bradyarrhythmias, asystole, or pulseless electrical activity, cumulatively accounting for 20–30% of events in various studies.[8] Electrically organized ventricular tachycardia (VT), with loss of effective blood flow, is the least common, accounting for less than 10% of

| TERM | DEFINITION | QUALIFIERS | MECHANISMS |
|------|------------|------------|------------|
| **Sudden Cardiac Death** | **Irreversible** cessation of all biological functions; onset of terminal event **sudden** and **unexpected** | **None** | **Extended** loss of cardiac mechanical function, usually secondary to cardiac arrest |
| **Cardiac Arrest** | **Abrupt cessation** of cardiac mechanical function, which **may be reversible** by an intervention | Spontaneous conversions occur rarely | VF, VT, asystole, PEA, bradycardia, mechanical factors |
| **Cardio-vascular Collapse** | **Sudden loss of effective blood flow**, due to cardiac or peripheral factors; may require interventions or reverse spontaneously | **Non-specific** term: includes cardiac arrest and transient events | Same as "Cardiac Arrest," plus vaso-depressor syncope and other causes of **transient** loss of blood flow |

Figure 1. Definition of sudden cardiac death, cardiac arrest, and cardiovascular collapse. The language used to describe sudden death and cardiac arrest is commonly imprecise. Sudden death is literally and biologically an irreversible event, whereas "survival from cardiac arrest" is a more accurate description of the outcome of a successful resuscitation. The terms death, cardiac arrest, and cardiovascular collapse have different meanings and mechanisms, and reflect different cardiac electrophysiological and hemodynamic states. VF = ventricular fibrillation; VT = ventricular tachycardia; PEA = pulseless electrical activity.

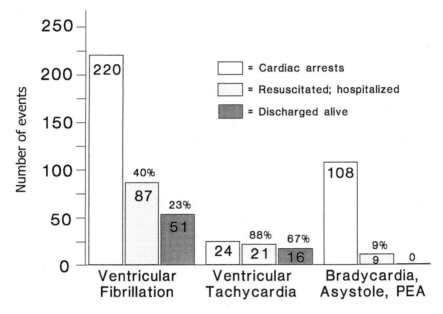

Figure 2. Mechanisms of sudden cardiac death and related survival rates. Among 352 out-of-hospital cardiac arrest victims, ventricular fibrillation was the mechanism identified during initial fire rescue contact in 220 (62%), ventricular tachycardia in 24 (7%), and bradycardia/asystole/pulseless electrical activity in 108 (31%). The rates for successful resuscitation and hospitalization, and for discharge alive, are provided for each category of cardiac arrest. (From Myerburg RJ, Castellanos A. Cardiac arrest and sudden cardiac death. In: Braunwald E (ed). Heart Disease (5th Edition). W.B. Saunders Company, Philadelphia, 1997, pp 742–779; reproduced with permission of the publisher.)

the events, and perhaps even fewer. However, it is likely that many episodes of ventricular fibrillation begin as an organized VT.

The best intervention outcomes occur among patients who are still having sustained organized tachyarrhythmias at the time of intervention, and the worst are with bradyarrhythmias, asystole or pulseless electrical activity, in which survival rates approach zero (Figure 2). Ventricular fibrillation outcomes are intermediate, with major potential benefit residing in the combination of numbers and potential effectiveness. Prognosis for survival from out-of-hospital ventricular fibrillation is a function of both severity of underlying disease and response time to the initial intervention.

## Epidemiology and Survival

An understanding of the epidemiology of sudden cardiac death is a key link among the strategies intended for primary prevention of cardiac arrest. Without it, impact on the cumulative problem will be impeded by limits of post facto responses to cardiac arrests. Unfortunately, initial enthusiasm regarding community-based emergency rescue systems, as originally designed,[9,10] has dampened as the systems have expanded. It is recognized that various factors leading to delayed response time have resulted in outcomes not as favorable as originally anticipated.

In the original studies from Miami, Florida,[9] and Seattle, Washington,[10] survival rates of cardiac arrest victims to hospital discharge were 14% and 11%, respectively. These figures improved over the ensuing years as a result of refinement of procedures, to eventually achieve peak survival rates between 25% and 35%.[8,11] However, since then, data from a variety of sources suggest that overall throughout the United States, and likely in Western Europe as well, the mean survival rates for out-of-hospital cardiac arrest victims are less than 10%, and possibly less than 5%. These estimates are based on data from those communities in which rescue systems exist and report their data. Cumulative data for the entire community-based cardiac arrest/sudden death problem are likely to be even less. These observations have led to systems developed with anticipated faster response time, such as police vehicle-based systems,[12,13] which offer some hope for improvement for the future. However, major impacts on the problem of sudden cardiac death will require not only response systems that are better than those currently available, but also the ability to recognize the victim at risk in advance of the event and take preventive measures. In order to address this issue, it is important to gain insight into several aspects of clinical epidemiology. These include population dynamics of cardiac arrest and sudden cardiac death (conventional epidemiology), the relationship between index events and the time-dependent risk of sudden cardiac arrest, the role of specific disease states in conditioning the risk of sudden cardiac death, the role of transient pathophysiological changes in triggering cardiac arrest, and the impact of predetermining factors for identification of the patient in whom a given set of circumstances will trigger a cardiac arrest. The latter is referred to as response risk or predetermination, and may, at least in part, relate to genetic characteristics of individuals at risk.[14]

## Incidence, Prevalence, and Population Dynamics

The early epidemiological studies on sudden cardiac death treated this entity as part of the complex of expression of coronary artery disease. Based on the fact that approximately 80% of all sudden cardiac deaths in the Western Hemisphere are a consequence of coronary artery disease, this epidemiological approach to the problem was reasonable. Since there were approximately 600,000 coronary heart disease deaths in the United States annually, and approximately 50% of the deaths were sudden cardiac deaths, the estimate of 300,000 sudden cardiac deaths per year emerged. The recent decrease in mortality from coronary heart disease,[15] countered by the fact that other causes of sudden death are not included in the *coronary* heart disease figures, supports the widely quoted estimate of 300,000 of sudden *cardiac* deaths annually in the United States.

The 50% distribution between sudden and nonsudden deaths derives from several studies. A 26-year follow-up of 5,209 men and women in the Framingham, Massachusetts, population who were 30–59 years of age and free of identified heart disease at baseline observation, demonstrated that sudden cardiac death accounted for 46% of the coronary heart disease deaths among men and 34% among women.[16] *The incidence* of sudden cardiac death increased with age, but the *proportion* of coronary heart disease deaths that were sudden and unexpected was greater in the younger age groups. Pooled data from Albany, New York, and Framingham, Massachusetts (4,120 men) identified sudden cardiac death as the initial and terminal manifestation of coronary heart disease in more than one-half of all sudden death victims.[17] In the Tecumseh, Michigan, study of 8,641 subjects, 46% of all coronary heart disease deaths occurred within 1 hour of onset of acute symptoms[18]; and in the Yugoslavian cardiovascular disease study, involving 6,614 men, age 35–62 and free of coronary disease at entry, 75% of all coronary deaths occurred suddenly. Two of every 3 victims had had no documented coronary events prior to death.[19]

The incidence of sudden cardiac death within the United States represents an estimate for the total population which is composed of subgroups at varying levels of risk. When sudden cardiac death is analyzed in terms of the absolute number of events annually within defined subpopulations, it is clear that the highest risk clinical subgroups, such as patients with low ejection fractions, a history of heart failure, and survivors of out-of-hospital cardiac arrests, do not generate the majority of sudden cardiac death events.[20] Thus, subgroups with the highest case fatality rates have the lowest population attributable risk. In contrast, the larger population subgroups, with much lower relative fatality rates, generate the largest absolute numbers of sudden cardiac death events because of the size of the population pools from which the events emerge. The magnitude of risk, expressed as incidence, is compared to the total number of events annually under 6 different conditions in Figure 3. These estimates are based on published epidemiological and clinical data. [7,20,21] When the 300,000 sudden cardiac deaths that occur annually among an unselected adult population in the United States are expressed as a fraction of the total adult population, the overall incidence is 0.1–0.2% per year. When the more easily identified high-risk subgroups are removed from this total population base, the calculated incidence for the remaining population decreases and

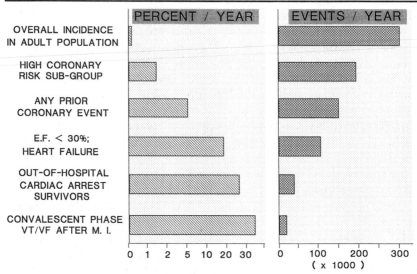

Figure 3. Sudden cardiac deaths among population subgroups. Estimates of incidence (percent per year) and total number of sudden cardiac deaths per year are shown for the overall adult population in the United States and for higher risk subgroups. The overall estimated incidence is 0.1% to 0.2% per year, totaling more than 300,000 deaths per year. Within subgroups identified by increasingly powerful risk factors, the increasing incidence is accompanied by progressively decreasing total numbers. Practical interventions for the larger subgroups will require identification of higher risk clusters within the groups. EF = ejection fraction; MI = myocardial infarction; VT/VF = ventricular tachycardia/ventricular fibrillation. The horizontal axis for the incidence figures is nonlinear; see text for details. (From Myerburg RJ, et al.[20]; reproduced with permission of the American Heart Association.)

the identification of specific individuals at risk becomes more difficult. Based on these estimates, a preventive intervention designed for the general adult population would have to be applied to the 999/1,000 people who will not have an event during the course of a year in order to reach and potentially influence the unidentified 1/1,000 who will. A model of such limited efficiency prohibits the application of many active interventions and highlights the need for more sensitive and specific markers of risk, which can be applied to large segments of the general population.

This point has relevance for both public health considerations and clinical therapeutics. The public health relevance of this point lies within the relationship between the size of the denominator in any population pool and the number of events occurring within that subgroup. For example, with escalation from high coronary risk subgroups without prior clinical events (risk = 1–2%/year, see Figure 3), to those with prior coronary events, low ejection fraction, and heart failure, or survival after out-of-hospital cardiac arrest, the probability of identifying individuals at higher risk becomes progressively greater, but the absolute number of individuals who can be identified for interventions decreases with each escalation. The relevance for clinical therapeutics embodies a distinction between therapeutic efficacy and efficiency.[12] *Efficacy* refers to the probability that an intervention will provide benefit to an affected individual or subgroup, regardless of the size of the population pool. It is usually expressed as an estimated or measured *relative reduction of event rates* compared to an untreated (placebo) group, without regard to the prevalence of the condition in the group (Figure 4). *Efficiency* is a measure of *absolute risk reduction,* considering the magnitude of the population, and recognizing that all members of a subset are exposed to adverse effects of the intervention, while only the affected members of

- **EFFICACY - Therapeutic benefit (or harm) expressed as a relative reduction (or increase) in risk caused an intervention.**

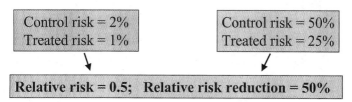

- **EFFICIENCY - Therapeutic benefit (or harm) expressed as absolute change in event rate in a treated population.**

| Control risk = 2% | Control risk = 50% |
| Treated risk = 1% | Treated risk = 25% |
| Absolute risk reduction = 1% | Absolute risk reduction = 25% |

**Figure 4.** Efficacy versus efficiency of interventions: relative versus absolute statistics. Efficacy refers to the relative benefit of an intervention as a result of an active treatment, compared to controls, regardless of the magnitude of risk among the untreated patients. Efficiency is an expression of the size of the treated population that can benefit, based on the magnitude of the risk at baseline. Since all treated patients are exposed to adverse effects of treatment, the importance of efficiency considerations relates to the number of patients who have the potential for benefit, in contrast to the potential for harm among the total group. Efficacy or relative risk is the same for change from a 2% control risk to a 1% treated risk as it is for a 50% control risk reducing to a 25% treated risk. In both instances, the relative risk is 0.5. Efficiency, in contrast, refers to the absolute differences, and the 2%/1% model provides a 1% benefit, whereas the 50%/25% model produces a 25% benefit.

the group may benefit. Interventions for prevention of sudden cardiac death among specific high-risk population subgroups (e.g., survivors of out-of-hospital cardiac arrest) provide a very efficient model because of high absolute event rates, while strategies for more general populations with much lower event rates are inherently inefficient,[22,23] even though they contain much greater absolute numbers of individuals at risk.

Age, heredity, gender, and race also contribute to subgroup behavior within the cumulative at risk population. Sudden cardiac death peaks initially between birth and 6 months of age in the form of the sudden infant death syndrome, and then becomes very infrequent throughout childhood, adolescence, and young adulthood. A second increase begins beyond the age of 40 years and peaks between the mid-50s and 70 years of age. The mean risk in the 35- to 64-year-old subgroup is 0.1–0.2% per year, while the risk is 100 times less in adolescents and young adults under the age of 30 (Figure 5).

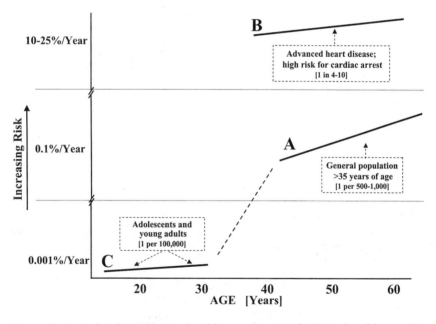

Figure 5. Age-related incidence of sudden cardiac death. Risk of sudden cardiac death as a function of age is demonstrated. For the general population over the age of 35 years (A) the risk of sudden cardiac death is approximately 0.1% to 0.2% per year. In contrast, a subgroup of that population with advanced heart disease and markers of high risk for cardiac arrest and sudden cardiac death may have a untreated risk of 25% per year or more (B). Adolescents and young adults (C) have an average risk of cardiac arrest of 1 in 100,000 or 0.001% per year. In addition to magnitude of risk, the general adolescent population has a different spectrum of etiological mechanisms compared to older adults (see text).

Hereditary aspects of the risk of sudden cardiac death were of limited interest until recently. While certain inherited disorders, particularly in the adolescent and young adult group, such as congenital long QT interval syndrome, hypertrophic cardiomyopathy, right ventricular dysplasia, and Brugada syndrome, are known to have patterns of familial distribution, it has recently been suggested that hereditary patterns might influence risk of sudden cardiac death due to coronary heart disease. Specifically, 2 large epidemiological surveys have suggested that sudden cardiac death as an expression of coronary heart disease may have specific patterns of risk distribution within families.[24,25] While cultural and familial environmental factors certainly might play a role,[24] it is also possible that hereditary influences on electrophysiological behavior of cardiac tissue under conditions of ischemia might be predetermined by hereditary patterns of ion channel behavior.[14,24] If sudden death can be identified as a specific expression of coronary artery disease subject to identifiable genetic patterns, a powerful impact on preventive strategies will emerge. It is still too early to speculate that this might be the case, but it is an area worthy of intensive investigation.

The risk of sudden cardiac death in middle life and early advanced years in men far exceeds that in women.[26] To a large extent this reflects the delayed onset of coronary artery disease in premenopausal women and the time for evolution of the disease in early postmenopausal women.[26] However, as the differences in prevalence of coronary artery disease between men and women decrease with advancing years, the differences in risk of sudden cardiac death also decrease. The same risk factors for sudden cardiac death operate in both women and men. In respect to race, the previously held notion that sudden cardiac death has a higher incidence among white males than other subgroups has been effectively challenged by recent studies demonstrating an excessive risk in black Americans, especially black males.[27,28]

## Time-Dependent Risk

Risk of death after surviving a major change in cardiovascular status is not linear over time.[29–32] Survival estimates for both sudden cardiac death and total cardiac mortality demonstrate that the highest secondary death rates occur during the first 6 to 18 months after an index event. By 18 to 24 months, the slopes of survival curves begin to approach the configuration of those describing a similar population that has remained free of interposed cardiovascular events (Figure 6). The configuration of survival curves may also be influenced by the magnitude of increased risk after an index event. The data from the Cardiac Arrhythmia Suppression Trial (CAST)[33, 34] demonstrate linear survival curves for the placebo population during long-term follow-up, while data from the multicenter postinfarction

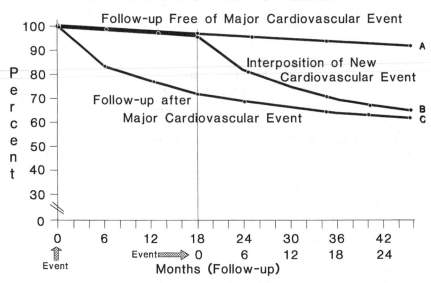

Figure 6. Time dependence of risk after cardiovascular events. Survival curves for hypothetical patients with known cardiovascular disease free of a major index event (curve A) and for patients surviving major cardiovascular events (curve C). Attrition is accelerated during the initial 6 to 24 months after the event. Curve B shows the dynamics of risk over time in low-risk patients with an interposed major event that is normalized to a time point (for example, 18 months). The subsequent attrition is accelerated for 6 to 24 months. (From Myerberg RJ, et al.[20]; reproduced with permission of the American Heart Association.)

program[29,30] demonstrated that subgrouping postmyocardial infarction patients according to increasing risk, based on interaction between premature ventricular contraction frequency and ejection fractions, results in progressively higher risk as the number and power of risk factors increased. The added mortality in the higher risk subgroups is expressed early. Thus, among the higher risk subgroups, time-dependent risk provides the greatest opportunity for effective intervention strategies in the early period after conditioning cardiovascular events. Mortality risk patterns having these characteristics have been observed among survivors of out-of-hospital cardiac arrest,[31] among patients with recent onset of heart failure, and those who have high-risk markers after myocardial infarction.[32] In contrast, data from one of the angiotensin-converting enzyme inhibitor trials (Survival and Ventricular Enlargement Trial, SAVE) suggested that mortality benefit, as a result of limiting the delayed onset of ventricular remodeling, is expressed late after the index event.[35] Similarly, a lipid-lowering trial in postmyocardial infarction patients (Cholesterol and Recurrent Events Study,

CARE)[36] also demonstrated late benefit, presumably because of influence on developing structural disease, rather than on shorter term risks.

Time as a dimension for estimating risk must be integrated into strategies designed for population interventions. Ignoring this characteristic of the clinical epidemiology of cardiac arrest and sudden death may preselect study groups that are composed of lower risk components. When merged into a population defined by high-risk characteristics, the predicted risk of the population is diluted by the time dynamics. The greater the increase in early mortality related to the index event, the greater is the potential for distortion of event rates caused by late entrants.

## Conditioning Risk: The Structural Basis of Sudden Cardiac Death

As shown in Figure 3, the presence of structural cardiac disease is a conditioning factor for increasing risk of sudden cardiac death. The magnitude of risk increases in relationship to the severity of underlying structural heart disease, but the mere presence of structural disease exerts a major influence on risk. In recent years, a distinction has emerged between structural preconditions for sudden cardiac death (Figure 7), and acute functional events responsible for the initiation of potentially fatal arrhythmias (Figure 8).[22,37] It is now generally agreed that: (1) established etiological states provide the cardiac substrate for the genesis of fatal arrhythmias, and (2) all structural abnormalities, and likely some functional ones as well, can serve this function. Moreover, new knowledge of the genetic control of ion channel function in cardiac myocytes in patients with congenital long QT interval syndrome[38] and other entities now defines structural abnormalities at a molecular level.

Coronary atherosclerosis and its major structural consequences—acute and healed myocardial infarction—constitute the most common structural bases of sudden death. Accounting for approximately 80% of events, it was the first category of disease to receive attention and initially was almost exclusively equated with cause of sudden death. More recently, insights have been emerging into other structural abnormalities, such as left ventricular hypertrophy and the cardiomyopathies. The role of left ventricular hypertrophy as a risk factor has been recognized in epidemiological studies[39,40] and clinical associations have been described.[41,42] New information on arrhythmogenic membrane channel and electrophysiological alterations of the hypertrophied myocardium is emerging,[43,44] providing insight into mechanisms by which this structural abnormality may contribute to the genesis of potentially fatal arrhythmias. The fact that regional hypertrophy is common after healing of myocardial infarction[45–47] carries

## ETIOLOGICAL BASIS OF SUDDEN CARDIAC DEATH

▷ CORONARY HEART DISEASE            80%
    - Acute ischemic events
    - Chronic ischemic heart disease

▷ CARDIOMYOPATHIES             10-15%
    - Dilated cardiomyopathies
    - Hypertrophic cardiomyopathies

▷ VALVULAR / INFLAMMATION / INFILTRATION   ±5%

▷ SUBTLE, POORLY-DEFINED LESIONS

▷ LESIONS OF MOLECULAR STRUCTURE

                                       → ? %

▷ FUNCTIONAL ABNORMALITIES

▷ "NORMAL" HEARTS - IDIOPATHIC VF

Figure 7. Etiological basis for potentially fatal arrhythmias. Structural heart disease establishes the long-term basis of risk for the best management of potentially fatal arrhythmias. It is the conditioning substrate that allows functional abnormalities to initiate a potentially fatal arrhythmia under specific conditions. Collectively, coronary artery disease and the myopathies account for 90% to 95% of the structural causes of sudden cardiac death in the United States. All of the remaining causes listed account for the remainder. Genetically determined molecular abnormalities at an ion channel level of structure can now be identified. (From Myerberg RJ, et al.[37]; reproduced with permission of the American Journal of Cardiology.)

further implications for the role of hypertrophy-related electrical disturbances in the generation of life-threatening arrhythmias.

The proportion of sudden cardiac deaths caused by the various etiologies approximates the prevalence estimates of various cardiac diseases. Thus, 80% of sudden cardiac deaths are associated with coronary artery disease, 10–15% with the various cardiomyopathies, and only small fractions by the less common disorders (see Figure 7). However, the small numbers of less common diseases often provide excellent models for understanding pathophysiology and commonly affect younger individuals without a variety of co-morbid states. Their recognition clinically is important beyond their numbers because the affected individuals can often survive long term if the condition is recognized and therapy is initiated before an unexpected fatal arrhythmic event.

Since coronary heart disease accounts for approximately 80% of sudden

# TRANSIENT RISK FACTORS

- ## Ischemia and Reperfusion
  - \> Ischemic Ventricular Tachycardia/Fibrillation
  - \> Initiation of Monomorphic VT by Ischemia
  - \> Reperfusion Arrhythmias

- ## Systemic Inciting Factors
  - \> Hemodynamic Dysfunction
  - \> Hypoxemia, Acidosis
  - \> Electrolyte Imbalance

- ## Neurophysiologic Interactions
  - \> Central and Systemic Factors
  - \> Local Cardiac Factors - Transmitters/Receptors

- ## Toxic Cardiac Effects
  - \> Idiosyncratic Proarrhythmia
  - \> Dose-dependent Proarrhythmia
  - \> Transient Proarrhythmic Risk

Figure 8. Triggering events for cardiac arrest. The four general categories listed include most of the functional factors responsible for initiating cardiac arrest. These factors are responsible for initiating electrophysiological disturbances that interact with structural preconditions for cardiac arrest. They may also contribute to maintenance of life-threatening arrhythmias after their initiation. (From Myerberg RJ, et al.[37]; reproduced with permission of the American Journal of Cardiology.)

cardiac deaths in Western societies,[7] most of the major studies of risk factors have focused on this etiological category. Data from multiple studies have demonstrated a concordance between risk factors for coronary atherosclerosis, total cardiovascular mortality, and sudden death.[6,15,48,49] In most studies, approximately 50% of all deaths related to coronary heart disease are sudden and unexpected, although proportions of sudden-to-nonsudden deaths may vary as a function of the severity of left ventricular dysfunction and functional impairment.[50] Among patients having cardiomyopathies, those with better preserved functional capacity (functional Classes 1 and 2) have lower total death rates, but the fraction of all deaths that are sudden and unexpected is higher among Class 4 patients, total death rates are higher, but the fraction of sudden deaths is lower. There is a *competing risk* between sudden and nonsudden deaths, which implies that the extent to which arrhythmic mortality improvement will influence total mortality may be limited by the frequency of other mechanisms of death.[14,22,51]

For patients with coronary heart disease, the evolution of the structural abnormalities that condition risk are the physical expression of conventional coronary risk factors. The magnitude of risk relates well to the number of risk factors present. In the Framingham study,[16] there was a 14-fold increase in risk from the lowest risk decile to the highest risk decile; and in the Yugoslavian cardiovascular disease study, the probability of sudden cardiac death was 11 times higher in the top quintile than in the bottom quintile of multivariate risk distribution.[19] Thus, risk factors such as age, family history, gender, cigarette smoking, the hypertension/hypertrophy complex, hyperlipidemias, and the other conventional coronary risk factors provide easily identifiable markers for sudden death risk. These markers may be viewed as static because of their potential to be continuously present over time. Their limitation is that they primarily identify the risk of developing the underlying disease responsible for sudden death, rather than for the pathophysiological event responsible for its expression. The ability of conventional risk factors to identify high-risk subgroups in epidemiological terms is unquestioned, and it is likely that for some of these risk factors, active preventive interventions will influence risk and significantly alter the number of events occurring among the population. However, their application to individual patients is limited because the absolute event rate predicted by risk factors alone is limited.[23] Since pathophysiological susceptibility does not necessarily equate with structural heart disease risk (see below), the ability of these long-term risk factors to identify specific individuals who will manifest cardiac arrest is limited. Therefore, while conventional risk factors relate well to the anatomic basis for cardiac arrest and sudden death and provide important preventive opportunities, they lack the specific focus required for efficient preventive strategies in large subgroups and in individual patients.

A higher power of risk is provided by the presence of specific structural cardiac abnormalities. Once established, they constitute the substrate upon which triggering events can initiate unstable cardiac electrophysiological disturbances (Figure 8). The clinical recognition of structural disease defines individual risk much more specifically than do the conventional risk factors (Figure 3). At a different level of resolution, specific myocardial pathways that form the myocardial structural support for life-threatening arrhythmias (i.e., potential reentrant circuits) have been well studied.[40] These might provide a much more specific anatomic description of risk but lack direct clinical or epidemiological accessibility short of extensive and costly testing techniques.

## Transient Risk Factors

In regard to the mechanism of onset of ventricular tachycardia/ventricular fibrillation as causing sudden cardiac death, transient risk indicates *a time-limited* and often *unpredictable* event or state that has the potential to initiate or allow the initiation of unstable electrophysiological properties in the heart (Figures 8 and 9). The term "unstable" is used to indicate an increased probability of transition from a normal or benign cardiac rhythm to potentially fatal ventricular tachyarrhythmias. The transient nature of these events makes their prospective elucidation a difficult clinical and epidemiological chore, and the concept of transient risk as an epidemiological measure is being developed.[52,53] An observation of cardiovascular event rates after a major environmental disaster provided a unique insight into transient risk. An analysis of cardiac and sudden deaths at the time of the 1994 Los Angeles earthquake revealed that there was a clustering of events on the day of the earthquake, with a proportional reduction in expected rates for 1–2 weeks subsequently, followed by a return to baseline rates.[54] An interpretation is that the intense acute en-

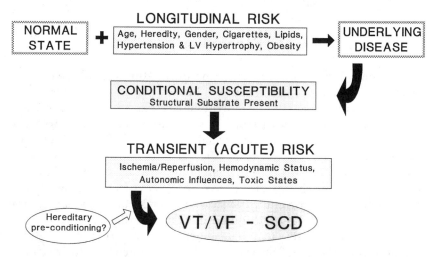

Figure 9. Long-term risk factors versus transient risk. Longitudinal risk refers to those epidemiological risk factors that predict the evolution of the disease states predisposing to the event (i.e., the conditioning factors). Transient or acute risk refers to those factors that are directly related to electrophysiological instability at a specific point in time. The latter may also be interpreted in terms of the individual susceptibility to the adverse influences of the transient risk factor, as suggested by recent epidemiological surveys indicating specificity of sudden death risk as an expression of coronary artery disease in families. (Modified from Myerburg RJ, Kessler KM, Kimura S, Bassett AL, Cox MM, et al. Life-threatening ventricular arrhythmias: the link between epidemiology and pathophysiology. From Zipes DP, Jalife J (eds). Cardiac Electrophysiology: From Cell to Bedside. WB Saunders, Philadelphia, 1995, pp 723–731; reproduced with permission of the publisher.)

vironmental stress advanced in time events that were impending when an appropriate trigger occurred.

The development of a base of experimental information on the role of myocardial ischemia in creating an electrophysiological risk of ventricular tachyarrhythmias first led to the concept of an initiating or transitional event, in which the role of premature ventricular contractions in the initiation of sustained arrhythmias could be defined by a predictable set of circumstances.[55] Subsequently, other functional perturbations received attention. Intense functional changes alone may destabilize this system in the absence of structural abnormalities, but the vast majority of cardiac arrests occur in hearts with preceding structural abnormalities. As shown in Figures 6 and 8, the major functional influences or categories of transient risk factors may be separated into 4 groups: (1) ischemia and reperfusion, (2) systemic abnormalities, (3) autonomic changes, and (4) cardiotoxic factors, including the general problem of proarrhythmia. While each of these categories can be viewed as clinical events or pathophysiological influences, they are now also being modeled and applied as measurable epidemiological risk factors.[52,53]

## Transient Ischemia and Reperfusion

Ischemia occurring at the onset and during the early phase of acute myocardial infarction has a clearly established clinical and experimental association with potentially fatal arrhythmias. However, the majority of sudden death victims and survivors of out-of-hospital cardiac arrest do not have acute transmural myocardial infarctions.[56,57] Specifically, approximately 80% of sudden deaths due to coronary heart disease are *not* associated with acute myocardial infarction,[57] and it is assumed that transient acute ischemia is one of the major triggering factors. However, its transient nature has precluded systematic clinical and epidemiological studies. Unstable angina pectoris and silent myocardial ischemia also appear to have the capability to initiate potentially fatal arrhythmias,[58–62] but clinical documentation of these mechanisms is limited.[62] Both are associated with a statistical increase in the risk of sudden cardiac death when they accompany preexisting coronary artery disease.

Clinical and epidemiological data demonstrating associations between ischemia and potentially fatal arrhythmia are paralleled by experimental data that demonstrate adverse effects of ischemia, especially in the presence of a prior myocardial infarction. For example, a study in dogs with healed myocardial infarction was designed to determine the arrhythmogenic effects of graded reductions in blood flow through a noninfarct-related artery. The study demonstrated that lesser decreases in blood flow resulted in inducible VT or spontaneous ventricular fibrillation in the presence of a prior myocardial infarction compared to controls without a prior infarction.[63] In addition, the epidemiological impact of left ventricular hypertrophy, especially in the presence of coronary artery disease and prior myocardial infarction, is paralleled by observations of specific ion channel abnormalities in hypertrophied myocytes, some of which become manifest primarily during ischemia. These observations include differences in ATP-sensitive $K^+$ channels during ischemia in the hypertrophied myocardium compared to normal hearts, and between endocardium and epicardium in normal hearts,[64] as well as changes in $Ca^{++}$ and $K^+$ currents under conditions of metabolic inhibition as a surrogate for ischemia.[65] Thus, some of the epidemiological factors that increase risk of sudden death are paralleled by abnormalities at the level of membrane channels which could serve as an explanation for increased risk. While the study of the interaction between epidemiology and membrane physiology is only in its infancy, these relationships warrant further exploration.

The electrophysiological consequences of reperfusion of ischemic muscle are beginning to be clarified. Reperfusion appears to induce electrical instability by several different mechanisms, both reentrant[65] and triggered activity.[44] The former is characterized by rapid electrical activity, which may be due to abrupt changes in refractoriness,[66] while the latter is likely due to generation of afterdepolarizations, which are experimentally sensitive to $Ca^{++}$ blockade.[67] Hypertrophied myocytes appear to be more prone to generate reperfusion-induced early afterdepolarizations and triggered activity than are normal myocytes, apparently due to depressed delayed rectifier current $(I_K)$ in the hypertrophied myocyte.[44] In situ studies of the frequency of ventricular fibrillation during ischemia and reperfusion in previously hypertrophied hearts support the potential clinical relevance of such data.[68]

## Systemic Factors in Transient Risk

Acute or subacute systemic abnormalities modulate chronic structural cardiac abnormalities, influencing electrophysiological stability and susceptibility to life-threatening arrhythmias.[69] Among the larger studies of survivors of out-of-hospital cardiac arrest, small subgroups have had recognizable reversible systemic abnormalities that contribute to life-threatening arrhythmias. When transient systemic factors can be identified *and* predictably controlled, no other preventive interventions against recurrences are required.[51] Hypoxemia, acidosis, and electrolyte imbalances all may contribute to destabilization[70-72]; these factors are clinically recognizable and reversible with appropriate therapy. Clues regarding the mechanisms by which these forms of transient risk may influence electrophysiology are beginning to evolve. For instance, in myocytes from globally hypertrophied hearts, conductance through ATP-sensitive $K^+$-channels may be increased by a reduction in pH.[73] When a hypertrophied heart becomes regionally ischemic and acidotic, this characteristic may cause dispersion of electrophysiological properties, thereby predisposing to reentrant ventricular arrhythmias. Chronic electrolyte disturbances, most prominently hypokalemia associated with long-term use of diuretics, are associated with an increased risk of cardiovascular mortality.[71] Hypokalemia as a cause or contributor to the initiation of polymorphic VT and torsades de pointes is well recognized,[72,74] most commonly in patients with chronically abnormal hearts and in the presence of Class I antiarrhythmic drugs and other proarrhythmic substances.

Transient hemodynamic dysfunction in patients with abnormal hearts is likely among the most common systemic inciting factors, but is one that is difficult to study clinically in a controlled manner. Severe acute or subacute hemodynamic deterioration may cause a secondary cardiac arrest, which has long been known to carry a very high short-term mortality rate.[70,75] However, the less well-defined relationship between *chronically* impaired left ventricular function, *acute modulations* in hemodynamic status, and predisposition to ventricular tachycardia/ventricular fibrillation is an important focus for the future. It has been shown experimentally that volume loading of isolated perfused canine left ventricles shortens refractory periods[76,77] and regional disparity in hearts with prior myocardial infarction has been demonstrated.[77] Stretch-induced modulation of membrane channels may play a role in such changes. Clinical studies to define such mechanisms have been limited to date.

## Autonomic Fluctuations and Transient Risk

Central nervous system, peripheral systemic, and local cardiac neurophysiological factors are receiving increasing attention as markers for identifying high-risk subgroups and for elucidating mechanisms of fatal arrhythmias.[78] At a local myocardial level, experimental observations[78-84] and limited clinical data[85-92] suggest that prior myocardial infarction and other cardiac abnormalities predisposing to sudden cardiac death are accompanied by changes in cardiac autonomic function. Several patterns of altered regional responses to sympathetic stimulation have been reported in different myocardial infarction models.[79-81] Regionally altered beta-adrenoceptor numbers and changes in coupling proteins and in adenylate cyclase activity have been observed in hearts with healed myocardial infarction.[84] Experimental and clinical imaging studies have also shown disruption of myocardial sympathetic innervation after acute myocardial infarction, with apparent reinnervation after convalescence.[79,81,86,89]

At a systemic level, qualitative and quantitative estimates of neurophysiological alterations that may modulate cardiac activity have been proposed as a means of identifying subgroups at increased risk for sudden death. Changes in heart rate variability or baroreceptor sensitivity have been studied in selected subgroups. Among myocardial infarction survivors[85–89] and survivors of out-of-hospital cardiac arrest, altered heart rate variability has been suggested as a marker for risk. Power spectrum analysis of heart rate variability in the frequency domain has suggested specific patterns that identify high-risk subgroups[85] and short-term frequency domain patterns differ before the onset of sustained VT compared to nonsustained VT.[87] A blunted baroreceptor response to phenylephrine infusion has also identified increased risk for VT[88] and sudden death[88,89] after myocardial infarction. An association between sinus node rate immediately following the onset of sustained VT and the electrophysiological and hemodynamic stability of the ventricular tachycardoa has been reported.[92] In patients with stable VT, sinus node rate during ventriculoatrial dissociation increases progressively during the first 30 seconds of VT. When VT is unstable, sinus node rate increases more rapidly during the initial 5 seconds of VT, and then decreases abruptly. A role for autonomic dysfunction, either as a cause or a consequence of the arrhythmia pattern, has been suggested.

## Effects of Toxic Substances on the Heart

Classic proarrhythmic responses—torsades de pointes—may occur with any of the Class I-A antiarrhythmic drugs, as well as the Class III drugs. More subtle, but possibly quite important, is the emerging number of clinically used substances that are not used as antiarrhythmic drugs, but which may induce similar proarrhythmic responses. These include diverse categories of medications, such as erythromycin, pentamidine, haloperidol, a number of the psychotropic drugs, and terfenadine.[93] In addition, limited clinical data suggest an effect on QT interval and the risk of torsades de pointes in the susceptible individual for such diverse other substances as organic phosphate insecticides, cocaine,[94] and probucol.[95] For many of these substances, limited data at this time suggest that the offending substances prolong QT intervals by an effect on repolarizing currents, such as the delayed rectifier current $I_K$ ($I_{kR}$).[93,94] The combination of an inherent ability of a substance to prolong action potential duration and specific patterns of individual susceptibility to this effect may explain the sporadic occurrence of these responses. It follows that identification of an offending channel effect, coupled with the ability to identify individual susceptibility, might provide a method to identify risk prospectively. Unfortunately, since such events are more common in patients with underlying heart disease, the distinction between a proarrhythmic response and a confounding clinical arrhythmia caused by the underlying disease is difficult at the present time.

## Response Variables: Preconditioned Risk

The concept of *response risk* is an attempt to introduce principles of epidemiology and genetics to the disciplines of cardiac electrophysiology and myocardial cell membrane function.[14] It refers to the mechanisms by which a specific individual, who has a conditioning risk factor, is susceptible to arrhythmogenesis when exposed to a transient functional risk influence. Based on the premises that the conditioning factors create a persistent substrate for arrhythmic risk and the transient functional factors serve an initiating role (see Figure 7), the epidemiological question focuses on the identification of those subjects whose inherent physiological characteristics make the initiation of electrophysiological instability more likely when these conditions are met.[24, 25] It requires clinically identifiable, genetically based or acquired individual differences in the responses of membrane channels and receptors. That such conditions exist in nature has been shown clinically in the long QT interval syndrome.[38] Abnormalities of both potassium ($I_{KR}$, $I_{KS}$) and sodium ($I_{Na}$) channels have been identified in genetic variants of long QT interval syndromes in humans.[96] A parallel concept, not yet worked out genetically, is the clinical model of "idiosyncratic" proarrhythmic responses to Class I-A antiarrhythmic drugs, which is expressed as excessive prolongation of repolarization and generation of torsades de pointes. This response occurs in 1% to 3% of the exposed population that appears to have the specific susceptibility. Exaggerated depression of $I_{kR}$ may create individual susceptibility upon exposure,[97] while the arrhythmia itself may be mediated electrophysiologically by $I_{Ca,L}$.[98] The ability to identify abnormal response characteristics of specific channels or receptors, under a variety of pathophysiological conditions, holds the promise of identifying individuals at risk for potentially fatal arrhythmias under conditions of specific substance exposures. This extends beyond proarrhythmic effects of antiarrhythmic drugs to include factors such as the response of specific channels to ischemia and reperfusion[43, 97, 98] and the response of previously conditioned hearts to stimuli in the environment (e.g., cocaine) which can influence specific ion channel function.[94]

In summary, therefore, the ability to identify specific individuals at risk for responding abnormally to a specific transient stimulus will provide increasing power for epidemiological approaches and yield greater resolution of risk within large population groups.[24,25]

## References

1. Weiss S. Instantaneous "physiologic" death. N Engl J Med 1940; 223:793.
2. Spain DM, Bradess VA, Mohr C. Coronary atherosclerosis as a cause of unexpected and unexplained death: an autopsy study from 1949–1959. JAMA 1960; 174:384.
3. Burch GE, DePasquale NP. Sudden, unexpected, natural death. Am J Med Sci 1965; 249:86.
4. Kannel WB, Doyle JT, McNamara PM, et al. Precursors of sudden coronary death: factors related to the incidence of sudden death. Circulation 1975; 51:606.
5. Gillum RF. Sudden coronary deaths in the United States, 1980–1985. Circulation 1989; 79:756–765.
6. Report of the Working Group on Arteriosclerosis of the National Heart, Lung, and Blood Institute (Volume 2). Patient Oriented Research—Fundamental and Applied, Sudden Cardiac Death. DHEW, NIH Publication #83–2035, U.S. Government Printing Office, Washington, DC, 1981, pp 114–122.
7. Myerburg RJ, Castellanos A. Cardiac arrest and sudden cardiac death. In: Braunwald E (ed). Heart Disease: A Textbook of Cardiovascular Medicine, 5th edition. WB Saunders Publishing Co., NY, 1997, Chapter 24, pp 742–779.
8. Myerburg RJ, Kessler KM, Zaman L, et al. Survivors of prehospital cardiac arrest. JAMA 1982; 247:1485.
9. Liberthson RR, Nagel EL, Hirschman JC, Nussenfeld SR. Prehospital ventricular fibrillation: prognosis and follow-up course. N Engl J Med 1974; 291:317.
10. Baum RS, Alvarez H, Cobb LA. Survival after resuscitation from out-of-hospital ventricular fibrillation. Circulation 1974; 50:1231–1235.
11. Cummins RO, Ornato JP, Thies WH, Pepe PE. Improving survival from sudden cardiac arrest: the chain of survival concept. A statement for heart professionals from the Advanced Cardiac Life Support Subcommittee and the Emergency Cardiac Care Committee, American Heart Association. Circulation 1991; 83:1832.
12. Waalewijn RA, de Vos R, Koster RW. Out-of-hospital cardiac arrests in Amsterdam and its surrounding areas: results from the Amsterdam resuscitation study (ARREST) in 'Utstein' style. Resuscitation 1998; 38:157.
13. White RD, Hankins DG, Bugliosi TF. Seven years' experience with early defibrillation by police and paramedics in an emergency medical services system. Resuscitation 1998; 39:145.
14. Myerburg RJ, Kessler KM, Castellanos A. Epidemiology of sudden cardiac death: population characteristics, conditioning risk factors, and dynamic risk factors. In: Spooner PM, Brown AM, Catterall WA, et al (eds). Ion Channels in the Cardiovascular System. Futura Publishing Co., Armonk, NY, 1994, pp 15–33.
15. Epstein FH, Pisa Z. International comparisons in ischemic heart disease mortality. Decline in Coronary Heart Disease Mortality. DHEW, NIH Publication No. 79-1610, Washington, D.C., U.S. Government Printing Office, 1979, pp 58–88.
16. Kannel WB, Thomas HE. Sudden coronary death: the Framingham study. Ann NY Acad Sc 1982; 382: 3–21.
17. Doyle JT, Kannel WB, McNamara RM, Quikenton R, Gordon T. Factors related to suddenness of death from coronary heart disease: combined Albany-Framingham studies. Am J Cardiol 1976; 37:1073–1078.

18. Chiang B, Perlman HV, Fulton M, Ostrander ID, Epstein RH. Predisposing factors in sudden cardiac death in Tecumseh, Michigan: a prospective study. Circulation 1970; 41:31–37.
19. Demirovic J. Risk factors in the incidence of sudden cardiac death and possibilities for its prevention. Doctoral thesis, University of Belgrade Press, Belgrade, Yugoslavia, 1985.
20. Myerburg RJ, Kessler KM Castellanos A. Sudden cardiac death: structure, function, and time-dependence of risk. Circulation 1992; 85(Suppl I):1-2–10.
21. Myerburg RJ, Demirovic J. Epidemiologic considerations in cardiac arrest and sudden cardiac death: etiology and prehospital and posthospital outcomes. In: Podrid RJ, Kowey PR. Cardiac Arrhythmia: Mechanisms, Diagnosis, and Management. Williams & Wilkins, Baltimore, MD, Chapter 44, 1995, pp 964–1003.
22. Myerburg RJ, Kessler KM, Castellanos A. Sudden cardiac death: epidemiology, transient risk, and intervention assessment. Ann Intern Med 1993; 119:1187–1197.
23. Myerburg RJ, Mitrani R, Interian A Jr, Castellanos A. Interpretation of outcomes of antiarrhythmic clinical trials: design features and population impact. Circulation 1998; 97:1514.
24. Friedlander Y, Siscovick DS, Weinmann S, et al. Family history as a risk factor for primary cardiac arrest. Circulation 1998; 97:155.
25. Jouven X, Desnos M, Guerot C, Ducimetiere P. Predicting sudden death in the population: the Paris Prospective Study I. Circulation 1999; 99:1978.
26. Kannel WB, Thomas HE. Sudden coronary death: the Framingham study. Ann NY Acad Sci 1982; 382:3.
27. Becker L B, Han BH, Mayer PM, et al. Racial differences in the incidence of cardiac arrest and subsequent survival. N Engl J Med 1993; 329:600.
28. Gillum RF. Sudden cardiac death in Hispanic Americans and African Americans. Am J Public Health 1997; 87:1461.
29. Bigger JT, Fleiss JL, Kleiger R, Miller JP, Rolnitzky LM, and the Multicenter Post-Infarction Research Group. The relationships among ventricular arrhythmias, left ventricular dysfunction, and mortality in the 2 years after myocardial infarction. Circulation 1984; 69:250–258.
30. Bigger JT. Antiarrhythmic therapy: an overview after myocardial infarction. Am J Cardiol 1984; 53:8B–16B.
31. Furukawa T, Rozanski JJ, Nogami A, Moroe K, Gosselin AJ, et al. Time-dependent risk of and predictors for cardiac arrest recurrence in survivors of out-of-hospital cardiac arrest with chronic coronary artery disease. Circulation 1989; 80:599–608.
32. Schechtman KB, Bipone RJ, Kleiger RE, Gibson RS, Schwartz DJ, et al., and the Diltiazem Reinfarction Study Research Group. Risk stratification of patients with non-Q wave myocardial infarction. Circulation 1989; 80:1148–1158.
33. The Cardiac Arrhythmia Suppression Trial (CAST) Investigators. Preliminary report: effect of encainide and flecainide on mortality in a randomized trial of arrhythmia suppression after myocardial infarction. N Engl J Med 1989; 331:406–412.
34. Echt DS, Liebson PR, Mitchell B, Peters RW, Obias-Manno D, et al., and the CAST Investigators. Mortality and morbidity in patients receiving encainide, flecainide, or placebo. The Cardiac Arrhythmias Suppression Trial. N Engl J Med 1991; 324:781–788.
35. Pfeffer MA, Braunwald E, Moye LA, Basta L, Brown EJ Jr, et al., and the SAVE Investigators. The effect of captopril on mortality and morbidity in patients with left ventricular dysfunction after myocardial infarction: results of the survival and ventricular enlargement trial. N Engl J Med 1992; 327:669–677.

36. Sacks FM, Pfeffer MA, Moye LA, Rouleau JL, Rutherford JD, et al., for the Cholesterol and Recurrent Events Trial Investigators. The effect of pravastatin on coronary events after myocardial infarction in patients with average cholesterol levels. N Engl J Med 1996; 335:1001–1009.
37. Myerburg RJ, Interian A Jr, Mitrani RM, Kessler KM, Castellanos A. Frequency of sudden cardiac death and profiles of risk. Am J Cardiol 1997; 80:10F–19F.
38. Priori SG, Barhanin J, Hauer RNW, et al. Genetic and molecular basis of cardiac arrhythmias: impact on clinical management. Circulation 1999; 99:518.
39. Kannel WB, Thomas HE. Sudden coronary death: the Framingham Study. Ann NY Acad Sci 1982; 38: 3–21.
40. Cupples LA, Gagnon DR, Kannel WB. Long- and short-term risk of sudden coronary death. Circulation 1992; 85(Suppl I):I-11–18.
41. Anderson KP. Sudden death, hypertension, and hypertrophy. J Cardiovasc Pharm 1984; 6(Suppl III):S498–S503.
42. Messerli FH, Ventura HO, Elizardi DJ, Dunn FG, Frohlich ED. Hypertension and sudden increased ventricular ectopic activity in left ventricular hypertrophy. Am J Med 1984; 77:18–22.
43. Furukawa T, Myerburg RJ, Furukawa N, Kimura S, Bassett AL. Ionic mechanism of increased susceptibility of hypertrophied feline myocytes to metabolic inhibition. Circulation 1990; 82(Suppl III):III-522.
44. Furukawa T, Bassett AL, Kimura S, Furukawa N, Myerburg RJ. The ionic mechanism of reperfusion-induced early afterdepolarizations in feline left ventricular hypertrophy. J Clin Invest 1993; 91:1521–1531.
45. Ginzton LE, Conant R, Rodrigues DM, Laks MM. Functional significance of hypertrophy of the non-infarcted myocardium after myocardial infarction in humans. Circulation 1989; 80: 816–822.
46. Cox MM, Berman I, Myerburg RJ, Smets MJD, Kozlovskis PL. Morphometric mapping of regional myocyte diameters after healing of myocardial infarction in cats. J Mol Cell Cardiol 1991; 23:127–135.
47. Yuan F, Pinto JMB, Li Q, Wasserlauf BJ, Yang X, et al. Characteristics of $I_k$ and its response to quinidine in experimental healed myocardial infarction. J Cardiovasc Electrophysiol 1999; 10:844–854.
48. Kannel WB, Doyle JT, McNamara PM, Quickenton P, Gordon T. Precursors of sudden coronary death: factors related to the incidence of sudden death. Circulation 1979; 51:606–613.
49. Kuller LH. Sudden death: definition and epidemiologic considerations. Prog Cardiovasc Dis 1980; 23:1–12.
50. Kjekshus J. Arrhythrnias and mortality in congestive heart failure. Am J Cardiol 1990; 65:I-42-I-48.
51. Myerburg RJ, Kessler KM, Kimura S, Castellanos A. Sudden cardiac death: future approaches based on identification and control of transient risk factors. J Cardiovasc Electrophysiol 1992; 3:626–640.
52. Muller JE, Tofler GH, Stone PH. Circadian variation and triggers of onset of acute cardiovascular disease. Circulation 1989; 79:733–743.
53. Maclure M. The case-crossover design: a method for studying transient effects on the risk of acute events. Am J Epidemiol 1991; 133:144–153.
54. Leor J, Poole WK, Kloner RA. Sudden cardiac death triggered by an earthquake. N Engl J Med 1996; 334:413–419.
55. Rosen MR, Janse MJ, Myerburg RJ. Arrhythmias induced by coronary artery occlusion: What are the electrophysiological mechanisms? In: Hearse D, Manning A, Janse M (eds). Life-Threatening Arrhythmias During Ischemia and Infarction. Raven Press, NY, 1987, Chapter 2, pp 11–47.

56. Baum RS, Alvarez H, Cobb LA. Survival after resuscitation from out-of-hospital ventricular fibrillation. Circulation 1974; 50:1231–1235.
57. Myerburg RJ, Kessler KM, Zaman L, Conde CA, Castellanos A. Survivors of prehospital cardiac arrest. J Am Med Assoc 1982; 247:1485–1490.
58. Gottlieb SO, Weisfeldt MI, Ouyang P, Mellits ED, Gerstenblith. Silent ischemia as a marker for early unfavorable outcomes in patients with unstable angina. N Engl J Med 1986; 314:1214.
59. Weintraub RM, Aroesty JM, Paulin S, Levine RH, Markis JE, et al. Medically refractory unstable angina pectoris. 1. Long-term follow-up of patients undergoing intra-aortic balloon counterpulsation and operation. Am J Cardiol 1979; 43:877.
60. Mulcahy R, Awadhi AHA, deBuitieor M, Tobin G, Johnson H, et al. Natural history and prognosis of unstable angina. Am Heart J 1985; 109:753.
61. Nademanee K, Intarachot V, Josephson MA, Rieders D, Mody FV, et al. Prognostic significance of silent myocardial ischemia in patients with unstable angina. J Am Coll Cardiol 1987; 1:1–9.
62. Myerburg RJ, Kessler KM, Mallow SM, Cox M, deMarchena E, et al. Potentially fatal arrhythmias in patients with silent myocardial ischemia due to coronary artery spasm. N Engl J Med 1992; 326:1451–1455.
63. Furukawa T, Moroe K, Mayrovitz HN, Sampsell R, Myerburg RJ. Arrhythmogenic effects of graded coronary blood flow reduction superimposed upon prior myocardial infarction in dogs. Circulation 1991; 84:368–377.
64. Furukawa T, Kimura S, Furukawa N, Bassett AL, Myerburg RJ. Role of cardiac ATP-regulated potassium channels in differential responses of endocardial and epicardial cells to ischemia. Circ Res 1991; 68:1693–1702.
65. Coronel R, Wilms-Schopman FJG, Opthof T, Cinca J, Fiolet JWT, et al. Reperfusion arrhythmias in isolated perfused pig hearts: inhomogeneities in extracellular potassium, ST and TO potentials and transmembrane action potentials. Circ Res 1992; 71:1131–1142.
66. Ideker RE, Klein GJ, Harrison L, Smith WM, Kasell J, et al. The transition to ventricular fibrillation induced by reperfusion after ischemia in the dog: a period of organized epicardial activation. Circulation 1981; 63:1371–1379.
67. Priori SG, Mantica M, Napolitano C, Schwartz PJ. Early afterdepolarization induced in vivo by reperfusion of ischenic myocardium. Circulation 1990; 81:1911–1920.
68. Koyha T, Kimura S, Myerburg RJ, Bassett AL. Susceptibility of hypertrophied rat hearts to ventricular fibrillation during acute ischemia. J Mol Cell Cardiol 1988; 20:159–168.
69. Myerburg RJ, Kessler KM, Castellanos A. Pathophysiology of sudden cardiac death. PACE 1991; 14(Part II):935–943.
70. Packer M. Sudden unexpected death in patients with congestive heart failure: a second frontier. Circulation 1985; 72:681–685.
71. Multiple Risk Factor Intervention Trial Research Group. Multiple-risk factor intervention trial: risk factor changes in mortality results. J Am Med Assoc 1982; 248:1465–1477.
72. Gettes LS. Electrolyte abnormalities underlying lethal ventricular arrhythmias. Circulation 1992; 85(Suppl I):I-70–I-76.
73. Kimura S, Bassett AL, Xi H, Tomita F, Myerburg J. Characteristics of ATP-sensitive K$^+$ channels in hypertrophied cells: effects of pH. Circulation 1992; 86(Suppl I):I-92.
74. Jackman WM, Friday KJ, Anderson JL, Aliot EM, Clark K, et al. The long QT syndrome: a critical review, new clinical observations, and a unifying hypothesis. Prog Cardiovasc Dis 1988; 32 (2):115–172.

75. Robinson JS, Sloman G, Mathew TH, Goble AJ. Survival after resuscitation from cardiac arrest in acute myocardial infarction. Am Heart J 1965; 69:740–747.
76. Lab MJ. Contraction-excitation feedback in myocardium: physiologic basis and clinical relevance. Circ Res 1982; 50:757–766.
77. Calkins H, Maughan WL, Weissman HF, Sugiura S, Sagawa K, et al. Effect of acute volume load on refractoriness and arrhythmia development in isolated chronically infarcted canine hearts. Circulation 1989; 79: 687–697.
78. Schwartz PJ, La Rovere T, Vanoli E. Autonomic nervous system and sudden cardiac death: experimental basis and clinical observations for post-myocardial infarction risk stratification. Circulation 1992; 85(Suppl I):I-77–I-91.
79. Barber MJ, Mueller TM, Henry DF, Felton SJ, Zipes DP. Transmural myocardial infarction in the dog produces sympathectomy in non-infarcted myocardium. Circulation 1982; 67:787–796.
80. Gaide MS, Myerburg RJ, Kozlovskis PL, Bassett AL. Elevated sympathetic response of epicardium proximal to healed myocardial infarction. Am J Physiol 1983; 14:646–652.
81. Schwartz PJ, Billman GE, Stone HL. Autonomic mechanisms in ventricular fibrillation induced by myocardial ischemia during exercise in dogs with a healed myocardial infarction: an experimental preparation for sudden cardiac death. Circulation 1984; 69:780–790.
82. Kammerling JJ, Green FJ, Watanabe AM, Inoue H, Barber MJ, et al. Denervation supersensitivity of refractoriness in non-infarcted areas apical to transmural myocardial infarction. Circulation 1987; 76:383–393.
83. Schwartz PJ, Vanoli E, Stramba-Badiale M, De Ferrari GM, Billman GE, et al. Autonomic mechanisms and sudden death: new insights from analysis of baroreceptor reflexes in conscious dogs with and without a myocardial infarction. Circulation 1988; 78:969–979.
84. Kozlovskis PL, Smets MJD, Duncan RC, Bailey BK, Bassett AL, et al. Regional beta-adrenergic receptors and adenylate cyclase activity after healing of myocardial infarction in cats. J Mol Cell Cardiol 1990; 22:311–322.
85. Bigger JT, Fleiss JL, Steinman RC, Rolnitzky LM, Kleiger RE, et al. Frequency domain measures of heart period variability and mortality after myocardial infarction. Circulation 1992; 85:164–171.
86. Huikuri HV, Linnaluoto MK, Seppanen T, Airaksinen KEJ, Kessler KM, et al. Heart rate variability and its circadian rhythm in survivors of cardiac arrest. Am J Cardiol 1992; 70:610–615.
87. Huikuri HV, Valkama JO, Airaksinen KEJ, Seppanen T, Kessler M, et al. Frequency domain measures of heart rate variability before the onset of nonsustained and sustained ventricular tachycardia in patients with coronary artery disease. Circulation 1993; 87:1220–1228.
88. Le Rovere MT, Specchia G, Mortara A, Schwartz PJ. Baroreflex sensitivity, clinical correlates and cardiovascular mortality among patients with first myocardial infarction: a prospective study. Circulation 1988; 78:816–824.
89. La Rovere MT, Bigger JT Jr, Marcus FI, Mortara A, Schwartz PJ, for the ATRAMI (Autonomic Tone and Reflexes After Myocardial Infarction) Investigators. Baroreflex sensitivity and heart-rate variability in prediction of total cardiac mortality after myocardial infarction. Lancet 1998; 351:478–484.
90. Tull M, Minardo J, Mock BH, Weiner RE, Siddiqui AR, et al. SPECT with high purity 1-123-MIBG after transmural myocardial infarction (TMI), demonstrating sympathetic denervation followed by reinnervation in a dog model. J Nucl Med 1987; 28:669.

91. Huikuri HV, Cox M, Interian A Jr, Kessler KM, Castellanos A, et al. Efficacy of intravenous propranolol for suppression of inducibility of ventricular tachyarrhythmias with different electrophysiological characteristics in coronary artery disease. Am J Cardiol 1989; 64:1305–1309.
92. Huikuri HV, Zaman L, Castellanos A, Kessler KM, Cox M, et al. Changes in spontaneous sinus node rate as an estimate of cardiac autonomic tone during stable and unstable ventricular tachycardia. J Am Col Cardiol 1989; 13:646–652.
93. Woosley RL, Chen Y, Freiman JP, Gillis RA. Mechanism of cardiotoxic actions of terfenadine. JAMA 1993; 269:1532–1536.
94. Kimura S, Bassett AL, Xi H, Myerburg RJ. Early afterdepolarizations and triggered activity induced by cocaine: a possible mechanism of cocaine arrhythmogenesis.Circulation 1992; 85:2227–2235.
95. Gohn DC, Simmons TW. Polymorphic ventricular tachycardia (torsades de pointes) associated with the use of probucol. N Engl J Med 1992; 326:1435–1436.
96. Roden DM, George AL, Bennett PB. Recent advances in understanding the molecular mechanisms of the long QT syndrome. J Cardiol Electrophysiol 1995; 6:1023–1031.
97. Roden DK, Bennett PB, Snyders DJ, Balser JR, Hondeghem LM. Quinidine delays $I_k$ activation in guinea pig ventricular myocytes. Circ Res 1988; 62:1055–1058.
98. January CR, Riddle JM. Early afterdepolarizations: mechanisms of induction and block: a role for L-type $Ca^{++}$ current. Circ Res 1989; 64:977–990.

# 2

# The Classification of Sudden Death in Clinical Trials

*Luc J.L.M. Jordaens, MD*

## Introduction

Sudden cardiac death is an important problem for the epidemiologist. Its etiology remains a scientific enigma for the physiologist, and its therapy a major challenge for public health. Prevention of sudden death continues to be one of the traditional tasks of the cardiologist, and if he succeeds in this field, it will certainly not be because he is successful with antiarrhythmic drugs. However, there are several methodological difficulties with the approach of sudden death in clinical trials.

Indeed, while the clinical expression "sudden death" is often used in cardiology and by the general public, it should be pointed out that "sudden" in clinical trials is not always as sudden as the expression suggests. Therefore, we are facing a semantic problem that originates in the original literature on "sudden" death.[1] The adjective "sudden" means unexpected. It has the same roots as the French *soudain;* words come from the Latin *subitaneis,* derived from *sub-ire,* which means "to go stealthily." This aspect is related to the emotional side associated with the problem and also to the huge problems cardiologists are facing when they try to predict such an event in an individual.

The work of Hinkle and Thaler on the clinical classification of cardiac death is among the most quoted in this domain.[1] It is important to note that they divide cardiac deaths into only 2 categories: circulatory failure and arrhythmia. The word "sudden" is only secondary, and mostly used in the abstract and in the discussion. The descriptive term "instantaneous" is applied to 43% of the arrhythmic deaths, which accounts for 58% of all cardiac deaths. Nevertheless, another 20% of the patients with arrhythmic death died within 1 hour of onset of a terminal illness, which of course is most often ischemic in origin. If the old World Health Organization definition had been used in their study (death within 24 hours of the onset of new symptoms), a considerable additional number of patients with heart

From: Aliot E, Clementy J, Prystowsky EN (editors). *Fighting Sudden Cardiac Death: A Worldwide Challenge.* ©Futura Publishing Company, Armonk, NY, 2000.

failure death would have been classified as "sudden." Difficulties in classification are evident throughout their classic attempt, which was based on information related to the status of the circulation immediately before death. There is a surprisingly high number of arrhythmic deaths described in their series. In our registry on mortality after infarction, we could assign the category of sudden death to only about 1.7% of those who died in the first 2 years after infarction.[2] This illustrates that the incidence of sudden cardiac death today is probably much lower than during the years of their studies. Also, definitions are extremely important if we want to understand the impact of interventions on the general population (with general strategies) or on individual cardiac patients.

The goal of this chapter is to analyze the definitions used in some trials in cardiology in general, and in the field of cardiac arrhythmias in particular. Also, we will try to understand whether the used definition did lead to a correct classification of sudden death. I hope this chapter will lead to a better use of definitions in future clinical trials and to a better application of the great technology we have now for the prevention of sudden cardiac death (and all-cause death) of patients at risk.[3]

# The Definitions

## Sudden Cardiac Death

This is not the place to address the etiology of sudden death. The average victim from sudden death suffers from coronary artery disease (acute myocardial infarction, or old myocardial infarction with fatal arrhythmias). It is clear that noncardiac diseases can also cause sudden death, although this is not frequent. Noncardiac and uncommon cardiac causes are much more often the cause of sudden death in younger patients. Even when these generalizations are accepted, it becomes reasonable to speak in terms of "cardiac" sudden death to improve the accuracy.

"Sudden" has a meaning with a time frame attached to it, leaving no room for further reflection. "Sudden" implies that a thing happens unexpectedly, without announcement, and is unanticipated. It is suggested that the individual (by definition not a patient until that moment) drops dead without a warning.[4] This interpretation suggests that sudden death is instantaneous, without preceding symptoms. It is easy to understand that as several larger trials classified sudden cardiac death according to the definition of arrhythmic death as used by Hinkle and Thaler, this logical time frame most often is not respected. Therefore, most trials referring to this definition accept a large variety of prodromi or preterminal symptoms before death is declared as "sudden." The accepted time frame can vary from

1 to 24 hours. This imprecision is not acceptable if we want to assess antiarrhythmic strategies. It explains some of the confusion existing today when the value of drugs, in general, and amiodarone and/or defibrillators (ICDs), in particular, for the therapy of arrhythmia survivors or for the prevention of arrhythmias are discussed.

A very acceptable definition of sudden death is used in the U.S. Physicians' Health Study.[5,6] The 1-hour definition was used. The specificity for arrhythmic death was increased by excluding cases with collapse of the circulation before the pulse disappeared. If autopsy revealed other causes, patients were equally excluded. Unwitnessed deaths were considered only as possible sudden cardiac deaths if no conflicting information was obtained. Unexpected death during sleep is conventionally classified as sudden death.[6] It seems better to classify such cases as uncertain.[7]

## Arrhythmic Death

Sudden death is not equal to arrhythmic death. However, we need detailed information on arrhythmic death in clinical trials because this is what really matters. If a patient has an ICD and receives multiple shocks, goes to the hospital, has complications or cardiogenic shock, and dies 3 weeks later, he has arrhythmic death, even if he has had no more ventricular arrhythmias during the observation. The death mechanism, however, cannot be classified as sudden. On the other hand, if a patient has new-onset angina pectoris, takes flecainide on a regular basis for atrial fibrillation, and dies "suddenly" after 90 minutes, his death mechanism can be classified as arrhythmic, but not as sudden, even if he has documented ventricular fibrillation.[8] The cause of death will be classified as "cardiac, nonarrhythmic" in most trials, while the antiarrhythmic drug is the most likely killer. So, we will continue having dilemmas in death classification. Excluding patients who show ischemia or progressive heart failure within the final hour does not seem to be logical, as these symptoms may accompany arrhythmias.[7,9]

## Cardiac Arrest

Recent efforts have been made to improve reporting cardiac arrest and resuscitation.[10] This should be helpful in the interpretation of what leads to the cardiac arrest. Only a minority of patients with cardiac arrest are successfully resuscitated. If patients recover from resuscitation, the event should be taken into account, but it cannot be considered as cardiac death (this is done in many trials). The initial condition of the patient and the character of the arrhythmia leading to arrest may influence the outcome of the resuscitation attempt. Cardiac arrest can be precipitated by angina pectoris, infarction, and heart failure. These may all remain unnoticed after the patient's demise.

## Death Mechanism Information from Implantable Devices

The idea to obtain information from the memory of implantable devices (loop recorders, pacemakers, ICDs) is not new. Pratt analyzed a large database of patients equipped with an early generation ICD, which could produce telemetered electrograms of events as arrhythmias.[11] He tried to identify sudden cardiac death and associate it with the available electrograms, but learned that clinical and autopsy data often changed the diagnosis of "sudden cardiac death" to noncardiac causes (pulmonary embolism, aneurysms). Nevertheless, when tracings are properly used, and the correct interpretation is given, some extrapolations on "avoided" sudden death can be made, if it can be believed that fast ventricular arrhythmias are associated with a higher death risk.[12]

### Cardiac Death

In general cardiology trials, cardiac death remains the most important end-point. This is logical, but it seems that "cardiac" can have many variations, such as, cardiovascular and vascular (but as the heart in the embryo is a vessel, it is also "vascular"). Further, some additional definitions within the cardiac death classification are encountered (as coronary death), creating more uncertainty. Cardiac transplantation is usually censored; it is to be considered as the end of follow-up or death in statistics (and it means that other therapies fail).

### All-Cause Death

Finally, total death, or all-cause death, is not considered as a surrogate end-point, and is indeed the most reliable one if we want to create hard data on drugs and interventions. It is easy to produce large numbers, but often, death mechanisms are lacking.[3,13]

## Clinical Trials and Their (Hard ?) Mortality End-Points

The arrhythmia literature (at least that part concerning recent randomized drug trials and the randomized ICD studies) was reviewed and put into perspective with some pivotal cardiology papers[13–21] that have implications for arrhythmia treatment.

The studies are summarized in Tables 1–3, with the most important primary and secondary end-points. It is not surprising to see that early studies used the 24-hour World Health Organization definition of sudden death.[14] It is really disappointing that not a single other general study (Table 1) was able to show in a prospective way (i.e., with a predefined question) that sudden death rates were influenced.[13,15–21] This can be due to the liberal 24-hour definition in the early β-blocker study. A recent study often quoted to reduce sudden death was not announcing sudden death as a primary or secondary end-point, and did not use acceptable definitions.[20] Cardiac arrest is more often used than sudden death, and is a very common end-point (Table 2) in antiarrhythmic drug trials.[22–30] CAST, EMIAT, and CAMIAT combined cardiac arrest with arrhythmic death to gain more power. Sudden death was not addressed in these 3 important studies. All-cause death becomes the leading end-point (after the disappointing CAST results); sudden death within 1 hour is surprisingly used in only 2 trials studying amiodarone for heart failure.[25,26] and in one ICD trial.[4,31–37] Arrhythmic death with/without cardiac arrest becomes popular in more recent drug trials (as already mentioned), but also in ICD trials (Table 3), and is often used as the surrogate for all-cause death.[38]

## Conclusions

Several attempts to classify sudden cardiac death and to improve its definition have been undertaken recently by task forces and with the idea that devices could be helpful for our understanding.[10,12] The European Society for Cardiology is trying to constitute a new task force to study the problem of sudden death again, as this is the common end-point of several cardiac and noncardiac diseases and conditions. The impact of prophylactic ICD implantation justifies all efforts in this direction.[4,37] The confusion that exists with respect to drug efficacy for prevention of "sudden" death is based on weak reporting, faulty definitions, and wrong classifications. Studies with all-cause mortality are more important than those focusing on sudden death, certainly in a time that devices can record the primary events. Arrhythmic death is not well understood, and electrograms can play a role in the understanding of its mechanism (this is often prevented by poor programming of devices). The fact that ICDs reduce total mortality is enough to justify their use. From a human point of view this is more important than a postulated role in the prevention of instantaneous death. Indeed, sudden death should be considered as a blessing for mankind, while this cannot be said for cardiac death.

## Table 1

### End-Points in Randomized Pivotal Drug Trials in Cardiology, if Possible in Relation with Arrhythmia End-Points

| Trial | Sudden Death Instantan. (1); < 1 hour (2); <24 hours (3) | Arrhythmic Death (1); Cardiac Arrest (2) | Recurrent VF (1); Cardiac Arrest (2) | Cardiac Death | All-Cause Death | Hospital Admission | Cost (1); QOL (2); Heart Failure (3) | Other Arrhythmias (1); Shocks (2) |
|---|---|---|---|---|---|---|---|---|
| Timolol Norvegian (14) | S(3) | S(2) | S(2) | S | P | | | |
| VHEFT 1[15] | S(?) | | | | P | | | |
| SSSS[16] | | | | | | | | |
| SAVE[17] | | | | S | P | S | | |
| Carvedilol[18] | | | | | P | P | S(3) | |
| TRACE[13] | | | | | P | | | |
| PRAISE[19] | | | | | S | S | | |
| CIBIS II[20] | | | | | S | | | |
| HOPE[21] | | | T(2) | P | S | S | S(3) | |

P = primary; S = secondary; T = tertiary; Instantan = instantaneous; QOL = quality of life; VF = ventricular fibrillation. The number between brackets refers to the above-mentioned item or condition. Other abbreviations from the trials are explained by the cited references.

Table 2

End-Points in Randomized Antiarrhythmic Drug Trials

| Trial | Sudden Death Instantan (1); < 1 hour (2) | Arrhythmic Death (1); Cardiac Arrest (2) | Recurrent VF (1); Cardiac Arrest (2) | Cardiac Death | All-Cause Death | Hospital Admission | Cost (1); QOL (2); Heart Failure (3) | Other Arrhythmias (1); Shocks (2) |
|---|---|---|---|---|---|---|---|---|
| CAST[22] | | P(1 or 2); S(1) | | S | S | | | |
| CASCADE[23] | | S(1 or 2) | | P | S | S | S(1,2,3) | S(1) |
| ESVEM[24] | | S(1) | | S | S | | | P(1) |
| GESICA[25] | S(2) | | | S | P | S | S(3) | S(1) |
| CHF-STAT[26,27] | S(2) | | S(1,2) | S | P | | | |
| SWORD[28] | | | | S | P | | | |
| EMIAT[29] | | S(1 or 2); S(1) | | S | P | | | |
| CAMIAT[30] | | P(1 or 2); S(1) | | S | S | | | T(1) |

P = primary; S = secondary; T = tertiary; Instantan = instantaneous; QOL = quality of life; VF = ventricular fibrillation. The number between brackets refers to the above-mentioned item or condition. Other abbreviations from the trials are explained by the cited references.

## Table 3
### End-Points in Randomized Device Trials

| Trial | Sudden Death Instantan (1); < 1 hour (2) | Arrhythmic Death (1); Cardiac Arrest (2) | Recurrent VF (1); Cardiac Arrest (2) | Cardiac Death | All-Cause Death | Hospital Admission | Cost (1); QOL (2); Heart Failure (3) | Other Arrhythmias (1); Shocks (2) |
|---|---|---|---|---|---|---|---|---|
| MADIT[4] | | S(1) | | S | P | | | |
| AVID[31] | | | | S | P | | | |
| CABG-Patch[32] | | | | | P | | S(1,2) | |
| CIDS[33] | | P | S(1) | S | S | | | S(1) |
| DCE[34] | | | | | P | S | P(3); S(3) | P; S(2) |
| CASH[35,36] | S(1) | | S(2) | | P | | | S |
| MUSST[37] | | P(1,2) | | S | S | | | |

P = primary; S = secondary; T = tertiary; Instantan = instantaneous; QOL = quality of life; VF = ventricular fibrillation. The number between brackets refers to the above-mentioned item or condition. Other abbreviations from the trials are explained by the cited references.

# References

1. Hinkle LE, Thaler HT. Clinical classification of cardiac deaths. Circulation 1992; 65:457–464.
2. Jordaens L, Tavernier R, and the Mirracle's Investigators. The actual therapy and in-hospital mortality of acute myocardial infarction in Flanders. Acta Cardiol 1997; 52:397–410.
3. Moss AJ, Hall WJ, Cannom DS, et al. Improved survival with an implanted defibrillator in patients with coronary disease at high risk for ventricular arrhythmia. N Engl J Med 1996; 335:1933–1940.
4. Epstein SE, Quyyumi AA, Bonow RO. Sudden cardiac death without a warning. N Engl J Med 1989; 321:320–324.
5. Albert CM, Hennekens CH, O'Donnell CJ, et al. Fish consumption and risk of sudden cardiac death. J Am Med Assoc 1998; 297:23–28.
6. Multicenter Postinfarction Research Group. Risk stratification and survival after myocardial infarction. N Engl J Med 1983; 309:331–336.
7. Escobedo LG, Zack MM. Comparison of sudden and nonsudden coronary deaths in the United States. Circulation 1996; 93:2033–2036.
8. Greenberg HM, Dwyer EM Jr, Hochman JS, et al. Interaction of ischaemia and encainide/flecainide treatment: a proposed mechanism for the increased mortality in CAST I. Br Heart J 1995; 74:631–635.
9. Hartikainen JEK, Malik M, Staunton A, et al. Distinction between arrhythmic and non-arrhythmic death after acute myocardial infarction based on heart rate variability, signal-averaged electrocardiogram, ventricular arrhythmias and left ventricular ejection fraction. J Am Coll Cardiol 1996; 28:296–304.
10. European Resuscitation Council, American Heart Association, Heart and Stroke Foundation of Canada, et al. Recommended guidelines for uniform reporting of data from out-of-hospital cardiac arrest (new abridged version). Br Heart J 1992; 67:325–333.
11. Pratt CM, Greenway PS, Schoenfeld MH, et al. Exploration of the precision of classifying sudden cardiac death: implications for the interpretation of clinical trials. Circulation 1996; 93:519–524.
12. Böcker D, Bansch D, Heinecke A, et al. Potential benefit from implantable cardioverter-defibrillator therapy in patients with and without heart failure. Circulation 1998; 98:1636–1643.
13. Torp-Pedersen C, Kober L, for the TRACE study group. Effect of ACE inhibitor trandolapril on life expectancy of patients with reduced left-ventricular function after acute myocardial infarction. Lancet 1999; 354:9–12.
14. Pedersen TR, for the Norwegian Multicenter Study Group. The Norwegian multicenter study of timolol after myocardial infarction. Circulation 1983; 67:49–53.
15. Cohn JN, Archibald DG, Phil M, et al. Effect of vasodilator therapy on mortality in chronic congestive heart failure. N Engl J Med 1986; 314:1547–1552.
16. Scandinavian Simvastatin Survival Study Group. Randomised trial of cholesterol lowering in 4444 patients with coronary heart disease: the Scandinavian Simvastatin Survival Study (4S). Lancet 1994; 344:1383–1389.
17. Pfeffer MA, Braunwald E, Moyé LA, et al. Effect of captopril on mortality and morbidity in patients with left ventricular dysfunction after myocardial infarction. N Engl J Med 1992; 327:669–677.
18. Packer M, Bristow MR, Cohn JN, et al. The effect of carvedilol on morbidity and mortality in patients with chronic heart failure. N Engl J Med 1996; 334:1349–1355.

19. Packer M, O'Connor CM, Ghali JK, et al. Effect of amlodipine on morbidity and mortality in severe chronic heart failure. N Engl J Med 1996; 335:1107–1114.
20. CIBIS-II Investigators and Committees. The Cardiac Insufficiency Bisoprolol Study II (CIBIS-II): a randomised trial. Lancet 1999; 3539–3513.
21. The Heart Outcomes Prevention Evaluation Study Investigators. Effects of an angiotensin-converting-enzyme inhibitor, ramipril, on death from cardiovascular causes, myocardial infarction, and stroke in high risks. N Eng J Med 1991; 32:1371–1372.
22. Cardiac Arrhythmias Suppression Trial (CAST). Preliminary report: effect of encainide and flecainide on mortality in a randomized trial of arrhythmia suppression after myocardial infarction. N Engl J Med 1989; 321:406–412.
23. The Cascade Investigators. Cardiac arrest in Seattle: conventional versus amiodarone drug evaluation (the CASCADE study). Am J Cardiol 1991; 67:578–584.
24. Mason JW, for the Electrophysiologic Study Versus Electrocardiographic Monitoring Investigators. A comparison of electrophysiologic testing with Holter monitoring to predict antiarrhythmic-drug efficacy for ventricular tachyarrhythmias. N Engl J Med 1993; 329:445–451.
25. Doval HC, Nul DR, Grancelli HO, et al. Randomised trial of low-dose amiodarone in severe congestive heart failure. Lancet 1994; 344:493–498.
26. Singh SN, Fletcher RD, Fisher S, et al. Veterans Affairs congestive heart failure antiarrhythmic trial. Am J Cardiol 1993; 72:99F–102F.
27. Singh SN, Fletcher RD, Fisher SG, et al. Amiodarone in patients with congestive heart failure and asymptomatic ventricular arrhythmia. N Engl J Med 1995; 333:77–82.
28. Waldo AL, Camm AJ, Deruyter H, et al. Survival with oral d-sotalol in patients with left ventricular dysfunction after myocardial infarction: rationale, design, and methods (the SWORD trial). Am J Cardiol 1995; 75:1023–1027.
29. Julian DG, Camm AJ, Frangin G, et al. Randomised trial of effect of amiodarone on mortality in patients with left-ventricular dysfunction after recent myocardial infarction. Lancet 1997; 349:667–674.
30. Cairns JA, Connolly SJ, Roberts R, et al. Randomised trial of outcome after myocardial infarction in patients with frequent or repetitive ventricular premature depolarisations: CAMIAT. Lancet 1997; 349:675–682.
31. The Antiarrhythmics versus Implantable Defibrillators (AVID). Investigators. A comparison of antiarrhythmic-drug therapy with implantable defibrillators in patients resuscitated from near-fatal ventricular arrhythmias. N Engl J Med 1997; 337:1576–1583.
32. Bigger JT Jr, for the Coronary Artery Bypass Graft Patch Trial Investigators. Prophylactic use of implanted cardiac defibrillators in patients at high risk for ventricular arrhythmias after coronary-artery bypass graft surgery. N Engl J Med 1997; 27;337:1569–1575.
33. Connolly SJ, Gent M, Roberts RS, et al. Canadian Implantable Defibrillator Study (CIDS): study design and organization. Am J Cardiol 1993; 72:103F–108F.
34. Wever EF, Hauer RN, van Capelle FL, et al. Randomized study of implantable defibrillator as first-choice therapy versus conventional strategy in postinfarct sudden death survivors. Circulation 1995; 91:2195–2203.
35. Siebels J, Cappato R, Ruppel R, et al. Preliminary results of the Cardiac Arrest Study Hamburg (CASH). Am J Cardiol 1993; 72:109F–113F.
36. Cappato R. Secondary prevention of sudden death: the Dutch study, the antiaarrhythmics versus implantable defibrillator trial, the cardiac arrest study

Hamburg, and the Canadian implantable defibrillator study. Am J Cardiol 1999; 83:68–73.

37. Buxton AE, Lee KL, Fisher JD, et al. A randomized study of the prevention of sudden death in patients with coronary artery disease. N Engl J Med 1999; 341:1882–1890.

38. Gottlieb SS. Dead is dead. Lancet 1997; 349:662–663.

# 3

# How Genetics May Help to Understand and Prevent Sudden Cardiac Death

*Ketty Schwartz, PhD*

## Introduction

At the beginning of this decade, it was difficult to find a cardiologist who thought that genes could be important players in the pathogenesis of cardiac arrhythmias and sudden deaths. Table 1 shows where we are now. It is adapted from a paper by Priori et al.[1] that was the outcome of a workshop convened by the Study Group of the Molecular Basis of Arrhythmias of the Working Group on Arrhythmias of the European Society of Cardiology. During this workshop, we tried to answer the questions that clinical cardiologists managing arrhythmias are faced with due to the rapidly expanding knowledge of medical genetics. In recent years, the genes responsible for all of the cardiac arrhythmias listed in Table 1 have been mapped on the human genome and, for some of them, characterized. For example, the gene responsible for X-linked dilated cardiomyopathy is dystrophin, for the Barth syndrome, it is G4.5. Contractile protein defects are the origin of familial hypertrophic cardiomyopathy, and 5 different ionic channels are responsible for the long QT syndromes (Romano-Ward autosomal dominant, Romano-Ward recessive, and Jervell and Lange-Nielsen). One of these ionic channels, *SCN5A*, encoding the sodium channel, is also responsible for a form of idiopathic ventricular fibrillation. It is a real explosion of knowledge, and the molecular mechanisms that predispose a patient with or without cardiac pathology to arrhythmias are beginning to be understood. This chapter focuses on 2 pathologies: familial hypertrophic cardiomyopathy and Emery-Dreifuss muscular dystrophy, which we now propose to call a new form of autosomal dominant cardiomyopathy with conduction defects. For these 2 pathologies, very unexpected results were found through the use of molecular genetics.

From: Aliot E, Clementy J, Prystowsky EN (editors). *Fighting Sudden Cardiac Death: A Worldwide Challenge*. ©Futura Publishing Company, Armonk, NY, 2000.

---

**Table 1**

**Inherited Arrhythmogenic Disorders Where the Disease
Gene and/or the Disease Locus Have Been Identified**

---

- X-linked dilated cardiomyopathy
- Barth syndrome
- Autosomal dominant dilated cardiomyopathy
- Conduction defect and dilated cardiomyopathy
- Familial hypertrophic cardiomyopathy
- Progressive familial heart block type I
- Long QT syndrome Romano-Ward type
- Long QT syndrome Jervell and Lange-Nielsen type
- Arrhythmogenic right ventricular cardiomyopathy
- Naxos disease
- Familial idiopathic ventricular fibrillation

---

Adapted from Priori et al.[1]

## Familial Hypertrophic Cardiomyopathy

Familial hypertrophic cardiomyopathy was first described in the middle of the 19th century by Edmée Felix Alfred Vulpian,[2] a neurologist who worked in the hospital La Salpêtrière in Paris. One of his students, Henry Liouville, stated *"l'importance clinique considérable que leur connaissance complète nous semble devoir comporter, lorsque l'attention des médecins sera plus spécialement attirée sur eux." Alfred Vulpian called what he saw at the organ level "rétrécissement sous aortique." The attention of the physicians was attracted to this disease more than 1 century later, on the other side of the Atlantic, and with the advent of echocardiography, its clinical characteristics were precisely described, more specifically in Bethesda. It was precisely redefined by the task force from the World Health Organization and the International Society and Federation of Cardiology.[3]

Hypertrophic cardiomyopathy[4] is transmitted as an autosomal dominant disease. Its clinical phenotype is characterized by unexplained and inappropriate clinical left and/or right ventricular hypertrophy, which may be severe (4 to 5 cm), mild, or even absent. Characterization of the distribution of left ventricular hypertrophy is arbitrary, but by convention hypertrophy is considered to be either asymmetric septal hypertrophy, concentric, or predominantly distal ventricular. Any pattern of hypertrophy, however, may be seen including hypertrophy confined to the poste-

---

*The great clinical impact that their complete knowledge will have, when physicians will pay sufficient attention to them.

rior or free wall. Characteristic histological features include myocyte disarray surrounding areas of increased loose connective tissue. Clinically, there is marked hemodynamic heterogeneity among patients with familial hypertrophic cardiomyopathy. Systolic function may be hyperdynamic (with or without obstruction), "normal," or impaired (10–15%). Diastolic dysfunction is the usual physiological abnormality, although the precise abnormality of ventricular filling and compliance is extremely variable. Familial hypertrophic cardiomyopathy-related arrhythmias occur both at the ventricular and the atrial level. Importantly, sudden cardiac death in familial hypertrophic cardiomyopathy is not necessarily caused by ventricular arrhythmias. Atrial fibrillation in the presence of an accessory pathway, bradyarrhythmias, and ischemia may all lead to sudden death.

None of the previous hypotheses of the pathophysiological mechanisms would have predicted that defects in sarcomeric genes could be a possible molecular basis for the disease. The results of molecular genetic studies have nevertheless shown that all mutations found so far concern sarcomeric proteins[5-7]: 3 myofilament proteins, the β-myosin heavy chain (β-MyHc), the ventricular myosin essential light chain 1 (MLC-1s/v), and the ventricular myosin regulatory light chain 2 (MLC-2s/v); 4 thin-filament proteins, cardiac troponin T (cTnT), cardiac troponin I (cTnI), α-tropomyosin (α-TM) and cardiac α-actin; 1 myosin-binding protein, the cardiac myosin-binding protein C (cMyBP-C); and, finally, the third filament protein, titin. The schematic localization of these proteins is shown in Figure 1. These genes certainly do not represent the whole spectrum of familial hypertrophic cardiomyopathy disease genes since an additional locus was reported,[8] and one might reasonably hypothesize that disease genes yet to be identified include additional components of the sarcomere.

In a panel of 48 families or probands analyzed in France and coming from different countries, we found that the disease gene was *MYH7* in 19 of them, and that the cardiac myosin-binding protein C gene was the disease gene in 33 of them. We found a total of 40 different mutations, some of them yet unpublished. There is a striking genetic heterogeneity, without any predominant mutation. On the contrary, it appears as if each family has its own mutation.

One of the main questions now is to determine whether this large genetic heterogeneity can account for the large phenotypic heterogeneity of the disease, and more specifically for the high incidence of sudden deaths occurring in some families. The results obtained thus far must be considered as very preliminary, because the available data relate to only a few hundred individuals, and it is obvious that although a given phenotype may be apparent in a small family, examining large or multiple

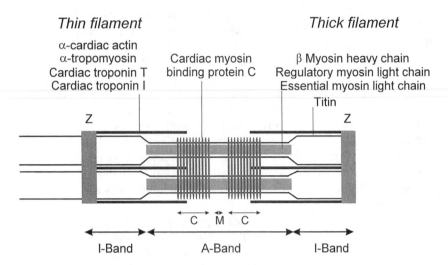

Figure 1. Schematic representation of the cardiac sarcomere and of the disease genes in hypertrophic cardiomyopathy. (Adapted with permission from Bonne G, et al.[5])

families with the same mutation is required before drawing unambiguous conclusions. There are, nevertheless, several emerging concepts: (1) TNNT2 mutations appear to be associated with usually mild or moderate hypertrophy and a high incidence of sudden death; (2) MYBPC3 mutations are now associated with a mild phenotype in young subjects, a delayed age at the onset of symptoms, and a favorable prognosis under 40 years of age; (3) as for MYH7 mutations, the prognosis and hypertrophy may vary considerably with the mutation. In a recent study, we examined 76 genetically affected subjects from 9 families with 7 mutations.[9] Detailed clinical, ECG, and echocardiographic parameters were analyzed. An intergene analysis was performed by comparing the MYBPC3 group to 7 mutations in the β-myosin heavy chain gene (β-MHC) group (n=52). There was no significant phenotypic difference among the different mutations in the MYBPC3 gene. However, in the MYBPC3 group compared with the β-MHC group: (1) prognosis was significantly better, and no deaths occurred before the age of 40 years; (2) the age at onset of symptoms was delayed (41±19 versus 35±17years); and (3) before 30 years of age, the phenotype was particularly mild because penetrance was low, maximal wall thicknesses lower, and abnormal T waves less frequent. Similar conclusions were drawn by Niimura et al.[10] These findings could be particularly important for the purpose of clinical management and genetic counseling in familial hypertrophic cardiomyopathy.

# Autosomal Dominant Emery-Dreifuss Muscular Dystrophy: A New Form of Autosomal Dominant Cardiomyopathy With Conduction Defects?

In 1902, Cestan and LeJonne,[11] working in the Neurological Clinic of the Hospital La Salpêtrière, described a disease that they called *"myopathie avec rétractions familiales." They stated that **"les deux cas que nous publions, observés à la clinique de notre maître le Professeur Raymond, nous ont parus remarquables, d'abord à cause de l'intensité de la généralisation du processus de rétraction, ensuite et surtout par le caractère familial de ce processus, fait qui nous a paru jusque là signalé par aucun auteur."

In 1966, Emery examined a large Virginia family affected with an X-linked muscular dystrophy.[12] Members of this family had been reported earlier by Dreifuss and Hogan[13] as having a possible benign form of Duchenne-type muscular dystrophy (DMD), but after detailed clinical, electrophysiological, and biochemical analysis, Emery realized that the disease observed in the Dreifuss family was quite distinct from both DMD and BMD (Becker type, the benign allelic form of DMD): the unusual elbow and spine contractures, the proximal arm and distal leg pattern of weakness, and the essential cardiac features were first described in the Emery report. Later on, similar manifestations were described in other families, until 1979, when Rowland suggested the term "Emery-Dreifuss muscular dystrophy" for this distinctive disease. Families show X-linked recessive inheritance (X-EDMD: OMIM no. 310300), or autosomal dominant form (AD-EDMD: OMIM no. 181350). Emery has summarized the clinical triad of X-EDMD as follows: (1) early contractures, often before there is any significant weakness, of the elbows, Achilles tendons, and posterior neck (with limitation initially of neck flexion but later of forward flexion of the entire spine); (2) slowly progressive muscle wasting and weakness with a humeroperoneal distribution early in the course of the disease, and later, weakness also affecting the proximal limb-girdle musculature; and (3) a cardiomyopathy usually presenting as an atrioventricular conduction block, ranging from sinus bradycardia, prolongation of the PR interval to complete heart block, which is often life threatening. Importantly, the cardiac conduction defects often cause sudden death, and appropriate implantation of a cardiac pacemaker is recommended. Voit et

---

*Myopathy with familial contractures.

**The 2 cases that we publish, observed in the clinic of our master Professor Raymond, are remarkable, first because the intensity of the generalization of the process of retraction, and secondly and mainly because of the familial aspect of this process, which has never been reported before.

al.[14] performed a detailed cardiological follow-up study of patients with EDMD, and found 4 main features: (1) impairment of impulse-generating cells; (2) conduction defects with atrial preponderance; (3) increased atrial and ventricular heterotopia; and (4) functional impairment of ventricular myocardium. Lethal cardiac involvement may also occur in female carriers, and, therefore, careful cardiological follow-up examinations are recommended. Variations in clinical severity within families may be seen.

Mutations in *EMD*, the gene encoding emerin, are responsible for the X-linked form.[15] We have mapped the locus for EDMD-AD on chromosome 1q11–q23 in a large French pedigree and found that 4 other small families were potentially linked to this locus. This region contains the lamin A/C gene (*LMNA*), a candidate gene encoding 2 proteins of the nuclear lamina, lamins A and C, through alternative splicing.[16,17] We identified 4 mutations in *LMNA* that co-segregate with the disease phenotype in the 5 families: 1 nonsense mutation and 3 missense mutations.[18] These results were the first to identify mutations in a component of the nuclear lamina as a cause of inherited muscle disorder. Together with mutations in *DMD*, they underscore the potential importance of the nuclear envelope components in the pathogenesis of neuromuscular disorders. These results also underscored the potential importance of proteins of the nuclear envelope in the development of dilated cardiomyopathy with conduction defect and in the etiology of sudden death. Indeed, in the large French pedigree, there were 3 nuclei of patients presenting only with the cardiac symptoms, without any skeletal muscle involvement.[19] In a routine clinical cardiologist practice, these patients would have been diagnosed as having dilated cardiomyopathy, and the link with the skeletal myopathy observed in other members of the family would certainly not have been noticed.

## Conclusion

It is clear that the genetic and molecular bases of cardiac arrhythmias are beginning to be revealed and that completely unexpected genes seem now to be involved in the pathogenesis of these life-threatening diseases. There is no doubt that, in the near future, most genes responsible for inherited arrhythmogenic conditions will be identified, and that this will produce results applicable to the successful clinical management of patients and their families.

## *References*

1. Priori SG, Barhanin J, Hauer RN, et al. Genetic and molecular basis of cardiac arrhythmias: impact on clinical management. Study Group on the Molecular

Basis of Arrhythmias of the Working Group on Arrhythmias of the European Society of Cardiology. Eur Heart J 1999; 20:174–195.

2. Vulpian A. Contribution à l'étude des rétrécissements de l'orifice ventriculo-aortique. Archiv Physiol 1868; 3:220–222.

3. Richardson P, McKenna W, Bristow M, et al. Report of the 1995 World Health Organisation/International Society and Federation of Cardiology task force on the definition and classification of cardiomyopathies. Circulation 1995; 93:841–842.

4. Schwartz K, Carrier L, Guicheney P, et al. Molecular basis of familial cardiomyopathies. Circulation 1995; 91:532–540.

5. Bonne G, Carrier L, Richard P, et al. Familial hypertrophic cardiomyopathy: from mutations to functional defects. Circ Res 1998; 83:579–593.

6. Mogensen J, Klausen IC, Pedersen AK, et al. α-cardiac actin is a novel disease gene in familial hypertrophic cardiomyopathy. J Clin Invest 1999; 103:R39–R43.

7. Satoh M, Takahashi M, Sakamoto T, et al. Structural analysis of the titin gene in hypertrophic cardiomyopathy: identification of a novel disease gene. Biochem Biophys Res Comm 1999; 262: 411–417.

8. MacRae CA, Ghaisas N, Kass S, et al. Familial hypertrophic cardiomyopathy with Wolff-Parkinson-White syndrome maps to a locus on chromosome 7q3. J Clin Invest 1995; 96:1216–1220.

9. Charron P, Dubourg O, Desnos M, et al. Genotype-phenotype correlations in familial hypertrophic cardiomyopathy: a comparison between mutations in the cardiac protein-C and the β-myosin heavy chain genes. Eur Heart J 1998; 19:139–145.

10. Niimura H, Bachinski LL, Sangwatanaroj S, et al. Mutations in the gene for cardiac myosin-binding protein C and late-onset familial hypertrophic cardiomyopathy. N Engl J Med 1998; 338:1248–1257.

11. Cestan R, LeJonne. Une myopathie avec rétractions familiales. Nouvelle iconographie de la Salpétrière 1902; 15:38–52.

12. Emery AEH, Dreifuss FE. Unusual type of benign X-linked muscular dystrophy. J Neurol Neurosurg Psychiat 1966; 29:338–342.

13. Dreifuss FE, Hogan GR. Survival in X-chromosomal muscular dystrophy. Neurology 1961; 11:734–737.

14. Voit T, Krogmann O, Lenard HG, et al. Emery-Dreifuss muscular dystrophy: disease spectrum and differential diagnosis. Neuropediatrics 1988; 19: 62–71.

15. Bione S, Maestrini E, Rivella S, et al. Identification of a novel X-linked gene responsible for Emery-Dreifuss muscular dystrophy. Nat Genet 1994; 8:323–327.

16. Lin F, Worman HJ. Structural organization of the human gene (LMNB1) encoding nuclearlamin B1. Genomics 1995; 27:230–236.

17. Wydner KL, McNeil JA, Lin F, et al. Chromosomal assignment of human nuclear envelope protein genes LMNA, LMNB1, and LBR by fluorescence in situ hybridization. Genomics 1996; 32:474–478.

18. Bonne G, Di Barletta MR, Varnous S, et al. Mutations in the gene encoding lamin A/C cause autosomal dominant Emery-Dreifuss muscular dystrophy. Nat Genet 1999; 21:285–288.

19. Bonne G, Di Barletta MR, Varnous S, et al. Genetic localisation of autosomal dominant Emery-Dreifuss muscular dystrophy. IX International Congress on Neuromuscular Diseases. Muscle Nerve 1998; (Suppl 7): S65.

# 4

# Autonomic Nervous System and Sudden Cardiac Death

*Hugh Calkins, MD*

## Introduction

In the United States, sudden cardiac death resulting largely from sustained ventricular arrhythmias is responsible for approximately 300,000 deaths annually. The overall incidence of sudden death in the adult population has been estimated to be 0.1% to 0.2% per year. Sudden death is the most common and often the initial manifestation of coronary heart disease and is responsible for one-half of the mortality from cardiovascular disease in the United States.

The precise cause of sudden death remains incompletely understood. However, there is increasing evidence to support the concept that sudden death is an "electrical accident" that results from a complex interplay between anatomic and functional substrates, modulated by transient triggering events that further disturb the electrical milieu[1] (Figure 1). Compelling evidence now exists that implicates the autonomic nervous system in the cause of sudden cardiac death. Heightened sympathetic activity has been shown to favor the development of cardiac arrhythmias, whereas increased vagal tone is thought to be protective. The mechanisms by which the autonomic nervous system promotes and/or triggers the development of cardiac arrhythmias remain incompletely understood. The purpose of this chapter is to review the current body of knowledge having to do with various aspects of the interaction between the autonomic nervous system and the occurrence of sudden death.

## Evidence Supporting an Interaction Between the Autonomic Nervous System and Sudden Death

John MacWilliam is credited with proposing that ventricular fibrillation was the mechanism of sudden death in humans in 1889.[2,3] He notes

From: Aliot E, Clementy J, Prystowsky EN (editors). *Fighting Sudden Cardiac Death: A Worldwide Challenge.* ©Futura Publishing Company, Armonk, NY, 2000.

## Etiology of Sudden Cardiac Death

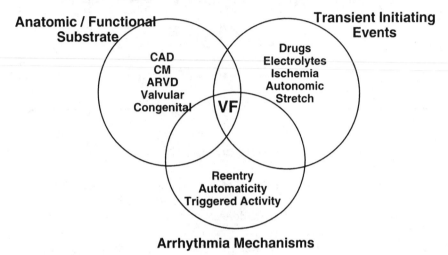

**Figure 1.** Venn diagram showing interaction of various anatomic/functional and transient factors that modulate potential arrhythmogenic mechanisms capable of causing sudden cardiac death.

that " . . . sudden cardiac failure does not usually take the form of a simple ventricular standstill in diastole . . . It assumes, on the contrary, the form of violent, though irregular and incoordinated, manifestations of ventricular energy. Instead of quiescence, there is tumultuous activity, irregular in its character and wholly ineffective."[3] MacWilliam was also the first to propose the concept that sudden cardiac death typically occurred in the setting a structural heart disease but that important precipitating factors were also involved.[3,4] In his classic paper of 1889, MacWilliam cited Gairdner, who wrote: "It is plainly out of the question to suppose that a chronic, and in its very nature gradually advancing lesion like fatty degeneration or disease of the coronary vessels, is the direct and immediate cause of death which occurs in a moment."[3] He clearly recognized that fixed coronary artery disease or preexisting myocardial or valvular disease alone, while causing symptoms, did not account completely for the occurrence of sudden death and that additional transiently occurring factors were required. In a subsequent paper, entitled "Blood Pressure and Heart Action in Sleep and Dreams," he further developed the concept that the central nervous system plays a role in sudden death. These observations and hypotheses that were initially developed 100 years ago are now widely accepted underpinnings of our current concepts of sudden cardiac death and are commonly referred to as the "arrhythmia genesis triangle." This popular clinical model illustrates the arrhythmic mechanisms of sudden cardiac death and describes the notion that ventricular arrhythmias occur in the setting of an abnormal myocardial substrate, usually associated with fibrosis or scarring from a prior myocardial infarction in the presence of certain modulating factors known to provoke ventricular arrhythmias (ischemia, hypokalemia, autonomic nervous system activation).[5]

There exists a large body of data that directly or indirectly implicates the autonomic nervous system, particularly the sympathetic nervous system in the precipitation of sudden cardiac death. These data include the results of animal studies,[6–17] and more recently the results of clinical studies that have identified a link between the time of day and risk of sudden death.[18–26] It was demonstrated more than 70 years ago that ventricular arrhythmias could be invoked in normal animals by stimulating certain areas in the hypothalamus.[7] These observations were subsequently confirmed by others.[8] Other investigators demonstrated that stimulation of the posterior hypothalamus resulted in a 10-fold increase in the incidence of ventricular fibrillation associated with acute coronary occlusion.[9] This effect was blocked by beta blockade but not vagotomy, consistent with the notion that this response was due to sympathetic activation.[10] Further insights have been provided by Skinner and Reed who reported that cryogenic blockade of the thalamic gating mechanisms or its output from the frontal cortex of the brain delayed or prevented ventricular fibrillation during stress in pigs.[11] Thus it appears that the central nervous system plays a critical role in triggering cardiac arrhythmias. In other models it was shown that aversive conditioning of dogs resulted in a 3-fold increase in the occurrence of spontaneous ventricular fibrillation. This effect was blocked by beta blockade, indicating a primary role of the sympathetic nervous system in stress-induced changes in cardiac vulnerability.[12,13] Further experiments using this model revealed that vagal blockade with atropine resulted in a marked increase of vulnerability induced by an adversive environment.[14] A clinical correlate of these observations are the clinical reports that cerebral vascular disease and intracranial hemorrhage can produce pronounced cardiac repolarization abnormalities and life-threatening arrhythmias.[15,16] Additional clinical evidence for the importance of neural triggers in the development of life-threatening arrhythmias results from the observation that sudden cardiac death occurs in a circadian pattern, with a peak in death rates in the early morning[18–23] (Figure 2). These studies have shown that this phenomenon is the consequence of a centrally mediated increase in sympathetic activity and a decrease in parasympathetic activity in the early morning hours prior to awakening. Another factor in this diurnal variation in the incidence of sudden cardiac death likely re-

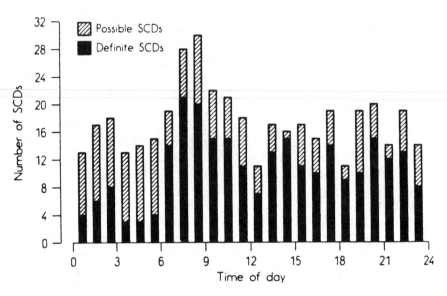

**Figure 2.** Bar graph showing time of definite (n=264) and possible (n=165) sudden cardiac death (SCD) in the Framingham Heart Study. The circadian pattern of all definite sudden cardiac deaths was characterized by a trough period during the night. A 3-fold increase in the number of sudden deaths was observed in the early morning between 7 AM and 9 AM. (From Willich SN, et al.[24] with permission.)

sults from an adrenergically mediated increase in platelet aggregability leading to adrenergically mediated thrombosis that is exacerbated by arising.[22,25,26]

## Pattern of Autonomic Innervation in the Heart

The autonomic nervous system regulates body functions that can proceed independently of volitional activity, and is composed of afferent, efferent, and central integrating structures. The 2 divisions of this system, the sympathetic and parasympathetic components, are made up of preganglionic and postganglionic neurons. The cell bodies of the preganglionic neurons are located in the brain or spinal cord whereas postganglionic neurons are located in the autonomic ganglia. The preganglionic sympathetic neurons are located in the thoracic and upper lumbar spinal cord whereas those of the parasympathetic nervous system are located in the brainstem and sacral spinal cord (Figure 3). The synaptic sites for sympathetic fibers are located in paravertebral or prevertebral ganglia whereas the synaptic sites of parasympathetic fibers are located in peripheral (terminal) ganglia.

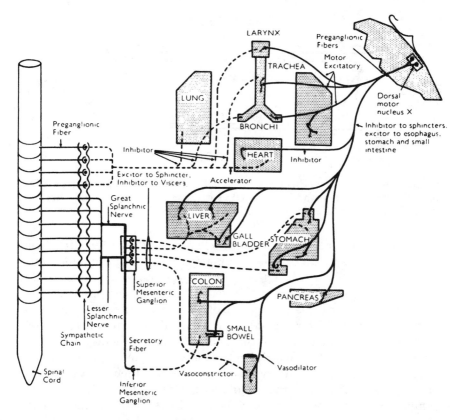

**Figure 3.** Diagram to show the pre- and postganglionic fibers of the autonomic innervation of the thoracic and abdominal viscera. Dotted lines: postganglionic fibers of the thoracolumbar (sympathetic) division. Short solid lines on viscera: postganglionic fibers of the craniosacral (parasympathetic) division.

The heart, like other viscera, is innervated by both sympathetic and parasympathetic fibers. Over the past decade, many of the details concerning the precise pattern of innervation of the heart have been elucidated.[27–39] Zipes and colleagues have demonstrated that sympathetic afferent and efferent fibers to the ventricle cross at the atrioventricular groove and travel in the superficial subepicardium throughout most of their course, predominantly along with the larger coronary arteries[27–30] (Figure 4). In contrast, afferent and efferent vagal fibers cross the atrioventricular groove in the superficial subepicardium and then dive intramurally to become located in the subendocardium.[31–35] Vagal efferent fibers crossing the atrioventricular groove are likely postganglionic axons with ganglion cells located in the atria.[36] Innervation patterns to the right ventricle are similar to those of the left ventricle.[37] Efferent

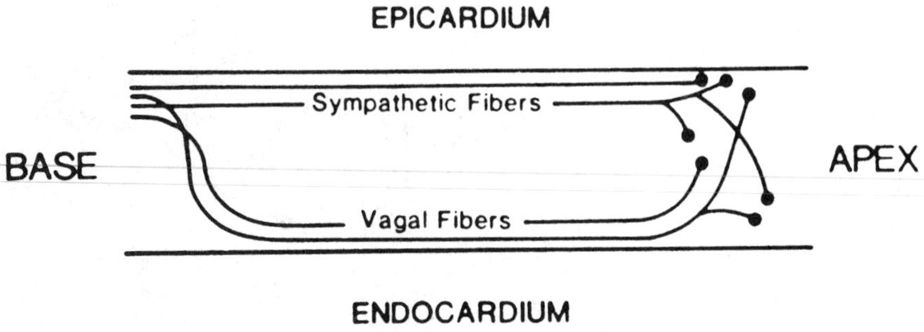

**EPICARDIUM**

**ENDOCARDIUM**

Figure 4. Schematic diagram of functional pathways of afferent and efferent sympathetic and vagal innervation to the left ventricle. Sagittal view from the left ventricle. (From Barber MJ, Zipes D, et al.[32] with permission.)

sympathetic axons to the right ventricle are located in the superficial subepicardium and are oriented perpendicular to the right lateral atrioventricular groove or the left anterior descending artery. Myocardial sites near the right coronary artery receive efferent sympathetic innervation mainly from the lateral margin of the right ventricle near the atrioventricular groove. More septal myocardial sites, located near the left anterior descending artery, receive efferent sympathetic innervation from both the right lateral atrioventricular groove and regions near the left anterior descending artery. The innervation of the right ventricular outflow tract differs from the rest of the right and left ventricle. Efferent sympathetic innervation to the right ventricular outflow tract is both from the right lateral atrioventricular groove near the origin of the RCA and from regions near the left anterior descending artery. Some axons are located in the superficial subepicardium while others are located in the deep myocardium. Vagal efferent fibers to the right ventricle are located superficially at the right lateral atrioventricular groove and penetrate the myocardium quickly, so that at sites more than 1 cm from the atrioventricular groove, they are intramural. Myocardial sites close to the right coronary artery receive efferent vagal innervation predominantly from the lateral margin of the right ventricle near the atrioventricular groove. Myocardial sites close to the left anterior descending artery receive vagal innervation, partially from the right lateral atrioventricular groove as well as from regions near the left anterior descending artery. Pathways of vagal innervation to the right ventricular outflow tract are located deep in the myocardium, originating from the right lateral atrioventricular groove near the origin of the right coronary artery and from regions near the left anterior descending artery. The afferent pathways of right ventricular innervation have not been well established.

# Noninvasive Evaluation of Cardiac Autonomic Function

## Scintigraphic Imaging of Cardiac Sympathetic Innervation

In the past, evaluation of the sympathetic nervous system of the heart was limited to invasive procedures to determine the arteriovenous differences of plasma catecholamine concentrations or characterization of functional changes after surgical ligation of sympathetic nerves. Noninvasive scintigraphic evaluation of the pattern of sympathetic innervation of the heart has become posssible with the development of two catecholamine analogs: radioiodinated metaiodobenzylguanidine (MIBG) or C-11 hydroxyephedrine (HED).[40–50] HED is a norepinephrine analog that shares the same uptake-1 and vesicular storage mechanisms as naturally occurring norepinephrine.[46] When used in conjunction with positron emission tomography, HED allows quantitative noninvasive evaluation of the sympathic nervous system in the human heart.[41] Because HED is not metabolized by monoamine oxidase in the cytosol of sympathetic nerve terminals, retained HED activity reflects the uptake and storage of HED by adrenergic nerve terminals. Animal studies have confirmed that tissue retention of HED correlates closely with the concentration of norepinephrine in tissue,[50] and studies in transplant patients have demonstrated low nonspecific binding of HED.[47] Myocardial blood flow can be simultaneously assessed with positron emission tomography following injection of N-13 ammonia. The pattern of sympathetic innervation can then be displayed and analyzed using polar maps. The relative regional uptake of HED in each of 9 myocardial segments can be evaluated qualitatively by normalizing to maximal myocardial C-11 activity. The myocardial uptake of HED can also be evaluated by determining the HED retention index in each of the 9 regions of interest. The retention index of HED is determined by dividing the myocardial C-11 activity at 40 minutes by the integral of C-11 HED concentration in the arterial blood from the time of injection to 40 minutes later. This allows both the relative and absolute myocardial uptake of HED by the sympathetic nerve terminals to be evaluated.

## Heart Rate Variability

The evaluation of heart rate variability from long-term ECG recordings, which primarily reflects tonic parasympathetic tone, is another method for assessing the autonomic nervous system.[51] The beat-to-beat heart rate is not completely regular. This beat-to-beat variation in heart rate is based in part on the autonomic innervation of the sinus node. This variation, termed heart rate variability, has been shown to be a noninvasive marker of autonomic input into the heart. The analysis of heart rate variability can be performed in the time or the frequency domain. Time domain analysis calculates a number of variables that describe these beat-to-beat changes, including the standard deviation of all normal RR intervals in the entire 24-hour recording, the standard deviation of the mean value of all 5-minute segments of all normal RR intervals and the percent difference between adjacent normal RR intervals that exceed 50 ms. Frequency domain analysis examines the periodic oscillations of a given heart rate at various frequencies. It is accomplished by fast Fourier transform. Typically, these frequencies have been divided into 4 major groups: high, low, very low, and ultra low-frequency bands. These 4 bands are thought to each reflect different components of the autonomic nervous system. High frequency, which is in the 0.15–0.4 Hz range, is thought to represent the parasympathetic component of the autonomic nervous system.[52] Low frequency, which is in the 0.04 to 0.15 Hz range, is mediated by both the parasympathetic and sympathetic nervous system and is influenced by the baroreceptor system.[53] Very low frequency, which is in the 0.0033 to 0.04 Hz range and ultra-low frequency, which is in the $1.15 \times 10^{-5}$ to 0.0033 Hz range, are influenced by many factors, including thermoregulation and the renin angiotensin system. Total power is the sum of all of these individual components.

The potential prognostic importance of heart rate variability has been shown in both animal and clinical studies. In 1990, Hull and colleagues reported, in an animal model, that reduced heart rate variability was sensitive and specific in predicting susceptibility to ischemia-induced ventricular fibrillation.[54] The first large-scale clinical study was performed by Kleiger and colleagues.[55] Among 808 postinfarction patients, reduced heart rate variability had a higher mortality, independent of ejection fraction. These findings have been confirmed by others.[56] Other studies have shown that congestive heart failure is associated with autonomic dysfunction, which can be quantified by measuring heart rate variability. The prognostic value of heart rate variability has also been shown among patients with heart failure. The recently completed UK Heart trial examined the value of heart rate variability measures as an independent predictor of death in patients with heart failure.[57] Among 433 patients with Class 1–3 heart failure, SDNN, a measurement of heart rate variability, was identified as the most powerful predictor of the risk of death due to progressive heart failure but no sudden death per se.

## Measurements of Baroreflex Sensitivity

Baroreflex sensitivity, which predominantly measures reflex vagal activity, is another noninvasive method to assess the autonomic nervous system. The arterial baroreceptor control of heart rate has been studied by 3 techniques: (1) increasing blood pressure with a vasoconstricting agent such as phenylephrine, (2) lowering blood pressure with a vasodilator such as nitroprusside, and (3) direct stimulation of carotid baroreceptors with neck suction. The majority of studies that have examined the relationship between the autonomic nervous system and sudden cardiac death have focused on reflex parasympathetic tone using the phenylephrine method.[58] For example, Schwartz and colleagues have shown in their postinfarction dog model that baroreflex sensitivity was significantly reduced in dogs resistent to ischemia-induced ventricular fibrillation as compared to those who were susceptible.[58] Additional studies in humans revealed that baroreflex sensitivity is lower after myocardial infarction and that this reduction is transient.[59] Subsequent clinical studies have demonstrated that markedly reduced baroreflex sensitivity is associated with a higher mortality in postinfarction patients as compared to those with more normal baroreflex sensitivity.[60] The recently completed ATRAMI trial was designed to evaluate the independent prognostic value of measurements of heart rate variability and baroreflex sensitivity among postinfarction patients.[61] This study enrolled 1,284 patients with a recent myocardial infarction. Holter monitoring was done to measure heart rate variability and ventricular arrhythmias. Baroreflex sensitivity was determined using the phenylephrine method. During 21 months of follow-up there were 44 cardiac deaths. Low values of either heart rate variability (SDNN < 70 ms) or baroreflex sensitivity (< 3 ms per mm Hg) carried a significant multivariate risk of cardiac mortality. The 2-year mortality was 17% when both were reduced as compared with 25% when both were preserved. The observation that the prognostic value of measurements of heart rate variability and baroreflex sensitivity were independent and significantly added to the prognostic value of the ejection fraction and ambient ventricular arrhythmias demonstrates that prognostic value of an analysis of vagal reflexes.

The observation that low heart rate variability is a risk factor for sudden death after myocardial infarction suggests that an imbalance in autonomic tone, caused either by high sympathetic activity or concomitant low vagal activity, or both, plays a role in precipitating sudden cardiac death in humans.[55,62,63] However, the mechanism by which sympathovagal imbalance may precipitate sudden death remains uncertain.

## Potential Mechanism

There are likely to be a large number of mechanisms by which abnormalities or fluctuations of autonomic tone or function may be linked to sudden death. Central to these relationships is the well-established link between increased sympathetic tone and increased risk for sudden death.

## Interaction Between Sympathetic Tone and Increased Myocardial Ischemia

Shown in Figure 5 is a model proposed by a National Heart Lung and Blood Workshop, which outlines the interaction between and role of acute and chronic risk factors in the development of acute cardiovascular events such as a myocardial infarction or ventricular fibrillation.[22] An increase in sympathetic tone is central to these interactions. Increased sympathetic tone plays a role in plaque disruption and thrombosis, which lead to ischemia. Increased sympathetic tone may also directly cause electrical instability.

## Creation of Increased Dispersion of Refractoriness Due to Denervation and Denervation Supersensitivity

There is an increasing body of literature to suggest that transient or permanent myocardial injury may disrupt autonomic neural transmission, which may ultimately increase propensity for the development of cardiac arrhythmias. Much of this work has been performed by Zipes and colleagues who have been interested in this topic for more than a decade. Some of the more important findings that have been reported by this laboratory will be briefly summarized. One set of studies from this laboratory explored and validated the hypothesis that transmural myo-

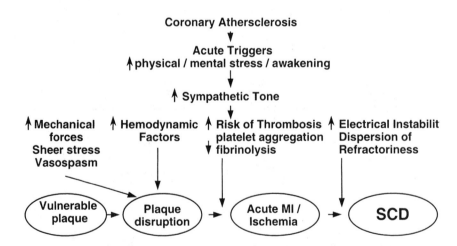

Figure 5. Schematic drawing showing the interactions between chronic and acute risk factors in the precipitation of ischemia, myocardial infarction (MI), and sudden cardiac death (SCD). (Adapted from Muller JE, et al.[22] with permission.)

cardial infarction or ischemia could interrupt sympathetic and vagal transmission over axons located within the infarction and produce sympathetic and vagal denervation at noninfarcted sites apical to the infarction. Barber et al. reported that transmural myocardial infarction in dogs produces sympathectomy in noninfarcted myocardium apical to the infarction.[38] These investigators also demonstrated that transmural myocardial infarction produces heterogeneous loss of efferent sympathetic innervation in noninfarcted apical sites as early as 5–10 minutes after coronary occlusion, with more complete denervation occurring over time.[64]

Other studies demonstrated the presence of denervation supersensitivity as manifested by an exaggerated shortening of refractoriness during both norepinephrine and isoproterenol infusions with an upward and leftward shift in the dose-response curves in denervated regions of the left ventricle.[65,66] Subsequent studies demonstrated the arrhythmogenic relevance of these findings in dog models and the protective effects of beta blockade.[67] The authors speculated that beta adrenergic blockade may reduce the incidence of sudden cardiac death after myocardial infarction in part by attenuating the effects of denervation supersensitivity and the resultant increased dispersion of refractoriness.[67] A second set of studies explored and confirmed the hypothesis that ischemia or infarction may cause afferent denervation.[68] These authors demonstrated that several minutes after creation of transmural (but not nontransmural) myocardial ischemia, the sympathetic reflex elicited from the epicardium of the ischemic area or apical to it becomes interrupted or attenuated when the myocardial blood flow in the epicardium decreases to approximately 40% or less of the control value.[68] Because afferent sympathetic fibers appear to mediate cardiac pain sensation, the authors speculated that in some patients a subset of episodes of myocardial ischemia affecting the subepicardium may be "silent" as a result of "autodenervation" due to an ischemia-induced decrease in sympathetic nerve traffic. A third set of studies demonstrated that the cardiac response to ischemia or infarction is influenced by the "myocardial history." In this study, the authors demonstrated that four 5-minute episodes of coronary occlusion and reperfusion preserve the efferent sympathetic response during the first hour of subsequent sustained ischemia and preserve the efferent vagal response for at least 3 hours without an increase in collateral blood flow to the ischemic myocardium.[69] A fourth set of studies was performed, which tested and validated the hypothesis that substances in the pericardial sack can modulate autonomic neural transmission to the heart as both vagal and sympathetic nerves are located superficially in the subepicardium during at least some part of their course. Zipes and colleagues went on to demonstrate that pericardial prostaglandins produce an antisympa-thetic action.[70,71] They went on to provide evidence that the increase in pericardial prostaglandin production in response to increased sympa-thetic tone may act as a negative feedback control mechanism regulat-ing sympathetic stimulation of the heart. When efferent sympathetic in-put to the heart is heightened or plasma which bathe the cardiac sympathetic nerves and limit efferent sympathetic input to the heart and further release of catecholamines. Because cardiac pericardial prostaglandins do not affect cardiac responses to vagal stimulation, they may act to suppress arrhythmia development in various situations such as myocardial ischemia. A fifth and most recent study assessed the ef-fects of a right ventricular myocardial infarction on efferent sympathetic and vagal innervation of viable myocardium. This study revealed that right ventricular myocardial infarction causes sympathetic and vagal denervation at viable sites in the right ventricular outflow tract, lateral, and, to a lesser extent, septal sides of the viable peri-infarct area.[72]

Sympathetic denervation can be evaluated in humans, as noninva-sive scintigraphic evaluation of the pattern of sympathetic innervation of the human heart is possible with either radioiodinated metaiodobenzyl-guanidine (MIBG) or C11-hydroxyephedrine (HED), as noted above. With these agents, scintigraphic evidence of sympathetic neural dys-function has been demonstrated in patients with coronary artery dis-ease[42-44,49] and in patients with idiopathic dilated cardiomyopathy.[45,49] We were the first to determine if scintigraphic evidence of sympathetic neural dysfunction correlates with measurements of ventricular refrac-toriness and to determine if the phenomenon of denervation supersensi-tivity can be demonstrated in humans by evaluating the change in re-fractoriness during a catecholamine infusion in regions of myocardium with and without scintigraphic evidence of sympathetic neuronal dys-function.[49] The study was performed in 11 patients with a history of sus-tained ventricular tachycardia or sudden death who were referred for placement of an implantable defibrillator (7 men, 51 ± 18 years). Preop-erative scintigraphic evaluation of the pattern of sympathetic innerva-tion was performed with HED in conjunction with positron emission to-mography. At the time of surgery, ventricular refractoriness was determined in regions of myocardium demonstrating normal and re-duced HED retention in the baseline state and during an infusion of nor-epinephrine. Scintigraphic evaluation demonstrated regions of reduced HED retention in each patient. Shown in Figure 6 are blood flow and HED images obtained in a normal volunteer. Myocardial blood flow and HED retention are homogeneous throughout the entire left ventricle. Fig-ure 7 shows an example of a patient with coronary artery disease. This 60-year-old man with a history of a prior anterior wall myocardial in-

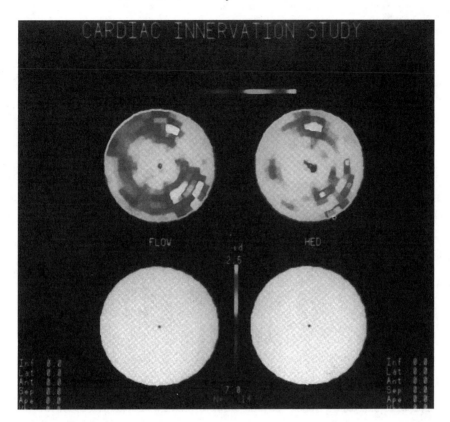

**Figure 6.** Polar map of relative tracer distribution generated from circumferential profile analysis of short-axis left ventricular images for blood flow (left) and [11]C-hydroxyephedrine (HED) (right) in a normal volunteer. Upper panel: Maps of normalized count data. The relative amount of tracer uptake is displayed using a gray scale. Both myocardial flow and HED are homogeneous throughout the ventricle. Lower panel: Data in this patient compared with a normal database obtained from 14 volunteers. The homogeneous white throughout demonstrates that the tracer retention in this volunteer is within 2.5 SDs of the normal control population. (From Calkins H, et al.[49] with permission.)

farction presented with sudden death. Regional myocardial perfusion was reduced in the anterior wall, consistent with a prior anterior wall myocardial infarction. The corresponding scintigraphic images demonstrate a more extensive area of reduced HED retention that extends in a circumferential fashion beyond the region of myocardium that demonstrated reduced myocardial perfusion. Figure 8 shows a representative image obtained from a 31-year-old man with sudden death who was subsequently demonstrated to have an idiopathic dilated cardiomyopathy. Regional myocardial blood flow in this patient demonstrated a small per-

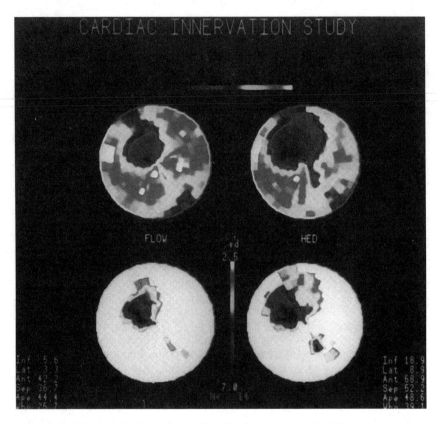

**Figure 7.** Polar map of relative tracer distribution in a patient with a previous myocardial infarction. Short-axis left ventricular images for blood flow are shown in the left panel and for $^{11}$C-hydroxyephedrine (HED) uptake are shown in the right panel. The upper panels show polar maps of normalized count data, and the lower panels show polar maps of relative tracer uptake. A gray scale is used. Both myocardial flow and HED uptake are markedly reduced in the anteroapical region. The extent of the area of reduced HED uptake is greater than the area of reduced myocardial flow. Lower maps compare the data in this patient with a normal database. The regions of the myocardium in which myocardial flow and HED retention differ by more than 2.5 SDs of the control population are shown as a gray scale. In this patient, 26% of the left ventricle demonstrates abnormal blood flow (left lower) and 39% of the left ventricle demonstrates abnormal HED retention (right lower). This example demonstrates neuronal injury exceeding the area of abnormal blood flow after infarction. (From Calkins H, et al.[49] with permission.)

fusion abnormality in the midinferolateral wall, consistent with fibrosis. The corresponding HED images show heterogeneous areas of reduced HED retention in parts of the anterior, lateral, and inferior walls of the left ventricle. Overall, among patients with coronary artery disease in this study, the region of myocardium demonstrating reduced HED re-

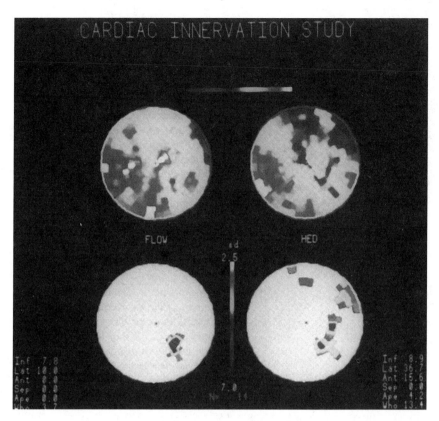

**Figure 8.** Polar maps from a patient with an idiopathic dilated cardiomyopathy arranged. These polar maps show a small blood flow abnormality in the inferolateral wall representing 4% of the left ventricle (left), consistent with myocardial fibrosis. Corresponding [11]C-hydroxyephedrine (HED) maps (right) show heterogeneous abnormalities in parts of the anterior, lateral and inferior walls that occupy 13% of the left ventricle. (From Calkins H, et al.[49] with permission.

tention was similar in size to the region demonstrating decreased perfusion (matched defect) in 4 patients. The region of reduced HED retention was larger than the region demonstrating reduced perfusion in 3 patients (mismatched defect). In the 4 patients without coronary artery disease, the region of reduced HED retention was larger than the region demonstrating reduced perfusion in 3 patients. The effective refractory period in regions of myocardium that demonstrated reduced HED retention was significantly longer than in areas of myocardium demonstrating normal HED retention ($273 \pm 32$ versus $243 \pm 32$ ms) (Figure 9). Norepinephrine shortened the effective refractory period in regions of myocardium demonstrating normal and reduced HED retention to a similar degree (Figure 9). Thus a clear correlation between scintigraphic evi-

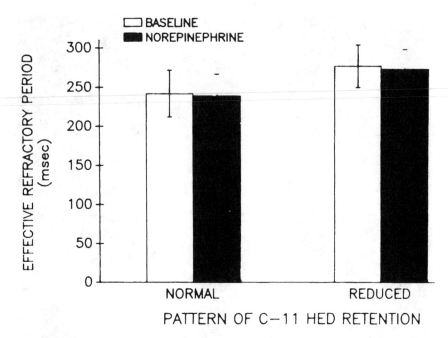

Figure 9. Bar graph of mean effective refractory period in regions of myocardium demonstrating normal and reduced [11]C-hydroxyephedrine (HED) uptake in the baseline state and during an infusion of norepinephrine. The mean baseline effective refractory period in areas of myocardium that demonstrated reduced HED was longer than in areas that demonstrated normal HED retention ($p<0.001$). Norepinephrine resulted in shortening of the effective refractory period at both types of sites ($p<0.05$). (From Calkins H, et al.[49] with permission.)

dence of sympathetic neuronal dysfunction and ventricular refractoriness in the human heart was shown.

## Conclusion

In conclusion, sudden cardiac death can be considered an electrical accident that develops in a small subset of individuals who have both an abnormal underlying myocardial substrate and who are exposed to other transient precipitating factors such as electrolyte abnormalities, ischemia, myocardial stretch, and fluctuations in autonomic tone and function. There is compelling evidence to suggest that activation of the sympathetic nervous system increases the probability of developing sudden cardiac death whereas high vagal tone may be protective. Further studies will be needed to determine if interventions other than beta blockade, which are designed specifically to alter autonomic tone and/or function, may reduce the risk of sudden death in the future.

# References

1. Zipes DP, Wellens HJJ. Sudden cardiac death. Circulation 1998; 98:2334–2351.
2. De Silva RA. John MacWilliam, evolutionary biology and sudden cardiac death. J Am Coll Cardiol 1989; 14:1843–1849.
3. MacWilliam JA. Cardiac failure and sudden death. Br Med J 1889; 1:6–8.
4. MacWilliam JA. Blood pressure and heart action in sleep and dreams. Br Med J 1923; 2:1196–1200.
5. Kennedy HL. Beta blockade, ventricular arrhythmias, and sudden cardiac death. Am J Cardiol 1997; 80(9B):29J–34J.
6. Lown B, Verrier RL. Neural activity and ventricular fibrillation. N Engl J Med 1976; 294:1165–1170.
7. Levy AG. The exciting causes of ventricular fibrillation in animals under chloroform anesthesia. Heart 1912; 4:319.
8. Hockman CH, Mauck HP, Hoff EC. ECG changes resulting from cerebral stimulation: II. A spectrum of ventricular arrhythmias of sympathetic origin. Am Heart J 1966; 68:98.
9. Satinsky J, Kosowsky B, Lown B, et al. Ventricular fibrillation induced by hypothalamic stimulation during coronary occlusion (abstract). Circulation 1971; 44:11–60.
10. Verrier RL, Calvert A, Lown B, et al. Effect of acute blood pressure elevation on the ventricular fibrillation threshold. Am J Physiol 1974; 226:893.
11. Skinner JE, Reed JC. Blockade of frontocortical-brain stem pathway prevents ventricular fibrillation of ischemic heart. Am J Physiol 1981; 240:H156.
12. Matta RJ, Lawler JE, Lown B. Ventricular electrical instability in the conscious dog: effects of psychological stress and beta adrenergic blockade. Am J Cardiol 1976; 38:594.
13. Verrier RL, Lown B. Influence of neural activity on ventricular electrical stability during acute myocardial ischemia and infarction. In: Sandoe E, Julian DC, Bell JW (eds). Management of Ventricular Tachycardia: Role of Mexiletine. International Congress Series No. 458. Excerpta Medica, Amsterdam, 1978, p 133.
14. Verrier RL, Lown B. Behavioral stress and cardiac arrhythmias. Annu Rev Physiol 1984; 46:155–176.
15. Cropp GJ, Manning GW. Electrocardiographic changes simulate myocardial ischemia and infarction associated with spontaneous intracranial hemorrhage. Circulation 1960; 22:25.
16. Hugenholtz PG. Electrocardiographic abnormalities in cerebral disorders: report of six cases and review of the literature. Am Heart J 1962; 63:451.
17. Schwartz PJ, Billman GE, Stone HL. Autonomic mechanisms in ventricular fibrillation induced by myocardial ischemia during exercise in dogs with healed myocardial infarction: an experimental preparation for sudden cardiac death. Circulation 1984; 69(4):790–800.
18. Muller JE, Stone PH, Turi ZG, et al. Circadian variation in the frequency of onset of acute myocardial infarction. N Engl J Med 1985; 313:1313.
19. Muller JE, Tofler GH, Stone PH. Circadian variation and triggers of onset of acute cardiovascular disease. Circulation 1989; 79:733.
20. Tofler GH, Brezinski D, Schafer AI, et al. Concurrent morning increase in platelet aggregability and the risk of myocardial infarction and sudden cardiac death. N Engl J Med 1987; 316:1514.
21. Peckova M, Fahrenbruch CE, Cobb LA, Hallstrom AP. Circadian variations in the occurrence of cardiac arrests; initial and repeat episodes. Circulation 1998; 98:31–39.

22. Muller JE, Kaufmann PG, Luepker RV, Weisfeldt ML, Deedwania PC, et al. Mechanisms precipitating acute cardiac events. Circulation 1997; 96:3233–3239.
23. Barry J, Campbell S, Yeung AC, et al. Waking and rising at night as a trigger of myocardial ischemia. Am J Cardiol 1991; 67:1067.
24. Willich SN, Levy D, Rocco MB, Tofler GH, Stone PH, et al. Circadian variation in the incidence of sudden cardiac death in the Framingham Heart Study population. Am J Cardiol 1987; 60:801–806.
25. Folts JD, Gallagher K, Rowe GG. Blood flow reduction in stenosed canine coronary arteries: vasospasm or platelet aggregation? Circulation 1982; 65:248.
26. Raeder EA, Verrier RL, Lown B. Influence of the autonomic nervous system on coronary blood flow during partial stenosis. Am Heart J 1982; 104:249.
27. Martins JB, Zipes DP. Epicardial phenol interrupts refractory period responses to sympathetic but not vagal stimulation in canine left ventricular epicardium and endocardium. Circ Res 1980; 47:33–40.
28. Randall WC, Szentivanyi M, Pace JB, Wechsler JS, Kaye MP. Patterns of sympathetic nerve projections onto the canine heart. Circ Res 1968; 22:315–323.
29. Geis WP, Kaye MP. Distribution of sympathetic fibers in the left ventricular epicardial plexus of the dog. Circ Res 1968; 23:165–170.
30. Randall WC, Armour JA. Regional vagosympathetic control of the heart. Am J Physiol 1974; 227:444–452.
31. Kent KM, Epstein SE, Cooper T, Jacobowitz DM. Cholinergic innervation of the canine and human ventricular conduction system. Circulation 1974; 50:948–955.
32. Barber MJ, Mueller TM, Davies BG, Zipes DP. Phenol topically applied to left ventricular epicardium interrupts sympathetic but not vagal afferents. Circ Res 1984:55:532–544.
33. Takahashi N, Barber MJ, Zipes DP. Efferent vagal innervation of the canine left ventricle. Am J Physiol 1985; 248 (Heart Circ Physiol 17):H89–H97.
34. Inoue H, Mahomed Y, Zipes DP. Surgery for Wolff-Parkinson-White syndrome interrupts efferent vagal innervation to the left ventricle and to the atrioventricular node in the canine heart. Cardiovasc Res 1988; 22:163–170.
35. Chilson DA, Peigh P, Mahomed Y, Zipes DP. Encircling endocardial incision interrupts efferent vagal-induced prolongation of endocardial and epicardial refractoriness in the dog. J Am Coll Cardiol 1985; 5:290–296.
36. Blomquist TM, Priola DV, Romero AM. Source of intrinsic innervation of canine ventricles: a functional study. Am J Physiol 1987; 252(Heart Circ Physiol):H638–H644.
37. Ito M, Zipes DP. Efferent sympathetic and vagal innervation of the canine right ventricle. Circulation 1994:90:1459–1468.
38. Barber MJ, Mueller TM, Henry DP, et al. Transmural myocardial infarction in the dog produces sympathectomy in noninfarcted myocardium. Circulation 1983; 67:787.
39. Dae MW, O'Connell W, Botvinick EH, Ahearn T, Yee E, et al. Scintigraphic assessment of regional cardiac adrenergic innervation. Circulation 1989; 79:634–644.
40. Sisson JC, Lynch JJ, Johnson J, Jaques S, Wu D, et al. Scintigraphic detection of regional disruption of adrenergic neurons in the heart. Am Heart J 1988; 116:67–76.
41. Schwaiger M, Kalff V, Rosenspire K, Haka MS, Molina E, et al. Noninvasive evaluation of sympathetic nervous system in human heart by positron emission tomography. Circulation 1990; 82:457–464.
42. Stanton MS, Tuli MM, Radtke NL, Heger JJ, Miles WM, et al. Regional sympa-

thetic denervation after myocardial infarction in humans detected noninvasively using I-123-metaiodobenzylguanidine. J Am Coll Cardiol. 1989; 14:1519–1526.

43. Wharton JM, Friedman IM, Greenfield RA, Vitullo RN, Strauss HC, et al. Quantitative perfusion and sympathetic nerve defect size after myocardial infarction in humans. J Am Coll Cardiol 1992; 19:264A.

44. Allman K, Hutchins G, Wolfe E, Allman C, Wieland D, et al. [11]C-Hydroxyephedrine myocardial retention following acute myocardial infarction. Circulation 1991; 11:423.

45. Henderson EB, Kahn JK, Corbett JR, Jansen DE, Pippin JJ, et al. Abnormal I-123 metaiodobenzylguanidine myocardial washout and distribution may reflect myocardial adrenergic derangement in patients with congestive cardiomyopathy. Circulation 1988; 78:1192–1199.

46. Wieland DM, Hutchins GD, Rosenspire KC, Haka MS, Sherman PS, et al. [C-11]Hydroxyephedrine (HED): a high specific activity alternative to F-18 fluorometaraminol (FMR) for heart neuronal imaging. J Nucl Med 1989; 30:767.

47. Schwaiger M, Hutchins GD, Kalff V, Rosenspire K, Haka MS, et al. Evidence for regional catecholamine uptake and storage sites in the transplanted human heart by positron emission tomography. J Clin Invest 1990; 87:1681–1690.

48. Calkins H, Lehman M, Allman K, Schwaiger M. Scintigraphic pattern of regional cardiac sympathetic innervation in patients with familial long QT syndrome using positron emission tomography. Circulation 1993; 87:1616–1621.

49. Calkins H, Allman K, Bolling S, Kirsch M, Wieland D, et al. Correlation between scintigraphic evidence of regional sympathetic neuronal dysfunction and ventricular refractoriness in the human heart. Circulation 1993; 88:172–179.

50. Fuller RW, Snoddy HD, Perry KW, Bernstein JR, Murphy PJ. Formation of a-methylnorepinephrine as a metabolite of alphametaraminol in guinea pigs. Biochem Pharmacol 1981; 30:2831–2836.

51. Barron HV, Lesh MD. Autonomic nervous system and sudden cardiac death. J Am Coll Cardiol 1996; 27:1053–1060.

52. Berger RD, Akselrod S, Gordon D, Cohen RJ. An efficient algorithm for spectral analysis of heart rate variability. IEEE Trans Biomed Eng 1986; 33:900–904.

53. Kamath MV, Ghista DN, Fallen EL, Fitchett D, Miller D, et al. Heart rate variability power spectrogram as a potential noninvasive signature of cardiac regulatory system response, mechanisms, and disorders. Heart Vessels 1987; 3:33–41.

54. Hull SSJ, Evans AR, Vanoli E, et al. Heart rate variability before and after myocardial infarction in conscious dogs at high and low risk of sudden death. J Am Coll Cardiol 1990; 16:978–985.

55. Kleiger RE, Miller JP, Bigger JTJ, Moss AJ. Decreased heart rate variability and its association with increased mortality after acute myocardial infarction. Am J Cardiol 1987; 59:256–262.

56. Odemuyiwa O, Poloniecki J, Malik M, et al. Temporal influences on the prediction of postinfarction mortality by heart rate variability: a comparison with the left ventricular ejection fraction. Br Heart J 1994; 71:521–527.

57. Nolan J, Batin PD, Andrews R, Lindsay SJ, Brooksby P, et al. Prospective study of heart rate variability and mortality in chronic heart failure: results of the United Kingdom heart failure evaluation and assessment of risk trial (UK-Heart). Circulation 1998; 98:1510–1516.

58. Schwartz PJ, Vanoli E, Stramba BM, De FGM, Billman GE, et al. Autonomic mechanisms and sudden death: new insights from analysis of baroreceptor reflexes in conscious dogs with and without a myocardial infarction. Circulation 1988; 78:969–979.

59. Schwartz PJ, Zaza A, Pala M, Locati E, Beria G, et al. Baroreflex sensitivity and its evolution during the first year after myocardial infarction. J Am Coll Cardiol 1988; 12:629–636.
60. La Rovere MT, Specchia G, Mortara A, Schwartz PJ. Baroreflex sensitivity, clinical correlates, and cardiovascular mortality among patients with a first myocardial infarction: a prospective study. Circulation 1988; 78:816–824.
62. Schwartz PJ, La Rovere MT, Vanoli E. Autonomic nervous system and sudden cardiac death: experimental basis and clinical observations for post-myocardial infarction risk stratification. Circulation 1992; 85:177–191.
63. Pozzati A, Pancaldi LG, DiPasquale G, Pinelli G, Bugiardini R. Transient sympathovagal imbalance triggers "ischemic" sudden death in patients undergoing electrocardiographic Holter monitoring. J Am Coll Cardiol 1996; 27:847–852.
64. Inoue H, Zipes DP. Time course of denervation of efferent sympathetic and vagal nerves after occlusion of the coronary artery in the canine heart. Circ Res 1988:62:1111.
65. Kammerling JM, Green FJ, Watanabe AM, et al. Denervation supersensitivity of refractoriness in noninfarcted areas apical to transmural myocardial infarction. Circulation 1987; 76:383.
66. Martins JB. Time course of sympathetic denervation supersensitivity in canine ventricular recovery. Am J Physiol 1988; 25(Heart Circ Physiol 24):H577–H586.
67. Inoue H, Zipes DP, Results of sympathetic denervation in the canine heart: supersensitivity that may be arrhythmogenic. Circulation 1987:75:877.
68. Inoue H, Skale BT, Zipes DP. Effects of myocardial ischemia and infarction on cardiac afferent sympathetic and vagal reflexes in the dog. Am J Physiol 1988; 255(Heart Circ Physiol 24):H26–H35.
69. Miyazaki T, Zipes DP. Protection against autonomic denervation following acute myocardial infarction by preconditioning ischemia. Circ Res 1989; 64:437–448.
70. Miyazaki T, Pride HP, Zipes DP. Prostaglandins in the pericardial fluid modulate neural regulation of cardiac electrophysiologic properties. Circ Res 1990; 66:163–175.
72. Elvan A, Zipes DP. Right ventricular infarction causes heterogeneous autonomic denervation of the viable peri-infarct area. Circulation 1998; 97:484–492.

# 5

# Apoptosis and Sudden Cardiac Death

*Ziad Mallat, MD, PhD, Bénédicte Hugel, PhD,*
*Guy Lesèche, MD,*
*Jean-Marie Freyssinet, PhD, and*
*Alain Tedgui, PhD*

## Introduction

Sudden cardiac death is the most common manifestation of coronary heart disease and is responsible for approximately 50% of the mortality from cardiovascular disease in developed countries.[1] At least 80% of patients who experience sudden cardiac death have atherosclerotic coronary artery disease as the underlying anatomic substrate.[1] Autopsy studies have reported that a recent occlusive coronary thrombus was found in 15% to 64% of victims of sudden cardiac death, caused by ischemic heart disease, with many hearts showing plaque fissuring, hemorrhage, and thrombosis.[2] In hearts with healed myocardial infarction, active coronary lesions are identified in 46% of cases. Therefore, atherosclerotic plaque disruption (rupture or erosion) with or without thrombosis is a frequent pathological finding in subjects victims of sudden cardiac death.[3,4] We propose here that apoptotic cell death may play a major role in the combination of events leading to sudden cardiac death, and will focus on obstructive coronary artery disease as the underlying substrate. The role of apoptotic death in arrhythmogenic right ventricular dysplasia (ARVD) and paroxysmal arrhythmias has been addressed elsewhere.[5]

## Definition of Apoptosis

Vascular pathologists have long been intrigued by the observation of a form of active vascular cell death within the arterial wall in atherosclerosis[6,7] in the absence of overt necrosis. Rational explanations for these observations may now be at hand after the description by Kerr and col-

From: Aliot E, Clementy J, Prystowsky EN (editors). *Fighting Sudden Cardiac Death: A Worldwide Challenge.* ©Futura Publishing Company, Armonk, NY, 2000.

leagues in the early 1970s of a novel form of cell death distinct from necrosis, which they designated "apoptosis" (from the Greek word for falling).[8]

In contrast to the cellular and organelle swelling and to the blebbing and membrane rupture associated with the classic form of induced cell death or "oncosis," apoptosis was initially described in cells that are programmed to die on the basis of characteristic morphology.[8] Cells undergoing apoptosis show cell shrinkage, chromatin margination, and condensation with subsequent internucleosomal fragmentation of DNA, membrane redistribution of phospholipids,[9] and budding (emission of pseudopodia), with maintenance of membrane integrity. They tend to break off into apoptotic bodies that are recognized and rapidly engulfed by professional macrophages or adjacent neighboring cells without inducing an inflammatory response. However, cell corpses that escape phagocytosis and remain free undergo secondary necrosis.

Apoptosis can be initiated by *intrinsic signals* during normal development, for example. This occurs when cells activate an internal program of self-destruction (cell suicide, programmed cell death) in response to an internal clock, withdrawal of survival factors, changes in hemodynamic parameters, or loss of contact. Every cell already contains all the components of the suicide machinery and is ready to engage in self-destruction unless it is actively signaled not to do so.

On the other hand, apoptosis can be initiated by a wide variety of *extrinsic signals* such as cytokines, hormones, oxidized lipids, chemotherapeutic, ionizing, or viral agents. In contrast to the more chronic and progressive loss of cells that occurs during normal development, apoptosis triggered by extrinsic signals is generally more acute and massive. Therefore, the capacity for removal of apoptotic cells may be overcome and secondary necrosis of unremoved apoptotic cells is frequent. This may lead to chronic accumulation of cellular debris with the potential for inducing inflammatory and/or autoimmune responses.[10–12]

# Role of Apoptosis in Sudden Death Related to Obstructive Coronary Artery Disease

## Apoptosis and Plaque Rupture

Pathoanatomic examination of intact and disrupted plaques indicates that atherosclerotic plaques at risk of rupture are rich in lipid, have a high macrophage content (which produces matrix metalloproteinases degrading collagen and other extracellular matrix proteins) and a thin fibrous cap poor in smooth muscle cells.[13] Therefore, relative cell densities of inflammatory cells and smooth muscle cells greatly determine the plaque vulnerability to rupture. The thinness of the fibrous cap is the physical measurement that appears to promote the greatest vulnerability to rupture.[14,15] The mechanism of plaque rupture likely involves both apoptotic and necrotic mechanisms of cell death.

## Apoptosis of Vascular Smooth Muscle Cells

After decades of intensive research on the mechanisms of vascular smooth muscle cell (VSMC) proliferation, recent studies have been undertaken to understand the mechanisms and roles of smooth muscle cell survival/apoptosis in normal vessel development and pathology. Thus, VSMC growth is now viewed as the result of the opposing effects of cell proliferation and apoptosis.

Observations that cell death occurs in atherosclerosis have already been made by Virchow,[6] and experimental studies in cholesterol-fed swine undertaken by Thomas et al.[7] more than 20 years ago showed that cell death is a major event occurring during atherosclerotic plaque development. More recently, Parkes et al. observed that plaque-derived smooth muscle cells (p-SMC) are characterized by *c-myc* overexpression and have a growth disadvantage in culture in comparison with VSMCs from normal arteries, especially under low serum conditions.[16] On the basis of these results, it has been suggested that cell death by apoptosis may occur in human atherosclerosis. Bennett et al. have subsequently demonstrated that deregulated expression of *c-myc* in VSMCs induces apoptosis[17] and that human p-SMCs have a markedly elevated rate of apoptosis in vitro. This was the first indication that programmed cell death (apoptosis) may occur in human atherosclerosis.[18] The balance between pro- and anti-apoptotic proteins in atherosclerosis is in favor of the former, suggesting that p-SMCs are programmed to die and effectively undergo apoptosis when additional proapoptotic stimuli are present (inflammatory cells and cytokines).

Subsequently, several studies have shown evidence for in situ apoptotic cell death in animal and human atherosclerotic plaques.[19-25] The distribution of apoptosis is heterogeneous within the plaque, suggesting that some regions of the plaque may show substantially higher levels of cell death, possibly predisposing to plaque rupture (and vessel occlusion or plaque progression). Death of VSMCs by apoptosis occurs more frequently in regions with a high density in macrophages, suggesting that these cells may participate in the induction of apoptosis. Apoptosis of VSMCs may be extremely harmful because it may weaken the fibrous cap by decreasing the synthesis of extracellular matrix and therefore may lead to plaque rupture.

*Apoptosis of Inflammatory Cells*

Although all cell types are involved, macrophages and T-lymphocytes form the bulk of apoptotic cells in human plaques.

Death of T-lymphocytes and macrophages by apoptosis may be viewed as beneficial if apoptosis is not accompanied by an inflammatory reaction. Indeed, removal of these cells from the plaque could attenuate the inflammatory response, and decrease the synthesis of matrix metalloproteinases and the consequent breakdown of the extracellular matrix, therefore favoring plaque stabilization. It may also be argued that apoptotic death of any cell type in the plaque may favor plaque regression over plaque progression. However, removal of apoptotic cells from the atherosclerotic tissue may not be very efficient, leaving unremoved apoptotic bodies with potentially high immunogenic properties. Moreover, unremoved apoptotic cells are prone to undergo secondary necrosis and this may lead to accumulation of extracellular lipids and to perpetuation of the inflammatory response.

The rate of apoptotic cell death in the plaque (2–10%)[21,26,27] may, in many instances, exceed the reported rate of cell proliferation (<1%).[28,29] In the light of observations that human atherosclerotic plaques are generally more prone to progression rather than regression, this finding suggests that apoptosis may actually be implicated in natural plaque progression (rather than regression), through development of the acellular lipid core, for example. Indeed, foam cell apoptosis (and secondary necrosis) has frequently been identified at the edges of the lipid core, suggesting that it may actively contribute to its formation.

Foam cell apoptosis within the plaque leads to lipid accumulation within the artery (and may greatly reduce the reverse transport of cholesterol) and is likely to contribute to plaque progression and vulnerability.

## Apoptosis and Plaque Erosion

Plaque rupture of a thin fibrous cap overlying a lipid core is not necessarily the only final common pathway in the formation of coronary thrombi. Several recently reported consistent studies[30,31] have shown that atherosclerotic plaque erosion without plaque rupture is an important predisposing substrate for acute coronary syndromes and sudden cardiac death. Eroded plaques differ from ruptured plaques in that they have a base rich in proteoglycans and smooth muscle cells. These lesions are more often seen in younger individuals and in women, have less luminal narrowing and less calcification, and less often have foci of macrophages and T cells compared with plaque ruptures. Although risk factors predisposing to plaque erosion have been identified,[31] the precise mechanisms responsible for this process remain unknown. We hypothesized that one mechanism may be apoptotic death of luminal endothelial cells.[32]

In mature vessels, endothelial cell turnover is under the tight control of cell proliferation and cell apoptosis. Since the vascular endothelium is involved in various physiological processes, endothelial cell apoptosis (and dysfunction) may constitute an initial step in a variety of pathological situations such as atherosclerosis. As for other cell types, it has been hypothesized that interactions of endothelial cells with their microenvironment may be critical for their survival.

Vascular endothelial cells are continuously exposed to a range of hemodynamic forces that have a great impact on their cellular structure and function. Variations in blood flow play an important role in vessel growth or regression and in the focal development of atherosclerosis. A link between mechanical stimulation and cell survival or death has been therefore suggested by several groups. Human umbilical vein endothelial cells cultured under static conditions undergo a basal low level of apoptosis.[33] The empty space left between cells induces proliferation of adjacent cells so that an equilibrium state is reached with low levels of apoptosis and proliferation. Exposure to flow in a perfusion chamber or in an ex vivo organ culture directly inhibits the apoptotic process and indirectly supresses proliferation, leading to a "truly" quiescent monolayer.[33] Shear stress-dependent release of nitric oxide has been shown to account for the shear stress-dependent anti-apoptotic activity.[34]

Despite the major potential implications of endothelial cell apoptosis in atherosclerotic plaque development and stability, little is known about the occurrence of endothelial cell apoptosis in human atherosclerosis and on its relation to blood flow. Using carotid human atherosclerotic plaques, which are validated models to study interactions between low or oscillatory shear stress and atherosclerosis, we provided the first in vivo evidence that blood flow exerts a direct influence on endothelial cell survival or death by apoptosis in human atherosclerosis.[32] Luminal endothelial cell apoptosis was observed in 60% of plaques examined. In these plaques, we found a 7-fold increase in luminal endothelial cell apoptosis in the downstream parts of plaques where low shear and oscillatory shear prevail in comparison with the upstream parts ($p < 0.001$). This suggests that relatively large areas of endothelial erosion may occur in the distal part of atherosclerotic plaques. Given the high procoagulant and proadhesive potentials of apoptotic endothelial cells (see below) and the propensity of denuded vessel segments to increased vasospasm and platelet aggregation, this may lead to substantial lumen thrombosis favoring plaque progression and the occurrence of acute coronary syndromes. Our results suggest that in vivo local shear stress influences endothelial cell apoptosis and may be a major determinant of plaque erosion and thrombosis.

## Apoptosis and Thrombosis

Phosphatidylserine exposure on the outer cell surface is a hallmark of apoptosis.[9] Phosphatidylserine exposure at the surface of activated platelets is essential for normal hemostasis as demonstrated by the bleeding tendency in Scott syndrome patients, presenting a defect of phosphatidylserine transbilayer migration and membrane microparticle shedding.[35,36] However, it is also conceivable that a sustained accessibility of phosphatidylserine at the surface of apoptotic cells or of released apoptotic microparticles may be thrombogenic, for various reasons. In addition to its direct procoagulant potential in the tenase and prothrombinase enzyme complexes, phosphatidylserine plays an important role in the initial phase of coagulation by increasing the catalytic efficiency of the tissue factor/factor VIIa complex.[37] We have shown that apoptosis induced in THP-1 monocytic cell line by 2 oxysterols ($7\beta$-hydroxycholesterol and 25-hydroxycholesterol) significantly enhanced the activity of tissue factor constitutively expressed by these cells. This occurs strictly through phosphatidylserine externalization with no de novo protein synthesis.[38] Microparticles can also become a source of aminophospholipid substrates for secretory phospholipase $A_2$ to generate lysophosphatidic acid, a potent proinflammatory lipid mediator and platelet agonist.[39] Like activated platelet-derived microparticles,[40] apoptotic membrane fragments may well carry bioactive metabolites making them actors of transcellular communication or activation, or modulators of cell-cell interactions. This procoagulant and proaggregant potential of apoptotic cells may be deleterious in atherosclerosis since it may be involved in determining plaque thrombogenicity following plaque rupture and may therefore favor the occurrence of acute ischemic events and infarction.

Flynn et al. have shown that thrombin generation is increased at the contact of plaque-derived smooth cells undergoing apoptosis in culture,[41] and Bombeli et al. have shown that apoptotic endothelial cells are procoagulant and proadhesive in vitro.[42,43] Moreover, we have recently observed significant extracellular tissue factor expression around apoptotic cells in some regions of human atherosclerotic plaques, suggesting that tissue factor may be shed from apoptotic cells via apoptotic microparticles.[44] To examine whether apoptosis may be involved in tissue factor activity in vivo, we examined advanced human atherosclerotic plaques for the presence of shed membrane apoptotic microparticles (captured by biotinylated annexin V insolubilized onto streptavidin-coated microtitration plaques) and determined the procoagulant potential of these microparticles.[44] We found that high levels of shed membrane microparticles of monocytic and lymphocytic origins are produced in the atherosclerotic plaques and are associated with increased tissue factor activity. Interestingly, removing the microparticles from the supernatants resulted in a 97% reduction in tissue factor activity, indicating that almost all of the tissue factor activity of plaque extracts is associated with the shed membrane microparticles.[44] These experiments provide direct evidence that apoptosis is involved in the increased thrombogenic potential of human atherosclerotic plaques.

In general, arterial thrombosis is considered to arise from the interaction of tissue factor in the vascular wall with platelets and coagulation factors in circulating blood. However, there is some evidence that acute thrombosis may be initiated by circulating tissue factor originating from monocytes and neutrophils.[45] Therefore blood-borne tissue factor may be thrombogenic and may propagate thrombus at the site of vascular injury. A major source of blood-borne tissue factor could be circulating apoptotic microparticles with potent procoagulant activity due to the presence of phosphatidylserine at the surface of these shed particles.[38] Preliminary experiments in our laboratory show that plasma levels of procoagulant microparticles are increased in patients with acute coronary syndromes and may be associated with coronary reocclusion.[46]

## Apoptosis in Acute Ischemic Myocardium

Abrupt closure of the coronary lumen by a thrombus formed on contact with a disrupted plaque leads to acute and profound myocardial ischemia, especially in the absence of functional coronary collaterals. Recent studies in animals and humans have shown that cardiomyocyte death by apoptosis may play an important role in myocardial cell loss following acute myocardial infarction.[47,48]

Although no study has specifically addressed the role of apoptosis in the genesis of fatal ventricular arrhythmias following acute myocardial infarction, apoptotic death could contribute to these manifestations through various mechanisms. The heterogeneous distribution of apoptotic cardiomyocytes, especially in the border zone of the infarct, may be a potential substrate for the generation of excessive electrical heterogeneity, setting the base for the initiation of reentrant ventricular arrhythmias and ventricular fibrillation. Another mechanism could be Fas-mediated arrhythmogenicity.[49] Expression of Fas, a cell surface death receptor, is upregulated during hypoxia, and it has recently been shown that Fas ligation on cultured cardiomyocytes induces an increase in resting potential, an increase in action potential amplitude, and an increase in action potential duration.[49] Fas ligation also induced early and delayed afterdepolarizations as well as arrhythmogenic activity.

Ischemia-reperfusion has also been shown to induce apoptotic death of cardiomyocytes as well as upregulation of the Fas-Fas ligand system. These processes may therefore contribute to arrhythmogenicity and sudden death related to obstructive, but not thrombotic, coronary artery disease. This may apply, for example, to sudden death due to complete heart block following abrupt and intermittent closure of small arteries supplying the sinus node and/or the His bundle.

Finally, apoptosis and Fas-mediated arrhythmogenicity may also be relevant to the pathogenesis of myocarditis or other inflammatory myocardium responsible for sudden cardiac death.

## Environmental Stress, Catecholamines and Apoptosis

Environmental and physical stress have been proposed as risk factors for sudden cardiac death.[1] They enhance platelet adhesiveness and aggregability and it has been shown that circulating catecholamines may modulate coronary thrombosis in vivo. Besides these effects, several studies have recently reported proapoptotic properties for catecholamines, especially in cardiomyocytes.[50] These properties, in the context of acute ischemia or severe myocardial dysfunction, may greatly contribute to the onset of sudden cardiac death.

## Inflammatory Balance, Apoptosis, and Sudden Death

There are several lines of evidence suggesting that the inflammatory reaction may play an important role in the combination of events leading to sudden cardiac death.

Atherosclerosis is a chronic inflammatory disease of the arterial wall.[51] Inflammation plays a major role in atherosclerotic plaque disruption and thrombosis,[52] and therefore greatly influences the occurrence of acute coronary syndromes and their related mortality, including sudden death. Moreover, inflammation characterizes other disease states responsible for sudden cardiac death, including myocarditis, arrhythmogenic right ventricular dysplasia, and heart failure.

Proinflammatory cytokines with proapoptotic potential such as IL-1, TNF-$\alpha$, and IFN-$\gamma$ are present in the human plaque and may be involved in the local induction of the apoptotic process, although no studies have been performed showing direct correlation between their expression and the occurrence of apoptosis. However, one of their mediators, inflammatory nitric oxide (NO), produced as the result of upregulation of inducible NO synthase (NOS II), may exert potent cell cytotoxicity. We have recently found a positive association between NOS II expression and TUNEL labeling for apoptotic cells in advanced human atherosclerosis.[27] Upregulation of NOS II has also been reported in patients with heart failure and is thought to contribute to cardiomyocyte apoptosis in this setting. Moreover, increased production of inflammatory NO has potent depressive effects on myocardial contractility.[53] Taken together, the available data suggest that an imbalance in favor of proinflammatory cytokines may exacerbate the cell damage and significantly contribute to the occurrence of sudden death. Control of the inflammatory reaction (using anti-inflammatory cytokines) should be beneficial in preventing the occurrence of sudden cardiac death.

## Conclusion

Determination of the levels of cell proliferation and death in the human cardiovascular system and knowledge of the molecular mechanisms involved in these processes may shed important light on the pathophysiology of a variety of cardiovascular diseases and stimulate the development of interventions selectively aimed at cell death to prevent disease progression.

## *References*

1. Zipes DP, Wellens HJ. Sudden cardiac death. Circulation 1998; 98:2334–2351.
2. Roberts WC, Kragel AH, Bertz D, et al. Coronary arteries in unstable angina pectoris, acute myocardial infarction and sudden cardiac death. Am Heart J 1994; 127:1588–1593.
3. Davies MJ. Anatomic features in victims of sudden coronary death: coronary artery pathology. Circulation 1992; 85(Suppl):I19–24.
4. Theroux P, Fuster V. Acute coronary syndromes: unstable angina and non–Q-wave myocardial infarction. Circulation 1998; 97:1195–1206.
5. James TN. Normal and abnormal consequences of apoptosis in the human heart. Ann Rev Physiol 1998; 60:309–325.
6. Virchow R. Cellular pathology as based upon physiological and pathological histology. In: Classics of Medicine Library. Birmingham, AL, 1858, p 361.
7. Thomas WA, Reiner JM, Florentin FA, Lee KT, Lee WM. Population dynamics of arterial smooth muscle cells. V. Cell proliferation and cell death during initial three months in atherosclerotic lesions induced in swine by hypercholesterolemic diet and intimal trauma. Exp Mol Pathol 1976; 24:360–374.
8. Kerr JFR, Wyllie AH, Currie AR. Apoptosis: a basic biological phenomenon with wide-ranging implications in tissue kinetics. Br J Cancer 1972; 26:239–257.
9. Martin SJ, Reutelingsperger CPM, McGahon AJ, Rader JA, van Schie RCA, et al. Early redistribution of plasma membrane phosphatidylserine is a general feature of apoptosis regardless of the initiating stimulus: inhibition by overexpression of Bcl-2 and Abl. J Exp Med 1995; 182:1545–1556.
10. Casciola-Rosen LA, Anhalt G, Rosen A. Autoantigens targeted in systemic lupus erythematosus are clustered in two populations of surface structures on apoptotic keratinocytes. J Exp Med 1994; 179:1317–1330.

11. Tan EM. Autoimmunity and apoptosis. J Exp Med 1994; 179:1083–1086.
12. Rosen A, Casciola-Rosen L, Ahearn J. Novel packages of viral and self-antigens are generated during apoptosis. J Exp Med 1995; 181:1557–1561.
13. Mann JM, Davies MJ. Vulnerable plaque: relation of characteristics to degree of stenosis in human coronary arteries. Circulation 1996; 94:928–931.
14. Loree HM, Tobias BJ, Gibson LJ, et al. Mechanical properties of model atherosclerotic lesion lipid pools. Arterioscler Thromb 1994; 14:230–234.
15. Burke AP, Farb A, Malcom GT, et al. Plaque rupture and sudden death related to exertion in men with coronary artery disease. JAMA 1999; 281:921–926.
15a. Fadok VA, Savill JS, Haslett C, Bratton DL, Doherty DE, et al. Different populations of macrophages use either the vitronectin receptor or the phosphatidylserine receptor to recognize and remove apoptotic cells. J Immunol 1992; 149:4029–4035.
16. Parkes JL, Cardell RR, Hubbard FCJ, et al. Cultured human atherosclerotic plaque smooth muscle cells retain transforming potential and display enhanced expression of the myc protooncogene. Am J Pathol 1991; 138:765–775.
17. Bennett MR, Evan GI, Newby AC. Deregulated expression of the c-myc oncogene abolishes inhibition of proliferation of rat vascular smooth muscle cells by serum reduction, interferon-$\gamma$, heparin, and cyclic nucleotide analogues and induces apoptosis. Circ Res 1994; 74:525–536.
18. Bennett MR, Evan GI, Schwartz SM. Apoptosis of human vascular smooth muscle cells derived from normal vessels and coronary atherosclerotic plaques. J Clin Invest 1995; 95:2266–2274.
19. Geng Y-J, Libby P. Evidence for apoptosis in advanced human atheroma : colocalization with interleukin-1$\beta$-converting enzyme. Am J Pathol 1995; 147:251–266.
20. Han DKM, Haudenschild CC, Hong MK, et al. Evidence for apoptosis in human atherogenesis and in a rat vascular injury model. Am J Pathol 1995; 147:267–277.
21. Kockx MM, Demeyer GRY, Muhring J, et al. Distribution of cell replication and apoptosis in atherosclerotic plaques of cholesterol-fed rabbits. Atherosclerosis 1996; 120:115–124.
22. Björkerud S, Björkerud B. Apoptosis is abundant in human atherosclerotic lesions, especially in inflammatory cells (macrophages and T cells), and may contribute to the accumulation of gruel and plaque instability. Am J Pathol 1996; 149:367–380.
23. Hegyi L, Skepper JN, Cary NR, et al. Foam cell apoptosis and the development of the lipid core of human atherosclerosis. J Pathol 1996; 180:423–442.
24. Mallat Z, Ohan J, Lesèche G, et al. Colocalization of CPP-32 with apoptotic cells in human atherosclerotic plaques. Circulation 1997; 96:424–428.
25. Cai W, Devaux B, Schaper W, et al. The role of Fas/APO 1 and apoptosis in the development of human atherosclerotic lesions. Atherosclerosis 1997; 131:177–186.
26. Bauriedel G, Schluckebier S, Hutter R, et al. Apoptosis in restenosis versus stable-angina atherosclerosis: implications for the pathogenesis of restenosis. Arterioscler Thromb Vasc Biol 1998; 18:1132–1139.
27. Mallat Z, Heymes C, Ohan J, et al. Expression of interleukin-10 in human atherosclerotic plaques: relation to inducible nitric oxide synthase expression and cell death. Arterioscler Thromb Vasc Biol 1999; 19:611–616.
28. Gordon D, Reidy MA, Benditt EP, et al. Cell proliferation in human coronary arteries. Proc Natl Acad Sci USA 1990; 87:4600–4604.
29. Brandl R, Richter T, Haug K, et al. Topographic analysis of proliferative activ-

ity in carotid endarterectomy specimens by immunocytochemical detection of the cell cycle-related antigen Ki-67. Circulation 1997; 96:3360–3368.

30. Farb A, Burke AP, Tang AL, et al. Coronary plaque erosion without rupture into a lipid core: a frequent cause of coronary thrombosis in sudden coronary death. Circulation 1996; 93:1354–1363.

31. Burke AP, Farb A, Malcom GT, et al. Coronary risk factors and plaque morphology in men with coronary disease who died suddenly. N Engl J Med 1997; 336:1276–1282.

32. Tricot O, Mallat Z, Lesèche G, et al. Distribution of apoptosis in human carotid atherosclerosis: relation to flow direction (abstract). AHA meeting, 1999.

33. Kaiser D, Freyberg MA, Friedl P. Lack of hemodynamic forces triggers apoptosis in vascular endothelial cells. Biochem Biophys Res Commun 1997; 231:586–590.

34. Dimmeler S, Haendeler J, Nehls M, et al. Suppression of apoptosis by nitric oxide via inhibition of interleukin-1 beta-converting enzyme (ICE)-like and cysteine protease protein (CPP)-32-like proteases. J Exp Med 1997; 185: 601–607.

35. Aupeix K, Toti F, Satta N, et al. Oxysterols induce membrane procoagulant activity in monocytic THP-1 cells. Biochem J 1996; 314:1027–1033.

36. Weiss HJ. Scott syndrome: a disorder of platelet coagulant activity. Sem Hematol 1994; 31:312–319.

37. Bach R, Rifkin DB. Expression of tissue factor procoagulant activity: regulation by cytosolic calcium. Proc Natl Acad Sci USA 1990; 87:6995–6999.

38. Aupeix K, Hugel B, Martin T, et al. The significance of shed membrane particles during programmed cell death in vitro, and in vivo, in HIV-1 infection. J Clin Invest 1997; 99:1546–1554.

39. Fourcade O, Simon MF, Viode C, et al. Secretory phospholipase A2 generates the novel lipid mediator lysophosphatidic acid in membrane microvesicles shed from activated cells. Cell 1995; 80:919–927.

40. Barry OP, Pratico D, Savani RC, et al. Modulation of monocyte-endothelial cell interactions by platelet microparticles. J Clin Invest 1998; 102:136–144.

41. Flynn PD, Byrne CD, Baglin TP, et al. Thrombin generation by apoptotic vascular smooth muscle cells. Blood 1997; 89:4378–4384.

42. Bombeli T, Karsan A, Tait JF, et al. Apoptotic vascular endothelial cells become procoagulant. Blood 1997; 89:2429–2442.

43. Bombeli T, Schwartz BR, Harlan JM. Endothelial cells undergoing apoptosis become proadhesive for nonactivated platelets. Blood 1999; 93:3831–3838.

44. Mallat Z, Hugel B, Ohan J, et al. Shed membrane microparticles with procoagulant potential in human atherosclerotic plaques: a role for apoptosis in plaque thrombogenicity. Circulation 1999; 99:348–353.

45. Giesen PL, Rauch U, Bohrmann B, et al. Blood-borne tissue factor: another view of thrombosis. Proc Natl Acad Sci USA 1999; 96:2311–2315.

46. Mallat Z, Benamer H, Hugel B, et al. Elevated circulating levels of procoagulant microparticles in patients with acute coronary syndromes (abstract). AHA meeting, 1998.

47. Saraste A, Pulkki K, Kallajoki M, et al. Apoptosis in human acute myocardial infarction. Circulation 1997; 95:320–323.

48. Olivetti G, Quaini F, Sala R, et al. Acute myocardial infarction in humans is associated with activation of programmed myocyte cell death in the surviving portion of the heart. J Mol Cell Cardiol 1996; 28:2005–2016.

49. Felzen B, Shilkrut M, Less H, et al. Fas (CD95/Apo-1)-mediated damage to ventricular myocytes induced by cytotoxic T lymphocytes from perforin-

deficient mice: a major role for inositol 1,4,5-trisphosphate. Circ Res 1998; 82:438–450.
50. Colucci WS. The effects of norepinephrine on myocardial biology: implications for the therapy of heart failure. Clin Cardiol 1998; 21(12 Suppl 1):I20–I24.
51. Ross R. Atherosclerosis: an inflammatory disease. N Engl J Med 1999; 340:115–126.
52. Lee RT, Libby P. The unstable atheroma. Arterioscler Thromb Vasc Biol 1997; 17:1859–1867.
53. Sawyer DB, Colucci WS. Nitric oxide in the failing myocardium. Cardiol Clin 1998; 16:657–664.

# 6

# Spatiotemporal Organization of Ventricular Fibrillation Increases During Global Ischemia in the Isolated Rabbit Heart

*Jay Chen, BSc, Ravi Mandapati, MD,
Omer Berenfeld, PhD, Moussa Mansour, MD, and
José Jalife, MD*

## Introduction

Ventricular fibrillation (VF) is known to slow down[1] after its onset. Some reports also describe an increase in temporal organization of electrical activity at various stages during VF evolution. Huang et al.[2] showed that VF in the in-situ heart becomes more organized 10–40 sec after its onset. Witkowski et al.[3] reported that, in Langendorff-perfused hearts, VF was most organized at initiation with activation patterns becoming more chaotic over time. The basic mechanism underlying the changes in VF organization were not ascertained in those studies. We have previously demonstrated that under conditions of global ischemia, VF slows down and appears to organize.[4] However, changes in VF organization were not quantified in that study. Defibrillation procedures have been shown to be more successful in organized arrhythmias[5,6]; however, with the passage of time, VF is more difficult to terminate[7] despite seeming to become more organized. It is therefore important to establish whether VF organization does indeed increase with the passage of time and to determine the mechanisms underlying such a change.

Global ischemia is known to accompany the natural evolution of VF and most likely influences the activation patterns during the progression of VF.[4,8] In this study, global ischemia was induced during VF in the Langendorff-perfused rabbit heart to mimic the natural evolution of the ar-

From: Aliot E, Clementy J, Prystowsky EN (editors). *Fighting Sudden Cardiac Death: A Worldwide Challenge.* ©Futura Publishing Company, Armonk, NY, 2000.

rhythmia. We hypothesized that a decrease in tissue excitability slows the frequency of activation by periodic sources responsible for VF, leading to a reduction in frequency-dependent fibrillatory conduction, thereby increasing VF organization.

It was our objective to (1) demonstrate that, under conditions of global ischemia, spatiotemporal organization increases during VF, and (2) quantify the changes in organization that modulate the natural course of VF. The overall results demonstrate that global ischemia and the consequent decrease in tissue excitability are major factors causing VF organization and may be a possible explanation as to why defibrillation becomes less successful with the progression of VF despite an increase in its organization.

# Methods

## Langendorff-Perfused Rabbit Heart

New Zealand rabbits (~2 kg) were anesthetized with sodium pentobarbital (60 mg/kg). The chest was opened through a midline incision, and the heart was rapidly removed and connected to a Langendorff apparatus.[8,9] The coronary arteries were continuously perfused through a cannula in the aortic root with warm (36.5 ± 1°C) HEPES-Tyrode's solution under a pressure head of 70 mm Hg. The solution consisted of the following (mM): HEPES, 15; NaCl, 148; KCl, 5.4; $CaCl_2$, 1.8; $MgCl_2$, 1.0; $NaHCO_3$, 5.8; $NaH_2PO_4$, 0.4; glucose, 5.5; and albumin, (40 mg/L). The solution was saturated with 100% oxygen and its pH was 7.4. The heart was immersed in a rectangular temperature-controlled chamber full of warm HEPES-Tyrode's solution that was continuously replenished by the coronary sinus outflow. Care was taken to maintain the epicardial and endocardial temperatures equal and constant at 36.5 ± 1°C. The sinus node was excised and the atrioventricular node was ablated using a portable high-temperature cautery. Following this, 2 mL of HEPES-Tyrode's solution containing the voltage-sensitive dye di-4-ANEPPS (15 μg/mL) dissolved in DMSO was perfused through the coronaries for 1–2 min.

## High-Resolution Optical Mapping

Details about the experimental setup have previously been described.[8,9] Briefly, the light from a tungsten-halogen lamp was filtered (520/535 nm) and then shone on the epicardial surface of the vertically hanging heart. A 50-mm objective lens was used to collect the emitted light with a depth of field of approximately 8 mm. The emitted light was transmitted through an emission filter (645 nm) and projected onto a CCD video camera (Cohu 5600). The video images (typically $50 \times 150$ pixels or 1,500 pixels/cm$^2$) of the left ventricular epicardial surface, with the left anterior descending coronary artery facing the light source and the camera, were acquired with an A/D frame grabber (Epix). A noninterlace mode was used with a speed of 240 frames/sec (4.17-ms sampling interval). The mapping area was approximately 40% of the entire epicardial surface of the ventricle. In the absence of filtering, the spatial resolution was approximately 0.15 mm.[10] To reveal the transmembrane signal, the background fluorescence was subtracted from each frame. Low-pass spatial filtering (weighted average of 15 neighboring pixels) was applied to improve the signals, which resulted in an effective spatial resolution of less than 0.5 mm (for details see Baxter et al).[10] All the optical recordings were approximately 3–4 sec in duration. During VF there was minimal motion of the heart; nevertheless, an adjustable glass wall was used to gently compress and restrain the heart against the fixed wall of the chamber that faced the camera. Such a procedure eliminated motion artifacts almost completely, and thus electromechanical uncoupling agents were not used in these experiments.

## Electrocardiographic and Frequency Analysis

The Tyrode solution bathing the heart was used as a volume conductor for recording the bipolar ECG. Horizontal ECG recordings were obtained using 2 unipolar electrodes immersed in the chamber at equidistant locations from the heart's surface.[8,9] The signals were bandpass filtered at 0.05–1,000 Hz (Gould 2400S) and displayed continuously on a digital oscilloscope (Tektronix 2214). Episodes of interest were acquired at a sampling interval of 0.4 ms over 4-sec periods, digitized, and transferred to a personal computer. Pseudo-electrocardiograms (pseudo-ECGs) were constructed from optical recordings by integrating the transmembrane fluorescence signal over the entire mapped region of the ventricle.[8,9] To measure the frequency content of the activity during individual episodes of VF, fast Fourier transformation (FFT) was performed on ECGs using Welch's method[11] with a frequency resolution of about 1.0 Hz. All spectral analyses were carried out in the Matlab environment (Matlab, The MathWorks, Inc., Natick, MA).

# Specific Experimental Protocols

## Effects of Global Ischemia on VF Organization

VF was induced by burst pacing at 50 Hz. Three min later, simultaneous optical recordings and ECGs were obtained. VF was defined as the global volume conducted ECG showing rapid irregular activity and the optical recordings showing complex activity. Two to 3 sets of simultaneous optical and ECG recordings were obtained for control VF. No-flow global ischemia was then induced by stopping flow in the aortic cannula and quickly replacing the oxygenated HEPES-Tyrode solution in the chamber with HEPES-Tyrode solution saturated with 100% $N_2$ (pH 6.8).[8,12] Optical mapping data and corresponding bipolar ECG data were obtained at 5 min of global ischemia. Immediately following this recording, reperfusion was started by opening flow in the aortic cannula and replacing the HEPES-Tyrode solution in the chamber with HEPES-Tyrode solution saturated with 100% $O_2$ (pH 7.4). Optical and bipolar ECG data were obtained at 5 min of reperfusion. Epicardial temperature was maintained constant at 36.5 ± 1°C throughout the experiment.

## Effects of Global Ischemia on Tissue Excitability

In 5 additional hearts effects of global ischemia on tissue excitability were measured. The heart was paced at a basic cycle length of 300 ms ($S_1$) and premature stimuli ($S_2$) up to a maximum of 10 times diastolic threshold[13] were applied to the LV epicardial surface using a suction electrode at decreasing intervals of prematurity during control and 5 min of global ischemia.

## Dominant Frequency Maps

To reveal hidden organization behind the complex propagation patterns during VF, we constructed dominant frequency (DF) maps from our optical recordings using spectral decomposition methods. This technique has been described elsewhere.[14-16] Succinctly, spectral analysis of each 7,500 pixels' electrical activity over the entire 4-sec optical movie was performed. The frequency at which the maximum power was generated was assigned to be the DF. The DF of each pixel was pictorially represented in a DF map, where the DF of each pixel was denoted on a color scale from 1 to 30 Hz. It was found that the DFs tend to cluster in contiguous regions, termed hereafter as "domains." The accuracy of such a spatial distribution of DFs was assessed by subtracting the DF power of each pixel by one-half of its standard error (based on the $\chi^2$ distribution function[16]). The maximum power frequency was then calculated again. If the new maximum power frequency shifted to a different frequency, then the DF of that pixel was considered to be nonreliable. This provided the uncertainty of the location of the domain boundary to be typically less than 1.0 mm. Thus, discrete domains of DFs were considered significant only when their area exceeded a 1% cutoff of the total mapped area. All spectral analyses were performed in the Matlab programming environment (The MathWorks Inc., Natick, MA).

## Approximate Entropy Algorithm

Approximate entropy (ApEn) was used to determine the degree of organization of ECGs. ApEn was calculated by methods previously described.[17–19] ApEn is a statistical measure of variability, expressing the logarithmic likelihood that data points that are of a certain deviation (r) over a defined number of observations (m) remain the same distance between incremental comparisons. More regularity is associated with smaller values of ApEn and greater irregularity with larger values of ApEn. Approximate entropy was calculated for >1,000 points. Values of m=2 and r=0.1 were used.

## Two-Dimensional Phase Maps

We quantified the density of wavelets during VF using a recently developed technique, 2-dimensional phase mapping,[20] which highlights the formation of wavebreaks and the resulting singularity points. Briefly, 2-dimensional phase maps were constructed by plotting $F(t+\tau)$ versus $F(t)$ for a given pixel from our optical signals with $\tau = -2$. This allowed a new parameter, the phase $\theta(t)$, to be defined as the angle of the coordinate [$F(t)$, $F(t+\tau)$] around the mean fluorescence ($F_{mean}$) for that pixel; $\theta(t)$ was computed as atan($F[t+\tau]-F_{mean}$, $F[t]-F_{mean}$). The value of $\theta(t)$, with values between $-\pi$ and $\pi$, was visually represented as a continuous color scheme from red to violet. Then the fluorescence of each pixel over time was remapped as a 2-dimensional phase map, $\theta(t)$. A singularity point was defined as the point where all phases converged. The resulting 2-dimensional phase maps, one for each sequential frame of the optical recording, were replayed as a series of phase maps where wavebreaks, with resulting formation of phase singularity points and wavelets,[20–22] could rigorously be identified and followed from frame to frame.

## Statistical Analysis

These data are presented as mean ± standard error of the mean (SEM) for group comparisons and as mean ± standard deviation of the mean (SDM) for individual group statistics. Comparisons were performed using standard analysis of variance (ANOVA). A $p<0.05$ was considered to be statistically significant.

# Results

## Electrocardiographic and Frequency Analysis

The ECG of VF and its corresponding frequency spectra in the same experiment under conditions of control, 5 min of global ischemia, and 5 min of reperfusion, are shown in Figure 1. During control VF (1A), the ECG was irregular and its corresponding FFT showed multiple peaks with a dominant frequency at 10.1 Hz. At 5 min of no-flow global ischemia (1B), the optical pseudo-ECG became more organized and the DF of the arrhythmia slowed down to 8.1 Hz. Reversible changes in the disorganization of the electrogram and DF were seen when reperfusion of oxygenated Tyrode solution was initiated (2C). The DF at 5 min of reperfusion was 11.8 Hz. Similar changes were seen in all experiments; quantification of the same parameters from all 6 experiments is presented in panel D. The DF decreased from $13.5 \pm 2.4$ Hz during control to $6.0 \pm 1.7$ Hz at 5 min of ischemia ($p < 0.05$) and increased to $13.6 \pm 2.1$ Hz at 5 min of reperfusion.

## Organization of Patterns of Activation During Global Ischemia

Activation patterns during VF became repetitive and organized during conditions of global ischemia as shown in Figure 2. Isochrone maps (2A) for 3 consecutive activation sequences during control VF show complex activity changing from beat to beat. At t=456 ms, 2 wavefronts are seen to enter the mapped region from opposite directions. These wavelets collide, coalesce, and then propagate in a different direction. At t=532 ms, repetitive activation of the 2 wavefronts shown at t=456 ms is seen, in conjunction with a breakthrough pattern of propagation. At t=600 ms, another breakthrough occurs at a different location and a second wavefront is seen to enter the mapped region from the left ventricular free wall. In contrast, under conditions of no-flow global ischemia (2B), the propagation patterns became more organized as a single wavefront propagated upward relatively undisturbed in a spatially and temporally similar fashion for the 3 consecutive activation sequences shown. Such spatially and temporally organized activity (spatiotemporal periodicity[23]) persisted for 34 activations. During reperfusion (2C), the propagation patterns of wavefronts returned to a similar level of complexity as during control VF (2A). At t=64 ms, a breakthrough occurred with a second wavefront entering the mapped region from the left ventricular free wall. At t=120 ms, the same breakthrough repeated itself and 2 separate wavefronts entered the mapped region from the left and right ventricular free walls. Finally at

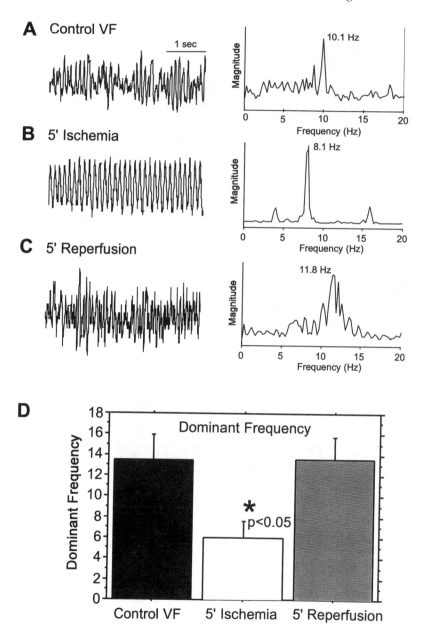

Figure 1. Effects of global ischemia on the VF dominant frequency. A–C: ECGs and corresponding frequency spectra during the same episode of VF. D: Quantification of change in VF dominant frequency (DF) under conditions of control VF, 5 min (') of ischemia, and 5 min of reperfusion for all 6 experiments. See text for details. *p<0.05.

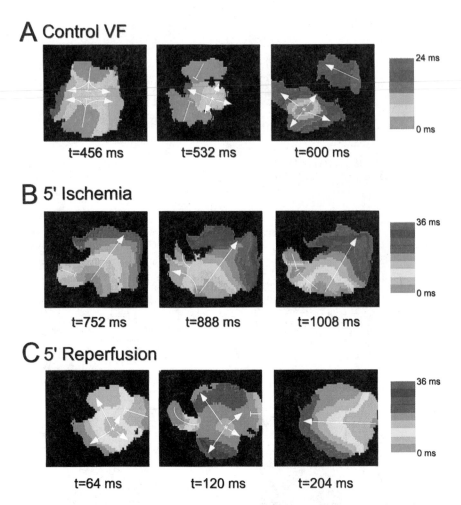

**Figure 2.** A–C: Isochrone maps of 3 sequential activation sequences of VF during control VF, 5 min (') global ischemia, and 5 min of reperfusion from the same episode. Lines denote the path of the excitation wave, where red is the first site to be activated and purple the last. See text for details.

t=204 ms, a single wavefront entered the mapping field of view from the left ventricular free wall and propagated toward the right ventricle. In addition to the greater number of repetitive activations during ischemia, the propagation away from such periodic sites was relatively uniform with lesser breakup of activity. Global ischemia significantly increased the duration of repetitive activity in all 6 experiments. The duration of repetitive spatiotemporally periodic activity increased from $3 \pm 0.7$ activations during control to $36 \pm 2.4$ activations at 5 min of global ischemia ($p < 0.001$).

## Dominant Frequency Maps

Dominant frequency maps are a tool that enables us to look at arrhythmia organization in the frequency domain and are useful in revealing hidden organization during VF. DF maps under conditions of control VF, 5 min of no-flow global ischemia, and 5 min of reperfusion were constructed for all 6 experiments. A representative example is shown in Figure 3. A DF map

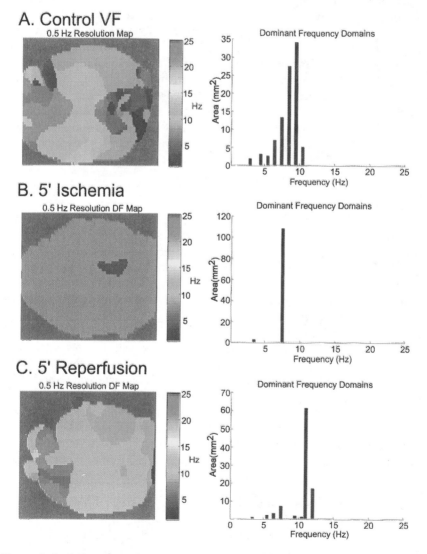

Figure 3. A–C: Dominant frequency (DF) maps during conditions of control VF, 5 min (') of global ischemia, and 5 min of reperfusion. See text for details.

during control VF (3A) is shown along with the corresponding areas of domains at each dominant frequency. In this specific example, there were a total of 13 domains; the density of domains (# of domains/area) was 10.25/cm$^2$ and the % area of the largest domain was 28.0%. Under conditions of 5 min of global ischemia (3B), the DF map clearly became more organized. Only 2 domains were seen; the density of domains decreased to 1.8/cm$^2$ and the % area of the largest domain increased to 94.8%. During reperfusion (3C), the arrhythmia returned toward its original level of complexity; 12 domains were seen; the density of domains increased to 12.3/cm$^2$, and the % area of the largest domain decreased to 17.0%. In Figure 4, the density of domains and % area of the largest domain during conditions of control VF, 5 min of global ischemia, and 5 min of reperfusion are shown for all 6 experiments. The domain density (4A) significantly changed from 11.5 $\pm$ 1.4 cm$^2$ to 3.2 $\pm$ 1.1 cm$^2$ ($p < 0.05$) to 13.4 $\pm$ 3.8 cm$^2$ under conditions of control VF, 5 min of global ischemia, and 5 min of reperfusion, respectively. The % area of the largest domain (4B) increased from 34.0 $\pm$ 6.7% during control VF to 83.9 $\pm$ 4.5% during 5 min of global ischemia and decreased again to 28.2 $\pm$ 8.5% during 5 min of reperfusion.

## Approximate Entropy

To further quantify changes in VF organization, the degree of organization of the ECGs was studied using the approximate entropy (ApEn) algorithm.[17–19] In Figure 5, a representative example of optical pseudo-ECGs and their ApEn values from the same episode of VF are shown under conditions of control VF, 5 min of no-flow global ischemia, and 5 min of reperfusion. In panel A, during control VF, the ECG was irregularly irregular, characteristic of ventricular fibrillation, with an ApEn value of 0.47. At 5 min of global ischemia (5B), the ECG became more regular and organized, reflected by an ApEn value of 0.36. During 5 min of reperfusion (panel C), the ECG returned to its original disorganized state, characteristic of VF, with a corresponding ApEn value of 0.54. Quantification of such changes in all 6 experiments showed that the global ischemia significantly increased organization in the ECG as shown in panel D. The ECG ApEn significantly changed from 0.49 $\pm$ 0.04 during control VF to 0.33 $\pm$ 0.042 during 5 min of global ischemia to 0.51 $\pm$ 0.03 during 5 min of reperfusion.

## Global Ischemia-Induced Change in Density of Wavelets

The isochrone and dominant frequency maps during global ischemia suggested that activity became more organized with a decrease in breakup of propagating waves. As a result one would expect to see a decrease in

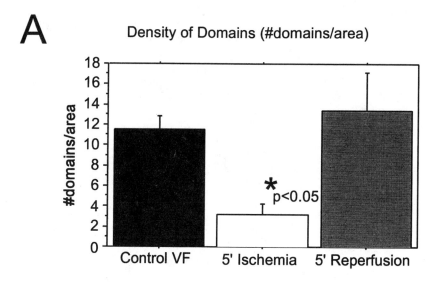

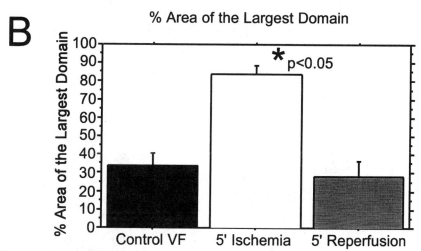

Figure 4. Quantification of dominant frequency domain organization during control VF, 5 min (') of global ischemia, and 5 min of reperfusion. A: Density of domains (# domains/cm $^2$) for all 6 experiments. B: % area of the largest domain for all 6 experiments. See text for details. *p<0.05.

the density of VF wavelets under conditions of global ischemia. To this aim, we used phase mapping in an effort to monitor the formation of phase singularities (PSs) resulting from wavebreaks,[20–22] and thus accurately identify and count wavelets that are formed as a result of the interaction of wavefronts with obstacles in their paths. The mean number of

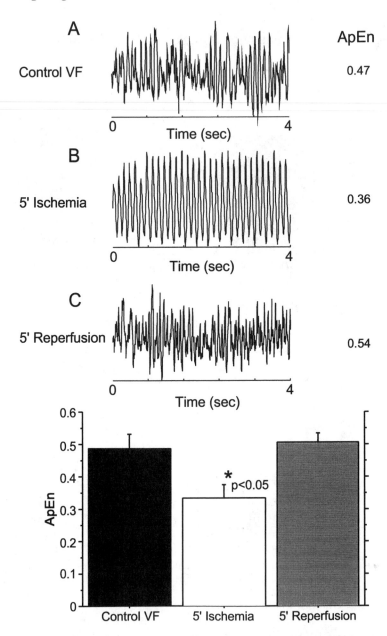

Figure 5. A–C: A representative example of ECGs and their corresponding ApEn values. Greater regularity is associated with smaller values of ApEn and higher irregularity with larger values of ApEn. D: ApEn for all 6 experiments under conditions of control VF, 5 min (=) of global ischemia, and 5 min of reperfusion. See text for details. *$p<0.05$.

wavelets/frame was obtained from the number of wavelets observed per frame in 50 consecutive frames (200 ms). Density of wavefronts was obtained by dividing the mean number of wavelets in each frame by the surface area of the entire mapping region.

As shown in Figure 6, the density of wavelets during control was $1.23 \pm 0.18/cm^2$ and decreased to $0.55 \pm 0.03 /cm^2$ at 5 min of ischemia ($p<0.002$). Reperfusion resulted in reversal of the changes with an increase in the density of wavefronts to a value near control ($1.04 \pm 0.13/cm^2$).

## Effects of Ischemia on Excitability and Refractoriness

The underlying assumption in our study is that the basic mechanism leading to changes in activation patterns of VF during global ischemia is a decrease in tissue excitability. To demonstrate that global ischemia did indeed reduce tissue excitability, in a set of 5 hearts, we examined the effects of ischemia on the strength-interval relationship, the results of which are shown in Figure 7. As expected, during global ischemia, there was a shift of the curve to the right and upward, which is consistent with an increase in refractoriness and a decrease in excitability.

## Discussion

This study quantifies the increase in spatiotemporal organization that occurs during ventricular fibrillation in the setting of no-flow global

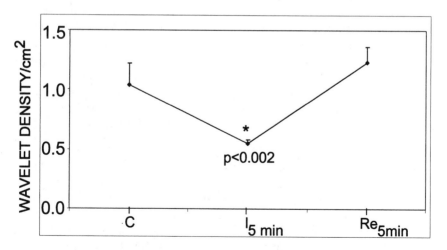

Figure 6. Density of VF wavelets (# wavelets/cm²) during control, 5 min of global ischemia and reperfusion. *p<0.05.

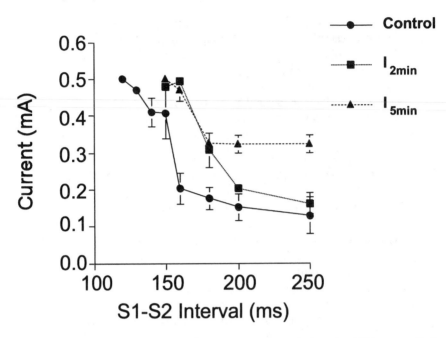

Figure 7. Strength interval relationship at a pacing cycle length of 300 ms studied using a standard $S_1$–$S_2$ protocol for 5 hearts. The minimum amount of current (mA) needed to capture the tissue is plotted against $S_1$–$S_2$ intervals. Values are shown as mean ±SD.

ischemia. During global ischemia, the ECG became more organized, the dominant frequency of VF decreased, and distribution of DF domains became more homogeneous (and hence more organized). VF activation patterns became more repetitive with decreased breakup of activity. Furthermore, reperfusion of oxygenated Tyrode solution reversed changes in spatiotemporal organization. Overall, our results demonstrate that ischemia-induced decrease in excitability on its own can increase VF organization. This might explain the decreased success of defibrillation procedures as VF progresses, despite an increase in organization.

## The Evolution of Spatiotemporal Organization During VF

Organization during various stages of VF has previously been described, but reports vary as to timing of organizational changes or to the basic underlying etiology. In 1934, Wiggers et al.[1] studied VF in in-situ dog hearts and found that during stage 4 of VF (2–3 min of its onset), the rate decreased and the electrical deflections of the electrocardiogram became more regular and periodic as time progressed. Recently, Witkowski et al.[3]

using isolated perfused dog hearts demonstrated that in the initial few seconds after VF induction, the arrhythmia seemed organized, with a pair of counter-rotating spiral waves being observed that later degenerated into multiple chaotically moving wavelets. Huang et al.[2] showed that the first few VF beats in the in-situ pig heart are organized, followed by chaotic activity which later seems to organize again by about 40 sec after induction. As VF was terminated by defibrillation, in Huang's work the arrhythmia was not studied beyond 40 sec after its onset.

## Organization During VF: Potential Relevance

Organization during VF evokes interest, as organized arrhythmias are potentially easier to defibrillate.[4–5] However, it is well known that success of defibrillation decreases as VF progresses,[6] and it is therefore important to establish whether organization does increase in VF with the passage of time and the underlying etiology. It has previously been shown that slowing of the rate as VF progresses is most likely caused by global ischemia because slowing of VF rate is prevented by perfusing the coronary arteries.[7] Furthermore, one may have expected that conditions of global ischemia would enhance heterogeneity of refractoriness and increase the degree of disorganization in VF. To gain better mechanistic insight into the basis of VF organization, the present study was conducted to determine whether global ischemia by itself does indeed increase VF organization.

## Ischemia-Induced VF Organization: Mechanism Underlying the Changes in Spatiotemporal Organization

We have demonstrated that global ischemia decreased the VF rate. This was accompanied by an increase in the organization of activation patterns that was quantified in terms of the duration of repetitive activity in the form of spatiotemporal periodicity, a decrease in density of DF domains, and a smaller ApEn value. Accompanying these changes was also a significant reduction in the density of wavefronts as measured by decrease in density of phase singularity points. These results suggest that a decrease in VF dominant frequency reduced the breakup of waves propagating away from periodic sources with more homogeneous propagation.

Recent work from our laboratory by Mandapati et al.[4] has shown that the core size of reentry during VF in the isolated rabbit heart increases under conditions of global ischemia. Similar results have also been reported by Rogers et al.[24,25] where during VF in an in-situ pig heart, the core size of rotors was seen to increase over time from 0–40 sec of VF. As the path length for reentry (i.e., core size) increased, the VF rate decreased. As shown in this study, tissue excitability is reduced by ischemia and most likely is the cause of an increase in core size owing to block of impulses at a lesser critical curvature.[26]

## Clinical Relevance

This study has implications for studies that seek to time defibrillation shocks or gauge effectiveness of drug therapy by using measures of organization.[4,5] Previous studies have shown that an increase in myocardial organization leads to a decreased energy requirement for successful defibrillation. Paradoxically, VF becomes more difficult to terminate as the arrhythmia progresses despite an increase in organization.[6] We attribute this paradox to the overall decreased excitability of the tissue as ischemia progresses during the natural evolution of VF. Overall, these results provide a quantitative understanding of the effects of global ischemia on the dynamics and spatiotemporal organization of VF, and suggest a possible explanation why an increase in organization in a setting of global ischemia is not a useful parameter to predict success of defibrillation.

## Conclusions

Overall, our study provides robust quantitative information about VF dynamics in control, as well as during ischemia and reperfusion. The results enhance our understanding of such dynamics and give insight into mechanisms causing the changes in activation patterns during the natural course of VF. It is to be hoped that such new knowledge could be the basis for improved strategies for defibrillation.

*Acknowledgements: This work was supported in part by a grant PO1-HL-39707 from the National Heart, Lung, and Blood Institute, NIH; AHA New York State Affiliate Fellowship awarded to Drs. Mandapati and Berenfeld. In addition, we would like to thank Jiang Jiang, Fan Yang, and Clara Wu for their technical assistance.*

## References

1. Wiggers CJ, Bell JR, Paine M. Studies of ventricular fibrillation caused by electric shock. II. Cinematographic and electrocardiographic observations of the natural process in the dog's heart: its inhibition by potassium and the revival of coordinated beats by calcium. Am Heart J 1930; 5:351–365.
2. Huang J, Rogers JM, KenKnight BH, Rollins DL, Smith WM, et al. Evolution of the organization of epicardial activation patterns during ventricular fibrillation. J Cardiovasc Electrophysiol 1998; 9:1291–1304.
3. Witkowski FX, Leon LJ, Penkoske PA, Giles WR, Spanol ML, et al. Spatiotemporal evolution of ventricular fibrillation. Nature 1998; 392:78–82.

4. Mandapati R, Asano Y, Baxter WT, Gray R, Davidenko JM, et al. Quantification of the effects of global ischemia on the dynamics of ventricular fibrillation in the isolated rabbit heart. Circulation 1998; 16:1688–1696.
5. Hsia PW, Fendelander L, Harrington G, Damiano RJ. Defibrillation success is associated with myocardial organization: spatial coherence as a new method of quantifying the electrical organization of the heart. J Electrocardiol 1996; 29(Suppl):189–197.
6. Dorian P, Newman D. Tedisamil increases coherence during ventricular fibrillation and decreases defibrillation energy requirements. Cardiovasc Res 1997; 33:485–494.
7. Yakaitis RW, Ewy A, Otto CW, Tarren DL, Moon TE. Influence of time and therapy on ventricular fibrillation in dogs. Crit Care Med 1980; 8:157–163.
8. Worley SJ, Swain JL, Colavita PG, Smith WM, Ideker RE. Development of an endocardial-epicardial gradient of activation rate during electrically induced sustained ventricular fibrillation in the dog. Am J Cardiol 1985; 55:813–820.
9. Gray RA, Jalife J, Panfilov AV, Baxter WT, Cabo C, et al. Nonstationary vortex-like reentry as a mechanism of polymorphic ventricular tachycardia in the isolated rabbit heart. Circulation 1995; 91:2454–2469.
10. Baxter WT, Davidenko JM, Loew LM, Wuskell JP, Jalife J. Technical features of a CCD camera system to record cardiac fluorescence data. Ann Biomed Eng 1997; 25:713–725.
11. Welch PD. The use of fast Fourier transform for the estimation of power spectra: a method based on time averaging over short, modified periodograms. IEEE Trans Audio Electracoust 1967; AU-15:70–73.
12. Yan GX, Kleber AG. Changes in extracellular and intracellular pH in ischemic rabbit papillary muscle. Circ Res 1992; 71:460–470.
13. Buxton AE, Josephson ME, Marchlinski FE, Miller JM. Polymorphic ventricular tachycardia induced by programmed stimulation: response to procainamide. J Am Coll Cardiol 1993; 21(1):90–98.
14. Jalifé J, Berenfeld O, Skanes AC, Mandapati R. Mechanisms of atrial fibrillation: mother rotors or multiple daughter wavelets, or both? J Cardiovasc Electrophysiol 1998;9(Suppl):S2–S12.
15. Berenfeld O, Mandapati R, Skanes AC, Chen J, Jalife J. Spatial organization of atrial activity decreases as atrial fibrillation frequency accelerates (abstract). PACE 1999; 22:703.
16. Kay SM. Modern Spectral Estimation: Theory and Application. Prentice Hall, New York, 1988, p 76.
17. Pincus SM. Approximate entropy as a measure of system complexity. Proc Natl Acad Sci USA 1991; 88:2297–2301.
18. Pincus SM. Goldberger AL. Physiological time-series analysis: what does regularity quantify? Am J Physiol 1994; 266(4 Pt 2):H1643–656.
19. Hamezi A, Toshiniko O, Lee M, Voroshilovsky O, Chen PS, et al. Approximate entropy as an index for ventricular fibrillation stratification: implications for mechanisms. JACC 1999; 33(Suppl): 1116–1180.
20. Gray RA. Pertsov AM, Jalife J. Spatial and temporal organization during cardiac fibrillation. Nature 1998; 392:75–78.
21. Winfree A. Electrical instability in cardiac muscle: phase singularities and rotors. J Theor Biol 1989; 138:393–405.
22. Chen J, Mandapati R, Skanes AC, Berenfeld O, Jalife J. Periodic epicardial breakthroughs and short-lived spiral waves in ventricular fibrillation (abstract). Circulation 1998; 17:250.
23. Skanes AC, Mandapati R, Berenfeld O, Davidenko JM, Jalife J. Spatiotemporal

periodicity during atrial fibrillation in the isolated sheep heart. Circulation 1998; 98:1236–1248.
24. Rogers JM, Unsui M, KenKnight BH, Ideker RE, Smith WM. The number of recurrent wavefront morphologies: a method for quantifying the complexity of epicardial activation patterns. Ann Biomed Eng 1997; 25:761–768.
25. Rogers JM, Huang J, Smith WM, Ideker RE. Incidence, evolution, and spatial distribution of functional reentry during ventricular fibrillation in pigs. Circ Res 1999; 84:945–954.
26. Cabo C, Pertsov AM, Baxter WT, Davidenko JM, Gray RA, et al. Wave front curvature as a cause of slow conduction and block in isolated cardiac muscle. Circ Res 1994; 75:1014–1028.

# 7

# The Role of Early Afterdepolarizations in Lethal Ventricular Arrhythmias

*Ralph Lazzara, MD, and Bela Szabo, MD*

## Introduction

Afterdepolarizations as mechanisms of cardiac arrhythmias have been studied extensively in recent years. Early afterdepolarizations (EADs), those defined as transient retardations or reversals of repolarization that may result in triggered firing, have been implicated convincingly as trigger mechanisms for ventricular tachyarrhythmias and sudden death in the long QT syndromes.[1] This chapter will highlight EADs and their role in the long QT syndromes with subsidiary comment on the possible roles of EADs in lethal arrhythmias in other clinical settings.

## Brief Historical Perspective

Afterdepolarizations were first observed in recordings of injury potentials on isolated strips of myocardium in the 1940s by Segers[2] and Bozler.[3] The phenomena excited little interest until 3 decades later when the demonstration that cardiac glycosides induced delayed afterdepolarization (DAD) in Purkinje fibers[4-6] generated interest in DAD. The distinction between EAD and DAD was defined by Cranefield.[7,8] EAD received scant attention until an association between EAD and the acquired and congenital long QT syndromes was suggested in 1983 based on observations in a canine model of $Cs^+$-blocked cardiac $K^+$ channels.[9] Since then, there has been an escalating interest in EAD: the settings for their generation, their ionic mechanisms, and their clinical relevance, especially in the long QT syndromes.

From: Aliot E, Clementy J, Prystowsky EN (editors). *Fighting Sudden Cardiac Death: A Worldwide Challenge.* ©Futura Publishing Company, Armonk, NY, 2000.

# Ionic Mechanisms of EADs

In the initial report postulating an association of EAD with the long QT syndromes,[9] a close link between EAD generation and prolonged repolarization produced by $Cs^+$ blockade of $K^+$ currents in canine myocardium was demonstrated. This link between EAD and prolonged repolarization has been abundantly reaffirmed since that report and it is universally accepted that prolongation of repolarization, either by reduction in outward currents or enhancement of inward currents, is the basic condition for EAD generation. A minor departure from this thesis is provided by the induction of EAD by adrenergic agonists ex vivo when EADs are generated without gross prolongation of repolarization.[10] The importance for EAD generation of reduced outward currents and/or enhanced inward currents during repolarization was pointed out by Cranefield when he defined EAD as distinct from DAD.[7,8]

Although there is agreement that reduced outward current and/or enhanced inward current causing prolonged repolarization provides the common settings in which EAD are generated, the actual transient flows of current that manifest directly as EAD have been debated. It has been emphasized that currents underlying EAD should be distinguished from currents responsible for triggered upstrokes (Figure 1). Among the various hypotheses for EAD-generating currents, 2 have gained ascendancy, both related to $Ca^{2+}$ transport.

One hypothesis proposed by January and co-workers relates EADs to L-type $Ca^{2+}$ current ($I_{CaL}$) flowing during repolarization as a "window current" within a range of membrane potential at which a fraction of channels have both activation and inactivation gates open.[12,13] This window current is postulated to increase when the membrane potential resides in the window range, about $-10$ mV, for long periods such as when repolarization is prolonged during the plateau. The increase in inward (depolarizing) current produces the EAD.

Zeng, Rudy, and associates[14] have examined a computer-based model of the guinea pig myocyte and derived information to support the $I_{CaL}$ hypothesis with the modification that enhancement of $I_{CaL}$ during prolonged repolarization near the plateau is due not only to window current enhancement but also to removal of $Ca^{2+}$-dependent inactivation and reopening of $Ca^{2+}$ channels. This removal is due to the decline of the $Ca^{2+}$ transient from sequestration of $Ca^{2+}$ by the sarcoplasmic reticulum during the prolonged repolarization.

Szabo and associates have obtained data that suggest that the current producing EAD is $Ca^{2+}$-activated Na:Ca exchange current ($I_{Na:Ca}$), related to spontaneous release of $Ca^{2+}$ during repolarization, in turn related to $Ca^{2+}$ loading because of prolonged repolarization.[11,15] Prolongation of the

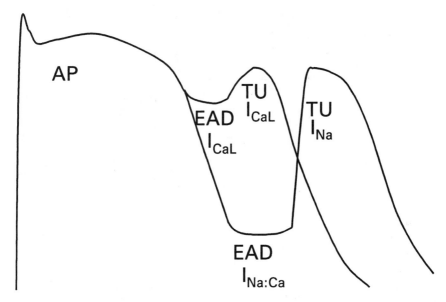

Figure 1. Action potential (AP) exhibiting EAD near the plateau with current generator presumed to be $I_{CaL}$ and a triggered upstroke (TU) with a current generator also presumed to be $I_{CaL}$ plus an EAD occurring at more negative membrane potential during phase III with current generator presumed to be $I_{Na:Ca}$ and a triggered upstroke generated by $Na^+$ current ($I_{Na:Ca}$). EAD and triggered upstrokes generated at different levels of membrane potentials may have different current generators.

plateau results in prolonged inflow of $Ca^{2+}$ through $Ca^{2+}$ channels and reduced extrusion of $Ca^{2+}$ by the Na:Ca exchanger, which operates better at more negative membrane potentials, leading to $Ca^{2+}$ loading of the cell and of the sarcoplasmic reticulum (Figure 2). This mechanism is akin to that thought to be the basis for DADs, which occur with $Ca^{2+}$ loading independent of prolonged repolarization. In the case of DAD, the spontaneous release of $Ca^{2+}$ occurs during diastole.

Since $I_{CaL}$ cannot be operative during later phases of repolarization (membrane potential more negative than $-40$ mV), EADs during much of phase III are more likely due to the Na:Ca exchange current mechanism, while EAD near plateau levels may be due to either mechanism. The great majority of EAD that have been recorded by the technique of monophasic action potentials in patients with acquired and congenital long QT syndromes appear during phase III,[16–32] apparently at levels of membrane potential more negative than the threshold of activation for $I_{CaL}$ (Figure 3). These observations in humans suggest that mechanisms for EADs in patients commonly are not dependent on $I_{CaL}$.

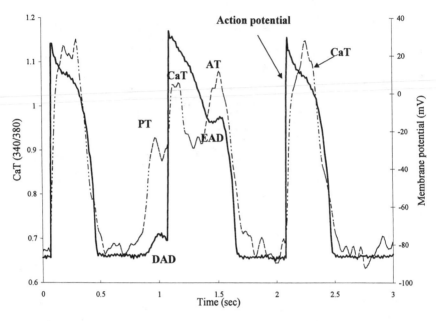

**Figure 2.** Action potentials and fluorescence recordings of cytosolic calcium (CaT, dashed line) recorded from a myocyte treated with isoproterenol ($2 \times 10^{-8}$M) generating both DAD and EAD. The cytosolic calcium shows a pretransient (PT) associated with the DAD and an aftertransient (AT) associated with but preceding in onset the EAD. The timing relationships indicate that the rise in intracellular $Ca^{2+}$ associated with EAD cannot be solely a consequence of calcium entering through L-type $Ca^{2+}$ channels opening during the EAD but reflect an internal process, most likely spontaneous $Ca^{2+}$ release from the sarcoplasmic reticulum.

## EADs and the Long QT Syndromes

Experimental models of the long QT syndromes involving reduction of repolarizing $K^+$ currents[9,33] or enhancement of persistent inward Na current during repolarization[34,35] have prominently manifested EADs as trigger mechanisms for ventricular tachyarrhythmias. Cells with normally prolonged repolarization, i.e., Purkinje cells and to a lesser extent M cells, are favored sites for EAD generation.[9,36,37] Accordingly, mapping of animal models has shown that the initiating beats of torsades de pointes begin focally in the endocardium.[38,39]

Recordings of monophasic action potentials in patients with long QT syndromes have readily demonstrated EADs at endocardial sites.[16–32] These EADs have shown responses that fit with experimental and clinical findings. These responses include accentuation of EADs after long diastole or during adrenergic stimulation, suppression by $Ca^+$ channel blockers, and correlation with T-U wave changes on the electrocardiogram.

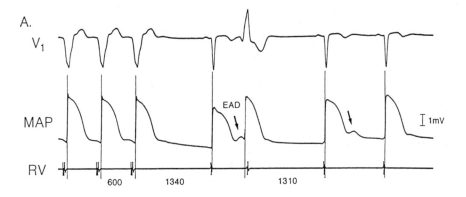

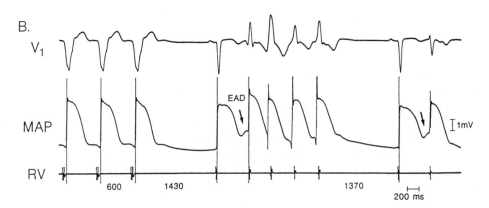

Figure 3. Monophasic action potential recordings of EADs in a patient with sporadic congenital long QT syndrome showing EADs generated relatively late during phase 3 with associated triggering. The EAD is more prominent in panel B compared with panel A and is followed by more triggered beats. The pause following a train of paced beats at cycle length of 600 ms was longer in panel B (1,430 ms) than in panel A (1,340 ms) indicating a pause dependence of EAD. (Reproduced by permission from J Cardiol Electrophysiol 1990; 1:198.)

While there is consensus that EADs are the trigger mechanisms for torsades de pointes, sustaining mechanisms for the ventricular tachycardias have not been consistent as observed in mapping studies in experimental animals. Both macroreentry involving M cell layers and repetitive focal firing have been implicated as sustaining mechanisms.[38,39]

Progress in clarification of the genetic defects of the congenital long QT syndrome has been remarkable in recent years.[40] The abnormal genes thus far identified produce reduction in the K$^+$ currents, I$_{Ks}$ and I$_{Kr}$, which are the major mediators of phase III repolarization, or (the most rare variant) enhancement of persistent Na current due to a defect in inactivation in the Na channel gene.[40] In the acquired long QT syndromes, reduction in $K^+$ currents, most commonly $I_{Kr}$, is the most frequent mechanism.[41,42] This current appears to be readily blocked by a diverse array of pharmacological agents including a number of agents whose primary therapeutic action is not targeted at the heart. These clinical scenarios are comparable to the common experimental models for EAD generation, satisfying the postulations of Cranefield as he defined EAD.

# EADs and Other Clinical Conditions Associated with Sudden Death

EADs have been described in experimental conditions associated with heart failure, hypertrophy, and ischemia/reperfusion.[43–47] Models of hypertrophy and heart failure have shown prolonged action potentials and propensity to generate both EADs and DADs. The transient outward current ($I_{to}$) has been shown to be reduced commonly along with other abnormalities including abnormalities of $Ca^{2+}$ transport.[43,48,49] Both animal models and failing human hearts have demonstrated mixed focal and reentrant mechanisms and a predominance of focal mechanisms in end-stage failing hearts.[50,51] The idea that nonreentrant mechanisms may be prevalent in failing hearts fits with the clinical observation that provocative stimulation during electrophysiology study is not a reliable means of inducing the clinical ventricular arrhythmias in idiopathic cardiomyopathy.

In ischemic heart disease, there is evidence for EAD generation and triggering in reperfusion arrhythmias. Compensatory hypertrophy could provide a substrate for triggering that could initiate reentrant mechanisms, up to now considered the prevalent mechanism in ischemically scarred hearts. Thus far, direct evidence for EAD generation in humans in vivo in heart failure, hypertrophy, and ischemia is lacking.

## Summary

The role of EADs as triggering mechanisms for arrhythmias in the long QT syndromes, both congenital and acquired, is well accepted. These syndromes represent global disorders of the myocardium. In the case of heart failure, hypertrophy, and ischemia/reperfusion, evidence for focal triggering is indirect and inconclusive but sufficient to warrant continued investigation.

## References

1. Roden DM, Lazzara R, Rosen M, Schwartz PJ, Towbin J, et al. Multiple mechanisms in the long-QT syndrome: current knowledge, gaps, and future direc-

tions. The SADS Foundation Task Force on LQTS. Circulation 1996; 94(8):1996–2012.

2. Segers M. Le role des potentials tardifs du coeur. Mem Acad R Med Belg Series II, Vol 1, fascile 7,1941, pp 1–30.

3. Bozler E. The initiation of impulses in cardiac muscle. Am J Physiol 1943; 138:273–282.

4. Davis LD. Effect of changes in cycle length on diastolic depolarization produced by ouabain in canine Purkinje fibers. Circ Res 1973; 32:206–214.

5. Rose MR, Gelband H, Hoffman, BF. Correlation between effects of ouabain on the canine electrocardiogram and transmembrane potentials of isolated Purkinje fibers. Circulation 1973; 47:65–72.

6. Ferrier GR, Saunders JH, Mendez C. A cellular mechanism for the generation of ventricular arrhythmias by acetylstrophanthidin. Circ Res 1973; 32:600–609.

7. Cranefield P. The Conduction of the Cardiac Impulse. Futura Publishing Company, Mount Kisco, NY, 1975, pp 272–277.

8. Cranefield P. Action potentials, afterpotentials, and arrhythmias. Circ Res 1977; 41:415–423.

9. Brachmann J, Scherlag BJ, Rosenshtraukh LV, Lazzara R. Bradycardia-dependent triggered activity: relevance to drug-induced multiform ventricular tachycardia. Circulation 1983; 68:846–856.

10. Volders PG, Kulscar A, Vos MA, Sipido KR, Wellens JH, et al. Similarities between early and delayed afterdepolarizations induced by isoproterenol in canine ventricular myocytes. Cardiovasc Res 1997; 34:348–359.

11. Szabo B, Sweidan R, Rajagopalan CV, Lazzara R. Role of $Na^+$:$Ca^{2+}$ exchange current in $Cs^+$-induced early afterdepolarizations in Purkinje fibers. J Cardiovasc Electrophysiol 1994; 5:933–944.

12. January CT, Riddle JM, Salata JJ. A model for early afterdepolarizations: induction with the $Ca^{2+}$ channel agonist Bay K 8644. Circ Res 1988; 62:563–571.

13. January CT, Riddle JM. Early afterdepolarizations: mechanism of induction and block: a role for L-type $Ca^{2+}$ current. Circ Res 1989; 64:977–990.

14. Zeng J, Rudy Y. Early afterdepolarizations in cardiac myocytes: mechanism and rate dependence. Biophys J 1995; 68:949–964.

15. Szabo B, Kovacs T, Lazzara R. Role of calcium loading in early afterdepolarizations generated by $Cs^+$ in canine and guinea pig Purkinje fibers. J Cardiovasc Electrophysiol 1995; 6:796–812.

16. Bonatti V, Finardi A, Botti G. Enregistrement des potentiels d'action monophasiques du ventricule droit dans un cas de QT long et alternance isolee de l'onde U. Arch Mal Coeur 1979; 72:1180–1186.

17. Bonatti V, Rolli A, Botti G. Recording of monophasic action potentials of the right ventricle in long QT syndromes complicated by severe ventricular arrhythmias. Eur Heart J 1983; 4:168–179.

18. Shimizu W, Ohe T, Kurita T, Takaki H, Aihara N, et al. Early afterdepolarizations induced by isoproterenol in patients with congenital long QT syndrome. Circulation 1991; 84:1915–1923.

19. Jackman WM, Szabo B, Friday KJ, Margolis PD, Moulton K, et al. Ventricular tachyarrhythmias related to early afterdepolarizations and triggered firing: relationship to QT interval prolongation and potential therapeutic role for calcium channel blocking agents. J Cardiovasc Electrophysiol 1990; 1:170–195.

20. Zhou JT, Zheng LR, Liu WY, Zhang GL, Zhao J, et al. Early afterdepolarizations in the familial long QTU syndrome. J Cardiovasc Electrophysiol 1992; 3:431–436.

21. Miwa S, Inoue T, Yokoyama M. Monophasic action potentials in patients with torsade de pointes. Jpn Circ J 1994; 58:248–258.

22. Shimomura K. Effects of verapamil and propranolol on early afterdepolarizations and ventricular arrhythmias induced by epinephrine in congenital long QT syndrome. J Am Coll Cardiol 1995; 26:1299–1309.
23. El-Sherif N, Zeiler RH, Craelius W, Gough WB, Henkin R. QTU prolongation and polymorphic ventricular tachyarrhythmias due to bradycardia-dependent early afterdepolarizations: afterdepolarizations and ventricular arrhythmias. Circ Res 1988; 63:286–305.
24. El-Sherif N, Bekheit SS, Henkin R. Quinidine-induced long QTU interval and torsade de pointes: role of bradycardia-dependent early afterdepolarizations. J Am Coll Cardiol 1989; 14:252–257.
25. Habbab MA, El-Sherif N. Drug-induced torsades de pointes: role of early afterdepolarizations and dispersion of repolarization. Am J Med 1990; 89:241–246.
26. Kurita T, Ohe T, Shimizu W, Suyama K. Aihara N, et al. Early afterdepolarizationlike activity in patients with class IA induced long QT syndrome and torsades de pointes. Pacing Clin Electrophysiol 1997; 20:695–705.
27. Ohe T, Kurita T, Aihara N, Kamakura S, Matsuhisa M, et al. Electrocardiographic and electrophysiologic studies in patients with torsade de pointe: role of monophasic action potentials. Jpn Circ J 1990; 54:1323–1330.
28. Shimizu W, Tanaka K, Suenaga K, Wakamoto A. Bradycardia-dependent dearly afterdepolarizations in a patient with QTU prolongation and torsade de pointes in association with marked bradycardia and hypokalemia. Pacing Clin Electrophysiol 1991; 14:1105–1111.
29. Kurita T, Ohe T, Shimizu W, Hotta D, Shimomura K. Early afterdepolarization in a patient with complete atrioventricular block and torsade de pointes. Pacing Clin Electrophysiol 1993; 126:33–38.
30. Shimizu W, Ohe T, Kurita T, Tokuda T, Shimomura K. Epinephrine-induced ventricular premature complexes due to early afterdepolarizations and effects of verapamil and propranolol in a patient with congenital long QT syndrome. J Cardiovasc Electrpohysiol 1994; 5:438–444.
31. Sato T, Hata Y, Yamamoto M, Morita H, Mizuo K, et al. Early afterdepolarization abolished by potassium channel opener in a patient with idiopathic long QT syndrome. J Cardiovasc Electrophysiol 1995; 6:279–282.
32. Shimizu W, Kurita T, Matsuo K. Suyama K, Aihara N, et al. Improvement of repolarization abnormalities by a $K^+$ channel opener in the LQT1 form of congenital long-QT syndrome. Circulation 1998; 97:1581–1588.
33. Patterson E, Szabo B, Scherlag BJ, Lazzara R. Early and delayed afterdepolarizations associated with cesium chloride-induced arrhythmias in the dog. J Cardiovasc Pharmacol 1990; 15:323–331.
34. Boutjdir M, El-Sherif N. Pharmacological evaluation of early afterdepolarizations induced by sea anemone toxi (ATX-II) in dog heart. Cardiovasc Res 1991; 25:815–819.
35. Shimizu W, Antzelevitch C. Cellular basis for the ECG features of the LQT1 form of the long-QT syndrome: effects of β-adrenergic agonists and antagonists and sodium channel blockers on transmural dispersion of repolarization and torsade de pointes. Circulation 1998; 98:2314–2322.
36. Boutjdir M, Restivo M, Wei Y, Stergiopoulos K, El-Sherif N. Early afterdepolarization formation in cardiac myocytes: analysis of phase plane patterns, action potential, and membrane currents. J Cardiovasc Electrophysiol 1994; 5:609–620.
37. Sicouri S, Antzelevitch C. Afterdepolarizations and triggered activity develop in a select population of cells (M cells) in canine ventricular myocardium: the

effects of acetylstrophanthidin and Bay K 8644. Pacing Clin Electrophysiol 1991; 14:1714–1720.

38. El-Sherif N, Caref EB, Yin H, Restivo M. The electrophysiological mechanism of ventricular arrhythmias in the long QT syndrome: tridimensional mapping of activation and recovery patterns. Circ Res 1996; 79:474–492.

39. Asano Y, Davidenko JM, Baxter WT, et al. Optical mapping of drug-induced polymorphic arrhythmias and torsade de pointes in the isolated rabbit heart. J Am Coll Cardiol 1997; 29:831–842.

40. Priori SG, Barhanin J, Hauer RN, Haverkamp W, Jongsma HJ, et al. Tenetic and molecular basis of cardiac arrhythmias: impact on clinical management parts I and II. Circulation 1999; 99:518–528.

41. Hohnloser SH, Singh BN. Proarrhythmia with class III antiarrhythmic drugs: definition, electrophysiologic mechanisms, incidence, predisposing factors, and clinical implications. J Cardiovasc Electrophysiol 1995; 6:920–936.

42. Priori SG. Exploring the hidden danger of noncardiac drugs. J Cardiol Electrophysiol 1998; 9:1114–1116.

43. Vermeulen JT. Mechanisms of arrhythmias in heart failure. J Cardiol Electrophysiol 1998; 9:208–221.

44. Ben-David J, Zipes DP, Ayers GM, et al. Canine left ventricular hypertrophy predisposes to ventricular tachycardia induction by phase 2 early afterdepolarizations after administration of Bay K 8644. J Am Coll Cardiol 1992; 20:1576–1584.

45. Vos MA, de Groot SHM, Verduyn SC, van der Zande J, Leunissen HDM, et al. Enhanced susceptibility for acquired torsade de pointes arrhythmias in the dog with chronic, complete AV block is related to cardiac hypertrophy and electrical remodeling. Circulation 1998; 98:1125–1135.

46. Priori SG, Mantica M, Napolitano C, et al. Early afterdepolarizations induced in vivo by reperfusion of ischemic myocardium: a possible mechanism for reperfusion arrhythmias. Circulation 1990; 81:1911–1920.

47. Vera Z, Pride HP, Zipes DP. Reperfusion arrhythmias: role of early afterdepolarizations studied by monophasic action potential recordings in the intact canine heart during autonomically denervated and stimulated states. J Cardiovasc Electrophysiol 1995; 6:532–543.

48. Beuckelmann DJ, Nabauer M, Erdmann E. Alterations of $K^+$ currents in isolated human ventricular myocytes from patients with terminal heart failure. Circ Res 1993; 73:379–385.

49. Kaab S, Nuss HB, Chiamvimonvat N, O'Rourke B, Pak PH, et al. Ionic mechanism of action potential prolongation in ventricular myocytes from dogs with pacing-induced heart failure. Circ Res 1996; 78:262–273.

50. Pogwizd SM. Nonreentrant mechanisms underlying spontaneous ventricular arrhythmias in a model of nonischemic heart failure in rabbits. Circulation 1995; 92:1034–1048.

51. Pogwizd SM, McKenzie JP, Cain ME. Mechanisms underlying spontaneous and induced ventricular arrhythmias in patients with idiopathic dilated cardiomyopathy. Circulation 1998; 98:2404–2414.

# 8

# Regional Differences in Electrophysiology of Ventricular Cells:

# Clinical Implications for Sudden Cardiac Death

*Charles Antzelevitch, PhD*

## Introduction

Recent studies have served to define the electrical heterogeneity that exists within the ventricular myocardium, pointing to the presence of at least 3 electrophysiologically distinct cell types: epicardial, endocardial, and M cells. Epicardial and M cells, but not endocardium, display action potentials with a notched or spike and dome morphology, the result of a prominent transient outward current ($I_{to}$)-mediated phase 1. M cells differ from endocardial and epicardial cells by the ability of their action potential to prolong disproportionately in response to a slowing of rate and/or to agents with Class III actions. This intrinsic electrical heterogeneity contributes to the inscription of the ECG as well as to the development of a variety of cardiac arrhythmias. The transmural dispersion of early and late repolarization is in large part responsible for the inscription of the J wave and T wave of the electrocardiogram. Full repolarization of epicardium is coincident with the peak of the T wave, and full repolarization of the M cells coincides with the end of the T wave. The interval between the peak and the end of the T wave may provide a valuable index of transmural dispersion of repolarization in the precordial leads. Regional differences in the response of the 3 cell types to pharmacological agents and/or patho-

Supported by grants from the National Institutes of Health (HL 47678), the American Heart Association, New York State Affiliate, and the Masons of New York State and Florida.

From: Aliot E, Clementy J, Prystowsky EN (editors). *Fighting Sudden Cardiac Death: A Worldwide Challenge.* ©Futura Publishing Company, Armonk, NY, 2000.

physiological states often results in amplification of intrinsic electrical heterogeneities, thus providing a substrate as well as a trigger for the development of reentrant arrhythmias, including torsades de pointes, commonly associated with the long QT syndrome (LQTS), and the polymorphic ventricular tachycardia/ventricular fibrillation (VT/VF) encountered in the Brugada syndrome. In the case of LQTS, a preferential prolongation of the M cell action potential contributes to the development of long QT intervals, wide-based or notched T waves, and a large transmural dispersion of repolarization, which provides the substrate for the development of a reentrant polymorphic VT with the characteristics of torsades de pointes. An early afterdepolarization-induced triggered beat is thought to provide the extrasystole that precipitates torsades de pointes. In the Brugada syndrome, early repolarization of the epicardial action potential is thought to undergo an abnormal abbreviation due to an all or none repolarization at the end of phase 1. Loss of the action potential dome in epicardium but not endocardium creates a dispersion of repolarization across the ventricular wall, resulting in a transmural voltage gradient, which manifests in the ECG as an ST segment elevation (or idiopathic J wave) and the development of a vulnerable window during which reentry can be induced. Under these conditions, loss of the action potential dome at some epicardial sites but not others gives rise to phase 2 reentry, which provides an extrasystole capable of precipitating VT/VF (or rapid torsades de pointes). Experimental models displaying these phenomena show ECG characteristics similar to those of the Brugada syndrome as well as those encountered during acute ischemia. In both LQTS and the Brugada syndrome, a mutation in an ion channel gene is responsible for the amplification of intrinsic electrical heterogeneities that give rise to a transmural dispersion of repolarization, thus creating an arrhythmogenic substrate capable of causing life-threatening cardiac arrhythmias.

## Regional Differences in the Electrical Activity of the Heart

A rapidly expanding base of knowledge has served to highlight regional differences in the electrical properties of cells that comprise the ventricular myocardium.[1] Electrical and pharmacological distinctions between endocardium and epicardium have been described in canine, feline, rabbit, rat and human hearts.[1-3] Distinctive electrophysiological and pharmacological characteristics have also been described for M cells residing in the deep structures of the canine, guinea pig, rabbit and human ventricles.[4-27]

The 3 ventricular myocardial cell types differ with respect to repolarization characteristics (Figures 1 and 2). Epicardium and M cells display a prominent transient outward current ($I_{to}$)-mediated phase 1, responsible

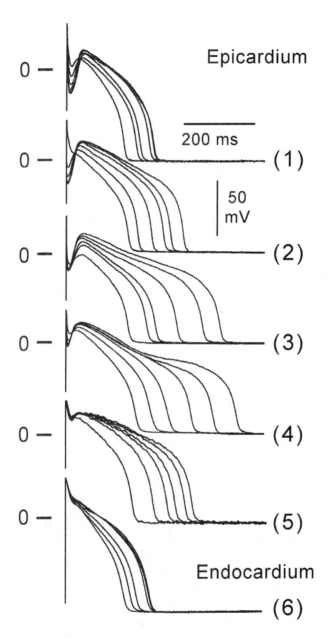

Figure 1. Transmembrane action potentials recorded from myocytes disaggregated from epicardial, midmyocardial, and endocardial regions of the canine left ventricle. Basic cycle lengths are varied over a range of 300 ms to 8,000 ms. Epicardial (cell 1) and endocardial (cell 6) were isolated from their respective tissues. M cells (longer action potentials) and transitional cells (cells 2–5) were isolated from the midmyocardial region. (From Liu DW, et al.[5] with permission.)

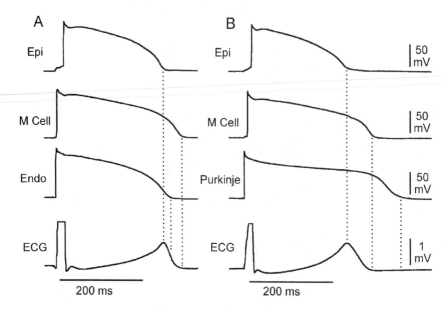

Figure 2. Action potentials from epicardium (Epi), M cell and subendocardial Purkinje were simultaneously recorded together with a transmural ECG. Repolarization of epicardium is coincident with the peak of the T wave of the ECG, whereas repolarization of the M cells is coincident with the end of the T wave. Although repolarization of the Purkinje fiber action potential occurs after that of the M cell, it does not register on the ECG. This is where we would expect to see a U wave if the density of the Purkinje system was greater. BCL = 2,000 ms. (Modified from Yan GX, et al.[25] with permission.)

for the action potential notch. The absence of a prominent notch in the endocardium is due to a much smaller $I_{to}$ in this tissue. Regional differences in $I_{to}$, first suggested on the basis of action potential data,[28] have now been demonstrated using whole cell patch clamp techniques to measure the ionic current in canine,[5] feline,[29] rabbit,[30] rat,[31] and human[32,33] ventricular myocytes. $I_{to}$ is not only larger in epicardium vs. endocardium, it is also much larger in right vs. left ventricular epicardium. Right ventricular epicardium therefore displays a much more prominent action potential notch.[34] The transmural gradient in the amplitude of the $I_{to}$-mediated action potential notch has been shown to underlie the inscription of the electrocardiographic J wave, also known as the Osborne wave.[35,36] Accentuation of this gradient is linked to the appearance of pathophysiological J waves, ST segment elevation, and the development of VT/VF in the Brugada syndrome as well as in experimental models of acute ischemia.[37–40]

The M cell is characterized by the ability of its action potential to prolong more than that of epicardium or endocardium in response to a slowing of rate and/or in response to action potential duration (APD)-prolonging agents (Figure 1).[6,15,41] Histologically, M cells are similar to epicardial and endocardial cells, although electrophysiologically and pharmacologically they appear to be a hybrid between Purkinje and ventricular cells (Table 1). The ionic basis for these features of the M cell include the presence of a smaller slowly activating delayed rectifier current $(I_{Ks})$[11] than in epicardium and endocardium, but a larger late sodium current (late $I_{Na}$).[42] Although the rapidly activating delayed rectifier $(I_{Kr})$ and inward rectifier $(I_{K1})$ currents are similar in the 3 cell types in the canine heart, transmural and apico-basal differences in the density of $I_{Kr}$ channels have been described in the 11-week-old ferret heart.[43] $I_{Kr}$ message and protein was found to be larger in the epicardium.

### Table 1

### Electrophysiological Distinctions among Epicardial, Endocardial, M Cells, and Purkinje Fibers Isolated from the Canine Heart

| | Purkinje | M | Epicardial | Endocardial |
|---|---|---|---|---|
| Long APD, steep APD-rate | Yes | Yes | No | No |
| Develop EADs in response to agents with class III actions | Yes | Yes | No | No |
| Develop DADs in response to digitalis, high $Ca^{2+}$, catecholamines | Yes | Yes | No | No |
| Display marked increase in APD in response to $I_{Kr}$ blockers | Yes | Yes | No | No |
| Display marked increase in APD in response to $I_{Ks}$ blockers | No | Yes | Yes | Yes |
| α1 Agonist-induced change in APD | ↑ | ↓ | ↔ | ↔ |
| $V_{max}$ | High | Intermediate | Low in surface tissues | |
| Phase 4 depolarization | Yes | No | No | No |
| Depolarize in $[K^+]_o < 2.5$ mM | Yes | No | No | No |
| Acceleration-induced EADs and APD prolongation in presence of $I_{Kr}$ block | No | Yes | No | No |
| Isoproterenol induces EADs and APD prolongation in presence of $I_{Kr}$ block | No | Yes | No | No |
| EADs sensitive to $[Ca^{2+}]_i$ | No | Yes | — | — |
| Develop DADs with Bay K 8644 | No | Yes | No | No |
| Found in bundles | Yes | No | No | No |

Modified from Antzelevitch C, et al.[1] with permission.
APD = action potential duration; EAD = early afterdepolarization; DAD = delayed afterdepolarization.

$I_{Kr}$ blockers, including d-sotalol, E-4031, almokalant, and erythromycin, produce a much greater prolongation of APD in M cells than in epicardium or endocardium (Table 1). In contrast, surface epicardial and endocardial tissues, when isolated from the canine left ventricle, show very little response. The preferential response of the M cell is due to its intrinsically smaller net repolarizing current. A similar preferential prolongation of the M cell APD is seen with agents that increase calcium current, $I_{Ca}$, such as Bay K 8644, as well as with agents that increase late $I_{Na}$ such as ATX-II and anthopleurin-A. An exception to this general rule applies to agents that block $I_{Ks}$, including azimilide, quinidine, pentobarbital, amiodarone and chromanol 293B. Chromanol 293B is the more specific of the $I_{Ks}$ blockers. In isolated tissues, chromanol 293B produces a similar prolongation of APD in the 3 transmural cell types. The situation is a bit more complicated for drugs affecting 2 or more ion channels, such as quinidine, pentobarbital, amiodarone, and azimilide. In the case of quinidine, relatively low therapeutic levels of the drug (3–5 μM), produce a marked prolongation of the M cell APD but not that of epicardium and endocardium, consistent with a predominant effect of the drug to block $I_{Kr}$ at this concentration.[44-47] At higher concentrations (10–30 μM) (Table 2), quinidine produces a further prolongation of the epicardial and endocardial action potential, consistent with an effect of the drug to block $I_{Ks}$, but abbreviates the APD of the M cell, due to its action to block late $I_{Na}$.[1]

M cells displaying the longest action potentials (at BCLs ≥2,000 ms) are usually localized in the deep subendocardium to midmyocardium in the anterior wall of the canine ventricle, although transitional cells are found throughout the wall.[24] M cells with the longest APD are generally found in the deep subepicardium to midmyocardium in the lateral wall [6] and throughout the wall in the region of the right ventricular outflow tracts.[1] M cells are also present in the deep layers of endocardial structures, including papillary muscles, trabeculae, and the interventricular septum.[9] Unlike Purkinje fibers, they are not found in discrete bundles. To the best of our knowledge, the first description of cells with an unusually long APD and rapid $V_{max}$ was made in a papillary muscle preparation. [48]

In the canine left ventricle, M cells with the longest action potentials reside in the deep subendocardium and transitions in $APD_{90}$ across the ventricular wall are fairly gradual due to geed electrotonic coupling of the cells throughout the wall except in the region between epicardium and deep subepicardium.[24] The sharp rise in $APD_{90}$ is due to a abrupt increase in tissue resistivity in this region. The increased tissue resistivity reduces electrotonic interaction, which allows cells in this region to exhibit more of their intrinsic properties. Thus, the degree of electrical heterogeneity across the intact ventricular wall depends on: (1) intrinsic action potential characteristics of neighboring cells; and (2) the extent to which they are

## Table 2

### Early Afterdepolarization (EAD)-Induced Triggered Activity and/or Prominent Action Potential Prolongation Recorded in Isolated Epicardial, M, and Endocardial Tissue Slices

|  | Epicardium | Endocardium | M cells |
|---|---|---|---|
| Quinidine (3–5 μM) | − | − | +++ |
| 4-Aminopyridine (2.5–5 mM) | − | − | +++ |
| Amiloride (1–10 μM) | − | − | ++ |
| Clofilium (1 μM) | − | − | +++ |
| Bay K 8644 (1 μM) | − | − | ++ |
| Cesium (5–10 mM) | − | − | ++ |
| Sotalol (100 μM) | − | − | +++ |
| Erythromycin (10–100 μg/ml) | − | − | +++ |
| E-4031 (1–5 μM) | − | − | +++ |
| ATX-II (10–20 nM) | +++ | ++ | ++++ |
| Quinidine (> 10 μM) | + | ++ | ++ |
| Azimilide (5–10 μM) | + | ++ | +++ |
| Chromanol 293B (10–100 μM) | +++ | +++ | +++ |

+/− Little to no response; ++++ Largest response
Modified from Antzelevitch C, et al.[1] with permission.

electrically coupled in the syncytium. These relationships are elegantly demonstrated in a moeling study by Viswanathan et al.[49] The shift in the position of the M cells from the deep subepicardium to the deep subendocardium appears to follow the transmural shift in the muscular layers that envelop the heart, as described by Streeter,[50,51] and more recently by Lunkenheimer and co-workers.[52]

Cells with the characteristics of M cells have been described in the canine, guinea pig, rabbit, and human ventricles.[4-26] Methodological considerations[1] have contributed to the inability of some studies to observe M cells in the ventricles of the pig, guinea pig, and rat.[16,53,54] Recent studies, while clearly demonstrating the presence of M cells in the ventricles of the canine heart in vitro, failed to delineate the unique cell type in vivo.[15,55] The combination of pentobarbital anesthesia, bipolar recording techniques, and use of high doses of quinidine, all of which suppress transmural dispersion of repolarization or prevent its accurate quantitation, may underlie the disparity.[1]

Amplification of transmural heterogeneities normally present in the early and late phases of the action potential can lead to the development of a variety of arrhythmias, including the Brugada and long QT syndromes.

# The Brugada Syndrome

The Brugada syndrome was first described as a clinical entity by Brugada and Brugada in 1992.[56] The syndrome is characterized by an ST segment elevation in the right precordial leads, $V_1$ to $V_3$, (unrelated to ischemia, electrolyte abnormalities, or structural heart disease) and a high risk of sudden cardiac death.[38,40,56–66]

The Brugada syndrome is most prevalent in males of Asian origin. The age for the first arrhythmic event ranges between 2 and 77 years, with a mean age of approximately 40.[58,65,66] A familial occurrence has long been recognized and an autosomal dominant mode of inheritance with variable expression has been described.[67] Although Brugada syndrome patients generally have structurally normal hearts, in some cases small amounts of lipid infiltration into the deep subepicardium can be detected. It is noteworthy that the Brugada syndrome is unrelated to any chromosomal loci thus far described for arrhythmogenic right ventricular dysplasia (ARVD).[68] The only gene mutations thus far linked to the Brugada syndrome are in the cardiac sodium channel gene, SCN5A.[69]

Chen et al. described several mutations in SCN5A at sites other than those known to contribute to the LQT3 form of the long QT syndrome (LQTS). Frameshift and deletion mutations lead to failure of the channel to express, thus importantly reducing $I_{Na}$ density.[69,70] Missense mutations cause a shift in the voltage- and time-dependence of activation, inactivation and reactivation. In the case of at least one missense mutation (T1620M), acceleration of the kinetics of inactivation of $I_{Na}$ provides the substrate for the syndrome, as discussed below.[71]

The Brugada syndrome is thought to be precipitated by an outward shift of the current active at the end of phase 1 of the right ventricular epicardial action potential (where $I_{to}$ is most prominent).[39,40]. Such a shift can cause all-or-none repolarization at the end of phase 1 and thus loss of the epicardial action potential dome, leading to marked abbreviation of the action potential. Pathophysiological conditions (e.g., ischemia, metabolic inhibition, hypothermia) and some pharmacological interventions cause loss of the dome and abbreviation of the action potential in canine and feline ventricular cells in which $I_{to}$ is prominent. Under ischemic conditions and in response to agents that block $I_{Na}$ or $I_{Ca}$ or activate $I_{K-ATP}$, canine ventricular epicardium exhibits an all-or-none repolarization as a result of the rebalancing of currents flowing at the end of phase 1 of the action potential. Failure of the dome to develop occurs when outward currents (principally $I_{to}$) overwhelm the inward currents (chiefly $I_{Ca}$), resulting in a marked abbreviation of the action potential. This occurs when $I_{to}$ remains strong, and inward current is reduced or outward current is augmented. In the case of the T1620M mutation of SCN5A, which has been linked to the Brugada syndrome, the contribution of $I_{Na}$ to the early part of the action potential is severely reduced due to an acceleration of the kinetics of inactivation of the current.[71]

Loss of the action potential dome in epicardium but not endocardium creates a voltage gradient during phases 2 and 3 of the action potential that manifests as an ST segment elevation. Studies involving the arterially perfused right ventricular wedge preparation provide direct evidence in support of the hypothesis that loss or depression of the action potential dome in epicardium but not endocardium underlies the development of a prominent ST segment elevation in the Brugada syndrome and other syndromes associated with an ST segment elevation.[37,39]

Heterogeneous loss of the epicardial action potential dome also leads to the development of a marked dispersion of repolarization within the ventricular epicardium. Propagation of the action potential dome from sites at which it is maintained to sites at which it is lost causes local reexcitation by a mechanism termed phase 2 reentry, leading to the development of a very closely coupled extrasystole, capable of initiating circus movement reentry.[72] Phase 2 reentry has been observed in canine epicardium exposed to: (1) $K^+$ channel openers such as pinacidil; [73] (2) sodium channel blockers such as flecainide; [74] (3) increased $[Ca^{2+}]$; [75] (4) metabolic inhibition; [76] and (5) simulated ischemia.[72] $I_{to}$ block with 4-aminopyridine restores electrical homogeneity and abolishes reentrant activity in all cases.

Phase 2 reentry induces circus movement reentry in isolated sheets of right ventricular epicardium.[72] More recent studies have demonstrated these phenomena in the intact wall of the canine right ventricle (Figure 3).[3,77] The arrhythmia often takes the form of a polymorphic VT, resembling a rapid torsades de pointes, which in some cases cannot be readily distinguished from VF. Investigators in the field have long appreciated the fact that circus movement reentry is more often than not precipitated by an extrasystole. The mechanism proposed not only provides the substrate for the development of circus movement reentry in the form of epicardial and transmural dispersion of repolarization, but also the phase 2 reentrant extrasystole that triggers the VT/VF episode.

A prominent $I_{to}$ is a prerequisite for phase 2 reentry. Agents that inhibit $I_{to}$, including 4-aminopyridine and quinidine, are effective in restoring the action potential dome, and thus electrical homogeneity, and in aborting all arrhythmic activity in experimental models of this syndrome.[3,78] Class IA and IC antiarrhythmic agents that block $I_{Na}$, but little to no $I_{to}$ (flecainide, ajmaline, and procainamide), exacerbate or unmask the Brugada syndrome, whereas those with actions to block both $I_{Na}$ and $I_{to}$ (quinidine and disopyramide) can exert an ameliorative effect.[39] The anticholinergic effects of quinidine and disopyramide may also contribute to

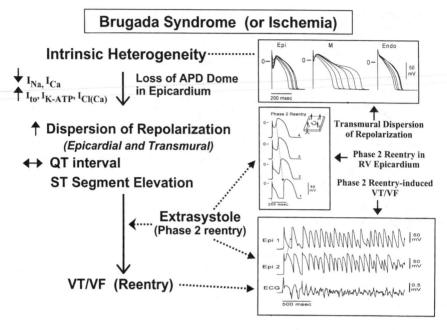

Figure 3. Proposed cellular and ionic mechanisms for the Brugada syndrome. (The middle inset is modified from Lukas A, et al.[72] with permission.)

their effectiveness. In the clinic, amiodarone and β blockers have been shown to be without effect.[58] The only therapeutic measure with proven effectiveness is the implantable cardioverter defibrillator. These findings highlight the need for a cardioselective $I_{to}$ blocker, which may prove to be effective in the Brugada syndrome as well as other syndromes associated with an ST segment elevation.

## The Long QT Syndrome

Amplification of intrinsic heterogeneities of ventricular repolarization also contribute to the development of the LQTS. The congenital and acquired (drug-induced) long QT syndromes are characterized by the development of long QT intervals in the ECG, abnormal T waves, and an atypical polymorphic tachycardia known as torsades de pointes.[79–83] Genetic linkage studies have identified several forms of the congenital long QT syndrome caused by mutations in ion channel genes located on chromosomes 3, 7, 11, and 21. Mutations in KvLQT1 and minK (KCNE1) are responsible for defects in the slowly activating delayed rectifier potassium current ($I_{Ks}$) which underlies the LQT1 and LQT5 forms of LQTS, whereas mutations in HERG and *SCN5A* are responsible for defects in the rapidly activating component of the delayed rectifier potassium current ($I_{Kr}$) and sodium current ($I_{Na}$) that underlie the LQT2 and LQT3 syndromes. Mutations in a minK-related protein, MiRP1, which associates with HERG to form the $I_{Kr}$ channel, are responsible for the LQT6 form of LQTS.[84]

The electrophysiological, electrocardiographic, and pharmacological characteristics of the LQT1, LQT2, and LQT3 syndromes have been studied in the arterially perfused canine left ventricular wedge preparation. Simultaneous recordings of transmembrane activity from epicardial, M, and endocardial or Purkinje sites, together with a transmural ECG recorded along the same axis, permit correlation of transmembrane and electrocardiographic activity.[17,22–25,85] The wedge preparation is capable of developing and sustaining a variety of arrhythmias, including torsades de pointes. Pharmacological models that mimic the clinical congenital syndromes with respect to prolongation of the QT interval, T wave morphology, rate dependence of repolarization and response to antiarrhythmic drugs have been developed (Figure 4).[17,22–25]

Preferential prolongation of APD of cells in the M region underlie LQTS, contributing to the development of long QT intervals, abnormal T waves, and the development of torsades de pointes (Figures 4 and 5). Support for this hypothesis derives from a number of studies involving the arterially perfused wedge preparation.[17,22,24,25,85,86]

$I_{Ks}$ block with chromanol 293B was used to mimic LQT1 and the β adrenergic agonist, isoproterenol, was used to assess β adrenergic influence. $I_{Ks}$ block alone produced a homogeneous prolongation of repolarization and refractoriness across the ventricular wall and never induced arrhythmias. The addition of isoproterenol caused abbreviation of epicardial and endocardial APD but a prolongation or no change in the APD of the M cell, resulting in a marked augmentation of transmural dispersion of repolarization and the development of spontaneous and stimulation-induced torsades de pointes.[22] These changes give rise to a broad-based T wave and the long QT interval characteristics of LQT1. The development of torsades de pointes in the model requires β adrenergic stimulation, consistent with a high sensitivity of congenital LQTS, LQT1 in particular, to sympathetic stimulation.[81,87–92]

The $I_{Kr}$ blocker, d-sotalol, was used to mimic LQT2 and the most common acquired (drug-induced) form of LQTS. A greater prolongation of the M cell action potential and slowing of phase 3 of the action potential of all 3 cell types results in a low-amplitude T wave, long QT interval, large transmural dispersion of repolarization, and the development of spontaneous as well as stimulation-induced torsades de pointes (Figures 4 and 5). The addition of hypokalemia gives rise to low-amplitude T waves with a

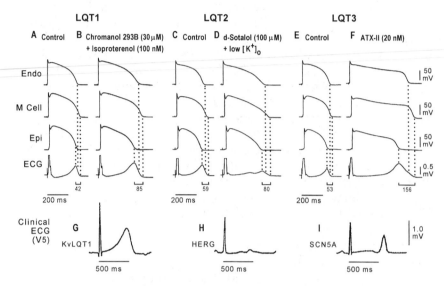

**Figure 4.** Transmembrane action potentials and transmural electrocardiograms (ECG) in the LQT1 (A and B), LQT2 (C and D), and LQT3 (E and F) models (arterially perfused canine left ventricular wedge preparations), and clinical ECG lead $V_5$ of patients with LQT1 (*KvLQT1* defect) (G), LQT2 (*HERG* defect) (H), and LQT3 (*SCN5A* defect) (I) syndromes. Isoproterenol + chromanol 293B—an $I_{Ks}$ blocker, d-sotalol + low $[K^+]_o$, and ATX-II, an agent that slows inactivation of late $I_{Na}$ are used to mimic the LQT1, LQT2, and LQT3 syndromes, respectively. Panels A-F depict action potentials simultaneously recorded from endocardial (Endo), M, and epicardial (Epi) sites together with a transmural ECG. BCL = 2,000 ms. In all cases, the peak of the T wave in the ECG is coincident with the repolarization of the epicardial action potential, whereas the end of the T wave is coincident with the repolarization of the M cell action potential. Repolarization of the endocardial cell is intermediate between that of the M cell and epicardial cell. Transmural dispersion of repolarization across the ventricular wall, defined as the difference in the repolarization time between M and epicardial cells, is denoted below the ECG traces. B: Isoproterenol (100 nM) in the presence of chromanol 293B (30 μM) produced a preferential prolongation of the APD of the M, resulting in an accentuated transmural dispersion of repolarization and broad-based T waves as commonly seen in LQT1 patients (G). D: d-Sotalol (100 μM) in the presence of low potassium (2 mM) gives rise to low-amplitude T waves with a notched or bifurcated appearance due to a very significant slowing of repolarization as commonly seen in LQT2 patients (H). F: ATX-II (20 nM) markedly prolongs the QT interval, widens the T wave, and causes a sharp rise in the dispersion of repolarization. ATX-II also produced a marked delay in onset of the T wave due to relatively large effects of the drug on the APD of epicardium and endocardium, consistent with the late-appearing T wave pattern observed in LQT3 patients (I). (Modified from Shimizu W, et al.[17,22] with permission.)

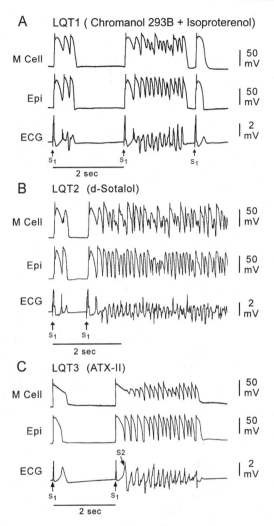

**Figure 5.** Polymorphic ventricular tachycardia displaying features of torsades de pointes in the LQT1 (A), LQT2 (B), and LQT3 (C) models (arterially perfused canine left ventricular wedge preparations). Isoproterenol + chromanol 293B, d-sotalol, and ATX-II are used to mimic the 3 LQTS syndromes, respectively. Each trace shows action potentials simultaneously recorded from M and epicardial (Epi) cells together with a transmural ECG. The preparation was paced from the endocardial surface at a BCL of 2,000 ms ($S_1$). A and B: Spontaneous torsades de pointes induced in the LQT1 and LQT2 models, respectively. In both models, the first groupings show spontaneous ventricular premature beat (or couplets) that fail to induce torsades de pointes, and a second grouping that show spontaneous premature beats that succeed. The premature response appears to originate in the deep subendocardium (M or Purkinje). C: Programmed electrical stimulation-induced torsades de pointes in the LQT3 model. ATX-II produced very significant dispersion of repolarization (first grouping). A single extrastimulus ($S_2$) applied to the epicardial surface at an $S_1$–$S_2$ interval of 320 ms initiates torsades de pointes (second grouping). (Modified from Shimizu W, et al.[17,22] with permission.)

deeply notched or bifurcated appearance, similar to those commonly seen in patients with the LQT2 syndrome.[17,25] Isoproterenol further exaggerates transmural dispersion of repolarization, thus increasing the incidence of torsades de pointes.[93]

LQT3 was mimicked using ATX-II, an agent that increases late $I_{Na}$, which helps to sustain the action potential plateau.[17] ATX-II markedly prolongs the QT interval, delays the onset of the T wave, in some cases also widening it, and produces a sharp rise in transmural dispersion of repolarization as a result of a greater prolongation of the APD of the M cell. The differential effect of ATX-II to prolong the M cell action potential is likely due to the presence of a larger late sodium current in the M cell.[42] ATX-II produces a marked delay in onset of the T wave because of a relatively large effect of the drug on epicardial and endocardial APD. This feature is consistent with the late-appearing T wave (long isoelectric ST segment) observed in patients with the LQT3 syndrome. Also in agreement with the clinical presentation of LQT3, the model displays a steep rate dependence of the QT interval and develops torsades de pointes at slow rates. Surprisingly, in the ATX-II model of LQT3, β adrenergic influence in the form of isoproterenol reduces transmural dispersion of repolarization by abbreviating the APD of the M cell more than that of epicardium or endocardium, and thus reduces the incidence of torsades de pointes. While the β adrenergic blocker propranolol is protective in LQT1 and LQT2 wedge models, it has the opposite effects in LQT3, acting to amplify transmural dispersion and promoting torsades de pointes.[93]

Torsades de pointes is a life-threatening atypical polymorphic ventricular tachycardia commonly associated with LQTS. Torsades de pointes has been reported in patients receiving potassium channel blockers like d-sotalol and quinidine, usually at slow heart rates or after long pauses. These conditions are similar to those under which these agents induce early afterdepolarizations (EADs) and triggered activity in isolated Purkinje fibers and M cells, suggesting a role for EAD-induced triggered activity in the genesis of torsades de pointes. While EADs may underlie the premature beat that initiates torsades de pointes, recent studies provide evidence in support of circus movement reentry as the mechanism responsible for the maintenance of the arrhythmia.[1,4,17,18,22,25,82,85,94,95] In the wedge, torsades de pointes develops spontaneously in all 3 models and can be readily induced by introduction of a single premature beat to the epicardial surface (the site of earliest repolarization).

The available data provide support for the hypothesis outlined in Figure 6. The hypothesis presumes the presence of electrical heterogeneity, principally in the form of transmural dispersion of repolarization, under baseline conditions. The intrinsic heterogeneity is amplified by agents that decrease net repolarizing current by reducing $I_{Kr}$ or $I_{Ks}$ or augmenting late

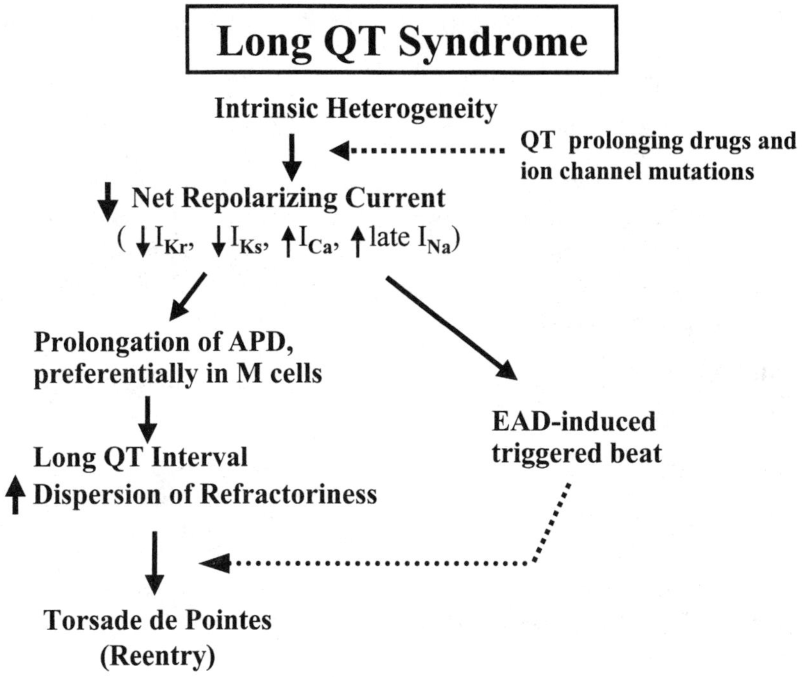

## Long QT Syndrome

**Intrinsic Heterogeneity**

↓ ◀·············· QT prolonging drugs and ion channel mutations

↓ **Net Repolarizing Current**

( ↓$I_{Kr}$, ↓$I_{Ks}$, ↑$I_{Ca}$, ↑late $I_{Na}$)

**Prolongation of APD, preferentially in M cells**

↓

**Long QT Interval**

↑ **Dispersion of Refractoriness**

**EAD-induced triggered beat**

↓ ◀··············

**Torsade de Pointes (Reentry)**

Figure 6. Proposed cellular and ionic mechanisms for the long QT syndrome.

$I_{Ca}$ or late $I_{Na}$ or by ion channel mutations that affect these currents and are responsible for the various forms of LQTS. $I_{Kr}$ blockers and LQT2 mutations or late $I_{Na}$ promoters and LQT3 mutations produce a preferential prolongation of the M cell action potential. As a consequence, the QT interval prolongs and is accompanied by a dramatic increase in transmural dispersion of repolarization, which creates a vulnerable window for the development of reentry. The decrease in net repolarizing current can also give rise to EAD-induced triggered activity in M and Purkinje cells, which are responsible for the extrasystole that triggers torsades de pointes. β adrenergic agonists serve to further amplify transmural heterogeneity (transiently) in the case of $I_{Kr}$ and LQT2, but to reduce it in the case of late $I_{Na}$ enhancers or LQT3.[93] $I_{Ks}$ blockers or LQT1 mutations cause a homogeneous prolongation of APD throughout the ventricular wall, leading to a prolongation of the QT interval but with no increase in transmural dispersion of repolarization. Under these conditions, torsades de pointes does not occur spontaneously nor can it be induced by programmed stimulation until a β adrenergic agonist is introduced. Isoproterenol dramatically increases transmural dispersion under these conditions by abbreviating

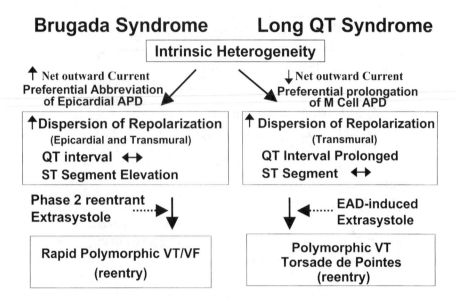

Figure 7. Similarities and differences in the mechanisms responsible for the development of arrhythmias in the Brugada and long QT syndromes.

the APD of epicardium and endocardium, thus creating a vulnerable window that an EAD-induced triggered response can capture to generate torsades de pointes, a circus movement arrhythmia.

## Conclusion

Regional differences in electrical activity contribute to the inscription of the ECG, and when amplified, to the development of a variety of cardiac arrhythmias displaying very different clinical phenotypes, but sharing a final common pathway in the precipitation of VT/VF. The Brugada and long QT syndromes share the ability to amplify the intrinsic heterogeneity that exists across the ventricular wall, in some cases by modifying the same gene (*SCN5A*) (Figure 7).

### References

1. Antzelevitch C, Shimizu W, Yan GX, Sicouri S, Weissenburger J, et al. The M cell: its contribution to the ECG and to normal and abnormal electrical function of the heart. J Cardiovasc Electrophysiol 1999; 10:1124–1152.
2. Antzelevitch C, Yan GX, Shimizu W. Transmural dispersion of repolarization and arrhythmogenicity: the Brugada syndrome vs. the long QT syndrome. J Electrocardiol 1999; 32(Suppl):158–165.

3. Antzelevitch C, Yan GX, Shimizu W, Burashnikov A. Electrical heterogeneity, the ECG, and cardiac arrhythmias. In: Zipes DP, Jalife J (eds): Cardiac Electrophysiology: From Cell to Bedside, 3rd ed. W.B. Saunders Co., Philadelphia, 1999, pp 222–238.
4. Antzelevitch C, Sicouri S. Clinical relevance of cardiac arrhythmias generated by afterdepolarizations: the role of M cells in the generation of U waves, triggered activity and torsade de pointes. J Am Coll Cardiol 1994; 23:259–277.
5. Liu DW, Gintant GA, Antzelevitch C. Ionic bases for electrophysiological distinctions among epicardial, midmyocardial, and endocardial myocytes from the free wall of the canine left ventricle. Circ Res 1993; 72:671–687.
6. Sicouri S, Antzelevitch C. A subpopulation of cells with unique electrophysiological properties in the deep subepicardium of the canine ventricle: the M cell. Circ Res 1991; 68:1729–1741.
7. Sicouri S, Antzelevitch C. Drug-induced afterdepolarizations and triggered activity occur in a discrete subpopulation of ventricular muscle cell (M cells) in the canine heart: quinidine and digitalis. J Cardiovasc Electrophysiol 1993; 4:48–58.
8. Sicouri S, Fish J, Antzelevitch C. Distribution of M cells in the canine ventricle. J Cardiovasc Electrophysiol 1994; 5:824–837.
9. Sicouri S, Antzelevitch C. Electrophysiologic characteristics of M cells in the canine left ventricular free wall. J Cardiovasc Electrophysiol 1995; 6:591–603.
10. Drouin E, Charpentier F, Gauthier C, Laurent K, Le Marec H. Electrophysiological characteristics of cells spanning the left ventricular wall of human heart: evidence for the presence of M cells. J Am Coll Cardiol 1995; 26:185–192.
11. Liu DW, Antzelevitch C. Characteristics of the delayed rectifier current ($I_{Kr}$ and $I_{Ks}$) in canine ventricular epicardial, midmyocardial and endocardial myocytes: a weaker $I_{Ks}$ contributes to the longer action potential of the M cell. Circ Res 1995; 76:351–365.
12. Weissenburger J, Nesterenko VV, Antzelevitch C. Intramural monophasic action potentials (MAP) display steeper APD-rate relations and higher sensitivity to Class III agents than epicardial and endocardial MAPS: characteristics of the M cell in vivo (abstract). Circulation 1995; 92:I-300.
13. Sicouri S, Quist M, Antzelevitch C. Evidence for the presence of M cells in the guinea pig ventricle. J Cardiovasc Electrophysiol 1996; 7:503–511.
14. Li GR, Feng J, Carrier M, Nattel S. Transmural electrophysiologic heterogeneity in the human ventricle (abstract). Circulation 1995; 92:I-158.
15. Anyukhovsky EP, Sosunov EA, Rosen MR. Regional differences in electrophysiologic properties of epicardium, midmyocardium and endocardium: in vitro and in vivo correlations. Circulation 1996; 94:1981–1988.
16. Rodriguez-Sinovas A, Cinca J, Tapias A, Armadans L, Tresanchez M, et al. Lack of evidence of M-cells in porcine left ventricular myocardium. Cardiovasc Res 1997; 33:307–313.
17. Shimizu W, Antzelevitch C. Sodium channel block with mexiletine is effective in reducing dispersion of repolarization and preventing torsade de pointes in LQT2 and LQT3 models of the long-QT syndrome. Circulation 1997; 96:2038–2047.
18. El-Sherif N, Caref EB, Yin H, Restivo M. The electrophysiological mechanism of ventricular arrhythmias in the long QT syndrome: tridimensional mapping of activation and recovery patterns. Circ Res 1996; 79:474–492.
19. Weirich J, Bernhardt R, Loewen N, Wenzel W, Antoni H. Regional- and species-dependent effects of $K^+$-channel blocking agents on subendocardium and mid-wall slices of human, rabbit, and guinea pig myocardium (abstract). Pflugers Arch 1996; 431:R 130.

20. Burashnikov A, Antzelevitch C. Acceleration-induced action potential prolongation and early afterdepolarizations. J Cardiovasc Electrophysiol 1998; 9:934–948.
21. Shimizu W, McMahon B, Antzelevitch C. Sodium pentobarbital reduces transmural dispersion of repolarization and prevents torsade de pointes in models of acquired and congenital long QT syndromes. J Cardiovasc Electrophysiol 1999; 10:156–164.
22. Shimizu W, Antzelevitch C. Cellular basis for the electrocardiographic features of the LQT1 form of the long QT syndrome: effects of beta-adrenergic agonists, antagonists and sodium channel blockers on transmural dispersion of repolarization and torsade de pointes. Circulation 1998; 98:2314–2322.
23. Shimizu W, Antzelevitch C. Cellular and ionic basis for T wave alternans under long QT conditions. Circulation 1999; 99:1499–1507.
24. Yan GX, Shimizu W, Antzelevitch C. Characteristics and distribution of M cells in arterially-perfused canine left ventricular wedge preparations. Circulation 1998; 98:1921–1927.
25. Yan GX, Antzelevitch C. Cellular basis for the normal T wave and the electrocardiographic manifestations of the long QT syndrome. Circulation 1998; 98:1928–1936.
26. Balati B, Varro A, Papp JG. Comparison of the cellular electrophysiological characteristics of canine left ventricular epicardium, M cells, endocardium and Purkinje fibres [in process citation]. Acta Physiol Scand 1998; 164:181–190.
27. Sicouri S, Moro S, Elizari MV. d-Sotalol induces marked action potential prolongation and early afterdepolarizations in M but not epicardial or endocardial cells of the canine ventricle. J Cardiovasc Pharmacol Ther 1997; 2:27–38.
28. Litovsky SH, Antzelevitch C. Transient outward current prominent in canine ventricular epicardium but not endocardium. Circ Res 1988; 62:116–126.
29. Furukawa T, Myerburg RJ, Furukawa N, Bassett AL, Kimura S. Differences in transient outward currents of feline endocardial and epicardial myocytes. Circ Res 1990; 67:1287–1291.
30. Fedida D, Giles WR. Regional variations in action potentials and transient outward current in myocytes isolated from rabbit left ventricle. J Physiol (Lond) 1991; 442:191–209.
31. Clark RB, Bouchard RA, Salinas-Stefanon E, Sanchez-Chapula J, Giles WR. Heterogeneity of action potential waveforms and potassium currents in rat ventricle. Cardiovasc Res 1993; 27:1795–1799.
32. Wettwer E, Amos GJ, Posival H, Ravens U. Transient outward current in human ventricular myocytes of subepicardial and subendocardial origin. Circ Res 1994; 75:473–482.
33. Nabauer M, Beuckelmann DJ, Uberfuhr P, Steinbeck G. Regional differences in current density and rate-dependent properties of the transient outward current in subepicardial and subendocardial myocytes of human left ventricle. Circulation 1996; 93:168–177.
34. Di Diego JM, Sun ZQ, Antzelevitch C. $I_{to}$ and action potential notch are smaller in left vs. right canine ventricular epicardium. Am J Physiol 1996; 271:H548–H561.
35. Yan GX, Antzelevitch C. Cellular basis for the electrocardiographic J wave. Circulation 1996; 93:372–379.
36. Antzelevitch C, Sicouri S, Lukas A, Nesterenko VV, Liu DW, et al. Regional differences in the electrophysiology of ventricular cells. Physiological and clinical implications. In: Zipes DP, Jalife J (eds). Cardiac Electrophysiology: From Cell to Bedside. W.B. Saunders Co., Philadelphia,1995, pp 228–245.

37. Antzelevitch C. The Brugada syndrome. J Cardiovasc Electrophysiol 1998; 9:513–516.
38. Gussak I, Antzelevitch C, Bjerregaard P, Towbin JA, Chaitman BR. The Brugada syndrome: clinical, electrophysiological and genetic aspects. J Am Coll Cardiol 1999; 33:5–15.
39. Yan GX, Antzelevitch C. Cellular basis for the Brugada syndrome and other mechanisms of arrhythmogenesis associated with ST segment elevation. Circulation 1999; 82:430–437.
40. Antzelevitch C, Brugada P, Brugada J, Brugada R, Nademanee K, et al. The Brugada Syndrome. Futura Publishing Company, Inc., Armonk, NY, 1999, pp 1–99.
41. Antzelevitch C, Sicouri S, Litovsky SH, Lukas A, Krishnan SC, et al. Heterogeneity within the ventricular wall: electrophysiology and pharmacology of epicardial, endocardial and M cells. Circ Res 1991; 69:1427–1449.
42. Eddlestone GT, Zygmunt AC, Antzelevitch C. Larger late sodium current contributes to the longer action potential of the M cell in canine ventricular myocardium (abstract). PACE 1996; 19:II-569.
43. Brahmajothi MV, Morales MJ, Reimer KA, Strauss HC. Regional localization of ERG, the channel protein responsible for the rapid component of the delayed rectifier, $K^+$ current in the ferret heart. Circ Res 1997; 81:128–135.
44. Sicouri S, Moro S, Litovsky SH, Elizari MV, Antzelevitch C. Chronic amiodarone reduces transmural dispersion of repolarization in the canine heart. J Cardiovasc Electrophysiol 1997; 8:1269–1279.
45. Sun ZQ, Eddlestone GT, Antzelevitch C. Ionic mechanisms underlying the effects of sodium pentobarbital to diminish transmural dispersion of repolarization (abstract). PACE 1997; 20:11–16.
46. Conder ML, Smith MA, Atwal KS, McCullough JR. Effects of NE-10064 on $K^+$ currents in cardiac cells (abstract). Biophys J 1994; 66:A326.
47. Condor MD, Hess TA, Smith MA, D'Alonzo AJ, McCullough JR. The effects of NE-10064 on cardiac sodium channels (abstract). FASEB J 1994; 8(5) part 2:A609.
48. Solberg LE, Singer DH, Ten Eick RE, Duffin EG. Glass microelectrode studies on intramural papillary muscle cells. Circ Res 1974; 34:783–797.
49. Viswanathan PC, Shaw RM, Rudy Y. Effects of $I_{Kr}$ and $I_{Ks}$ heterogeneity on action potential duration and its rate-dependence: a simulation study. Circulation 1999; 99:2466–2474.
50. Streeter DD, Spotnitz HM, Patel DP, Ross J, Sonnenblick EH. Fiber orientation in the canine left ventricle during diastole and systole. Circ Res 1969; 24:339–347.
51. Streeter DD. Gross morphology and fiber geometry of the heart. In: Berne RM (ed). Handbook of Physiology. Section 2: The Cardiovascular System. Waverly Press, Inc., Baltimore, 1979, pp 61–112.
52. Lunkenheimer PP, Redmann K, Scheld HH, Dietl K-H, Cryer C, et al. The heart muscle's putative secondary structure: functional implications of a band-like anisotropy. Technol Health Care 1997; 5:53–64.
53. Bryant SM, Wan X, Shipsey SJ, Hart G. Regional differences in the delayed rectifier current ($I_{Kr}$ and $I_{Ks}$) contribute to the differences in action potential duration in basal left ventricular myocytes in guinea pig. Cardiovasc Res 1998; 40:322–331.
54. Shipsey SJ, Bryant SM, Hart G. Effects of hypertrophy on regional action potential characteristics in the rat left ventricle: a cellular basis for T-wave inversion? Circulation 1997; 96:2061–2068.

55. Anyukhovsky EP, Sosunov EA, Gainullin RZ, Rosen MR. The controversial M cell. J Cardiovasc Electrophysiol 1999; 10:244–260.
56. Brugada P, Brugada J. Right bundle branch block, persistent ST segment elevation and sudden cardiac death: a distinct clinical and electrocardiographic syndrome. A multicenter report. J Am Coll Cardiol 1992; 20:1391–1396.
57. Brugada J, Brugada P, Robert R. Genetics of cardiovascular disease with emphasis on atrial fibrillation. J Cardiovasc Electrophysiol 1999; 3:7–13.
58. Brugada J, Brugada R, Brugada P. Right bundle-branch block and ST-segment elevation in leads $V_1$ through $V_3$. A marker for sudden death in patients without demonstrable structural heart disease. Circulation 1998; 97:457–460.
59. Aizawa Y, Tamura M, Chinushi M, Naitoh N , Uchiyama H, et al. Idiopathic ventricular fibrillation and bradycardia-dependent intraventricular block. Am Heart J 1993; 126:1473–1474.
60. Aizawa Y, Tamura M, Chinushi M, Niwano S , Kusano Y, et al. An attempt at electrical catheter ablation of the arrhythmogenic area in idiopathic ventricular fibrillation. Am Heart J 1992; 123:257–260.
61. Bjerregaard P, Gussak I, Kotar Sl, Gessler JE. Recurrent synocope in a patient with prominent J-wave. Am Heart J 1994; 127:1426–1430.
62. Martini B, Nava A, Thiene G, Buja GF, Canciani B, et al. Ventricular fibrillation without apparent heart disease: description of six cases. Am Heart J 1989; 118:1203–1209.
63. Miyazaki T, Mitamura H, Miyoshi S, Soejima K, Aizawa Y, et al. Autonomic and antiarrhythmic drug modulation of ST segment elevation in patients with Brugada syndrome. J Am Coll Cardiol 1996; 27:1061–1070.
64. Kasanuki H, Ohnishi S, Ohtuka M, Matsuda N, Nirei T, et al. Idiopathic ventricular fibrillation induced with vagal activity in patients without obvious heart disease. Circulation 1997; 95:2277–2285.
65. Nademanee K. Sudden unexplained death syndrome in southeast Asia. Am J Cardiol 1997; 79(6A):10–11.
66. Marcus FI. Idiopathic ventricular fibrillation. J Cardiovasc Electrophysiol 1997; 8:1075–1083.
67. Corrado D, Nava A, Buja G, Martini B, Fasoli G, et al. Familial cardiomyopathy underlies syndrome of right bundle branch block, ST segment elevation and sudden death. J Am Coll Cardiol 1996; 27:443–448.
68. Ahmed F, Li D, Karibe A, Gonzalez O, Tapscott T, et al. Localization of a gene responsible for arrhythmogenic right ventricular dysplasia to chromosome 3p23. Circulation 1998; 98:2791–2795.
69. Chen Q, Kirsch GE, Zhang D, Brugada R, Brugada J, et al. Genetic basis and molecular mechanisms for idiopathic ventricular fibrillation. Nature 1997; 392:293–296.
70. Alings M, Wilde AAM. Brugada syndrome: clinical data and suggested pathophysiological mechanism. Circulation 1999; 5:666–673.
71. Dumaine R, Towbin JA, Brugada P, Vatta M , Brugada J, et al. Ionic mechanisms responsible for the electrocardiographic phenotype of the Brugada syndrome are temperature dependent. Circ Res 1999; 85:803–809.
72. Lukas A, Antzelevitch C. Phase 2 reentry as a mechanism of initiation of circus movement reentry in canine epicardium exposed to simulated ischemia: the antiarrhythmic effects of 4-aminopyridine. Cardiovasc Res 1996; 32:593–603.
73. Di Diego JM, Antzelevitch C. Pinacidil-induced electrical heterogeneity and extrasystolic activity in canine ventricular tissues. Does activation of ATP-regulated potassium current promote phase 2 reentry? Circulation 1993; 88:1177–1189.

74. Krishnan SC, Antzelevitch C. Flecainide-induced arrhythmia in canine ventricular epicardium. Phase 2 Reentry? Circulation 1993; 87:562–572.
75. Di Diego JM, Antzelevitch C. High [$Ca^{2+}$]-induced electrical heterogeneity and extrasystolic activity in isolated canine ventricular epicardium. Phase 2 reentry. Circulation 1994; 89:1839–1850.
76. Antzelevitch C, Sicouri S, Lukas A, Di Diego JM, Nesterenko VV, et al. Clinical implications of electrical heterogeneity in the heart: the electrophysiology and pharmacology of epicardial, M and endocardial cells. In Podrid PJ, Kowey PR (eds). Cardiac Arrhythmia: Mechanism, Diagnosis and Management. William & Wilkins, Baltimore, MD, 1995, pp 88–107.
77. Antzelevitch C, Shimizu W, Yan GX, Sicouri S. Cellular basis for QT dispersion. J Electrocardiol 1998; 30(Suppl):168–175.
78. Yan GX, Antzelevitch C. Cellular basis for the Brugada syndrome and other mechanisms of arrhythmogenesis associated with ST segment elevation. Circulation 1999; 100:1660–1666.
79. Schwartz PJ, Periti M, Malliani A. The long QT syndrome. Am Heart J 1975; 89:378–390.
80. Moss AJ, Schwartz PJ, Crampton RS, Locati EH, Carleen E. The long QT syndrome: a prospective international study. Circulation 1985; 71:17–21.
81. Zipes DP. The long QT interval syndrome: a Rosetta stone for sympathetic related ventricular tachyarrhythmias. Circulation 1991; 84:1414–1419.
82. Shimizu W, Ohe T, Kurita T, Kawade M, Arakaki Y, et al. Effects of verapamil and propranolol on early afterdepolarizations and ventricular arrhythmias induced by epinephrine in congenital long QT syndrome. J Am Coll Cardiol 1995; 26:1299–1309.
83. Roden DM, Lazzara R, Rosen MR, Schwartz PJ, Towbin JA, et al. The SADS Foundation Task Force on LQTS, Antzelevitch C, Brown AM, Colatsky TJ, Crampton RS, Kass RS, et al. Multiple mechanisms in the long-QT syndrome: current knowledge, gaps, and future directions. Circulation 1996; 94: 1996–2012.
84. Abbott GW, Sesti F, Splawski I, Buck ME, Lehmann MH, et al. MiRP1 forms I$_{Kr}$ potassium channels with HERG and is associated with cardiac arrhythmias. Cell 1999; 97:175–187.
85. Antzelevitch C, Sun ZQ, Zhang ZQ, Yan GX. Cellular and ionic mechanisms underlying erythromycin-induced long QT and torsade de pointes. J Am Coll Cardiol 1996; 28:1836–1848.
86. Shimizu W, Antzelevitch C. Characteristics of spontaneous as well as stimulation-induced torsade de pointes in LQT2 and LQT3 models of the long QT syndrome (abstract). Circulation 1997; 96:I-554.
87. Schwartz PJ. The idiopathic long QT syndrome: progress and questions. Am Heart J 1985; 109:399–411.
88. Moss AJ, Schwartz PJ, Crampton RS, Tzivoni D, Locati EH, et al. The long QT syndrome: prospective longitudinal study of 328 families. Circulation 1991; 84:1136–1144.
89. Crampton RS. Preeminence of the left stellate ganglion in the long Q-T syndrome. Circulation 1979; 59:769–778.
90. Timothy KW, Zhang L, Meyer KJ, Vincent GM. Differences in precipitators of cardiac arrest and sudden death in chromosome 11 versus 7 genotype long QT syndrome patients (abstract). Circulation 1996; 94: I-204.
91. Ali RH, Zareba W, Rosero SZ, Moss AJ, Schwartz PJ, et al. Adrenergic triggers and non-adrenergic factors associated with cardiac events in long QT syndrome patients (abstract). PACE 1997; 20:1072.

92. Schwartz PJ, Malteo PS, Moss AJ, Priori SG, Wang Q, et al. Gene-specific influence on the triggers for cardiac arrest in the long QT syndrome (abstract). Circulation 1997; 96:I-212.
93. Shimizu W, Antzelevitch C. Differential effects of β-adrenergic agonists and antagonists on transmural dispersion of repolarization and torsade de pointes in LQT1, LQT2 and LQT3 models of the long QT syndrome (abstract). Circulation 1998; 98:I-10.
94. El-Sherif N, Chinushi M, Caref EB, Restivo M. Electrophysiological mechanism of the characteristic electrocardiographic morphology of torsade de pointes tachyarrhythmias in the long-QT syndrome: detailed analysis of ventricular tridimensional activation patterns. Circulation 1997; 96 :4392–4399.
95. Akar FG, Yan GX, Antzelevitch C, Rosenbaum DS. Optical maps reveal reentrant mechanism of torsade de pointes based on topography and electrophysiology of mid-myocardial cells (abstract). Circulation 1997; 96(8):I-355.

# 9

# Nonfibrillatory Sudden Cardiac Death:

## Role of Bradycardia

*Jean-Jacques Blanc, MD, and*
*Jacques Mansourati, MD*

## Introduction

Sudden cardiac death (SCD) is generally considered as the direct consequence of ventricular fibrillation (VF) or ventricular tachycardia (VT). Actually, if ventricular arrhythmias remain the major cause of SCD, bradycardia also plays an important role. The relationship between bradycardia and SCD seems obvious: a sudden and prolonged asystole leading to cerebral anoxia and death. However, if this scenario exists, relations between SCD and bradycardia are much more complex and subtle. In some cases bradycardia is not at all concerned: mainly when suddenly a ventricular premature beat initiates, without major changes in heart rate, a VF. But except in this situation the potential role of bradycardia in SCD has to be discussed.

## Bradycardia is the Trigger

In that case, bradycardia is generally only relative and this is perfectly illustrated by the so-called "long-short phenomenon."

For example, a premature beat induces a compensatory pause and the following ventricular premature beat induces VT or VF. In this situation the relative bradycardia due to the first premature beat has been the "trigger" for the second to induce the lethal arrhythmia. The pause has been necessary to destabilize the ventricular repolarization in such a way that the next extrasystole found an "excitable gap." The literature is very scarce in series reporting the exact influence of this phenomenon in patients with SCD. Among the 13 patients with a SCD while on Holter monitoring re-

From: Aliot E, Clementy J, Prystowsky EN (editors). *Fighting Sudden Cardiac Death: A Worldwide Challenge.* ©Futura Publishing Company, Armonk, NY, 2000.

ported by Milner,[1] only 1 had a "long-short phenomenon." For Leclercq et al.,[2] bradycardia before a lethal ventricular arrhythmia is more frequent although relative: in 45% of their 49 patients, they calculated a pause exceeding 125% of the mean 5 preceding beats just before initiation of VF. If in patients with VF the previous phenomenon seems relatively unfrequent, it is constant in patients with torsades de pointes.[2]

The role of bradycardia as a trigger of ventricular arrhythmia is more obvious in cases of complete atrioventricular (AV) block complicated by torsades de pointes. In that case bradycardia prolongs markedly the repolarization (very long QT interval) and ventricular premature beats initiate torsades de pointes. This arrhythmia is generally self-terminated but in some instances may perpetuate or degenerate into VF, leading to death. In this situation torsades de pointes is the terminal arrhythmia but bradycardia clearly has the key role as acceleration of the ventricular rhythm, for example, by cardiac pacing immediately removes the ventricular arrhythmia.

## Bradycardia is the Marker

In many cases of patients dying while being monitored, a progressive sinus or junctional bradycardia ending in asystole is registered. In those cases, as noted by Myerburg,[3] resuscitation maneuvers are always unsuccessful (Table 1). This failure is easily explained by the anatomic lesions found in such cases (Table 2) and bradycardia is only the electrical translation of a mechanical arrest.[4] It should be stressed that even after VT or VF, asystole is always the terminal "electrical" event and that may explain also why those patients could not be resuscitated.

## Bradycardia is the Killer

Only in that case could bradycardia be directly responsible for SCD. Although many efforts were directed to avoid this complication of bradycardia, it seems relatively exceptional. Figure 1 shows the results obtained

### Table 1

### Survival Rates According to the Preadmission Arrhythmia

| Preadmission Diagnosis | % Survival at Admission | % Survival at Discharge |
| --- | --- | --- |
| VT | 88% | 67% |
| VF | 40% | 28% |
| Asystole | 9% | 0% |

VT = ventricular tachycardia; VF = ventricular fibrillation.
From Myerburg RJ, et al.[3] with permission.

## Table 2

## Main Diagnosis Leading to Sudden Cardiac Death Associated with a Progressive Bradycardia (Electromechanical Dissociation)

Valvular occlusion
- left atrial myxoma (or other cardiac tumor)
- thrombosis of a valvular prothesis

Massive pulmonary embolism
Cardiac or aortic rupture
Massive myocardial destruction
- myocarditis
- amylosis
- coronary artery disease (the "last" branch is occluded)

in 10 series of the literature.[5,6] Among 218 patients with SCD during Holter monitoring, bradycardias were observed in only 17%. However, in that 17%, patients with electromechanical dissociation are included, and according to Leclercq et al.,[7] less than 10% of the patients with SCD and bradycardia have an abrupt asystole as the terminal electrical event. In half of these patients, Holter monitoring registered a complete atrioventricular (AV) block and in the other half, a complete sinoatrial (SA) block. This latter situation deserves some comments because the role of the autonomic nervous system should be more precisely defined. In 6 patients with cardiovascular collapse apparently in association with cardiac asystole re-

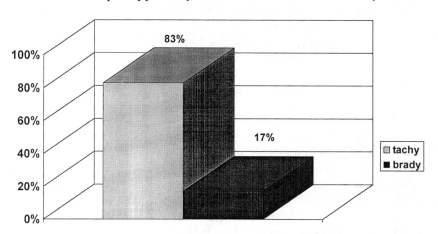

**Electral terminal activity**

Figure 1. Repartition of 218 patients who died during Holter monitoring according to the electrocardiographic terminal activity. (From Bayes de Luna A, et al.[5] and Olshausen KV, et al.[6] with permission.)

## Table 3

## Main Characteristics of Patients with Sudden Cardiac Death Supposed to Be the Consequence of Ventricular Tachycardia/Ventricular Fibrillation or Asystole (Brady)

|  | VT/VF | Bradycardia |
|---|---|---|
| N | 90 | 24 |
| Mean age (years) | 62 ± 11 | 68 ± 4 |
| Males | 77% | 42% |
| CHD | 93% | 57% |
| Antiarrhythmic drugs | 51% | 29% |

VT = ventricular tachycardia; VF = ventricular fibrillation; CHD = coronary heart disease. From Bayes de Luna A, et al.[5] with permission.

sulting in initiation of resuscitative measures, Milstein et al.[8] reported that tilt testing reproduced syncope in all patients, and was associated in 2 patients with a long SA block (16 and 22 sec). Other series have reported long asystole due to SA block during positive tilt testing, but to the best of our knowledge, no deaths were reported. However, if such asystole occurs in the absence of medical support, it may be responsible for SCD.

The comparison between the group of patients dying "from" VT-VF and the group dying "from" bradycardia reported by Bayes de Luna[5] showed that patients in this latter group are older, more frequently are women, had less coronary heart disease, and were less frequently treated by antiarrhythmic drugs (Table 3).

Finally, although precise epidemiological data are missing, bradycardia is the "killer" in probably less than 2% of the patients dying suddenly.

## Pathological Findings

Pathological examination is another possibility to explore the relation between objective abnormalities of the nodo-Hisian anatomy and sudden death. Among 1,000 patients with SCD, 111 had such abnormalities.[9] The main limitation of those studies is the absence of correlation between pathological findings and electrical activity just before death. Very exciting cases, sometimes clinically well documented, have been presented by James in a series of papers titled De subitaneis mortibus and published mainly in Circulation between 1973 and 1978.[10]

## Limitations of the Present Data

Precise analysis of the role of bradycardia in a patient with SCD requires a complete electrocardiographic sequence at least a few seconds before the event, i.e., Holter monitoring. But these data are insufficient to relate bradycardia to the disease leading to death. To achieve this level of patient history, previous ECG and precise knowledge of SCD circumstances (vasovagal conditions) are mandatory.

Finally, in case of progressive bradycardia, an autopsy is necessary to know which cardiac disease has been the cause of the electromechanical dissociation. With very few exceptions, all of these data are generally missing. These reasons explain why the present information concerning the role of bradycardia during SCD could not be considered as hard data.

## Conclusion

Finally, to summarize the available data, among 100 patients with SCD, bradycardia plays a role in about 60 cases: in 40 as a trigger and the bradycardia is relative, in 18 as a marker, and in only 2 as a "killer." In this latter situation the role of the autonomic nervous system ("neurocardiogenic death") is certainly not insignificant.

### *References*

1. Milner PG, Platia EV, Reid PR, Griffith LS. Ambulatory electrocardiographic recording at the time of fatal cardiac arrest. Am J Cardiol 1985; 56:588–659.
2. Leclercq JF, Maisonblanche P, Cauchemez B, Coumel P. Respective role of sympathetic tone and of cardiac pauses in the genesis of 62 cases of ventricular fibrillation recorded during Holter monitoring. Eur Heart J 1988; 9:1276–1283.
3. Myerburg RJ, Kessler KM, Castellamas A. Sudden cardiac death: structure, function and time-dependence of risk. Circulation 1992; 85(Suppl I) :1-2–1-10.
4. Wangs FS, Lien WP, Fong TE, Lin JL, Cherng JJ, et al. Terminal cardiac electrical activity in adults who die without apparent cardiac disease. Am J Cardiol 1986; 58:491–495.
5. Bayes de Luna A, Coumel P, Leclercq JF. Ambulatory sudden cardiac death: mechanisms of production of fatal arrhythmia on the basis of data from 157 cases. Am Heart J 1989; 117:151–159.
6. Olshausen KV, Witt T, Pop T, Treese N, Bethge KP, et al. Sudden cardiac death while wearing a Holter monitor. Am J Cardiol 1991; 67:381–386.
7. Leclercq JF, Coumel P, Maison-Blanche P, Cauchemez B, Zimmermann M, et al. Mise en évidence des mécanismes déterminants de la mort subite. Arch Mal C_ur 1986; 79:1024–1033.
8. Milstein S, Buetikofer J, Lesser J, Goldenberg IF, Benditt DG, et al. Cardiac asystole: a manifestation of neurally mediated hypotension-bradycardia. J Am Coll Cardiol 1989; 14:1626–1632.
9. Loire R, Tahib A. Unexpected sudden cardiac death: an evaluation of 1000 autopsies. Arch Mal C_ur 1996; 89:13–18.
10. James TN, Frogatt P, Atkinson WJ. De subitaneis mortibus XXX. Observations on the pathophysiology of the heart. Circulation 1978; 57:1221–1231.

# 10

# Sudden Cardiac Death:

# The Pathology Perspective

*Michael Davies, MD*

## Introduction

Pathology plays a major role in elucidating the causes of sudden death in subjects who have no known history of cardiac disease. Autopsies are also important in providing clues to the mechanisms that invoke the sudden onset of ventricular arrhythmias and sudden death in subjects with known prior cardiac disease. In either situation the pathologist must be aware of the probability and plausibility of the pathology found at autopsy being the cause of death. There are often pressures on the pathologist from the legal authorities or the family to provide a natural cause of death. The cause of death given by a pathologist must, however, be accurate, and if there is no structural abnormality of the heart this must be clearly stated.

Pathologists should adopt a sequential approach. The first step is to exclude extracardiac natural and unnatural disease. Ruptured cerebral artery aneurysms and dissection of the aorta can produce death within an hour or 2 of the onset of symptoms. Solvents and the use of cocaine can cause sudden death in circumstances in which it is not immediately apparent that the subject was abusing drugs. After these possibilities have been excluded, the pathologist can concentrate on the heart as the likely site of a disease causing sudden death.

## Vascular Causes of Sudden Death

In subjects over the age of 30, coronary atherosclerosis increasingly becomes the major cause of sudden natural death. There are, however, other rare vascular causes of sudden death, particularly in younger subjects. An examination of the heart in sudden death should specifically describe the coronary artery orifices. Normally 1 orifice is present in each of

From: Aliot E, Clementy J, Prystowsky EN (editors). *Fighting Sudden Cardiac Death: A Worldwide Challenge.* ©Futura Publishing Company, Armonk, NY, 2000.

the 2 forward-facing aortic sinuses (right and left). Anomalies in the coronary artery anatomy may be safe or dangerous. Dangerous anomalies fall into 2 clear groups.[1] In the first group, 1 artery arises in the aorta while the other ostium is in the pulmonary artery. An intramyocardial left-to-right shunt of blood develops and the arteries become dilated due to high flow. Sudden death may occur in early adult life after many years of normal exercise tolerance. The second dangerous group of anomalies occur when 2 coronary ostia arise in 1 aortic sinus. In such cases an arterial branch has to cross right to left or left to right depending on which sinus contains the ostia. If the crossing artery lies between the pulmonary and aortic trunk, the subject is at risk of sudden death.

Coronary ostia that arise from the aorta higher than their usual site and have to run through the media at an acute downward angle, as well as ostia that have a shelf-like fold of aortic wall at their upper border have been described as causing death[2] but these appearances can be found in control hearts in which there is a clear extracardiac cause of death. Kawasaki disease,[3] an isolated coronary arteritis in children, is instantly recognizable as huge dilated arteries containing thrombus. Spontaneous dissection of a coronary artery[4] is recognizable as a focal mass of red thrombus in an artery with minimal atherosclerosis, which either by naked-eye examination or under a microscope is shown to be a subadventitial hematoma rather than an intraluminal thrombus. Bridging where a layer of myocardium covers the epicardial surface of a major coronary artery is a contentious cause of sudden death. Up to 50% of control normal hearts have at least 1 or 2 cm of a bridged epicardial coronary artery covered by a layer of cardiac muscle.[5] Therefore most of these bridges must functionally be of no consequence. In vivo clinical reports based on very stringent criteria[6,7] do, however, show instances where compression of the artery within the bridge is associated with reversible myocardial ischemia. To ascribe a tunneled section of coronary artery as a cause of death with any degree of credibility requires additional evidence. This may take the form of a history of episodic anginal-type pain for a number of months before death or histological evidence of ischemic damage in the myocardium.

## Atherosclerotic Coronary Disease

The spectrum of the pathology found in the 85% of sudden natural deaths that are considered to be due to coronary artery disease is a good example of the range of probabilities for the arterial lesions being causative of death (Table 1). At one end of the spectrum the probability is 100% while at the other it is far below 50%. The figures for probability are rough esti-

## Table 1

### The Probability in Descending Order of Sudden Death Being Due to Ischemic Heart Disease When No Other Cause is Found Based on Macroscopic Examination in Hearts with Coronary Atherosclerosis

| | |
|---|---|
| • Pericardial tamponade—rupture of acute infarct-coronary thrombus | Certain |
| • Acute myocardial infarction/coronary thrombus | High Probability |
| • Coronary thrombosis alone | |
| • Healed previous infarct scar—no thrombus | |
| • No coronary thrombus—no myocardial scars | |
| ⨯ 3 vessels with > 50% stenosis | Medium Probability |
| ⨯ 2 | |
| ⨯ 1 | |
| • Stenosis < 50% alone | Low Probability |

mates and cannot be calculated accurately, but the important concept for pathologists is that the chance of being correct when ascribing death due to ischemic heart disease is a graded phenomenon. For example, apparently healthy males over 50 years of age in South London who die of clear noncardiac causes have a 10% incidence of at least 1 coronary artery with a high-grade stenotic lesion (Table 2). In giving a single-vessel stenosis as a cause of death in isolation, pathologists should remember that similar lesions are found in living subjects.

The data needed to assess probability of coronary disease being causative of sudden death are the presence of coronary thrombi, the presence and distribution of old and recent myocardial infarction, and the number of coronary arterial segments with a pinpoint lumen (<1 mm) equivalent to at least 50% diameter stenosis. Assessment of the lesser de-

## Table 2

### Sudden Death in Males Less than 69 Years of Age: Distribution of Coronary Stenosis

| Vessels with > 50% Stenosis | IHD Death | Non-IHD Death |
|---|---|---|
| *0 | 5 (2.4%) | 124 (85.5%) |
| ⨯1 | 53 (25.9%) | 15 (10.3%) |
| ⨯2 | 80 (39.0%) | 4 (2.8%) |
| ⨯3 | 67 (32.7%) | 2 (1.4%) |
| | 205 (100%) | 145 (100%) |

*Coronary thrombosis present. IHD = ischemic heart disease.

grees of coronary stenosis at autopsy is very subjective. The level at which the probability of coronary lesions being causal of death falls below the 50% chance level cannot be rigidly defined, but perhaps lies at the point of 1 major coronary artery having a significant stenosis. This concept assumes that the pathologist's estimate of disease severity in the coronary arteries approximates to that which angiography would have revealed in life. In reality, pathologists probably overestimate stenosis, further compounding the difficulties in giving coronary disease as the cause of death.

When thrombus is seen by naked-eye examination in a coronary artery, this provides good evidence of acute myocardial ischemia even if the artery is not completely occluded. Distal emboli of small clumps of platelets[8–10] from the thrombus cause microscopic foci of myocardial necrosis and, therefore, a substrate for reentry tachycardias even in the absence of acute infarction recognizable to the naked eye. Autopsy studies in which coronary angiography is carried out show that at least half of sudden deaths due to ischemic heart disease have an angiogram identical to

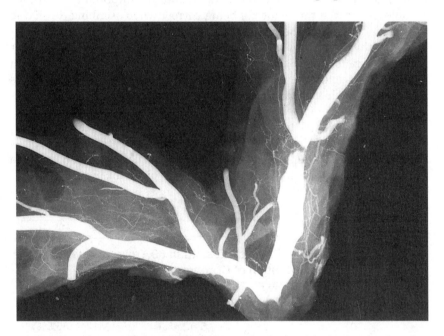

Figure 1. Postmortem angiogram in a subject who died suddenly shortly after playing squash. There is irregularity in the proximal segment of the left anterior descending coronary artery indicating the presence of nonstenosing plaques. In the more distal left anterior descending coronary artery just before a major branch there is an eccentric high-grade stenotic lesion with an irregular outline. Proximal to this there is a filling defect in the lumen indicating thrombosis.

those found in vivo in unstable angina (Figure 1). A major type II angiographic stenosis with an eccentric ragged outline is evident and an intraluminal filling defect indicating the presence of thrombus.

Occluding coronary thrombi can reasonably be expected to produce an area of regional myocardial necrosis, although due to the short interval between the onset of symptoms and death, there is often insufficient time for the infarction to be recognized by naked-eye examination. Despite the short time intervals, a significant proportion of sudden deaths from ischemic heart disease do have a well-established infarction, suggesting that the occlusion in the artery occurred some hours before the onset of any symptoms. Pericardial tamponade due to cardiac rupture may also cause sudden death. This is particularly found with type I rupture that occurs at the interface between the infarct and normal myocardium and develops within the first 6 hours unlike types II and III ruptures, which are through the infarct itself and require some days to develop.

Myocardial scars have the potential to cause reentry tachycardias and are therefore a substrate for sudden death. Ischemic scars that have expanded and become localized ventricular aneurysms are particularly associated with the survival of a subendocardial zone of myocytes arranged in complex circular configurations, providing an excellent basis for reentry.

The relative proportions of cases of sudden death due to coronary artery disease that are due to new acute ischemia compared to arrhythmias arising in a scarred and/or hypertrophied myocardium are very variable in the literature. Personal experience suggests that new arterial thrombotic lesions are present in over 70% of sudden ischemic deaths[11] but others find less than 30%.[12] The differences probably reflect case selection.[13] Any series that is biased toward subjects without prior known ischemic disease and includes subjects who have prodromal pain will record high frequencies of coronary thrombi. In contrast, series that include patients with known prior ischemic disease who die suddenly without prodromal pain will record lower frequencies of coronary thrombi.

The trigger initiating the coronary thrombosis that causes sudden death may be plaque rupture or endothelial denudation (erosion). Evidence is emerging that plaque rupture is the dominant mechanism in men and erosion is more important in women.[14,15]

The mechanism for sudden death in subjects without thrombus, without myocardial scars, and with stenosis equivalent to 50% or less by diameter is unknown. One postulate would be spasm of coronary arteries at the site of an eccentric coronary plaque in which a segment of normal media is retained. It is impossible to confirm or refute this by autopsy. Left ventricular hypertrophy often coexists with coronary artery disease and would be a potentiating factor in causing ventricular arrhythmias.

# Nonischemic Cardiac Causes of Sudden Death

Autopsy series throughout the United States and Europe consistently show that approximately 7–10% of sudden natural death is due to nonischemic cardiac disease that is easily recognized at autopsy by characteristic structural changes. There are innumerable other much rarer causes often reported in the literature as single case reports.

## Valve Disease and Sudden Death

Aortic valve calcific stenosis causing significant left ventricular hypertrophy is well recognized as a cause of sudden death. Nonstenotic noncalcified bicuspid valves occur in 1–2% of a normal population and cannot be taken in isolation to be causative of death. No mechanism is known that would link normally functioning bicuspid aortic valves to sudden death. Mitral valve prolapse (floppy mitral valve) is a contentious cause of sudden death. Floppy mitral valves with a minor degree of prolapse are very common in the normal population as shown by echocardiographic surveys of young subjects. A very small minority of subjects with such mitral valve prolapse have multiple ectopic ventricular beats and it is apparent that a small subgroup of this small subgroup can die suddenly.[16,17] For the pathologist, the difficulty is whether a mild or moderate degree of myxoid change with cusp expansion (floppy valve) is coincidental with or causative of sudden death. The argument for a causative role[18] is strengthened by a history of any cardiac arrhythmia or palpitations in life or by evidence of significant mitral regurgitation in the form of a dilated or hypertrophied left ventricle, ruptured chordae, or a large left atrium with jet lesions. The more severe the valve abnormality, the more likely is it to be a cause of sudden death.

## Myocardial Disease and Sudden Death

Acute myocarditis either due to viral infection or a drug hypersensitivity is a well-recognized cause of sudden death. It cannot, however, be diagnosed reliably without histological examination. Causal myocarditis will involve large areas of the myocardium and creates no difficulty in interpreting the histology, but if large numbers of blocks of any heart are taken, single foci of "myocarditis" that can be encompassed within a high-power microscopic field are very common even in normal hearts, i.e., where a clear noncardiac cause of death is present. Such foci must not be overinterpreted.

The genotype-phenotype relation in a number of familial cardiomyopathies is in a rapidly expanding phase and it has to be admitted that for the present these advances have made the pathologist's task harder rather than easier.

Familial hypertrophic cardiomyopathy (HCM) is due to at least 7 separate genes,[19] all encoding for different myofibrillary contractile proteins. The phenotype is expressed most clearly in the β heavy chain myosin gene defects and the cases originally described by Donald Teare[20] had mutations in this gene. Teare's original description emphasized asymmetric thickening of the left ventricular wall, particularly the septum. It rapidly became apparent that cases with symmetric left ventricular wall thickening were equally common. An increase in total heart weight with a thick LV wall (<2 cm) and a relatively small cavity became the hallmark for recognizing HCM by naked-eye examination. In hypertrophic cardiomyopathy, many cases develop left ventricular outflow tract obstruction in systole when the anterior cusp of the mitral valve moves anteriorly and hits the upper interventricular septum below the aortic valve. The impact over some years produces a subaortic localized patch of endocardial thickening on the septum that is specific for HCM.[21]

The histological marker of HCM is disarray of myocytes in which the cells run in circular whorls around a small focus of connective tissue. Disarray is, however, very rarely present throughout the left ventricle and is patchy, meaning that a single random histology block cannot exclude the diagnosis. Many cases of HCM have segments of myocardium that are totally normal.

The macroscopic appearances produced by the myofibrillary gene mutations are now recognized to be so wide that it is impossible by naked-eye examination at autopsy to exclude HCM. Widespread disarray and a risk of sudden death can be present in hearts in which the weight is not increased and the left ventricle is close to normal in shape.[22] This phenomenon is found particularly with some of the troponin T gene mutations. For the pathologist this means the left ventricle has to be studied by at least 8–10 separate histological blocks to exclude a myofibrillary gene defect cardiomyopathy.

Hearts are also encountered in which the left ventricle mass is increased considerably with some increase in myocardial fibrosis but no disarray is present on histology. The pathogenesis of such cases is widely debated and being intensely studied. The phenomenon is often encountered in subjects of Afro-Caribbean origin, and a left ventricle that can be described as "hocoid" but without disarray is a cause of sudden death. Similar hearts are seen in athletes and there is the inevitable question of the role of anabolic steroids in their causation. What seems likely is that a number of genes control left ventricular hypertrophy, and that mutations or polymorphisms in them can allow a disproportionate increase in left ventricular mass in response to exercise or mild hypertension, and there is a risk of sudden death. Infants of diabetic mothers develop a large thick-walled left ventricle, probably as a response to insulin-like growth factors.

The relation of left ventricular hypertrophy to sudden death means that pathologists should be better at objective assessment of heart size. Total heart weight at autopsy, however, is a meaningless figure unless equated to body size and a number of tables and equations allow adjustment to be made.[23] For myocardial hypertrophy to be credible as a cause of death, total heart weight should be at least outside the 95% confidence limits for body size.

Sudden death in subjects with good exercise tolerance and no known cardiac disease can also occur where there is no hypertrophy but widespread myocardial fibrosis is present on histology despite totally normal coronary arteries. Fibrosis may take the form of discrete linear scars or be diffuse and perimyocyte in distribution. It is tempting to ascribe this cause to previously healed myocarditis, implying there is no risk to other family members. The temptation should be avoided because although this may be true in some cases, in others a family member may subsequently die with identical pathology. The genetic basis is as yet unknown but the cases can be designated as idiopathic fibrosis or idiopathic myocardial fibrosis.

Fibrosis leads to dyshomogenicity in repolarization and is associated with abnormal QT dispersion, providing a plausible link to the onset of ventricular tachycardias. In areas of fibrosis the distribution of connexin43 on myocytes becomes abnormal, further potentiating reentry paths additional to the anatomic effects of scar tissue isolating strands and islands of myocardium.

Myotonic dystrophy is associated with marked cardiac involvement with left ventricular fibrosis and a high risk of sudden death, particularly during anesthesia. It is starting to be suspected, but as yet unproven, that families with myotonic dystrophy may have sudden deaths in subjects without skeletal muscle expression of the abnormal gene.

## Arrythmogenic Right Ventricular Dysplasia (ARVD)

This is another genetic cardiomyopathy with a high risk of sudden death in gene carriers.[24,25] At least 4 loci on separate chromosomes have been shown by linkage to be associated with the disease, but the candidate genes have not been identified and how the phenotype is produced is unknown. Studies of large families with the disease have shown the phenotype in the heart, which the pathologist has to recognize is wide. The easiest cases are where there are large areas of wall thinning producing aneurysmal bulges in the right ventricle. The thinned wall shows loss of myocytes and replacement by fibrofatty tissue. The areas of thinning may, however, be focal and small (1–2 sq cm) and one has to look at the right ventricle in some detail to find them.

The extremes of the phenotype are even more difficult; about 30% of cases of ARVD have some left ventricular involvement with foci of fibrofatty replacement of myocytes often in a band-like distribution on the posterior wall. Cases are seen in which the left ventricle is involved by this change in isolation and the right ventricle is normal. Whether this is part of the spectrum of ARVD is unknown at present. The most difficult cases are where there is simple adipose tissue infiltration of the right ventricular muscle without fibrosis. This is a common change in normal subjects, particularly women, and usually of no consequence. Studies of large families with known ARVD, however, suggest that occasional cases of sudden death occur when this simple picture of fatty infiltration in isolation in the right ventricle is found at autopsy. If pathologists ascribe sudden death as due to ARVD based on simple adipose infiltration in the right ventricle, there is going to be a huge increase in its frequency, which in most instances will be totally spurious. Once the genes are identified, these matters can be resolved but the phenotypic range of ARVD in the heart is not yet clearly defined.

## The Conduction System and Sudden Death

Patients with complete atrioventricular block or with preexcitation[26] (Wolff-Parkinson-White syndrome) do have a risk of sudden death, yet the number of cases who die in their very first syncopal attack must be very small. Unless there are prior ECG data, histological examination of the conduction system is time-consuming and rarely rewarding. The difficulty of such examinations is that normal hearts often contain minor anatomic abnormalities of the conduction system such as nodoventricular connections or small accessory masses of atrioventricular nodal tissue. The presence of these abnormalities in itself therefore cannot be taken as a cause of sudden death although many case reports in the literature do so.[27,28] It is, however, always worth looking at the atrioventricular nodal area with the naked eye to exclude the small benign tumor (atrioventricular nodal mesothelioma) that arises in the node.[29] It will be seen as a cystic nodule just anterior to the coronary sinus in the right atrium.

## Sudden Death with a Morphological Normal Heart

Sudden deaths do occur in young fit individuals in whom, despite taking adequate histology of the heart, no structural abnormality is found and in whom exhaustive toxicology is negative or shows therapeutic levels of prescribed medication. The frequency of such cases is not well defined. In England a study conducted specifically to answer this question suggested up to 200 cases occurred annually in a population of 35 million per year.[30]

It is being increasingly recognized that gene defects in ion channels in the myocyte lead to rhythm disturbances, ECG abnormalities, and a risk of sudden death but no morphological abnormality in the heart. Examples are the long QT and Brugada syndromes. The only way these conditions can be confirmed in a subject who has died suddenly are by ECGs taken earlier in the subject's life or by discovering other family members whose ECGs show the characteristic appearances. The frequency of the long QT syndrome as a cause of sudden death can only be approximated at the moment but it may be as much as 1 in 3 of all cases of sudden unexpected unexplained death in young subjects in which the heart is morphologically normal. Polymorphisms in the long QT genes are now being recognized that are associated with increased QT dispersion and may sensitize some individuals to therapeutic drug-induced ventricular tachycardia and therefore may be a risk of sudden death.[31]

It has also become apparent that sudden deaths occur in epileptic subjects without a clear cardiac morphological abnormality and in whom the final event was not related to a grand mal seizure.[32,33] The mechanisms are not clear but may be related to sympathetic overactivity in the prodromal phase of an epileptic attack, to alterations in the QT interval, and electrical stability of the heart related to therapeutic drugs or to cerebral neuronal arrest leading to respiratory arrest, hypoxia, and then VF. The phenomenon deserves far greater study and pathologists can help by recording deaths as due to sudden cardiac death in epilepsy to identify the cases. Rather similar sudden cardiac deaths with a normal heart can occur in subjects with marked fatty change in the liver.[34,35] Again the mechanisms are unclear. Blunt trauma to the anterior chest wall such as being hit by a cricket or hockey ball can invoke sudden VF without either acute structural damage to the sternum, pericardium, and myocardium or prior heart disease.[36]

# Conclusion

The pathologist has a valuable role to play in increasing the understanding of the causes of sudden death, particularly in excluding unnatural deaths due to drug abuse, including solvents or cocaine. The second role is in defining exactly what structural abnormality, if any, is present in the heart. The structural changes in the heart may be very specific such as hypertrophic cardiomyopathy or arrythmogenic dysplasia. If so, the diagnosis will help those who have to advise the family. The structural changes may, however, be nonspecific such as unexplained myocardial fibrosis that could be genetic or acquired following a viral myocarditis. The third and final role is to be honest and clear when there is no structural abnormality.[36] This group is likely to be heterogeneous in its pathogenesis and further genetic and family studies are needed to define what proportion are due to abnormalities in the long QT genes. In a family with a sudden death of a young person without cause despite detailed and expert examination of the heart, screening of all first-degree relatives by echocardiography and ECG examination is advisable if the family wishes it. In the future it will become possible to screen the DNA in these individuals for all the known mutations in the long QT, myofibrillary, and ARVD genes but this is probably 5 years away. The role of the pathologist can be summarized as the provider of an accurate phenotype to correlate with genetic or other studies in surviving family members.

## References

1. Roberts W. Major anomalies of coronary arterial origin seen in adulthood. Am Heart J 1986; 111:941–962.
2. Virmani R, Chun P, Goldstein R, Robinowitz M, McAllister H. Acute takeoffs of the coronary arteries along the aortic wall and congenital coronary ostial valve-like ridges: association with sudden death. J Am Coll Cardiol 1984; 3:766–771.
3. Fujiwara H, Hamashima Y. Pathology of the heart in Kawasaki disease. Paediatrics 1978; 61:100–107.
4. Basso C, Morgagni G, Thiene G. Spontaneous coronary artery dissection: a neglected cause of acute myocardial ischaemia and sudden death. Heart 1996; 75:451–454.
5. Ferreira AG Jr, Trotter SE, Konig B Jr, Decourt LV, Fox K, et al. Myocardial bridges: morphological and functional aspects. Br Heart J 1991; 66:364–367.
6. Swartz E, Klues H, von Dahl J, Klein I, Krebs W, et al. Functional characteristics of myocardial bridging: a combined angiographic and intracoronary Doppler flow study. Eur Heart J 1997; 18:434–442.
7. Tio R, van Gelder I, Boonstra P, Crijns H. Myocardial bridging in a survivor of sudden cardiac near-death: role of intracoronary Doppler flow measurements and angiography during dobutamine stress in the clinical evaluation. Heart 1997; 77:280–282.
8. Frink R, Ostrach L, Rooney P. Coronary thrombosis: ulcerated atherosclerotic plaques and platelet/fibrin microemboli in patients dying with acute coronary disease. A large autopsy study. J Inv Cardiol 1990; 2:199–210.
9. Falk E. Unstable angina with fatal outcome: dynamic coronary thrombosis leading to infarction and/or sudden death. Circulation 1985; 71:699–708.
10. Davies M, Thomas A, Knapman P, Hangartner R. Intramyocardial platelet aggregation in patients with unstable angina suffering sudden ischemic cardiac death. Circulation 1986; 73:418–427.
11. Davies M, Thomas A. Thrombosis and acute coronary artery lesions in sudden cardiac ischemic death. N Engl J Med 1984; 310:1137–1140.
12. Warnes C, Maron B, Roberts W. Massive cardiac ventricular scarring in first-

degree relatives with hypertrophic cardiomyopathy. Am J Cardiol 1984; 54:1377–1380.

13. Davies M, Bland J, Hangartner J, Angelini A, Thomas A. Factors influencing the presence or absence of acute coronary artery thrombi in sudden ischaemic death. Eur Heart J 1989; 10:203–208.

14. Burke AP, Farb A, Malcom GT, Liang Y, Smialek J, et al. Effect of risk factors on the mechanism of acute thrombosis and sudden coronary death in women. Circulation 1998; 43:267–271.

15. Davies MJ. The composition of coronary artery plaques. N Engl J Med 1997; 336:1312–1313.

16. Boudoulas H, Kligfield P, Wooley C. Mitral valve prolapse: sudden death. In: Boudoulas H, Wooley C (eds). Mitral Valve Prolapse and the Mitral Valve Prolapse Syndrome. Futura Publishing Co Inc, Mount Kisco, NY, 1988, pp 591–605.

17. MacMahon S, Roberts J, Kramer-Fox R, Zucker D, Roberts R, et al. Arrhythmias and sudden death in mitral valve prolapse. Am Heart J 1987; 113:1298–1307.

18. Farb A, Tang A, Atkinson J, McCarthy W, Virmani R. Comparison of cardiac findings in patients with mitral valve prolapse who die suddenly to those who have congestive heart failure from mitral regurgitation and to those with fatal noncardiac conditions. Am J Cardiol 1992; 70:234–239.

19. Burn J, Camm J, Davies M, Peltonen L, Schwartz P, et al. The phenotype/genotype relation and the current status of genetic screening in hypertrophic cardiomyopathy, Marfan syndrome, and the long QT syndrome. Heart 1997; 78:110–116.

20. Teare D. Asymmetrical hypertrophy of the heart in young patients. Br Heart J 1958; 20:1–8.

21. Davies M, McKenna W. Hypertrophic cardiomyopathy: pathology and pathogensis. Histopathology 1995; 26:493–500.

22. McKenna W, Stewart J, Niyannopoulos P, McGinty F, Davies M. Hypertrophic cardiomyopathy without hypertrophy: two families with myocardial disarray in the absence of increased myocardial mass. Br Heart J 1990; 63:287–290.

23. Kitzman D, Scholz D, Hagen P, Ilstrup D, Edwards W. Age-related changes in normal human hearts during the first 10 decades of life. Part II. Maturity: a quantitative anatomic study of 765 specimens from subjects 20 to 99 years old. Mayo Clin Proc 1988; 63:131–146.

24. Basso C, Thiene G, Corrado D, Angelini A, Nava A, et al. Arrhythmogenic right ventricular cardiomyopathy: dysplasia, dystrophy or myocarditis? Circulation 1996; 94:983–991.

25. Corrado D, Basso C, Thiene G, et al. Spectrum of clinicopathologic manifestations of arrhythmogenic right ventricular cardiomyopathy/dysplasia: a multicenter study. J Am Coll Cardiol 1997; 30:1512–1520.

26. Wiedermann C, Becker A, Hopferwieser T, Muhlberger V, Knapp E. Sudden death in a young competitive athlete with Wolff-Parkinson-White syndrome. Eur Heart J 1987; 8:651–655.

27. Bharati S, Lev M. The Cardiac Conduction System in Unexplained Sudden Death. Futura Publishing Co Inc, Mount Kisco, NY, 1990, pp 51–62.

28. James T, Froggatt P, Marshall T. Sudden death in young athletes. Ann Intern Med 1967; 67:1013–1021.

29 Subramanian R, Flygenring B. Mesothelioma of the atrioventricular node and congenital complete heart block. Clin Cardiol 1989; 12:3469–3472.

30. Davies M. Unexplained death in fit young people. BMJ 1992; 305:538–539.

31. Busjahn A, Knoblauch H, Faulbaber H-D, et al. QT interval is linked to 2 long QT syndrome loci in normal subjects. Circulation 1999; 99:3161–3164.

32. Lund A, Gormsen H. The role of anti-epileptics in sudden death in epilepsy. Acta Neurol Scand 1985; 72:444–446.
33. Nashef L, Brown S. Epilepsy and sudden death. Lancet 1996; 348:1324–1325.
34. Panos R, Sutton F, Young-Hyman P, Peters R. Sudden death associated with alcohol consumption. PACE 1988; 11:423–424.
35. Randall B. Fatty liver and sudden death. Hum Pathol 1980; 11:147–155.
36. Maron B, Poliac L, Kaplan J, Mueller F. Blunt impact to the chest leading to sudden death from cardiac arrest during sports activities. N Engl J Med 1995; 333:337–342.

# II

# Out-of-Hospital Sudden Cardiac Death

# 11

# Automated External Defibrillation in Europe

*Leo Bossaert, MD*

## Prehospital Sudden Death

The most important single cause of death in the adult population of the industrialized world is sudden cardiac arrest due to coronary disease. The first recorded rhythm in patients presenting with a sudden cardiovascular collapse is ventricular fibrillation (VF) in 75–80%.

In 1997 the World Health Organization (WHO) reported that of the 50 million deaths that occur each year worldwide, the leading causes of death were ischemic heart disease with 6.3 million deaths and cerebrovascular accidents with 4.4 million.[1]

A decline of age-adjusted total coronary death was observed in the United States and in most European countries in the past 20 years. However, due to increasing age of the population, the impact of the epidemic of ischemic heart disease will remain most important in the coming decades. In several central and Eastern European countries, there was no decline of coronary deaths or there was even an increase.[2–4] Although total mortality from coronary disease is decreasing, case fatality rate remained unchanged: at present, 28-day case fatality of acute myocardial infarction is still 45–50%. Two thirds of deaths from coronary disease occur in the prehospital phase and most victims do not survive long enough to receive medical help. Whereas in-hospital death is due mainly to the infarct size, prehospital death is due mainly to cardiac arrest from VF and ventricular tachycardia (VT). Both lethal pathways, lethal arrhythmias and lethal loss of functional myocardium, need a different interventional strategy during the first few hours after onset of symptoms.[5]

If any further impact is to be made on case fatality of acute coronary events, therapeutic strategies are needed that focus both on early patency of the obstructed coronary vessel and on early recognition and treatment of VF.

New technological developments in the field of automated external defibrillators have caused a major change in therapeutic strategies. Pa-

From: Aliot E, Clementy J, Prystowsky EN (editors). *Fighting Sudden Cardiac Death: A Worldwide Challenge.* ©Futura Publishing Company, Armonk, NY, 2000.

tients who have recovered from sudden cardiac death should receive appropriate therapeutic management, including coronary revascularization, antiarrhythmic drug treatment, and implantation of cardioverter-defibrillators (ICDs).

## Automated External Defibrillators (AEDs)

Defibrillation of the heart is the only effective treatment of VF and pulseless VT. The time between the onset of VF and the first defibrillating shock is the most important variable of the efficacy of this treatment.

Defibrillation used to be a medical treatment that could be delegated only to emergency care providers who were trained in advanced life support procedures. In order to achieve the earliest defibrillation possible in the prehospital setting, rescuers other than physicians need to have the ability to initiate this treatment. Technological developments of AEDs allowed the implementation of defibrillation by the first responding professional rescuer. AEDs eliminate the need for extensive training in rhythm recognition.

The introduction of AEDs allowed less-trained emergency medical technicians to deliver electric shocks in cases of out-of-hospital VF or VT, often several minutes before the arrival of the medical intervention team.

The term automated external defibrillator refers to external defibrillators that incorporate an automated rhythm analysis system. AEDs are attached to the patient by 2 adhesive pads to analyze the rhythm and to deliver the command to give a shock. The information is given by voice and/or on a visual display and the final delivery of the shock is triggered manually. The specificity of the diagnostic algorithm for VF is about 100%; sensitivity in case of coarse VF is about 90–92%, but is lower in case of fine VF. Failures of the diagnostic algorithm have been documented when using an AED in patients carrying an implanted pacemaker.

The new generation of AEDs uses new battery technology and some of them also use the new biphasic waveform technology. They are smaller, simpler, more reliable, and less inexpensive. This new generation of AEDs will stimulate widespread availability of defibrillators in ambulances, hospital wards, places of work, public places, and airplanes.[6]

## Results of AED Programs: Uniform Reporting According to the Utstein Style

Literature data on survival after cardiac arrest due to VF, where nonmedically qualified personnel use an AED, range between 0% and 54%.

These differences could be related to differences in characteristics of the treated population, differences in methodology and quality of registration, or real differences in the performance of the AED program.

The "Utstein style" for out-of-hospital and in-hospital cardiac arrest and resuscitation is a glossary of terms and reporting guidelines for description of cardiac arrest, resuscitation, the emergency medical services (EMS) system, and the outcome.[7,8]

Critical analysis of the reports on the efficacy of AED programs reinforce that reports of data on outcome from cardiac arrest must be as uniform as possible and should report on the performance of the several links of the chain of survival. Implementation of an AED program will be successful only if the other links in the chain of survival are well functioning. Several elements may be responsible for poor performance in the chain of survival: the delay in calling the EMS system, poor performance of the dispatch, long intervention times, poor performance of the rescuers of the first and second tier, and the subsequent treatment after hospital admission.[9]

## Results of AED Programs by Traditional Rescuers: Emergency Medical System Personnel

Recent reports from Sweden, Germany, Belgium, and the United States illustrated the potential clinical benefit of AED programs in terms of long-term survival.[10–15]

In 1999, Herlitz et al. published a survey of the survival data of 22 European EMS systems.[16] Survival to discharge from all types of cardiac arrest ranged between 6% and 23%. Survival from witnessed cardiac arrest of cardiac origin found in VF ranged between 13% and 55% (7 centers reported a survival rate of more than 30%). Part of these impressive differences might be explained by selection bias and by nonuniformity of definitions. But even taking this caveat into account, high survival rates were obtained in areas where the prevalence of bystander CPR is high, time to defibrillation is short, and the level of training, exposure, and experience of the first and second tier rescuers is high. This review explains also why the efficacy of AED programs is less satisfactory in areas where the efficacy of the other links of the chain of survival is poor. This was observed in areas of low population density where the number of interventions for a given EMS system (and therefore the experience of the crew) is limited.[17–19] These observations support the view that AEDs should not be implemented in EMS systems as an isolated intervention but should complement interventions that strengthen the other links of the chain of survival (early access to the EMS system, early basic CPR by the first witness, and early advanced life support).

# Results of AED Programs by Nontraditional Rescuers: Police, Aircraft Personnel, and the Public

## AEDs Used by Police

Roger White from Rochester, NY (USA) published some encouraging data obtained by equipping police cars with AEDs.[20,21] He compared the survival to hospital discharge in cardiac arrest patients presenting with VF or VT who had their first shock administered by a police officer or by a paramedic. Time delay from call to first defibrillation was not different in either group. There was good survival in 58% of patients who had the first shock administered by a police officer versus 43% where the first shock was given by a paramedic.[20, 21]

Other authors (Mosesso, et al.) confirmed that in case of out-of-hospital cardiac arrest, a policeman is frequently the first responder and that defibrillation by police results in shorter time to defibrillation and eventually improved survival.[22]

In 1999–2000, a prospective trial will investigate the efficacy of AED by police officers in Amsterdam (The Netherlands), and a similar investigation is under way also in Paris.

## AEDs on Commercial Aircraft

Recently, AEDs were installed on the commercial aircraft of several airline companies. Recent reports (O'Rourke 1997 and Page 1998) assessed the impact of making AEDs available for use on airline passengers with cardiac arrest.[23]

As many as 1,000 lives are lost annually from cardiac arrest in commercial aircraft. In the study by O'Rourke, AEDs were installed on international Qantas aircraft, and at major terminals, selected crew were trained in their use, and all crew members were trained in CPR. During a 64-month period, AEDs were used on 109 occasions: 63 times for monitoring an acutely ill passenger and 46 times for cardiac arrest. Long-term survival from VF was achieved in 26% (2 of 6 in aircraft and 4 of 17 in terminals). It was concluded that AEDs in aircraft and terminals, with appropriate crew training, are helpful in the management of cardiac emergencies. Costly aircraft diversions can be avoided in clearly futile situations, enhancing the cost-effectiveness of the program. At present, most commercial airline companies have decided to implement AED programs on international flights.[24]

## AEDs Used by the Public

The next logical step could be the implementation of AED programs in the community, with involvement of minimally trained lay individuals. Although this approach is technically feasible with the present technology and although this approach seems economically attractive, evaluation of effectiveness and cost are mandatory.[25,26]

For evaluating effectiveness and cost-effectiveness of implementation of AED programs by nontraditional rescuers in the community (public access defibrillation, PAD), randomized, controlled trials are needed.

## Defibrillation Energy and Waveforms

The output waveform of most conventional external defibrillators is half-sinusoidal or truncated exponential. Inspired by the experience of automatic ICDs, the use of biphasic waveforms has been introduced. Transthoracic biphasic external defibrillation has now been introduced in clinical practice. Biphasic waveforms have lower defibrillation thresholds than monophasic waveforms of the same duration. Biphasic waveforms require less energy and therefore capacitors and batteries can be simpler. Therefore, this new waveform technology could lead to lighter, simpler and cheaper defibrillators. Also, some reports suggest that less shock-induced myocardial damage occurs after biphasic shocks.

Further investigation is needed to define the optimum energy level and the optimum shape of the biphasic wave (voltage, slope, and duration of positive and of negative waves). It can be expected that in near future most major manufacturers of external defibrillators will use biphasic technology.

Scientific evidence endorsed that nonprogressive (150 J—150 J -150 J) impedance-adjusted biphasic waveform shocks for patients in out-of-hospital VF are safe, acceptable, and clinically effective. In a recently reported multicenter randomized comparison of 150 J biphasic and 200–360 J monophasic AEDs in out-of-hospital cardiac arrest, Schneider et al. demonstrated that 150 J impedance-compensating biphasic waveforms defibrillated at rates higher than 200–360 J monophasic shocks, resulting in more patients achieving restoration of spontaneous circulation. EMS system outcomes of survival to hospital admission and discharge were not statistically different.[27-31]

## Guidelines for the Use of AEDs

In case of sudden cardiac arrest, early defibrillation by the first responding professional rescuer is now well accepted as the standard of care. The European Resuscitation Council (ERC), the American Heart Association (AHA), and the International Liaison Committee on Resuscitation (ILCOR) have issued guidelines for the use of AEDs by the first responding member of the EMS system.

In 1997, ILCOR published international advisory statements relating to the early defibrillation strategy.[32,33] ILCOR recommended that all resuscitation personnel be authorized, trained, equipped, and directed to operate a defibrillator, if their professional responsibilities require them to respond to persons in cardiac arrest. This recommendation includes all first responding emergency personnel, in both the hospital and out-of-hospital settings. In some locations the medical profession will need to encourage medical and regulatory authorities to initiate changes in regulations and legislation.

Immediate defibrillation by first responders (defined as a trained individual acting independently in a medically controlled system) in the community offers a promising direction for the future evolution of early defibrillation. These may include police, security officers, lifeguards, airline attendants, railroad station officers, voluntary aides, and those assigned to provide first aid at their work place or in the community who are trained in the use of AEDs. Finally, ILCOR emphasized that early defibrillation initiatives will succeed only when implemented as part of the chain of survival concept.

In 1998 the European Resuscitation Council published guidelines for the use of AEDs by EMS providers and first responders and recommended that: (1) every ambulance in Europe that might respond to a cardiac arrest must carry a defibrillator with personnel trained and permitted to use it; (2) defibrillation should be one of the core competencies of doctors, nurses, and other health care professionals; (3) defibrillators should be available general hospital wards; (4) the feasibility and efficacy of allowing all those assigned to the management of cardiac arrest in the community to be trained and permitted to defibrillate should be investigated.

All first-responder defibrillation programs must operate within strict medical control by physicians qualified and experienced in emergency program management who will have responsibility for ensuring that each link in the chain of survival is in place and who have appropriate access to patient outcome information permitting systems using the Utstein template.[34,35] The guidelines for the use of automated external defibrillators are graphically represented in Figure 1.

Initial training in resuscitation involving AEDs should usually take approximately 8 hours. This is the usual amount of time that is required to achieve the competencies in knowledge of the chain of survival and defibrillation algorithms, basic life support, and defibrillation, and to allow practice and testing in simulated scenarios. Refresher training should be

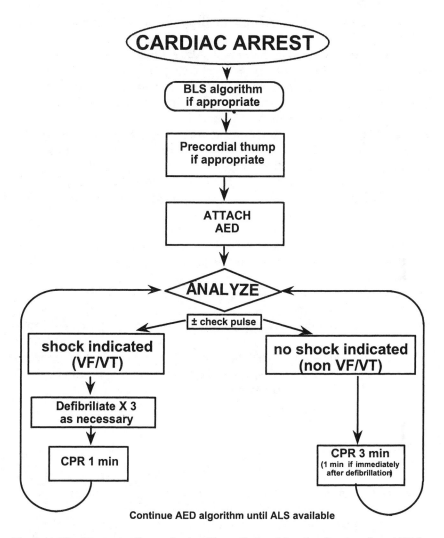

Figure 1. The European Resuscitation Council algorithm for the use of an AED by EMS providers and first responders. (From Resuscitation 1998; 37:91–94; with permission from ERC.[35])

carried out at least every 6 months. Specifically certified instructors working within a medically controlled system should give the training.

## Slow Implementation of AEDs in Europe.[6,36]

The first successful defibrillation of VF outside the hospital was achieved by the Belfast Mobile Coronary Care Unit in 1966 and first automated defibrillators appeared in Brighton and Seattle in the late 1970s.

After these early experiences with AEDs, the technology was further developed and implemented in several centers in the United States and Europe. In Europe, the strategy of early defibrillation with AEDs by ambulance personnel is now community-wide, implemented in UK and Scandinavia, and in parts of Germany and Belgium. Pilot experiences are emerging in many European countries. In some European countries, all ambulances are staffed with experienced nurses and/or doctors and are equipped with manual defibrillators.

As a result of these experiences, it was recognized that an early defibrillation program has the best chance of being successful if:

- the program is placed under medical control
- the time interval between cardiac arrest and first CPR is usually <4 min
- the time interval between cardiac arrest and defibrillation is usually <12 min
- there are a critical number of interventions
- there is a program of training and retraining
- there is a program for monitoring the performance of the program.

AED programs are only partially implemented in Europe and in the United States; less than 50% of ambulances are equipped with an AED. Major reasons for slow implementation are lack of awareness, organization, and legislation.

## Organization

In all European countries, the access to the EMS system is available with a specific telephone number. In 1991, the European Union published recommendation 396: the uniform European emergency telephone number 112 became available in 1997. This is actually the case in most European countries.

In the majority of European countries, doctors have an active role in prehospital emergency medical care, as part of the first or the second tier. In most parts of Scandinavia and in the United Kingdom, paramedics serve as members of the second tier.

Medical presence on the field could be one of the reasons for slow involvement of ambulance personnel in the act of defibrillation.

## Legislation

The "Code Napoleon" influenced law and organization in most European countries. However, due to historical, organizational, political, and religious reasons, legislation related to resuscitation and defibrillation is different in European countries. In countries where historically only ambulance personnel and paramedics were present on the field, the implementation of early defibrillation by ambulance personnel was easy. In countries, however, where medical presence was prominent in the second or even in the first tier, the introduction of defibrillation by first attending ambulance personnel was much slower.

The data in Table 1 indicate that in several European countries, law is a major or minor obstacle for nationwide implementation of AED programs by nonphysicians. Fortunately, awareness and, as a consequence, legal and regulatory aspects of defibrillation are changing rapidly.

The structure and organization of the EMS system in European countries and the legal background for defibrillation practice are summarized in Table 1.

## Conclusion

In the 21st century, cardiorespiratory arrest due to VF as a consequence of myocardial ischemia or infarction will continue to be a leading cause of sudden unexpected death in the community. Expanded public education of the recognition of the early symptoms and signs of a heart attack is likely to achieve a significant reduction in the present mortality and morbidity rates from of out-of-hospital heart attack.

Electrical defibrillation is the single most important therapy for the treatment of VF. The time interval between the onset of VF and the delivery of the first defibrillating shock is the main determinant of survival. To achieve the goal of early defibrillation, it is mandatory to allow for individuals other than doctors to defibrillate. Development of automated external defibrillators (AED) was a major breakthrough in the therapeutic possibilities and became widely available. Current AEDs are simple, reliable, and training in their use can be achieved in a short time, thus allowing implementation of defibrillation by nonphysicians.

Overwhelming scientific and clinical evidence reinforces early defibrillation as the standard of medical practice. The international scientific community (AHA, ERC, and the member organizations of ILCOR) has issued guidelines for the use of AEDs by the first responding rescuers.

In Scandinavia and UK, AEDs are now available in all front-line ambulances and ambulance personnel are trained in their use. However, in many European countries, early defibrillation with an AED by nonphysicians is not yet implemented on a nationwide basis due to a number of "real" and "perceived" obstacles such as law, structure, priorities, economics, tradition, and inertia.

Defibrillation with AEDs by other first responders such as police, air-

## Table 1

## EMS System in European Countries

| Country | 1st Tier | 2nd Tier | Emergency Phone | Who Is Allowed to Defibrillate |
|---|---|---|---|---|
| Austria | emt | md | 144 | md, emt-d |
| Belgium | emt-(d) | md | 100 (112) | md, rn, emt-d |
| Bulgaria | md | md | 150 | members of re-suscitation team |
| Croatia | md | — | 94 | md |
| Chechnya | emt | md | 155 | md, pm |
| Denmark | emt-(d) | (pm) | 112 | dr, rn, emt-d |
| Finland | emt-(d) | md | 112 | everybody trained |
| France | emt-(d) | md | 15 | md, rn, emt-d |
| Germany | emt-(d) | md | 112 | md, pm |
| Greece | emt | md (urban) | 166 | md (em-d) |
| Hungary | emt-(d) | rn/md | 04 | md, pm, emt-d |
| Iceland | emt-(d) | md | 112 | md, emt-d, rn |
| Ireland | emt | — | 999 | md, rn, pm |
| Italy | emt | (md) | 118 | md, rn |
| Macedonia | md | — | 94 | md |
| Malta | rn | md | 196 | md |
| Netherlands | rn | — | 112 | md, rn |
| Norway | emt-d | md/pm | 113 | md+ assistant in function |
| Poland | md | md | 999 | md, emt(*) |
| Portugal | md | — | 115 | md, emt(*) |
| Romania | emt, rn, md | — | 961 | md |
| Russia | md | — | 03 | md/representative |
| Slovakia | md, pm (emt) | -(md, pm, emt) | 155 | md, rn, emt-d, pm |
| Slovenia | md, rn, emt | — | 112 | md, rn, emt-d |
| Spain | emt, rn, md | — | 061 | md, rn no law |
| Sweden | emt-d (rn) | pm (md) | 112 | md, rn, emt-d |
| Switzerland | emt | (md) | 114 | md, rn, pm |
| Turkey | md, rn | — | 112 | md |
| UK | emt-(d) | (pm) | 999 | no law |
| Yugoslavia | md | md | 94 | md, rn, emt |

Figures between brackets indicate local variations in the country.
md = medical doctor; rn = nurse; pm = paramedic; emt = emergency medical technician; emt-d = emergency medical technician qualified for use of AED.
(*) In presence of a doctor.
For permission to defibrillate, the minimum training level is mentioned.

line, and security personnel was equally demonstrated to be effective. Medical supervision, however, remains a prerequisite for implementing any AED program, and AED programs are most effective if they are part of a well-functioning chain of survival.

## Recommendations

- The medical profession is urged to increase awareness of the public, of those responsible for emergency medical services and of those with regulatory powers, to permit changes in practice and legislation where necessary.
- It is essential to integrate the concept of early defibrillation into an effective emergency cardiac care system, which includes early access to the EMS systems, early CPR by the first witness, early defibrillation when indicated, and early advanced care.
- All emergency personnel should be trained and permitted to operate a defibrillator if their professional activities require that they respond to persons experiencing cardiac arrest. This includes all first-responding emergency personnel working in an organized EMS system, both in and outside the hospital.
- All emergency ambulances that respond to or transport cardiac patients should be equipped with a defibrillator.
- Defibrillation should be a core competence of all health care professionals including nurses, and defibrillators should be widely available on general hospital wards.
- All defibrillator programs must operate within medical control by qualified and experienced physicians. They should ensure that every link of the chain of survival is in place and should have access to all information required to permit system audit.
- To monitor the program, there must be appropriate registration of the interventions according to the Utstein style.

## *References*

1. Murray C, Lopez A. Mortality by cause for eight regions of the world: Global Burden of Disease Study. Lancet 1997; 349:1269–1276 and 1498–1504.
2. Chambless L, et al., for the WHO MONICA Project. Population versus clinical view of case fatality from acute coronary heart disease: results from the WHO MONICA project 1985–1990. Circulation 1997; 96:3849–3859.
3. Fox R. Trends in cardiovascular mortality in Europe. Circulation 1997; 96:3817
4. Hans S, Kesteloot H, Kromhout D. Coronary heart disease mortality in Europe: annual change from 1970 to 1992 in persons 45 to 74 years of age. Eur Heart J 1997; 18:1231–1248.
5. Arntz H, et al. The pre-hospital management of acute heart attacks: recom-

mendations of a task force of the European Society of Cardiology and the European Resuscitation Council. Eur Heart J 1998; 19:1140–1164.

6. Bossaert L. Electrical defibrillation: new technologies. Current Opinion Anaesthesiol 1999; 12:183–193.

7. Cummins R, et al. Special report: recommended guidelines for uniform reporting of data from out-of-hospital cardiac arrest. Resuscitation 1991; 22:91–26; Circulation 1991; 84,2:960–975; Ann Emerg Med 1991; 20(8):861–874, 1991; Br Heart J 1992; 67: 325–333.

8. Cummins R, et al. Recommended guidelines for reviewing, reporting and conducting research on in-hospital resuscitation, the "in-hospital Utstein style." Resuscitation 1997; 34:151–185.

9. Gallagher E, Lombardi G, Gennis P. Cardiac arrest witnessed by prehospital personnel: intersystem variation in initial rhythm as a basis for a proposed extension of the Utstein recommendations. Ann Emerg Med 1997; 30:76–81.

10. Holmberg M, Holmberg S, Herlitz J, Gardelov B. Survival after cardiac arrest outside hospital in Sweden: Swedish Cardiac Arrest Registry. Resuscitation 1998; 36:29–36.

11. Ladwig K, et al. Effects of early defibrillation by ambulance personnel on short- and long-term outcome of cardiac arrest survival: the Munich experiment. Chest 1997; 112:1584–1591.

12. Martens P, Calle P, Vanhaute O. Theoretical calculation of maximum attainable benefit of public access defibrillation in Belgium: Belgian Cardio Pulmonary Cerebral Resuscitation Study Group. Resuscitation 1998; 36:161–163.

13. Mols P, et al. Semi-automatic external defibrillation. Eur J Emerg Med 1994; 1:210–213.

14. Monsieurs K, De Cauwer H, Wuyts F, Bossaert L. A rule for early outcome classification of out-of-hospital cardiac arrest patients presenting with ventricular fibrillation. Resuscitation 1998; 36:37–44.

15. Calle P, et al. The effect of semi-automatic external defibrillation by emergency medical technicians on survival after out-of-hospital cardiac arrest: an observational study in urban and rural areas in Belgium. Acta Clin Belgium 1997; 52:72–83.

16. Herlitz J, et al. Resuscitation in Europe: a tale of five European regions. Resuscitation 1999; 41:121–131.

17. Becker L, Eisenberg M, Fahrenbruch C, Cobb L. Public locations of cardiac arrest: implications for public access defibrillation. Circulation 1998; 97:2106–2109.

18. Stapczynski J, Svenson J, Stone C. Population density, automated external defibrillator use, and survival in rural cardiac arrest. Acad Emerg Med 1997; 4:552–558.

19. Sweeney T, et al. EMT defibrillation does not increase survival from sudden cardiac death in a two-tiered urban-suburban EMS system. Ann Emerg Med 1998; 31:234–240.

20. White R, Asplin B, Bugliosi T, Hankins D. High discharge survival rate after out of hospital ventricular fibrillation with rapid defibrillation by police and paramedics. Ann Emerg Med 1996; 28:480–485.

21. White R. External defibrillation: the need for uniformity in analysing and reporting results. Ann Emerg Med 1998; 32:234–236.

22. Mosesso V, et al. Use of automated external defibrillators by police officers for treatment of out-of-hospital cardiac arrest. Ann Emerg Med 1998; 32:200–207.

23. O'Rourke M, Donaldson E, Geddes J. An airline cardiac arrest program. Circulation 1997; 96:2849–2853.

24. Page R, Hamdan M, McKenas D. Defibrillation aboard a commercial aircraft. Circulation. 1998; 97:1429–1430.
25. Nichol G, et al. Potential cost-effectiveness of public access defibrillation in the United States. Circulation. 1998; 97:1315–1320.
26. Weisfeldt M, et al. Public access defibrillation: a statement for healthcare professionals from the American Heart Association Task Force on Automatic External Defibrillation. Circulation 1995; 92:2763.
27. Cummins R, et al. Low energy biphasic waveform defibrillation: evidence-based review applied to emergency cardiovascular care guidelines. Circulation 1998; 97:1654–1667.
28. Kerber R, et al. Automatic external defibrillators for public access defibrillation: recommendations for specifying and reporting arrhythmia analysis algorithm performance, incorporating new waveforms, and enhancing safety. Circulation 1997; 95:1677–1682, and Biomed Instrum Technol 1997; 31:238–244.
29. Poole J, et al. Low-energy impedance-compensating biphasic waveforms terminate ventricular fibrillation at high rates in victims of out-of-hospital cardiac arrest. LIFE Investigators. J Cardiovasc Electrophysiol 1997; 8:1373–1385.
30. Reddy R, et al. Biphasic transthoracic defibrillation causes fewer ECG ST-segment changes after shock. Ann Emerg Med 1997; 30:127–134.
31. Schneider T, et al. Randomized comparison of 150 J biphasic and 200–360 J monophasic AEDs in out-of-hospital cardiac arrest victims. Eur Heart J 1999; 20:450.
32. Bossaert L, Callanan V, Cummins R. Early defibrillation: an advisory statement by the Advanced Life Support Working Group of the International Liaison Committee on Resuscitation. Resuscitation 1997; 34:113–115.
33. Kloeck W, et al. Early defibrillation: an advisory statement from the Advanced Life Support Working Group of the International Liaison Committee on Resuscitation. Circulation 1997; 95:2183–2185.
34. Bossaert L, et al. European Resuscitation Council guidelines for the use of automated external defibrillators by EMS providers and first responders. Resuscitation 1998; 37:91–94.
35. Robertson C, et al. The 1998 European Resuscitation Council guidelines for adult advanced life support. Resuscitation 1998; 37:81–90.
36. Bossaert L. Fibrillation and defibrillation of the heart. Br J Anaesthesia 1997; 79:203–213.

## 12

# The Maastricht Study:

# A Plea for New Approaches to Improve Results of Out-of-Hospital Resuscitation

*Hein J.J. Wellens, MD,*
*Jacqueline de Vreede-Swagemakers, MD,*
*Aimée Lousberg, MD, and*
*Anton M. Gorgels, MD*

## Introduction

Sudden cardiac death out of hospital continues to haunt us as a medical failure for several reasons. First, the majority of sudden death victims cannot be identified before the event. Second, no universally applicable successful preventive strategy is known, and third, only a minority of the sudden death victims can be resuscitated successfully.

During the past 2 decades, many millions of dollars have been spent to identify risk factors of sufficiently high predictive accuracy to recognize the population with known cardiac disease who are at high risk for dying suddenly. As will be discussed in this chapter, the results of the Maastricht study on sudden death out of hospital questions the wisdom of such an approach and argue in favor of optimizing our out-of-hospital resuscitation efforts.

## The Maastricht Study

As of 1992, all causes of sudden unexpected death out of hospital in the age group 20 to 75 years are carefully registered in the Maastricht area.[1] This is a population of approximately 135,000 persons. In the

From: Aliot E, Clementy J, Prystowsky EN (editors). *Fighting Sudden Cardiac Death: A Worldwide Challenge.* ©Futura Publishing Company, Armonk, NY, 2000.

Maastricht area, there is only 1 hospital, which means that in case of a previous hospital admission for a cardiac cause, information from that event can be retrieved easily. Maastricht has only 1 ambulance service, equipped with motivated personnel and adequate instrumentation for cardiac resuscitation. They carefully document in writing the circumstances of sudden death and the outcome of resuscitative efforts. All general practitioners in the area are regularly contacted to obtain information on cases of unwitnessed sudden death. All information is stored in a databank located in the Department of Cardiology of the Academic Hospital Maastricht.

# Important Findings of the Registry[1,2]

## The Incidence of Sudden Death Out of Hospital

In Maastricht, we found that the incidence of dying suddenly and unexpectedly out of hospital varies with age, gender, and presence or absence of a history of cardiac disease.

The occurrence of sudden death increases with advancing age, is more common in men than in women, and is 10 times more common when a previous history of cardiac disease is present. This means that in men over 55 years of age, 1/4 of all deaths occur suddenly and unexpectedly.

## Place of Sudden Death

As indicated in Table 1, approximately 80% of sudden deaths occurred at home and approximately 15% on the street or in a public place. This suggests that equipping the police or placing automatic defibrillators in public places will not result in a major increase in successful resuscitations.

## Presence and Severity of Known Heart Disease

Approximately 60% of sudden death victims were previously seen in hospital because of cardiac disease (which was more common in men than in women). When examining the hospital records, it was found that 20% of patients had a left ventricular ejection fraction of 30% or less, indicating that of the total group of sudden death victims (with or without a previous cardiac history) only approximately 10% had poor left ventricular function, a finding that is generally accepted as being a strong indicator of high risk for dying suddenly.

## Table 1
### Site of Sudden Cardiac Arrest (501 Consecutive Cases)

|                                      | No. | %    |
|--------------------------------------|-----|------|
| At home                              | 399 | 79.6 |
| On the street                        | 47  | 9.4  |
| Public place                         | 31  | 6.2  |
| Other places                         | 16  | 3.2  |
| At the general practioner's office   | 4   | 0.8  |
| At work                              | 4   | 0.8  |

# Witnessed and Unwitnessed Sudden Death

Forty percent of cases of sudden death were unwitnessed, resulting in the absence of resuscitation efforts. This stresses the necessity of developing reliable and affordable apparatus to document circulatory arrest and to sound a warning alarm.

## Activity at the Time of Sudden Death

As shown in Table 2, the majority of victims were at rest at the time of their sudden cardiac arrest. Only a few cases occurred during strenuous exercise. These observations are in agreement with the finding that 80% of sudden death cases take place at home.

## Resuscitation Attempts and Their Outcome

In Maastricht, 60% of cardiac arrest cases were witnessed. In 75% of these cases, resuscitation was attempted by the ambulance personnel.

## Table 2
### Activity at the Time of Sudden Cardiac Arrest

|                     | No. | %    |
|---------------------|-----|------|
| Lying/sleeping      | 144 | 32.0 |
| Sitting             | 138 | 30.7 |
| Standing/light work | 113 | 25.2 |
| At work             | 30  | 6.6  |
| In the bathroom     | 14  | 3.1  |
| Sports activity     | 11  | 2.4  |

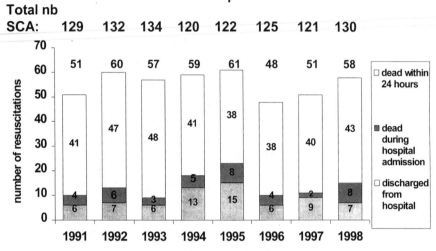

Figure 1. The number of cases of sudden cardiac arrest out of hospital and the number of cases in whom a resuscitation attempt was performed by ambulance personnel (advanced life support). Also indicated is the number of victims reaching the hospital alive and ultimately discharged alive from the hospital.

Twenty-five percent of the victims reached the hospital alive with 15% (approximately 7% of the total number of witnessed and unwitnessed cardiac arrest victims) discharged alive from hospital. As shown in Figure 1, these findings remained about the same over an 8-year period.

## Discussion

As shown in recent articles[3,4] and also in several chapters of this book, much effort and money is continuously put into identifying the characteristics of people dying suddenly from a cardiac arrest to make strategies possible to prevent the event from occurring or to enable successful resuscitation. While scientifically challenging, the sobering finding is the absence of such characteristics in the majority of cases of out-of-hospital sudden death.[5]

This indicates that it might be more rewarding to concentrate on efforts to improve results of resuscitation out of hospital. This means that the several components of the sequence—circulatory arrest to successful resuscitation—have to be controlled and improved. First, instrumentation has to be developed that continuously records cardiac rhythm and alarms the person and those around him of an ominous change in cardiac rhythmic activity. The same instrument should also be able to transmit the location of the victim to the center of advanced life support to bring experienced people and apparatus necessary for successful resuscitation to the victim as soon as possible. Because arrival of the advanced life support crew might take longer than the crucial 5 minutes when circulatory arrest results in serious brain damage, it is essential that the alarm brings people able to perform basic life support to the victim of circulatory arrest. This stresses the necessity of continuing education of the lay person, and especially family members of people with known heart disease, in the technique of basic life support.

The increasing availability and therefore more dense distribution of automated external defibrillators will obviously offer the ability to shorten the duration of circulatory arrest and to treat life-threatening ventricular arrhythmias.

The challenge for industry will be to develop the warning and localization systems described above and to do so at a reasonable price. The first stage will be to provide people with known heart disease with this equipment. Eventually, everybody willing to do so might be wearing such a device.

As pointed out elsewhere,[6] the challenge for cardiology in the coming decades will be to move from palliative to curative and ultimately to preventive therapy of cardiovascular diseases. Realistically, it will take several years to reach that goal. Sudden cardiac arrest kills many people whose hearts are "too good to die" and successful resuscitation will allow them a long and fruitful continuation of life. At the present time, it seems logical, therefore, to concentrate on measures to improve outcome of out-of-hospital resuscitation.

## Conclusion

To substantially reduce the number of victims dying suddenly out of hospital, it might be more rewarding to develop better warning and localization systems than to continue the search for the perfect test for risk stratification.

*Acknowledgement: The Maastricht Study is possible only because of the help of many. We gratefully acknowledge the support of the general practitioners of the area, the Health Service of Maastricht, and the Department of General Practice of the University of Maastricht.*

## References

1. De Vreede-Swagemakers JJM, Gorgels APM, Dubous-Arbouw W, Van Ree JW, Daemen MJAP, et al. Out-of-hospital cardiac arrest in the 1990's: a population-

based study in the Maastricht area on incidence, characteristics and survival. J Am Coll Cardiol 1997; 30:1500–1505.
2. De Vreede-Swagemakers JJM, Gorgels APM, Van Ree JW, Stijns RE, Wellens HJJ. Circumstances and causes of out-of-hospital cardiac arrest in sudden death survivors. Heart 1998; 79:356–361.
3. Wellens HJJ. Key references on sudden death. Circulation 1994; 90:2547–2553.
4. Zipes DP, Wellens HJJ. Sudden cardiac death. Circulation 1998; 98:2334–2351.
5. Demirovic J, Myerburg RJ. Epidemiology of sudden coronary death: an overview. Prog Cardiovasc Dis 1994; 37:39–48.
6. Wellens HJJ. The present and future of cardiology. Lancet (in press).

# 13

# European Resuscitation Council Guidelines for Resuscitation of the Adult Cardiac Arrest Victim

*Leo Bossaert*

## From the International Liaison Committee on Resuscitation (ILCOR) Policy Statements to the European Resuscitation Council (ERC) Model Guidelines

The European Resuscitation Council (ERC) was established in 1989 as an interdisciplinary council for resuscitation medicine and emergency medical care.

The objectives of the ERC are to improve standards of resuscitation in Europe and to coordinate the activities of European organizations with a major interest in cardiopulmonary resuscitation (CPR). The ERC pursues its objectives by: (1) producing guidelines and recommendations appropriate to Europe for the practice of CPR; (2) updating these guidelines in the light of critical review of CPR practice; (3) promoting audit of resuscitation practice by standardization of records of CPR attempts; (4) designing standardized teaching programs suitable for all levels of trainees in Europe; (5) promoting and coordinating appropriate research; (6) organizing relevant congresses and other scientific meetings in Europe; and (7) promoting political and public awareness of CPR requirements and practice in Europe.

In 1973, the American Heart Association (AHA) first published the *Standards for Cardiopulmonary Resuscitation and Emergency Cardiac Care*. At the time, only a few of the recommended measures were based on scientific evidence, but the medical world accepted them as the gold standard for resuscitation care. Since 1973, many national and supranational guide-

From: Aliot E, Clementy J, Prystowsky EN (editors). *Fighting Sudden Cardiac Death: A Worldwide Challenge.* ©Futura Publishing Company, Armonk, NY, 2000.

lines have been developed and published to complement the AHA standards. All new guidelines included detailed advice that was mostly scientifically unproven but was justified on the basis of clinical experience and tradition. Difficulties have arisen in relation to: medical considerations (examples: mouth-to-nose ventilation, ventilation volumes, pulse check, the Heimlich maneuver, availability of drugs); medico-legal issues (example: the role in resuscitation by nonphysicians); ethical and religious matters (notably in relation to DNAR orders); and linguistic problems (especially in Europe where more than 50 different languages are spoken).

In 1992–1996, the ERC presented *Guidelines for Basic, Advanced and Pediatric Life Support, for the Management of Peri-Arrest Arrhythmias, for the Basic and Advanced Management of the Airway and Ventilation during Resuscitation.* The guidelines were published in *Resuscitation,* which is the official journal of the ERC. They were translated in many languages and received wide acceptance and distribution throughout Europe.[1–8]

Against this background, ILCOR was founded in 1992 and comprises representatives of the AHA, the ERC, the Australian Resuscitation Council, the Resuscitation Council of Southern Africa, and the Resuscitation Council of Latin America. The mission of ILCOR is: "To provide a consensus mechanism by which the international science and knowledge relevant to emergency cardiac care can be identified and reviewed. This consensus mechanism will be used to provide consistent international guidelines for basic life support, pediatric life support, and advanced life support. These international guidelines will aim for a commonality supported by science for BLS [basic life support], PLS [pediatric life support], and ALS [adult life support]."

The constituent organizations agreed to make use of this resource so that all future guidelines will reflect the commonality of opinion that has evolved during the process. The first ILCOR advisory statements were published in 1997 in the journals *Resuscitation* and *Circulation.*[9–11]

In the time period after the publication of the ILCOR statements, the ERC has updated the 1992 Guidelines for Basic Life Support, Pediatric Life Support, and Advanced Life Support and adjusted them to the Advisory Statements of ILCOR. Because of the rapidly growing use of automated external defibrillators (AEDs) by ambulance personnel and by first responders, guidelines for the use of AEDs were also developed.

The ERC has closely followed the ILCOR statements in the 1998 *Model Guidelines,* which offer an authoritative supranational European model. These in turn may be adopted in toto by European national councils or adapted as necessary for specific national guidelines where medico-legal, ethical, religious, or medical considerations make it necessary to have local variations. These variations must be approved by the ERC in order to carry its name.[1–3]

# The ERC Guidelines for Adult Basic Life Support (BLS)

## The ILCOR Advisory Statements[9-11]

### Moving Toward Simplicity

Guidelines should be as simple as possible. After 30 years of public CPR education, most communities still do not train a sufficiently high proportion of the public to perform basic CPR. Increasing the efforts to teach CPR to the public is a vital priority for all communities.

There are many obstacles to lay CPR training. Psychomotor skills of CPR are too complex for the lay public, and retention of skills by people who do not use them regularly has been disappointing.

There is scientific uncertainty within the literature regarding how "good" CPR has to be in order to save a life. Any CPR (chest compression only) is clearly better than no CPR. Therefore, a simple, basic approach that can be effectively taught to the largest number of people will increase the number of individuals willing to attempt BLS.

### Circulatory Assessment

To date, all resuscitation councils require determination of absence of the carotid pulse as the diagnostic step that leads to the initiation of chest compression.

Recent studies suggest that the time needed to diagnose with confidence the presence or absence of a carotid pulse is far greater than the 5–10 seconds normally recommended. Even with prolonged palpation, 45% of carotid pulses may be pronounced absent even when present. Most of these studies were done in normotensive volunteers, a situation far different from finding a collapsed and cyanosed victim in the street who is likely to be hypotensive and vasoconstricted.

As a result of these studies, the BLS group considered that the carotid pulse check should be "de-emphasized" and that other criteria should be used to determine the need for chest compression in an unresponsive, apneic, adult patient. It was decided to use the expression "look for signs of life," which includes checking for movement as well as checking the carotid pulse. The rescuer should limit the time for this check to no more than 10 seconds. Therefore, the absence of any obvious signs of life, not necessarily the absence of the carotid pulse, should be sufficient indication to initiate chest compression.

## Volume and Rate of Ventilation

Rescue breathing is a well-accepted technique of airway management in BLS for the past 40 years. The volume of air required to be given with each inflation is usually quoted as 800–1,200 cc, with each breath taking 1–1.5 seconds.

Artificial ventilation without airway protection (such as tracheal intubation) carries a high risk of gastric inflation, regurgitation, and pulmonary aspiration. The risk of gastric inflation depends on the proximal airway pressure, which is determined by tidal volume and inflation rate, the alignment of the head and neck, and patency of the airway and the opening pressure of the lower esophageal sphincter (approximately 20 cm $H_2O$). It has recently been shown that a tidal volume of 400–500 cc is sufficient to give adequate ventilation in adult BLS because $CO_2$ production during cardiac arrest is very low. This recommendation overrules earlier guidelines and makes it necessary to recalibrate adult training mannequins. It is, however, consistent with the accepted teaching that the tidal volume should be that which causes the chest to rise.

## Call First–Call Fast

The optimum time during a CPR attempt to leave the victim and go for help will depend on whether the rescuer is alone, whether the victim has a primary respiratory or primary cardiac arrest, the distance to the nearest point of aid, and the facilities of the emergency medical service (EMS).

The importance of early defibrillation in the treatment of sudden cardiac death is now accepted. The 1992 AHA guidelines emphasized that the rescuer should, if no other help is available, leave an adult victim immediately after establishing unresponsiveness in order to call an ambulance or EMS system ("phone first"). The 1992 ERC guidelines advise that a shout for assistance should be made as soon as the victim is found to be unconscious, but that the lone rescuer should not leave to go for help until cardiac arrest is diagnosed by a pulse check ("phone fast"). Both the AHA and the ERC guidelines seek to ensure that a defibrillator reaches the victim at the earliest appropriate opportunity.

In children, respiratory arrest is far more common than cardiac arrest, and survival will depend mainly on the immediate delivery of effective rescue breathing, hence the recommendation of 1 minute of rescue support before leaving and phoning for help.

It is recognized that the result of the "call first–call fast" debate will vary in different parts of the world because of the different organization and functioning of EMS systems. For this reason, these advisory state-ments include 2 possible points in time when the lone rescuer may need to leave the victim to get help: after responsiveness is established, or after the airway has been opened but breathing has not resumed. In order to try to identify cases of primary respiratory arrest, "1 minute of resuscitation" is advised when dealing with children and victims of trauma and near drowning.

## Recovery Position

The airway of an unconscious victim who is breathing spontaneously is at risk of obstruction by the tongue and from inhalation of mucus and vomit. Placing the victim on the side helps to prevent these problems and allows fluid to drain easily from the mouth.

ILCOR agreed on 6 principles for recovery position in the unconscious breathing victim:

1. The position should be a true lateral with the head dependent;
2. The position should be stable;
3. Any pressure of the chest that impairs breathing should be avoided;
4. It should be possible to turn the victim onto the side and return to the back easily;
5. Good observation of and access to the airway should be possible;
6. The position should not give rise to injury to the victim.

## The ERC Guidelines for Adult Basic Life Support (Figure 1)[1]

### Sequence of Actions

1. Ensure *safety* of rescuer and victim.
2. *Check responsiveness:* shake the shoulders and ask: "Are you all right?"
3a. If victim responds by answering or moving:
   - Leave in the position in which you find the victim, check victim's condition, and get help if needed.
   - Reassess regularly.
3b. If victim does not respond:
   - Shout for help.
   - Open the airway by tilting the head and lifting the chin.
   - Avoid head tilt if trauma (injury) to the neck is suspected.
4. *Check breathing:* Keeping the airway open, check breathing (Figure 2).
   - Look for chest movements.

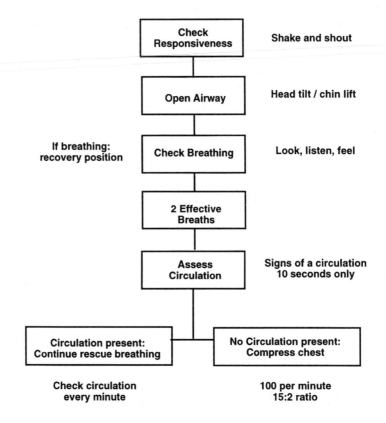

**Send or go for help as soon as possible according to guidelines**

Figure 1. The ERC guidelines for adult basic life support.

-     Listen for breath sounds.
-     Feel for air on your cheek.
-     Look, listen, and feel for 10 seconds before deciding that breathing is absent.

5a. If the victim is *breathing* (other than an occasional gasp):
-     Turn victim into the recovery position.
-     Check for continued breathing.

5b. If the victim is *not breathing:*
-     Send for help. If you are on your own, leave the victim and go for help; return and start rescue breathing.

- Turn the victim onto his back.
- Remove obstruction from the victim's mouth.
- Give 2 *effective* rescue breaths, each of which makes the chest rise and fall.
- Ensure head tilt and chin lift.
- Pinch victim's nose closed.
- Take a breath and place your lips around his mouth, with a good seal.
- Blow steadily into his mouth for about 1.5 to 2 seconds watching for his chest to rise (usually 400–600 mL).
- Maintaining open airway, take your mouth away from the victim and watch for his chest to fall as air comes out.
- Take another breath and repeat the sequence as above to give 2 effective rescue breaths (Figure 3).

6. Assess the victim for *signs of circulation:*
   - Look for any movement, including swallowing or breathing.
   - Check the carotid pulse.
   - Take *no more than 10 seconds* to do this.

7a. If you are confident that you can detect *signs of circulation* within 10 seconds:
   - Continue rescue breathing.
   - About every minute recheck for signs of circulation.

7b. If there are *no signs of circulation,* or you are unsure, start chest compression: Locate the lower half of the sternum.
   - Place the heel of one hand there, with the other hand on top of the first.
   - Interlock the fingers of both hands and lift them to avoid pressure over the victim's ribs.
   - Position yourself vertically above the victim's chest and, with your arms straight, press down on the sternum to depress it between 4–5 cm (Figure 4).
   - Release the pressure, without losing contact between the hand and sternum, then repeat at a rate of about 100 times a minute. Compression and release should take an equal amount of time.
   - Combine rescue breathing and chest compression, continuing compressions and breaths in a ratio of 15:2 (Figure 5).

8. Continue resuscitation until qualified help arrives, the victim shows signs of life, or you become exhausted.

## Recovery Position

There are different positions that fulfill most of the criteria recommended by ILCOR. National resuscitation councils and other major or-

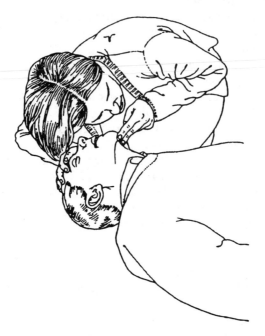

Figure 2. Open the airway; check breathing.

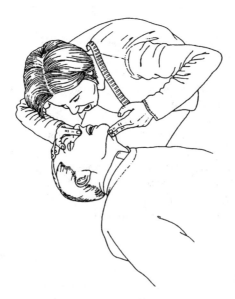

Figure 3. Give 2 effective breaths.

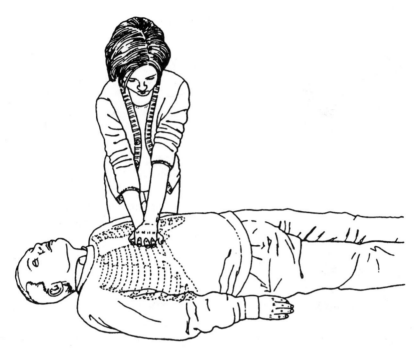

Figure 4. Compress the chest.

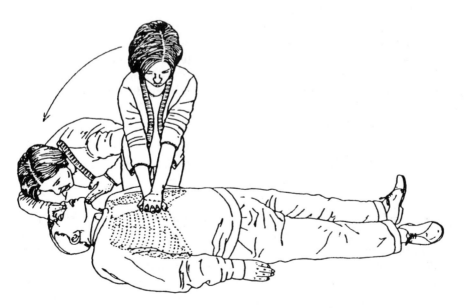

Figure 5. Rescue breathing and chest compression.

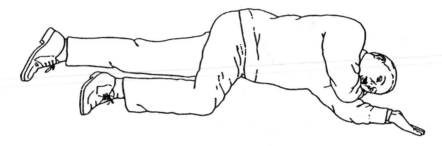

Figure 6. Recovery position.

ganizations should consider adopting one of the several available options so that training and practice can be consistent. The position recommended by the ERC is shown in Figure 6.

### When to Get Help

It is vital for rescuers to get help as quickly as possible.

- When there is more than one rescuer, one starts resuscitation and the other goes for help.
- A lone rescuer will have to decide whether to start resuscitation or to go for help first. This decision will be influenced by the availability of EMS and local practice.
- However, if the likely cause of unconsciousness is trauma (injury), drowning, or if the victim is an infant or a child, the rescuer should perform resuscitation for about 1 minute before going for help.
- If the victim is an adult, and the cause of unconsciousness is NOT trauma (injury) or drowning, the rescuer should assume that the victim has a heart problem and go for help immediately if it has been established that the victim is not breathing.

## The 1998 ERC Guidelines for Adult Advanced Life Support

The ERC recognized that the previous guidelines necessitated a level of rhythm recognition, interpretation, and subsequent decision making that some users found difficult. While automated external defibrillators (AEDs) ease some of these problems, the 1992 guidelines were not specifically designed for these devices. These 1998 guidelines are applicable to manual and automated external defibrillators. Decision making has been reduced to a minimum whenever possible. This increases clarity while still allowing individuals with specialist knowledge to apply their expertise.

The limitations of guidelines must be recognized. While much is known about the theory and practice of resuscitation, in many areas our ignorance is profound. Resuscitation practice remains as much an art as a science. Further, the interpretation of guidelines may differ according to the environment in which they are used. We acknowledge that individual resuscitation councils may wish to customize the details while accepting that the guiding principles are universal. Any such changes must be approved by the ERC if they are to be regarded by this organization as their official guidelines.[2]

## Specific ALS Interventions and Their Use in the ALS Algorithm

### Defibrillation

In adults, the most common arrhythmia at the onset of cardiac arrest is ventricular fibrillation (VF) or pulseless ventricular tachycardia (VT). The majority of eventual survivors come from this group. The *only* interventions that unequivocally improve long-term survival are basic life support and defibrillation. VF is a treatable rhythm, but the chances of successful defibrillation decline substantially with time. The amplitude and waveform of VF deteriorate rapidly, reflecting the depletion of myocardial high-energy phosphate stores. The rate of decline in success depends in part on the provision and adequacy of BLS. As a result, the priority is to minimize any delay between the onset of cardiac arrest and the administration of defibrillating shocks.

At present, the most commonly used transthoracic defibrillation waveforms are damped sinusoidal. Newer techniques such as biphasic waveforms may reduce the energy requirements for successful defibrillation. Automated biphasic waveform defibrillators are available and are being evaluated. Their use may increase the efficacy of individual shocks and reduce myocardial injury in patients with unusually high, or low, transthoracic impedance.

With conventional defibrillators, shocks are delivered in groups of 3, the initial sequence having energies of 200 J, 200 J, and 360 J. There is evidence that myocardial injury is greater with increasing energies.

Alternative waveforms and energy levels are acceptable if demonstrated to be of equal or greater net clinical benefit in terms of safety and efficacy. A pulse check is required after a shock only if a change in waveform to one compatible with cardiac output is produced. With modern defibrillators, charging times are sufficiently short for 3 shocks to be administered within 1 minute.

## Airway Management and Ventilation

Tracheal intubation remains the optimal procedure, but the technique can be difficult and regular experience and refresher training are required. The laryngeal mask airway offers an alternative to tracheal intubation. The pharyngotracheal lumen airway and the Combitube are alternatives but require more training and have specific problems in use.

During cardiac arrest and CPR, lung characteristics change because of an increase in dead space while the development of pulmonary edema reduces lung compliance. Oxygenation of the patient is the primary objective of ventilation, and the aim should be to provide inspired oxygen concentrations ($FiO_2$) of 1.0. Tidal volumes of 400–600 mL are adequate to make the chest rise and to eliminate $CO_2$.

Ventilation techniques vary from simple bag valve devices to the most sophisticated automatic ventilators which can provide an $FiO_2$ of 1.0, consistent tidal volumes, inspiratory flow rates, and respiratory frequencies that are adjustable on demand.

## CPR Techniques

The only change recommended in the technique of closed chest compression is that the rate should be 100/min. There have been and are ongoing trials of new techniques, most notably with active compression-decompression (ACD) CPR, but there are at present no clinical data showing unequivocal improvement in outcomes. To improve the scientific basis for future recommendations, the use of new techniques should be carefully evaluated by clinical trials before implementation into prehospital and in-hospital practice.

## Drug Delivery

The venous route remains the optimal method of drug administration during CPR. If already in situ, a central venous catheter can deliver drugs rapidly to the central circulation. If a central line is not present, the decision as to peripheral versus central cannulation will depend on the skill of the operator, the nature of the surrounding events, and available equipment. If a decision is made to attempt central venous cannulation, this must not delay defibrillation attempts, CPR, or airway security. When peripheral venous cannulation and drug delivery is performed, a flush of 20 mL of 0.9% saline is advised to expedite entry to the circulation.

The administration of drugs via a tracheal tube remains only a second-line approach because of impaired absorption and unpredictable pharmacodynamics. Agents that can be given by this route are adrenaline, lidocaine, and atropine. Doses of 2–3 times the standard IV dose diluted up to a total volume of at least 10 mL of 0.9% saline are currently recommended. Following administration, 5 ventilations are given to increase dispersion to the distal bronchial tree, thus maximizing absorption.

## Specific Drug Therapy

*Vasopressors:* Experimentally, adrenaline improves myocardial and cerebral blood flow and resuscitation rates in animals, and higher doses are more effective than the "standard" dose of 1 mg. There is no clinical evidence that adrenaline improves survival or neurological recovery in humans regardless of whether the standard dose or a high dose is used. Some clinical trials have reported slightly increased rates of spontaneous circulation with high-dose adrenaline but without improvement in overall survival rate. The reasons for the difference between experimental and clinical results are likely to reflect differences in underlying pathology and the relatively long periods of arrest before the ALS team is able to give adrenaline in the out-of-hospital clinical setting. It is also possible that higher doses of adrenaline may be detrimental in the post-resuscitation period. The indications, dosage, and time interval between doses for adrenaline remain unchanged. In practical terms, for non-VF/VT rhythms, each loop of the algorithm lasts 3 minutes and therefore adrenaline is given with every loop. For VF/VT rhythms, the process of rhythm assessment, 3 defibrillatory shocks followed by 1 minute of CPR will take 2–3 minutes. Thus, adrenaline should generally be given with each loop.

Caution should be used before routinely administering adrenaline in patients whose arrest is associated with solvent abuse, cocaine, and other sympathomimetic drugs.

The evidence regarding other vasopressors is limited. Experimentally, vasopressin leads to significantly higher coronary perfusion pressures, and preliminary data in relation to restoration of spontaneous circulation rates may be encouraging, but at present, no pressor agent other than adrenaline can be recommended.

*Antiarrhythmic Agents:* There is insufficient evidence to make firm recommendations on the use of any antiarrhythmic agent, although our knowledge of lidocaine is greater than that of the others. Pending the results of trials, it is recommended that no change be made in the previous recommendations with regard to lidocaine, bretylium, and other antiarrhythmic agents.

Atropine has a well-established role in the treatment of hemodynamically compromising bradyarrhythmias. Since any adverse effect is unlikely, its use can still be considered in a single dose of 3 mg IV. This dose is known to be sufficient to block vagal activity effectively in fit adults with a cardiac output.[4,5]

*Buffer Agents:* In previously healthy individuals, arterial blood gas analysis does not show a rapid or severe development of acidosis during cardiorespiratory arrest provided effective BLS is performed. The role of buffers in CPR is still uncertain.

Pending further studies, it is suggested that the judicious use of buffers be limited to severe acidosis as defined in the previous guidelines (arterial pH <7.1 and base excess <−10) and to certain special situations, such as cardiac arrest associated with hyperkalemia or following tricyclic antidepressant overdose. For sodium bicarbonate, a dose of 50 mmol (50 mL of an 8.4% solution) is appropriate, with further administration dependent on the clinical situation and repeat arterial blood gas analysis.

## Using the Universal Algorithm (Figure 7)

Each step that follows in the ALS algorithm assumes that the preceding one has been unsuccessful. A precordial thump may, in case of a witnessed event, precede the attachment of a monitor/defibrillator.

ECG monitoring then provides the link between BLS and ALS procedures. ECG rhythm assessment must always be interpreted within the clinical context as movement artifact, lead disconnection, and electrical interference can mimic rhythms associated with cardiac arrest.

Following this assessment, the algorithm splits into 2 pathways: VF/VT and other rhythms.

### VF/VT Rhythms

The first defibrillating shock must be given without any delay. If unsuccessful, it is repeated once and if necessary, twice. This initial group of 3 shocks should occur with successive energies of 200 J, 200 J, and 360 J. If VF/VT persists, further shocks are given with 360 J energies or the biphasic equivalent. A pulse check is performed if, after a defibrillating shock, a

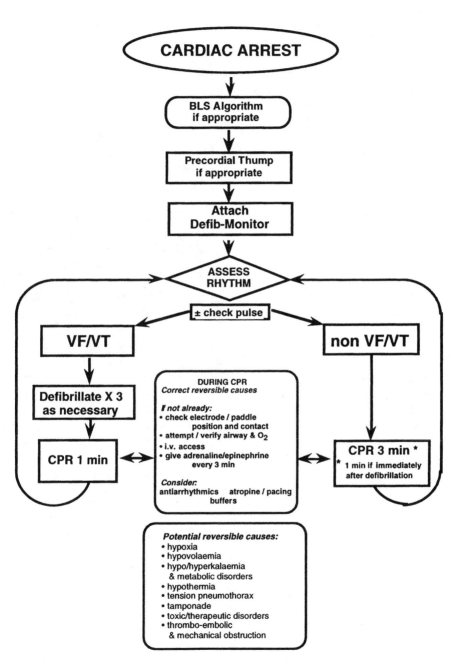

Figure 7. The universal adult life support algorithm.

change in waveform is produced that is compatible with output. If the monitor/defibrillator indicates that VF/VT persists, then further DC shocks are administered without a further pulse check.

It is important to note that after a shock, the ECG monitor screen will often show an isoelectric line for several seconds. This is commonly due to a transient period of electrical and/or myocardial "stunning," and does not necessarily mean that the rhythm has converted to asystole, because a coordinated rhythm or return of VF/VT may subsequently supervene. If the monitor screen of a manual defibrillator shows a "straight" line for more than 1 sweep immediately after a shock, 1 minute of CPR should be given without a new dose of adrenaline, and the patient should be reassessed. Only if the result of this reassessment is a non-VF/VT rhythm without a pulse should a new dose of adrenaline be administered and CPR given for a further 2 minutes before the patient is assessed again.

During defibrillation, no one should be in contact with the patient. Liquids, wet clothing, or the spreading of excess electrode gel can cause problems. Transdermal patches should be removed to prevent the possibility of electrical arcing. Paddle pads should be kept 12–15 cm away from implanted pacemakers. During manual defibrillation, the operator must give a command ("stand clear!") and check that this is obeyed before the shock is given.

Over 80% of individuals who will be successfully defibrillated have this achieved by 1 of the first 3 shocks. Subsequently, the best prospects for restoring a perfusing rhythm still remain with defibrillation, but at this stage, the search for and correction of potentially reversible causes or aggravating factors is indicated, together with an opportunity to maintain myocardial and cerebral viability with chest compressions and ventilation. During CPR, attempts can be made to institute advanced airway management and ventilation, venous access, and to administer drugs if appropriate to do so.

The time interval between the third and fourth shocks should not exceed 2 minutes. Although the interventions, which can be performed during this period, may improve the prospects for successful defibrillation, this is unproven, and it is well established that with the passage of time, the chances of success for defibrillating shocks diminish.

### "Looping" the Algorithm

For the patient with persistent VF/VT, potential causes or aggravating factors may include electrolyte imbalance, hypothermia, and drugs and toxic agents for which specific treatment may be indicated. Where it is appropriate to continue resuscitation, successive loops of the algorithm are followed, allowing further sequences of shocks, basic life support, and the ability to perform and secure advanced airway and ventilation techniques, oxygenation, and drug delivery. Antiarrhythmic drugs may be considered after the first 2 sets of 3 shocks, although maintaining the previous policy of deferring this treatment until 4 sets would be acceptable.

## Non-VF/VT Rhythms

If VF/VT can be positively excluded, defibrillation is not indicated as a primary intervention.

For patients in cardiac arrest with non-VF/VT rhythms, the prognosis is less favorable. The overall survival rate with these rhythms is approximately 10–15% of the survival rate with VF/VT rhythms, but the possibility of survival should not be disregarded. With the passage of time, all electrical rhythms associated with cardiac arrest deteriorate with the eventual production of asystole.

There are some situations where a non-VF/VT rhythm may be caused or aggravated by remediable conditions. During the search for and correction of these causes, CPR, together with advanced airway management, oxygenation, ventilation, and any necessary attempts to secure venous access, should occur, with adrenaline administered every 3 minutes.

The use of atropine for asystole was discussed above. Atropine 3 mg IV is given once, along with adrenaline 1 mg for asystole on the first loop. Pacing may play a valuable role in patients with extreme bradyarrhythmias, but its value in asystole is questionable, except in cases of AV block where P waves are seen. In patients where pacing is to be performed, but a delay occurs before it can be achieved, external cardiac percussion (known as "fist" or "thump" pacing) may generate QRS complexes with an effective cardiac output, particularly in cases where myocardial contractility is not critically compromised. Conventional CPR should be substituted immediately if QRS complexes with a discernable output are not being achieved.

After 3 minutes of CPR, the patient's electrical rhythm is reassessed. If VF/VT has supervened, the left-sided path of the algorithm is followed, otherwise loops of the right-sided path of the algorithm will continue for as long as it is considered appropriate for resuscitation to continue. Resuscitation should generally continue for at least 20–30 minutes from the time of collapse unless there are overwhelming reasons to believe that resuscitation is likely to be futile.

## Post-Resuscitation Care

The most vulnerable system for the ischemic/hypoxic damage occurring in association with cardiac arrest is the central nervous system (CNS). Approximately 1/3 of the patients who have return of spontaneous circulation die a neurological death, with 1/3 of long-term survivors having some degree of recognizable motor or cognitive deficits.

There are no new clinically validated treatment strategies for the cerebral damage sustained with cardiac arrest. Efforts should be directed to the avoidance and/or correction of hypotension, hypoxia, hypercarbia, electrolyte imbalance, and hypo- or hyperglycemia.

Many victims of cardiac arrest have features indicating that the event was precipitated by acute myocardial infarction. In these patients, there is an urgent need for appropriate management, including such aspects as thrombolysis or other methods for obtaining coronary reperfusion and maintaining electrical stability to reduce the chances of further episodes of cardiac arrest and to improve the overall prognosis. These aspects are covered by the publications on the Management of Acute Myocardial Infarction of the European Society of Cardiology and the ESC/ERC Task Force on the Prehospital Management of Myocardial Infarction.[8]

# ERC Guidelines for the Use of Automated External Defibrillators (AEDs) by EMS Providers and First Responders (Figure 8)

- Electrical defibrillation is the single most important therapy for the treatment of ventricular fibrillation. The time interval between the onset of ventricular fibrillation and the delivery of the first shock is clearly the main determinant of survival. Studies have shown that survival falls by approximately 7–10% for every minute after collapse for patients found in ventricular fibrillation. The ERC strongly endorses the concept of early defibrillation within the chain of survival. To achieve the goal of early defibrillation, it is mandatory to allow individuals other than physicians to defibrillate. The scientific and clinical evidence overwhelmingly reinforces this as the only acceptable strategy. Having accepted this principle, the medical profession is urged to bring pressure to bear on the public, those responsible for directing emergency services within the hospital and prehospital, and those with regulatory powers, to permit changes in practice and legislation where necessary.
- The purpose of the ERC is to produce guidelines for automated defibrillation performed by first responders other than physicians, defined as a trained individual acting independently within a medically controlled system. These include:
  - first responding professional or volunteer EMS personnel.
  - first responders other than EMS personnel prior to the arrival of the EMS.

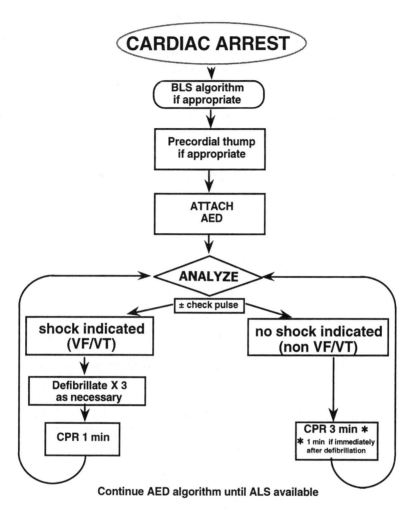

Figure 8. ERC guidelines for the use of AEDs by EMS providers and first responders.

- The ERC recommends
    - that every ambulance in Europe, which might respond to a cardiac arrest, must carry a defibrillator with personnel trained and permitted to use it.
    - that defibrillation should be one of the core competencies of doctors, nurses, and other health care professionals.
    - that defibrillators should be widely placed on general hospital wards.
    - to investigate the feasibility and efficacy of allowing all those assigned to the management of cardiac arrest in the community to be

trained and permitted to defibrillate. These first responders could include police, security officers, lifeguards, and volunteer first aiders.
- All first-responder defibrillation programs must operate within strict medical control by physicians qualified and experienced in emergency program management, who will have responsibility for ensuring that each link of the chain of survival is in place and who have appropriate access to patient outcome information permitting systems audit using the Utstein template.[12,13]

# Guidelines for the Use of Automated External Defibrillators

## Arrival of Rescuers

- If 2 EMS providers are available, one should rapidly approach the patient and start defibrillation sequence while the other requests backup help if appropriate, brings additional equipment to the arrest victim, and assists with CPR.
- Fetch AED and activate EMS: A single first responder should activate the EMS and get the defibrillator as rapidly as possible. In practice, it would be unusual for this person to have to leave the patient without anyone else being available to give CPR.
- Use mobile communications: It is essential that, when defibrillators are used, communications are available simultaneously to activate the other components of the chain of survival. When defibrillation is provided by basic life support EMS providers within a 2-tiered system, it is essential that they have access to mobile communications in order to contact the adult life support providers.

## Basic Life Support, If Appropriate

Check response, open airway and check for breathing, check circulation. Where an automated external defibrillator is immediately at hand, time should not be wasted performing the 2 ventilations after checking for breathing. Those trained in defibrillation should be taught to perform a pulse check, which is an important part of checking for signs of circulation. Where no defibrillator is available yet, the approved basic life support algorithm should be followed.

## Precordial Thump, If Appropriate

If the rescuer is trained in ALS and cardiac arrest is witnessed or monitored, a precordial thump may be given before the defibrillator is attached. Those trained only in BLS should not delay giving a precordial thump.

## Attach the Defibrillator

The carrying pouch with the AED must provide some strong scissors for cutting and a disposable razor for shaving chest hairs in order to obtain good electrode contact.

## Shock Indicated

When a shock is indicated, the priority is rapid defibrillation. Checking the pulse between the first 3 shocks is counterproductive because it interferes with proper rhythm analysis.

*After the first 3 shocks,* uninterrupted CPR should be given for 1 minute. There should be no "check pulse" or "analyze" prompts and the CPR interval (usually 4 cycles of 1-rescuer CPR) will be timed by the AED timer.

## No Shock Indicated

When no shock is indicated, the rhythm is likely to be either asystole or an organized but nonperfusing rhythm (electromechanical dissociation or pulseless electrical activity). In these circumstances, at the first analysis, uninterrupted CPR should be given for 3 minutes in line with the guidelines for ALS. During these 3 minutes there should be no "check pulse" or "press analyze" prompts, because these will interrupt the performance of CPR. CPR itself may produce an artifact, which may be recognized as a shockable rhythm.

When no shock is indicated for the first time after an episode of VF, the period of CPR before the next analysis is only 1 minute.

## Continue the AED Algorithm Until ALS Is Available

When no shock is indicated and no pulse is present, CPR should be uninterrupted and sustained either during transport to an ALS facility, until an ALS unit arrives, or until life is pronounced extinct according to local procedures.

If the AED is being used by ALS-trained EMS providers, they should then continue with the ALS algorithm (intubation, ventilation, IV access, drug delivery, etc.).

In persisting VF/VT, the course of action of the rescuers would be dictated by local policy. In some systems, it is unacceptable to move the patient until the arrival of ALS rescuers. In others, it is thought that, after a number of shocks (e.g., 12) when transport is available, it is permissible to move the patient to an advanced life support facility while continuing CPR.

## Training in the Use of AEDs

- Initial training in resuscitation involving AEDs should take about 8 hours. This is usually the amount of time that is required to achieve the competencies in knowledge of the chain of survival and defibrillation algorithms, BLS and defibrillation, and to allow practice and testing in simulated scenarios. Depending on previous training and experience in life support, the time taken to achieve competence with an AED might be considerably shorter.
- Refresher training should be carried out at least every 6 months. Reinforcement of the skills and knowledge learned is most important in the early stages of the program. Refreshment in the use of the equipment controls and the checking of the apparatus should be *at least* 6 monthly. The amount of time that is usually required for refresher training is 2 hours, depending on previous training and experience.
- Training should be given by specifically certified instructors working within a medically controlled system.
- Registration: The satisfactory completion of a course in the use of the AED (and the associated certification in competency) does not in itself imply any license to use the equipment or skills. The medical controller of the system who should be required to maintain a register of first responder providers should provide licensing.

## *References*

1. Handley A, Bahr J, Baskett P, Bossaert L, Chamberlain D, et al. The 1998 European Resuscitation Council guidelines for adult single rescuer basic life support. Resuscitation 1998; 37:67–80.
2. Robertson C, et al. The 1998 European Resuscitation Council guidelines for adult advanced life support. Resuscitation 1998; 37:81–90.
3. Bossaert L, et al. European Resuscitation Council guidelines for the use of automated external defibrillators by EMS providers and first responders. Resuscitation 1998; 37:91–94.
4. Chamberlain D, et al. Peri-arrest arrhythmias (management of arrhythmias associated with cardiac arrest): a statement by the Advanced Life Support Committee of the European Resuscitation Council, 1994. Resuscitation 1994; 28:151–159.
5. Chamberlain D, et al. Peri-arrest arrhythmias: notice of 1st update. Resuscitation 1996; 31:281.
6. Baskett P, et al. Guidelines for the basic management of the airway and ventilation during resuscitation. Resuscitation 1996; 31:187–200.

7. Baskett P, et al. Guidelines for the advanced management of the airway and ventilation during resuscitation. Resuscitation 1996; 31:201–230.

8. Arntz H, et al. The pre-hospital management of acute heart attacks: recommendations of a Task Force of the European Society of Cardiology and the European Resuscitation Council. Eur Heart J 1998; 19:1140–1164.

9. Handley A, Becker L, Allen M, Van Drenth A, Kramer E, et al. Single rescuer adult basic life support: an advisory statement by the Basic Life Support Working Group of the International Liaison Committee on Resuscitation.Resuscitation 1997; 34:101–108.

10. Kloeck W, et al. Early defibrillation: an advisory statement from the Advanced Life Support Working Group of the International Liaison Committee on Resuscitation. Circulation 1997; 95:2183–2185.

11. Bossaert L, Callanan V, Cummins R. Early defibrillation: an advisory statement by the Advanced Life Support Working Group of the International Liaison Committee on Resuscitation. Resuscitation 1997; 34:113–115.

12. Cummins R, et al. Special report: recommended guidelines for uniform reporting of data from out-of-hospital cardiac arrest. Resuscitation 1991, 22:1–26; Circulation 1991; 84,2:960–975.

13. Cummins R, et al. Recommended guidelines for reviewing, reporting and conducting research on in-hospital resuscitation: the "in-hospital Utstein style." Resuscitation 1997; 34:151–185.

# 14

# Evidence-Based Guidelines in Resuscitation:

## From Experiment to Guidelines

*Lance B. Becker, MD*

## Introduction

The American Heart Association (AHA), along with many other organizations, has been involved in the development of international guidelines for resuscitation for over 30 years.[1] The AHA first published guidelines on cardiopulmonary resuscitation in 1966.[2] Developing guidelines has evolved substantially since that time.[3] Currently there is a worldwide effort to develop evidence-based international guidelines. These are anticipated to be published in the year 2000. In this chapter, the *evidence evaluation process* used to develop these international evidence-based guidelines is described.

## Background and Overview of Guidelines Development

### Previous Guidelines Process

A prominent scientist involved in resuscitation guidelines once stated that final guidelines are not so much consensus but rather are heavily influenced by just one person—"the person who can stay awake the longest and talk the loudest." There is some truth to this observation. The major obstacle to guideline development is the problem that the available data on many subjects are inadequate. Yet while this science may be inadequate, practical matters make guidelines necessary, forcing panels of experts to make a compromise between what is known as fact and what is opinion (often strongly held). For example, in teaching cardiopulmonary resuscitation (CPR), students must be taught to perform a specific number of compressions per minute. Yet the data to support a rate of 80

From: Aliot E, Clementy J, Prystowsky EN (editors). *Fighting Sudden Cardiac Death: A Worldwide Challenge.* ©Futura Publishing Company, Armonk, NY, 2000.

versus something else is incomplete. Wouldn't 100 or 120 be better? But what if a person can't perform 120 per minute? What if a person can perform 100 for 1 minute but then becomes fatigued and performance drops to 60? While there are strong opinions on many of these issues, the real data to support these differences are marginal. However, despite these issues of data, practical guidelines must be created; otherwise no training will occur.

## The Knowledge Gap

The gap in our knowledge between what is fact and what is strongly held opinion is often quite large—and guidelines intended for broad implementation do not reflect this gap in knowledge. Moreover, our prior experience with guidelines suggests that they are often followed rigidly, sometimes with unintended results. The AHA's prior performance guidelines for students to demonstrate a 15:2 compressions-to-ventilation ratio was interpreted by the training network as the need to perform a "perfect strip" on a recording mannequin, which caused many students to fail the CPR course. As a result, many students felt that they might hurt a victim if they didn't do "perfect CPR." Some students, paradoxically, even felt more afraid to perform CPR than before they took the course. This result was never the intention of the scientists who thought that a 15:2 ratio was "about right."

## The Need for a Better Tool to Create Guidelines

Prior guidelines efforts have addressed this challenge by convening expert consensus panels and allowing the groups to interact to produce guidelines that are accepted as "consensus."[4] However, whether these were truly "consensus" remains debatable. The missing element in these guidelines was a clear indication of how strong (or weak) the scientific evidence really was on a topic. What is fundamentally different about the current guidelines process is that it indicates the strength of the science to support the guidelines. In 1992 the AHA added the "class of recommendation" to guidelines to indicate to readers the scientific strength of evidence that supported a guideline.[1] Example: Early defibrillation became a Class I recommendation, having the strongest science to support it. However, to summarize many papers into a single recommendation, there was still a need to assign an indicator of the quality of an individual paper. In response to this need, the AHA introduced the concept of the "level of evidence" to assign an indication of scientific strength to the multiple manuscripts that back up a guideline.

# The Need for Conservatism

Given these considerations, another important characteristic of the guidelines process is that it be conservative. Nothing irritates practitioners and the training networks more than changing 1 year to 1 instruction and then the following year changing the same guideline back to the prior instruction.

## Key Concepts on Producing Guidelines

Several important concepts emerge out of this discussion: (1) guidelines should be conservative, (2) decisions on practical guidelines must be made by experts based on the best available science, (3) the strength of the science that supports guidelines should be indicated on guidelines.

# The Guidelines Cycle: From Guidelines to Practice to Research and Back to Guidelines

It is important to understand that creating guidelines is one part of a much larger process—the overall evolution of the field of resuscitation. As described by Cummins (Figure 1), the cycle of guidelines development follows a cyclic pattern, repeating itself with a 4- to 8-year periodicity. With publication of new guidelines comes dissemination. Resuscitation guidelines are some of the most widely disseminated guidelines in the world. There is a broad base of educational programs, textbooks, video instructions, plus a whole training network that provides education to lay and professional students. These collective efforts reach well over 5 million students each year in the United States alone. It is this excellent dissemination process that makes resuscitation guidelines so unique and powerful as public health guidelines. Following dissemination (and education) comes community implementation—bystanders begin to actually use the recommended guidelines on victims of cardiac arrest. We still lack critical information on how well bystanders really perform many of our current guidelines. Following community implementation comes its effect on survival rates or the outcome of the guidelines. Research is performed at several points along this cycle. Research in basic science and animal laboratories describe mechanisms and physiology. Human trials describe effects of possible new therapies on outcomes. Research on educational techniques and epidemiological studies contribute additional data on success of strategies. All of this research is then collected in preparation for a new set of revised guidelines; such a new set of guidelines is scheduled for publi-

# Guidelines Cycle

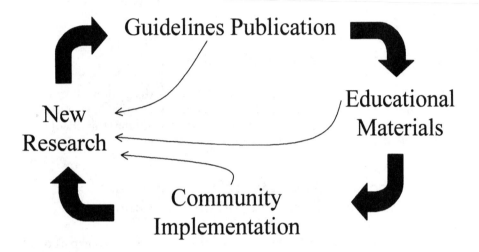

Guidelines Publication

New Research

Educational Materials

Community Implementation

cation in the year 2000. The cycle, with periodic updates and revisions, will repeat itself.

## The Evolving Evidence Evaluation Process

It is critical to note that this evidence evaluation process is not fixed in stone. It is still evolving rapidly, remains extremely dynamic, and continues to change in response to feedback from experts trying to use it.

## Role of Experts

Experts play a central role in this process and the selection of experts is critical to successful guidelines. The selection of a large number of international experts was guided by a review of the current literature in the field. For example, in preparation for the new guidelines in CPR, we reviewed over 1,600 papers published after 1990 on cardiac resuscitation guidelines with the selection of experts. In general, investigators with multiple reports were given priority as were more senior investigators. However, many younger investigators were invited to participate, as the evidence evaluation process is also a time to involve younger investigators in the larger community of researchers and many of the younger investigators had more available time than some senior researchers. In addition, recognized international authorities in the field were invited, as were international experts with expertise in training, research design, and education. Over 280 experts were identified and invited through this process.

## Worksheets

An important development for evidence-based guidelines was the creation of a worksheet for experts to complete that would (1) be simple to fill out yet (2) would answer the proper evidence evaluation questions. The worksheet was developed (see the Appendix for an abridged version) over a period of 3 years under the leadership of Richard Cummins, Mary Fran Hazinski, and Ahamed Idris, with input from the Emergency Cardiac Care committees of the American Heart Association. During this time there was continuous input and revision from the full membership of the Emergency Cardiac Care Committees (80 additional experts) as well as international input from the International Liaison Committee on Resuscitation (ILCOR) with 40 international experts. The worksheet allows an expert to go "step by step" through the evidence evaluation process, which includes: (1) a clear statement of the proposal to be considered; (2) gathering of the evidence that relates to that proposal; (3) assessing the "level of evidence" for individual study; (4) summarizing all the multiple studies that bear on a proposal according to quality; (5) assigning a "class of recommendation" to the proposal.

## "Level of Evidence" Versus "Class of Recommendation"

Level of evidence is a term used to describe the data that support or fail to support a proposal. Since it describes data, levels of evidence can be assigned to all the papers that apply to a proposal. We are currently using a scale of 8 various levels of evidence with level 1 being the best data and level 8 being the weakest data (see Levels of Evidence section in the Appendix). By summarizing the multiple levels of evidence, one can quickly develop an idea of the strength of the data to support a guideline. By contrast, the final step is to determine a class of recommendation for the guideline. Each guideline is given a single class of recommendation that helps readers understand how strong the overall data were to support that recommendation (see Class of Recommendation section in the Appendix). The classes of recommendation are currently: Class I (definitely helpful), Class II (acceptable), and Class III (possibly harmful). Class II is further divided into Class IIA (acceptable—probably helpful) and Class IIB (acceptable—possibly helpful).

## Participation by the Public

An important part of the process is a fair chance for anyone interested in the guidelines to have a forum to express their viewpoint. An overview of the last 5 years of guidelines development is listed in Figure 2. It is especially important for dissenting parties to be able to address specific concerns prior to the issuance of guidelines (in the past, when this was omitted, major deficiencies in the guidelines were identified only after the guidelines were published). To create this open forum for the public, the AHA sponsors 2 separate conferences devoted to the guidelines separated by 4 months. This provides 2 opportunities for feedback and revision of guidelines.

## The Role of International Experts and Participation

In addition, we are committed to having international guidelines because resuscitation is an international problem and because much of the best research is being done by international groups (rather than only in the United States).[5,6] The International Liaison Committee on Resuscitation (ILCOR) was developed in 1990 to facilitate this interaction.[6]

### Evidence Evaluation Process (AHA timetable)

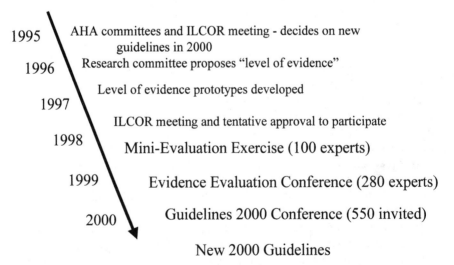

1995 — AHA committees and ILCOR meeting - decides on new guidelines in 2000

1996 — Research committee proposes "level of evidence"

Level of evidence prototypes developed

1997

ILCOR meeting and tentative approval to participate

1998 — Mini-Evaluation Exercise (100 experts)

1999 — Evidence Evaluation Conference (280 experts)

2000 — Guidelines 2000 Conference (550 invited)

New 2000 Guidelines

# APPENDIX 1
### SAMPLE ABRIDGEDWORKSHEET for PROPOSED
### Evidence-Based GUIDELINE RECOMMENDATIONS
(This ECC Worksheet Template developed by the AHA)

| Worksheet Author: | Chief Collaborator: |
|---|---|
| **Author's Home Resuscitation Council:**<br>AHA:___ ERC:___ CLAR:___ CHSF:___ RCSA:<br>___<br>ARC: ___ NZRC: ____ IAHF: ___ | **Collaborator's Home Resuscitation Council:**<br>AHA:___ ERC:___ CLAR:___ CHSF:___ RCSA: ___<br>ARC: ___ NZRC: ____ IAHF: ___ |
| **Home Subcommittee:**<br>BLS_____ ACLS _____ Peds RS ___<br>ProAd___ | **Collaborator's Home Subcommittee or Working Group:**<br>BLS_____ ACLS _____ Peds RS ____ Other _____ |
| Date Submitted to Subcommittee: 17 August 1999 | Date Worksheet ready to discuss: _____ |

**STEP 1: STATE THE PROPOSAL.** State: proposed new guideline; revision to current guideline; deletion of current guideline.

**Existing guideline, practice, or training activity**: State AHA/ILCOR published statements of the existing guidelines or practice to be revised, supplemented, or deleted. .

**Step 1A: Refine the question; state as a positive (or negative) hypothesis.** State proposed guideline recommendation as a specific, positive hypothesis. Use a single sentence if possible. Include type of patients; setting (in- /out-of-hospital); specific interventions (dose, route); specific outcomes (ROSC vs. hospital discharge).

**Step 1B: Gather the Evidence; define your search strategy.** Describe search results; describe best sources.

• List the major search terms used to search databases: condition/disease AND intervention of interest AND methodological terms AND database indexing terms (see L of E manuscript). Underline the most successful in terms of yield.

• List electronic databases searched (at least MEDLINE (http://igm.nlm.nih.gov/) and EMBASE E-mail: embase-europe@elsevier.nl In US: useembase-f@elsevier.com. http://elsevier.com/ (Excerpta Medica) {MEDLINE= free; mostly US publications; EMBASE= hourly charge; mostly European; 34% overlap of the two). Medline (PubMed)

• Summarize your yield from *hand-searches* of journals; ie. page through one or more journals for one or more years; include editorials, letters, review articles, abstracts, meeting summaries. Include hand-searches of bibliographies of all articles that meet inclusion criteria. Describe yield:

• Summarize the yield of any other sources, eg. investigator interviews, unpublished manuscripts, abstracts, book chapters, prepublication materials

• State major criteria you used to limit your search; state criteria for inclusion; state criteria for exclusion. Eg. only human studies with control group? no animal studies? n > minimal number? type of methodology? peer-reviewed manuscripts only? no abstract-only studies?

• Number of articles/sources meeting criteria for further review: List a citation marker for each study. If possible, please supply file of best references; ProCite 4.1 preferred as reference manager, though others are acceptable.

## STEP 2: ASSESS THE QUALITY OF THE STUDY

**Step 2A: Determine the Level of Evidence (strength of methodology.** For each article/source from step 1, assign a level of evidence based on study design and methodology (see definitions in table below).

### 1998 AHA-ECC Levels of Evidence Summary

| Level of Evidence | Definitions (See manuscript for full details) |
|---|---|
| Level 1 | One or more RCTs in which the lower limit of the CI for the treatment effect exceeds the minimal clinically important benefit |
| Level 2 | One or more RCTs in which the lower limit of the CI for the treatment effect overlaps the minimal clinically important benefit |
| Level 3 | Prospective, cohort of patients not randomized to an intervention; control or comparison group available |
| Level 4 | Historic, non-randomized, cohort or case-control studies |
| Level 5 | Case series: patients compiled in serial fashion, lacking a control group |
| Level 6 | An animal or mechanical model study. Level 6A study is well-designed; shows a homogeneous pattern of results. Level 6B study has less powerful design, demonstrates an equivocal or heterogeneous pattern of results |
| Level 7 | Reasonable extrapolations from existing data; quasi-experimental designs; pathophysiological and nonquantitative reasoning. |
| Level 8 | Rational conjecture (common sense); common practices accepted before evidence-based guidelines |

**Step 2A (continued) SORT THE STUDIES:** List the studies that you considered best met the original selection criteria for review, by their Level of Evidence. Use short citations or citation numbers so that articles can be identified specifically.

| Level of Evidence | Articles (use citation number or first author, date) |
|---|---|
| Level 1 | |
| Level 2 | |
| Level 3 | |
| Level 4 | |
| Level 5 | |
| Level 6 | |
| Level 7 | |
| Level 8 | |

**Step 2B: Critically assess each article/source in terms of research design and methods.** Was the study well executed? Suggested criteria appear in the table below. Assess design and methods and provide an overall rating. Ratings apply within each Level; a Level 1 study can be excellent or poor as a clinical trial, just as a Level 6 study could be excellent or poor as an animal study.

| | A. Excellent | B. Good | C. Fair | D. Poor | E. Unacceptable |
|---|---|---|---|---|---|
| | Highly appropriate sample or model, randomized, proper controls | More than adequate design; minimally biased | Adequate design, but possibly biased | Small or clearly biased population or model | Anecdotal, no controls, off target end-points |
| | Outstanding accuracy, precision, and data collection in its level | More than adequate in its class | Adequate under the circumstances | Weakly defensible; limited data or measures | Totally bogus |
| **Paper** Level 1 Level 2 Level 3 Level 4 Level 5 Level 6 Level 7 Level 8 | | | | | |

**Step 2C: Determine the <u>direction</u> of the results and the statistics: supportive? neutral? opposed?**

| DIRECTION of study by results & statistics: | SUPPORT the proposal | NEUTRAL | OPPOSE the proposal |
|---|---|---|---|
| **Results** | Outcome of proposed guideline is superior, to a clinically important degree, to current approach | Outcome of proposed guideline is no different from current approach | Outcome of proposed guideline is inferior to current approach |
| **Statistics** | Lower boundary of the 95% confidence interval exceeds minimal, clinically important benefit; OR odds ratio does not overlap 1; OR number needed to treat is acceptable. | Lower boundary of 95% CI does NOT exceed the minimal clinically important benefit; OR odds ratio overlaps 1; OR number needed to treat is borderline high. | Negative effects observed for proposed treatment; statistical significance not required. Odds ratio less than 1; or number needed to treat is unacceptably high.. |
| **Paper** Level 1 Level 2 Level 3 Level 4 Level 5 Level 6 Level 7 Level 8 | | | |

**Step 2D: Cross-tabulate assessed studies by a)** *level,* **b)** *quality,* **and c)** *direction;* **combine and summarize.** Exclude the *Poor* and *Unsatisfactory* studies. Sort the *Excellent, Good,* and *Fair* quality studies by both *Level and Quality of evidence;* and *Direction of support* in the summary grids below. Use citation marker (eg. author/date/source). In the *Neutral* or *Opposing* grid use bold font for *Opposing* studies to distinguish from merely neutral studies.

## Supporting Evidence

| Quality of Evidence | | | | | | | | |
|---|---|---|---|---|---|---|---|---|
| Excellent | | | | | | | | |
| Good | | | | | | | | |
| Fair | | | | | | | | |
| | Level of Evidence | | | | | | | |

## Neutral or Opposing Evidence

| Quality of Evidence | | | | | | | | |
|---|---|---|---|---|---|---|---|---|
| Excellent | | | | | | | | |
| Good | | | | | | | | |
| Fair | | | | | | | | |
| | 1 | 2 | 3 | 4 | 5 | 6 | 7 | 8 |
| | Level of Evidence | | | | | | | |

**SUMMARY of Step 2:**
**Enter the citation numbers of the critical studies selected by** Steps **1 and 2 that will provide the basis for** Step 3: *Determine the Class of Recommendation*

**Insert citation numbers of the critical studies:**

**Summarize core numeric data** from these critical studies in a 2x2 matrix, with **positive** vs. **negative** outcomes for the **intervention** vs **control** groups, if data are available. Combine outcome results from similar studies in the form of a meta-analysis if appropriate. (See manuscript for how to determine when meta-analysis is indicated.) Attach most critical tabulations.

**STEP 3. DETERMINE THE CLASS OF RECOMMENDATION.**
**Select from these summary definitions:**

| CLASS | CLINICAL DEFINITION | REQUIRED LEVEL OF EVIDENCE |
|---|---|---|
| **Class I**<br>*Definitely recommended.*<br>Definitive,<br>**excellent** evidence provides<br>support. | • Always acceptable, safe<br>• Definitely useful<br>• Proven in both efficacy & effectiveness<br>• Must be used in the intended manner for proper clinical indications. | • One or more Level 1 studies are present (with rare exceptions)<br>• Study results are consistently positive and compelling |
| **Class II:**<br>*Acceptable and useful* | • Safe, acceptable<br>• Clinically useful<br>• Not yet confirmed definitively | • Most evidence is positive<br>• Level 1 studies are absent, or inconsistent, or lack power<br>• No evidence of harm |
| • *Class IIa:* Acceptable and *useful*<br>**Good** evidence provides support | • Safe, acceptable<br>• Clinically useful<br>• Considered treatments of choice | • Generally higher levels of evidence<br>• Results are consistently positive |
| • *Class IIb:* Acceptable and *useful*<br>**Fair** evidence provides support | • Safe, acceptable<br>• Clinically useful<br>• Considered optional or alternative treatments | • Generally lower or intermediate levels of evidence<br>• Generally, but not consistently, positive results |
| **Class III:**<br>*Not acceptable, not useful,*<br>*may be harmful* | • Unacceptable<br>• Not useful clinically<br>• May be harmful. | • No positive high level data<br>• Some studies suggest or confirm harm. |
| **Indeterminate** | • Research just getting started.<br>• Continuing area of research<br>• No recommendations until further research | • Minimal evidence is available<br>• Higher studies in progress<br>• Results inconsistent, contradictory<br>• Results not compelling |

**STEP 3: DETERMINE THE CLASS OF RECOMMENDATION** State a **Class of Recommendation** for the Guideline Proposal. State either **a) the intervention**, and then the conditions under which the intervention is either Class I, Class IIA, IIB; or **b) the condition**, and then whether the intervention is Class I, Class IIA, or IIB. Both approaches may be necessary. (See manuscript for examples)

**EXPERT REVIEWER'S FINAL COMMENTS:** Summarize your final evidence integration and the rationale for the class of recommendation. Describe any mismatches between the evidence and your final Class of Recommendation. Mismatches refer to selection of a class of recommendation that is heavily influenced by other factors than just the evidence. For example, evidence is strong, but implementation difficult or expensive; evidence is weak, but future definitive evidence unlikely. Comment on contribution of animal or mechanical model studies to your final recommendation. Are results <u>within</u> animal studies homogeneous? Are animal results consistent with results from human studies? What is the frequency of adverse events? What is the possibility of harm? Describe any value or utility judgments you may have made, separate from the evidence. For example, evidence-supported interventions limited to in-hospital use because you think proper use is too difficult for pre-hospital providers.

**REFERENCES AND SUGGESTED EXPERTS**

## References

1. The Guidelines for Cardiopulmonary Resuscitation and Emergency Cardiac Care. By the Emergency Cardiac Care Committee of the American Heart Association. JAMA 1992; 268:2171–2295.
2. Cardiopulmonary Resuscitation. Conference Proceedings, May 23, 1966. Washington DC, National Academy of Sciences—National Research Council. JAMA 1966; 198:372–379.
3. Cummins R, Hazinski MF, Kerber R, Kudenchuk P, Becker L, et al. Low-energy biphasic waveform defibrillation: evidence-based review applied to emergency cardiovascular care guidelines. Circulation 1998; 97:1654–1667.
4. Handley AJ, Becker LB, Allen M, van Drenth A, Kramer EB, et al. Single-rescuer adult basic life support: an advisory statement from the Basic Life Support Working Group of the International Liaison Committee on Resuscitation. Circulation 1997; 15;95(8):2174–2179.
5. Cummins RO, Chamberlain DA. Advisory statements of the International Liaison Committee on Resuscitation. Circulation 1997; 95:2172–2173.
6. Chamberlain DA, Cummins RO. International emergency cardiac care: support, science, and universal guidelines. Ann Emerg Med 1993; 22:508–511.

# III

# Normal Heart, Sports, and Sudden Cardiac Death

# 15

# Sudden Cardiac Death in Young Athletes:

## Epidemiology, Screening, and Prevention

*Barry J. Maron, MD*

## Introduction

Sudden deaths of competitive athletes are personal tragedies with great impact on the lay and medical communities,[1] and are due to a variety of previously unsuspected cardiovascular diseases,[2-19] and occasionally low-energy chest blows.[20] Such events, particularly in young people, often assume a high public profile due to the widely held perception that trained athletes constitute the healthiest segment of our society; the occasional deaths of well-known elite athletes exaggerate this visibility.[1,21] These athletic field catastrophes have also substantially increased interest in the role and efficacy of preparticipation screening for the detection of cardiovascular disease.[22]

Therefore, with regard to young competitive athletes, this chapter will include an assessment of: (1) the epidemiology and the cardiovascular causes responsible for sudden death; (2) the strengths and limitations of preparticipation screening for early detection of these cardiovascular abnormalities as well as cost efficiency and feasibility issues, and medical-legal implications; and (3) consensus recommendations and guidelines for the most prudent, practical, and effective screening strategies, and criteria for sports eligibility and disqualification when cardiac abnormalities are known to be present. Given the large number of competitive athletes in the United States and in many other countries, and recent public health initiatives on physical activity and exercise, these issues have become particularly relevant.

From: Aliot E, Clementy J, Prystowsky EN (editors). *Fighting Sudden Cardiac Death: A Worldwide Challenge.* ©Futura Publishing Company, Armonk, NY, 2000.

## Definitions, Background, and General Considerations

The present considerations focus on the competitive athlete, previously described as one who participates in an organized team or individual sport requiring systematic training and regular competition against others, while placing a high premium on athletic excellence and achievement.[19] The purpose of screening, as described here, is to provide medical clearance for participation in competitive sports through routine and systematic evaluations intended to identify clinically relevant and preexisting cardiovascular abnormalities and thereby reduce the risks associated with organized sports. It should, however, be emphasized that raising the possibility of a cardiovascular abnormality on a standard screening examination is only the first tier of recognition after which referral to a specialist for further diagnostic investigation will probably be required. When a definitive cardiovascular diagnosis is made, the Consensus Panel Guidelines of Bethesda Conference #26[23] should be utilized to formulate recommendations for continued participation or disqualification from competitive sports.

American Heart Association guidelines[22] focus primarily on the potential for population-based screening of high school and collegiate student-athletes rather than on individual clinical assessments of athletes, and are designed to apply to competitors of all ages and both genders. These recommendations may also be extrapolated to athletes in youth, middle school, masters or professional sports, and in some instances to participants in intense recreational sporting activities. It should also be recognized that the overall preparticipation screening process extends well beyond the considerations described here (which are limited to the cardiovascular system), involving many other organ systems and medical issues.

Screening recommendations and eligibility/disqualification guidelines are predicated on the probability that intense athletic training is likely to increase the risk for sudden cardiac death (or disease progression) in trained athletes with clinically important underlying structural heart disease, although presently it is not possible to quantify that risk. Certainly, the vast majority of young athletes who die suddenly do so during athletic training or competition.[2-6] These observations support the proposition that physical exertion is an important trigger for sudden death, given the presence of certain underlying cardiovascular diseases. Finally, the early detection of clinically significant cardiovascular disease through preparticipation screening may well, in many instances, permit timely therapeutic interventions that may prolong life.

# Causes of Sudden Death in Athletes

A variety of cardiovascular abnormalities represent the most common causes of sudden death in competitive athletes.[2-19] The precise lesions responsible differ considerably with regard to age. For example, in youthful athletes (less than about 35 years of age) the vast majority are due to a variety of largely congenital cardiac malformations (Figures 1–3).[2-14] Indeed, virtually any disease capable of causing sudden death in young people may potentially do so in young competitive athletes. It should be emphasized that while these cardiovascular diseases may be relatively common

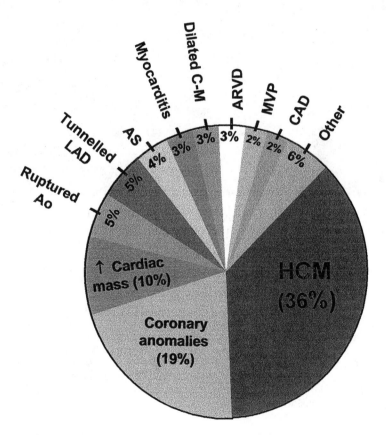

Figure 1. Causes of sudden cardiac death in young competitive athletes (median age, 17) based on systematic tracking of 158 athletes in the United States, primarily 1985–1995. Ao = aorta; LAD = left anterior descending; ARVD = arrhythmogenic right ventricular dysplasia; MVP = mitral valve prolapse; CAD = coronary heart disease; HCM = hypertrophic cardiomyopathy. (Adapted with permission of the American Heart Association from Maron BJ, et al.[22])

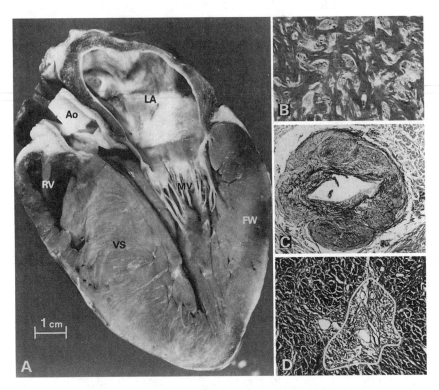

Figure 2. Morphological components of the disease process in HCM, the most common cause of sudden death in young competitive athletes. Panel A shows a gross heart specimen sectioned in a cross-sectional plane similar to that of the echocardiographic (parasternal) long axis; left ventricular wall thickening shows an asymmetrical pattern and is confined primarily to the ventricular septum (VS), which bulges prominently into the left ventricular outflow tract. Left ventricular cavity appears reduced in size. FW = left ventricular free wall. Panels B, C, and D show histologic features characteristic of left ventricular myocardium in hypertrophic cardiomyopathy. B: Markedly disordered architecture with adjacent hypertrophied cardiac muscle cells arranged at perpendicular and oblique angles. C: An intramural coronary artery with thickened wall, due primarily to medial hypertrophy, and apparently narrowed lumen. D: Replacement fibrosis in an area of ventricular myocardium adjacent to an abnormal intramural coronary artery. Ao = aorta; LA = left atrium; RV = right ventricle. (From Maron BJ, et al.,[29] reproduced with permission of The Lancet.)

among those young athletes dying suddenly, each is uncommon in the general population. Also, those lesions that are responsible for sudden death do not occur with the same frequency, with most being responsible for ≤5% of all such deaths (Figure 1). Such deaths occur most commonly in intense team sports, such as basketball and football, which also have high levels of participation.

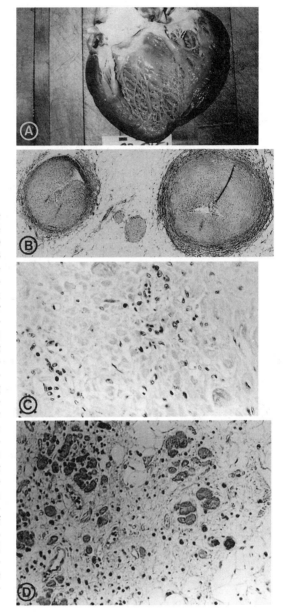

Figure 3. Cardiac morphologic findings at autopsy in 4 competitive athletes who died suddenly of causes other than hypertrophic cardiomyopathy. A: Gross specimen from an athlete with greatly enlarged ventricular cavities, consistent with dilated cardiomyopathy. B: Histologic section of the left anterior descending coronary artery (left) and a diagonal branch (right) showing severe (>95%) cross-sectional luminal narrowing by atherosclerotic plaque. C: Foci inflammatory cells consistent with myocarditis. D: Histologic section of right ventricular wall showing islands of myocytes within a matrix of fatty and fibrous replacement, characteristic of arrhythmogenic right ventricular dysplasia. (Adapted from Maron BJ, et al.,[3] reproduced with permission of the American Medical Association.)

## Hypertrophic Cardiomyopathy

The single most common cardiovascular abnormality among the causes of sudden death in young athletes is hypertrophic cardiomyopathy

(HCM), usually in the nonobstructive form,[3–5,8,11,12,14,24–30] and accounts for about 35% of these athletic field deaths[3] (Figures 1 and 2). HCM is a primary and familial cardiac disease with heterogeneous expression, complex pathophysiology, and a diverse clinical course for which well over 100 disease-causing mutations in 8 genes encoding proteins of the cardiac sarcomere have been reported,[27,29–34] including β-myosin heavy chain, cardiac troponin T and troponin-I, α-tropomyosin, essential and regulatory light chains of myosin, actin, and cardiac myosin-binding protein C. Within the general population, HCM is a relatively uncommon malformation occurring in about 0.2%.[35]

Not uncommonly, HCM is responsible for sudden cardiac death in young and asymptomatic individuals, and frequently occurs during moderate or severe exertion.[3,4,21–23] Indeed, the stress of intense training and competition (and associated alterations in blood volume, hydration, and electrolytes) undoubtedly increases that risk to some degree.[23] In HCM, particularly strenuous physical activity may act as a trigger mechanism (Figure 4) for generating potentially lethal ventricular tachyarrhythmias, given the underlying electrophysiologically unstable myocardial substrate

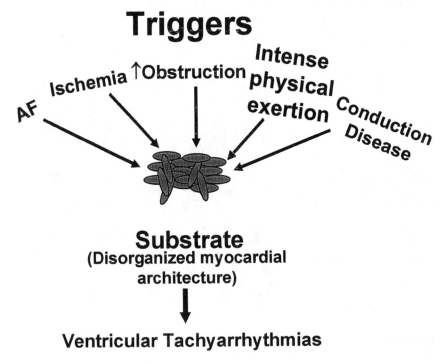

Figure 4. Proposed mechanisms by which sudden cardiac death may occur in athletes with hypertrophic cardiomyopathy.

comprised of replacement fibrosis (which is probably the consequence of ischemia) and disorganized cardiac muscle cell arrangement (Figure 2).

Disease variables that appear to identify those individuals at greatly increased risk include: prior aborted cardiac arrest or sustained ventricular tachycardia, family history or sudden or other premature HCM-related death (or high-risk genotype), multiple repetitive nonsustained ventricular tachycardia on ambulatory Holter ECG recording, recurrent syncope particularly in the young, massive degrees of left ventricular hypertrophy, and possibly hypotensive blood pressure response to exercise.[27,29] HCM patients judged to be at high risk for sudden death should be considered for primary prevention of sudden death with prophylactic cardioverter-defibrillator implants.[36]

While HCM may be suspected during preparticipation sports evaluations by the prior occurrence of exertion syncope, family history of HCM or premature cardiac death or the presence of a heart murmur, these features are relatively uncommon among all individuals affected by the disease.[22] Consequently, screening procedures limited to customary history and physical examination can not be expected to reliably and consistently identify HCM.

## Hypertrophic Cardiomyopathy and the Athlete's Heart

Some young athletes with segmental ventricular septal thickening (13–15 mm), consistent with a relatively mild morphological expression of HCM, may be difficult to distinguish from the physiological and benign form of left ventricular hypertrophy that represents an adaptation to athletic training (i.e., "athlete's heart").[37] Athletes within this morphological "gray zone" represent an important and not uncommon clinical problem in which the differential diagnosis between HCM and athlete's heart can often be resolved by noninvasive testing (Figure 3).[37] This distinction may have particularly important implications, given that young athletes with an unequivocal diagnosis of HCM are discouraged from participation in most competitive sports to minimize risk, with the possible exception of those sports considered to be of low intensity.[38] On the other hand, the improper diagnosis of cardiac disease in an athlete may lead to unnecessary withdrawal from athletics, thereby depriving that individual of the varied benefits of sports.

## Congenital Coronary Anomalies

The second most frequent cause of sudden death in young athletes is a variety of congenital coronary anomalies, primarily of wrong aortic sinus origin (occurring in about 20% of these deaths).[3] The most common of these lesions appears to be anomalous origin of the left main coronary artery from the right (anterior) sinus of Valsalva; [39,40] the mirror image malformation, anomalous right coronary artery from the left aortic sinus, has also been incriminated in these catastrophes[40] (Figure 4). Such malformations are difficult to recognize during life because they are often unassociated with symptoms (e.g., exertional syncope or chest pain) or alterations in the 12-lead or exercise ECG, and therefore diagnosis requires a high index of suspicion.[41] Indeed, occurrence of one or more episodes of exertional syncope in a young athlete necessitates the definitive exclusion of a coronary anomaly. It may also be possible to identify (or raise a strong suspicion of) anomalous coronaries of wrong sinus origin utilizing transthoracic or transesophageal echocardiography,[42–44] which can then lead to anatomic confirmation with coronary arteriography.

These coronary malformations should result in exclusion from intense competitive sports to reduce the potential risk of a cardiac event.[23] Also, wrong sinus anomalies are amenable to surgical correction with bypass grafting, which is the most common approach to restore distal coronary flow.[40,41] However, congenital coronary artery malformations cannot be reliably identified by standard screening for participation in athletics.

Myocardial ischemia in young people with coronary artery anomalies involving wrong sinus origin probably occur in infrequent bursts, cumulative with time, ultimately resulting in patchy myocardial necrosis and fibrosis; this process could predispose to lethal ventricular tachyarrhythmias by creating an electrically unstable myocardial substrate. Potential mechanisms that have been advanced include: (1) acute angled takeoff and kinking or flaplike closure at the origin of the coronary artery, or (2) compression of the anomalous artery between the aorta and the pulmonary trunk during exercise. Furthermore, the proximal portion of the artery may be intramural (i.e., within the aortic tunica media), which could further aggravate coronary obstruction, particularly with aortic expansion during exercise. Other coronary anomalies relevant to this problem include hypoplasia of the right coronary and left circumflex arteries, left anterior descending or right coronary artery from pulmonary trunk, virtual absence of the left coronary artery, and spontaneous coronary arterial intussusception and coronary artery dissection.[3–5,14]

Other less common causes of exercise-related sudden deaths in young athletes are myocarditis (Figure 3), idiopathic dilated cardiomyopathy (Figure 3), Marfan syndrome with aortic rupture, arrhythmogenic right ventricular dysplasia (Figure 3), sarcoidosis, mitral valve prolapse, aortic valve stenosis, atherosclerotic coronary artery disease (Figure 3), long QT syndrome, and possibly intramural (tunneled) coronary arteries.[3–7,11,14]

## Absence of Structural Heart Disease

Occasionally, athletes who die suddenly demonstrate no evidence of structural cardiovascular disease, even after careful gross and microscopic examination of the heart. In such instances (about 2% of 1 series),[3] it may not be possible to exclude noncardiac factors with certainty (e.g., drug abuse) or to know whether careful inspection of the specialized conduction system and associated vasculature with serial sectioning (which is not part of the standard medical examiners' protocol) would have revealed occult but clinically relevant abnormalities.[9,45,46] Although one can only speculate on the potential etiologies in many such deaths, it is possible that some are due to a primary arrhythmia in the absence of cardiac morphological abnormalities,[47] previously unidentified Wolff-Parkinson-White syndrome, rare diseases in which structural abnormalities of the heart are characteristically lacking at necropsy such as long QT syndrome[48–50] or possibly exercise-induced coronary spasm, or undetected segmental right ventricular dysplasia.[51]

Other medical problems that may occasionally cause sudden death in young people, such as ruptured cerebral aneurysm, sickle cell trait,[52] or bronchial asthma, have been excluded. Also, issues related to drug screening are not part of this discussion, although ingestion of agents such as cocaine may have important adverse cardiovascular consequences.[53–55] Screening for systemic hypertension has been addressed, although this disease is not regarded as an important cause of sudden unexpected death in young athletes.[56]

## Older Athletes

Of note, older and middle-aged athletes (over age 35) are involved in competitive long-distance running. The vast majority of deaths in such athletes are due to atherosclerotic coronary artery disease,[11,15–18,57] and only rarely to congenital cardiovascular diseases such as HCM or coronary artery anomalies.

## Mechanisms and Resuscitation

Although the precise mechanism ultimately responsible for sudden death in young athletes depends on the particular disease state involved, in the vast majority of instances, cardiac arrest results from electrical instability and ventricular tachyarrhythmias. In the case of HCM, the disorganized cardiac muscle cells distributed widely throughout the left ventricular wall probably represent the substrate for ventricular tachycardia/fibrillation when associated with a number of potential clinical triggers (including intense physical activity) (Figure 4). A clear exception to this model is Marfan syndrome in which sudden death is due to aortic rupture. Of note, regardless of the underlying mechanism, very few athletes with cardiovascular disease who collapse on the athletic field are successfully resuscitated.

It is possible that the routine presence of automatic external defibrillators at athletic events (and public access defibrillation) would lead to the survival of greater numbers of such athletes.[58] However, the great infrequency with which these events occur ultimately represents an obstacle to efficient resuscitation practice in the rare occasion of such an event. Therefore, it would appear equally important to emphasize the early detection of potentially lethal cardiovascular abnormalities through preparticipation screening[22] and the withdrawal of such athletes from intense training and competition.[23]

## Epidemiology, Prevalence, and Scope of the Problem

Relevant to the design of any screening strategy is the fact that sudden cardiac death in young athletes is a devastating but rather infrequent event, and only a small proportion of participants in organized sports in the United States are at risk.[22,59] Indeed, each of the lesions known to be responsible for sudden death in young athletes occurs infrequently in the general population, ranging from the relatively common (i.e., HCM) to the apparently very rare (e.g., coronary artery anomalies, arrhythmogenic right ventricular dysplasia, long QT syndrome, or Marfan syndrome). It is reasonable to estimate that all congenital malformations relevant to athletic screening may account for a combined prevalence of <0.5% in general athletic populations.

Also, the large reservoir of competitive athletes in the United States constitutes a major obstacle to screening strategies.[22,59] At present, there are approximately 5–6 million competitive athletes at the high school level (grades 9–12), in addition to lesser numbers of collegiate (500,000) and professional (5,000) athletes. This does not include an unspecified number of youth, middle-school, and masters level competitors for which reliable estimates are not presently available. Therefore, the total number of trained athletes in the United States every year is probably as high as 8 million.

While the prevalence of athletic field deaths due to cardiovascular disease is not known with certainty, current estimates for sudden cardiac death in United States high school and college-aged student-athletes is approximately 1:200,000/year,[4,59] although disproportionately higher in males than in females.[59] Considering such a relatively low prevalence, the heightened public awareness and intense interest in sudden deaths in athletes, often fueled by the news media, are perhaps disproportionate to their actual numerical impact as a public health problem.

## Ethical and Legal Considerations in Screening

Within a benevolent society, responsibility exists on the part of physicians to initiate prudent efforts to identify life-threatening diseases in athletes to minimize those cardiovascular risks associated with sports and to protect the health of such individuals.[1,22,23,60,61] Specifically, there is an implicit ethical obligation on the part of educational institutions (e.g., high schools and colleges) to implement cost-effective strategies to assure that student-athletes are not subject to unacceptable and unavoidable medical risks.[22] The libertarian view, held by some, that high school and college-aged athletes should be permitted to assume any specifically disclosed cardiovascular risk associated with sports as part of the overall uncertainty and risk of living is not ascribed to here. Despite sufficient resources, it is recognized that in professional sports, the motivation to implement cardiovascular screening may not presently exist due to the economic pressures in such sports environments, where athletic participation represents a vocation and the remuneration for services is often substantial.

The extent to which preparticipation screening can be supported at any level is mitigated by cost-efficiency considerations, practical limitations, and also by the awareness that it is not possible to achieve a "zero-risk" circumstance in competitive sports.[61,62] Indeed, there is often an implied acceptance of risk on the part of athletes; for example, as a society, we permit or condone many sports activities known to have intrinsic risks that cannot be controlled absolutely, e.g., automobile racing or mountain climbing, as well as more traditional sports such as football in which the possibility of serious traumatic injury exists.[61]

Although educational institutions and professional teams in the United States are required to use reasonable care in conducting their athletic programs, there is currently no clear legal precedent regarding their duty to conduct preparticipation screening of athletes for the purpose of detecting medically significant cardiovascular abnormalities.[22,62] Indeed, at present, no lawsuits have apparently been brought forward alleging negligence by the failure to either perform cardiovascular screening or to diagnose cardiac disease in young competitive athletes. In the absence of binding requirements established by state law or athletic governing bodies, most institutions and teams presently rely on the team physician (or other medical personnel) to determine appropriate medical screening procedures.

A physician who has medically cleared an athlete to participate in competitive sports is not necessarily legally liable for an injury or death caused by an undetected cardiovascular condition. Malpractice liability for failure to discover a latent, asymptomatic cardiovascular condition requires proof that a physician deviated from customary or accepted medical practice in his or her specialty in performing preparticipation screening of athletes, and furthermore that utilization of established diagnostic criteria and techniques would have disclosed the medical condition.

It should be emphasized that the law permits the medical profession to establish the appropriate nature and scope of preparticipation screening based on the exercise of its collective medical judgment. This necessarily involves the development of reliable diagnostic procedures in light of cost-benefit and feasibility factors. Of note, the American Heart Association recommendations for cardiovascular preparticipation screening of athletes described here[22] represent evidence of the proper medical standard of care; however, these guidelines will establish the legal standard of care only if generally accepted or customarily followed by physicians, or relied upon by courts in determining the nature and scope of the legal responsibility borne by sponsors of competitive athletes.[62-64]

While preparticipation examinations in United States high schools and colleges occur largely at the discretion of the examining physician and as customary practice, a considerably different circumstance has existed in Italy since 1971 in the form of benevolent government legislation ("Medical Protection of Athletic Activities Act") mandating preventive medical evaluations for all competitive athletes.[60] Unique to Italy, all citizens (ages 12–40) who are engaged in organized sports activities must obtain annual medical clearance from an approved physician stipulating that the athlete is free of cardiovascular abnormalities that could unacceptably increase the risk of sudden cardiac death during training or competition. Since 1982, more detailed guidelines for these preparticipation examinations have been formulated and include, as a minimum, history and physical examination, 12-lead ECG, and exercise and pulmonary function tests.

Echocardiography has been specifically required (since 1994) only in selected professional sports (i.e., soccer, boxing, and cycling). Under Italian law, the examining physician is primarily responsible for the accuracy of this clinical assessment and is the final arbiter of eligibility for sports by issuing the official certification of medical clearance. In the event of an incorrect or incomplete medical diagnosis that leads directly to the impaired health or the death of an athlete, the physician responsible for sanctioning athletic competition can be held accountable in criminal (as well as civil) court.

## Current Customary Screening Practices in the United States

It is important to clearly acknowledge the limitations of the preparticipation screening process currently in place for student-athletes in the

United States. Only in this way can an informed public be created that otherwise might harbor important misconceptions regarding the principles and efficacy of athletic screening. Currently, universally accepted standards for the screening of high school and college athletes are not available, nor are there approved certification procedures for the professionals who perform such screening examinations.[65] Some form of medical clearance by a physician or other trained health care worker, usually consisting of a history and physical examination, presently appears most customary for high school athletes.

However, there is no uniform agreement among the states as to the precise format of preparticipation medical evaluations. Indeed, 40% of all states either do not require this process, do not have recommended standard history and physical forms to serve as guides to examiners (of which some require only a signature to provide medical clearance), or have approved forms that are judged inadequate[65] when evaluated against the specific screening recommendations proposed by the aforementioned 1996 American Heart Association consensus panel.[22] These findings also emphasize that it is not possible at present to assume that medical clearance for sports competition precludes the possibility of underlying and potentially lethal cardiovascular disease. In a substantial proportion of states, nonphysician health care workers are sanctioned to perform preparticipation screening, including chiropractors (in 9 states) and nurse practitioners or physician assistants (in 20 states each).

## Expectations of Screening Strategies

Preparticipation screening by history and physical examination alone (without noninvasive testing) does not possess sufficient power to guarantee detection of many critical cardiovascular abnormalities in large populations of young trained athletes in high school or college[3] (Figure 5). Indeed, hemodynamically significant congenital aortic valve stenosis is probably the lesion most likely to be reliably detected during routine screening due to its characteristically loud heart murmur. Detection of HCM by the standard screening history or physical examination is unreliable because most patients have the nonobstructive form of this disease, characteristically expressed by only a soft heart murmur or none at all.[22,24–27,29] Furthermore, the majority of athletes with HCM do not experience syncope or have a family history of premature sudden death, and therefore this disease is not easily detected by the preparticipation personal history.[22] When symptoms such as chest pain or impaired consciousness are involved, the standard personal history conveys a generally low specificity for the detection of many cardiovascular abnormalities that lead to sudden cardiac death in young athletes.

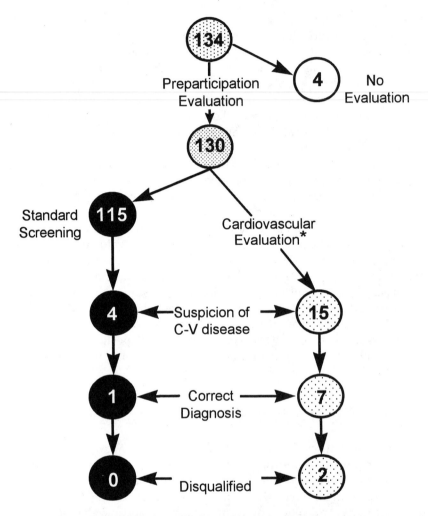

**Figure 5.** Flow-diagram showing impact of preparticipation medical history and physical examinations on the detection of structural cardiovascular disease (and causes of sudden death). * = cardiovascular evaluation with testing (independent of standard school or institutional preparticipation screening), performed in 15 athletes because of symptoms, family history, cardiac murmur, or physical findings suggestive of heart disease. (From Maron BJ, et al.,[3] reproduced with permission of the American Medical Association.)

It should also be emphasized that most of the lesions being considered here as potentially responsible for sudden death in young athletes may be particularly challenging to detect, even when echocardiography, ECG, or other noninvasive tests are incorporated into the standard screening process, e.g., a variety of congenital coronary anomalies (particularly anomalous origin of left main coronary artery from the right sinus of Valsalva).

Despite these major limitations, standard history and physical examination screening are theoretically of value by virtue of their capability for identifying (or raising the suspicion of) cardiovascular abnormalities in some at-risk athletes. For example, genetic diseases such as HCM, Marfan syndrome, and some cases of arrhythmogenic right ventricular dysplasia and premature atherosclerotic coronary artery disease can be suspected from the family history alone or by virtue of transient symptoms from the personal history; physical examination may identify the stigmata of Marfan syndrome, lesions associated with left ventricular outflow obstruction (aortic valvular stenosis and some patients with HCM) by a loud heart murmur, and systemic hypertension.

While there are few prospective data available that permit a direct assessment of the efficacy of large-scale athletic screening, a recent retrospective analysis of 134 young athletes who died suddenly from a variety of cardiovascular diseases showed that only 3% of those individuals exposed to standard preparticipation screening were suspected of having cardiac disease by virtue of these examinations, and less than 1% ultimately received an accurate diagnosis[3] (Figure 5).

Based on these observations, the preparticipation screening process as currently structured and carried out in United States high schools appears to lack sufficient power to consistently recognize clinically important cardiovascular abnormalities in many athletes. It is noteworthy that preparticipation screening in Italy (which routinely includes a 12-lead ECG) reports a contrasting experience; a not inconsequential number of HCM cases, similar in prevalence to that of HCM in the general population,[35] were identified over a 7-year period among approximately 33,000 consecutive athletes.[66]

## Potential Efficacy and Limitations of Noninvasive Screening Tests

The addition of noninvasive diagnostic tests to the screening process clearly has the potential to enhance the detection of certain cardiovascular defects in young athletes. For example, the 2-dimensional echocardiogram is the principal diagnostic tool for clinical recognition of HCM by virtue of demonstrating otherwise unexplained and asymmetric left ventricular wall thickening, the sine qua non of this disease.[24–29,67] Comprehensive and routine screening for HCM by genetic testing for a variety of known disease-causing mutations is not yet practical for large populations, given the substantial genetic heterogeneity of the disease, as well as the expensive and time-intensive methodologies involved.[27,29–34]

Echocardiography could also be expected to detect other relevant abnormalities associated with sudden death in young athletes such as valvular heart disease (e.g., mitral valve prolapse and aortic valvular stenosis), aortic root dilatation, and left ventricular dysfunction (associated with myocarditis or dilated cardiomyopathy). However, even such diagnostic testing cannot guarantee recognition of all important lesions, and some relevant cardiovascular diseases may be beyond detection with any screening methodology. For example, identification of many congenital coronary artery anomalies usually requires sophisticated laboratory examination including coronary arteriography, although it is possible in selected young athletes to raise a strong suspicion of important anomalies such as left main coronary artery from the right sinus of Valsalva with echocardiography.[41-44] Arrhythmogenic right ventricular dysplasia usually cannot be reliably diagnosed solely by echocardiography and ECG; the best available noninvasive test for this disease is probably magnetic resonance imaging, which unfortunately is both expensive and not universally available.[51,68]

Cost-efficiency issues are important when assessing the feasibility of applying expensive noninvasive testing to the screening of large athletic populations.[22,69-72] In the vast majority of instances, adequate financial and personnel resources are lacking for such endeavors. In those situations in which the full (i.e., unreduced) expense of testing would be the responsibility of administrative bodies such as a school, university, or team, the costs are probably prohibitive; for example, at present an echocardiographic study ranges from about $400 to $2,000 (average, about $600).[22] If the occurrence of hypertrophic cardiomyopathy in a young athletic population is assumed to be 1:500,[35] even at $500 per study it would theoretically cost $250,000 to detect even 1 previously undiagnosed case.

Screening protocols incorporating noninvasive testing at greatly reduced cost have been described.[22,69,72] However, these efforts have involved unique circumstances in which echocardiographic equipment was donated and professional expenses were waived for all but technician-related costs. Also, some investigators have suggested an inexpensive shortened-format echocardiogram for population screening (limited to parasternal views; about 2 minutes in duration).[69,72] While such individual initiatives should not be discouraged, it may also be noted that public service projects based largely on volunteerism usually cannot be sustained on a consistent basis.

An important limitation of preparticipation screening with 2-dimensional echocardiography is the potential for false positive or false negative test results. False positive results arise from the assignment of borderline values for left ventricular wall thicknesses (or particularly enlarged cavity size), which require formulation of a differential diagnosis between normal but extreme physiological adaptations of athlete's heart[73-78] and pathological conditions such as HCM or other cardiomyopathies.[37] Indeed, such clinical dilemmas (which may not always be definitively resolvable in individual athletes) generate emotional, financial, and medical burdens for the athlete, family, team, and institution by virtue of the uncertainty created and the requirement for additional testing. False negative screening results may occur in athletes with HCM when testing by echocardiography occurs at a point of incomplete phenotypic expression during adolescence.[79] For example, in young athletes with HCM less than 13–15 years old, left ventricular hypertrophy is often absent or mild, and therefore the echocardiographic findings may not yet be diagnostic at the time of preparticipation screening.

The 12-lead ECG has been proposed as a more practical and cost-efficient alternative to routine echocardiography for population-based screening.[66,80] Indeed, the ECG is abnormal in about 95% of patients with HCM,[81] may be abnormal in other potentially lethal structural lesions, and will usually identify the important (but uncommon) long QT syndrome.[48–50] However, of note, a substantial proportion of genetically affected relatives in families with long QT syndrome may not have phenotypic expression on the ECG.[48]

However, as a primary screening test, the ECG suffers in comparison to the echocardiogram by its lack of imaging capability for recognition of structural cardiovascular malformations. Also, the ECG has relatively low specificity as a screening test in athletic populations because of the high frequency with which ECG alterations occur in association with the normal physiological adaptations to training (athlete's heart).[82,83] Such false positive ECG test results substantially complicate the use of the 12-lead ECG as a primary screening tool in athletic populations. It can be anticipated that about 20–25% of athletes examined in the context of preparticipation screening will have ECG patterns that ultimately stimulate echocardiographic study.[80] Also of note is the fact that elite athletes not infrequently demonstrate distinctly abnormal ECG patterns consistent with pathological conditions, even in the absence of structural heart disease and without increased cardiac dimensions due to training.[82]

To date, there have been relatively few published reports of cardiovascular screening efforts in large athletic populations.[22,73,80,84] Most of these studies have implemented noninvasive testing (i.e., conventional or limited echocardiographic examination or 12-lead ECG) in young high school or college athletes. The populations subjected to screening ranged in size from 250 to 2,000 athletes, usually studied over a 1-year period. In general, these reports are consistent by virtue of describing the detection of very few definitive examples of potentially lethal cardiovascular abnormalities.

## Perspectives on Race and Gender

Hypertrophic cardiomyopathy is an important cause of sudden death in young African-American athletes and there is preliminary evidence that such catastrophes may be more common in black athletes compared to their white counterparts.[3,85] The substantial occurrence of HCM-related sudden death in young black male athletes contrasts sharply with the very infrequent reporting of black patients with HCM in hospital and clinic-based populations from tertiary referral centers.[24,25] Therefore, in African-Americans, HCM is most frequently encountered when the disease results in sudden and unexpected death during competitive athletics. These data emphasize the disproportionate access to subspecialty health care between the black and white communities in the United States that makes it less likely for young black male athletes to receive a relatively sophisticated cardiovascular diagnosis such as HCM. Consequently, African-American athletes with HCM are less likely to be identified or disqualified from competition to reduce their risk for sudden death, in accordance with the recommendations of Bethesda Conference #26.[23]

Sudden death on the athletic field is uncommon in young women[3] (comprising only about 10% of all such deaths); this disproportionality in women may be explained on the basis of lower participation rates or less severe training demands and cardiac adaptation[4,22] in some instances, but also because HCM is less commonly recognized clinically in women.[24-26,28-30] This observation also suggests the possibility that a measure of protection from sudden death is attributable in some physiological fashion to gender itself. Nevertheless, available data do not provide a compelling justification to construct specific screening algorithms, based on gender, race, or demographic subgrouping.

## Criteria for Eligibility and Disqualification

When a previously unsuspected cardiovascular abnormality is identified in a competitive athlete, whether by standard screening or other means, the following considerations arise: (1) the magnitude of risk for sudden cardiac death associated with continued participation in competitive sports and (2) the criteria to be implemented for determining whether that athlete would benefit from disqualification from athletics. In this regard, the 26th Bethesda Conference sponsored by the American College of Cardiology[23] offers prospective and consensus recommendations for athletic eligibility or disqualification, taking into account the severity of the cardiovascular abnormality as well as the nature of sports training and competition. The 26th Bethesda Conference recommendations[23] are predicated on the likelihood that intense athletic training will increase the risk for sudden cardiac death (or disease progression) in trained athletes with clinically important underlying structural heart disease, although it is not presently possible to quantify that risk precisely for individual participants. Nevertheless, it is presumed that the temporary or permanent withdrawal of selected athletes from participation in certain sports is prudent and likely to diminish the perceived risk.

## Other Risks of the Athletic Field Unrelated to Underlying Cardiovascular Disease: Commotio Cordis

Although sudden death in young athletes from unsuspected and largely congenital heart diseases has achieved great visibility, other unusual risks of organized or recreational sports activity leading to cardiovascular collapse have been more recently emphasized for the first time.[86–90] For example, although apparently uncommon, virtually instantaneous cardiac arrest may result from a relatively modest and nonpenetrating blow to the chest, in the absence of underlying cardiovascular disease or structural injury to the chest wall or heart itself.[86,87] This impact may, however, leave a contusion on the chest wall over the precordium in about one-third of cases (Figure 6). In such events, which have been referred to as commotio cordis ("disturbed or agitated heart motion"), blunt chest impact over the anatomic position of the heart is usually produced by a projectile (most commonly a baseball) or by bodily collision with another athlete. The chest blow is usually of low energy (with hockey pucks the exception) and not perceived as unusual for the sporting event, nor apparently of sufficient magnitude to result in death. A common scenario during competitive sports is that of a young baseball player struck in the chest (while batting) by a pitched ball thrown at about 40 mph from a distance of about 40 feet. Of note, these catastrophes have occurred in a variety of organized sports but just as commonly in purely recreational situations at home or on the playing field, with the fatal injuries often produced by close relatives (Figure 7).

Although the precise mechanisms responsible for a commotio cordis event are not known with certainty, a recently developed experimental model in juvenile swine closely simulates the clinical profile of this phenomenon and provides important insights.[88,89] This model demonstrates that a precordial blow can create devastating electrophysiological consequences largely by virtue of its precise timing (and location over the heart). When chest impact occurred with modest force (30 mph) during a very narrow window of 15–30 ms prior to the peak of the T wave (representing only about 1% of the overall cardiac cycle), and interfered with the vul-

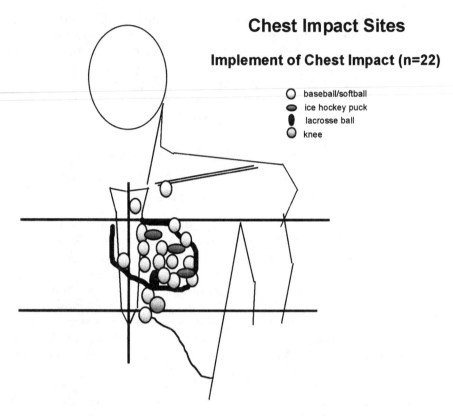

**Chest Impact Sites**

**Implement of Chest Impact (n=22)**

○ baseball/softball
◑ ice hockey puck
❚ lacrosse ball
◉ knee

Figure 6. Schematic representation of the location of impact points (contusions) on the anterior chest wall judged to be produced by projectiles such as baseballs or softballs, ice hockey pucks, lacrosse balls, or blunt bodily contact, identifiable in 22 victims of commotio cordis. Estimated contour of the heart is demarcated by the solid line. The lesions are either oval or circular contusions, abrasions, or bruises located in the mid-precordial area, usually to the left of the sternum, extending laterally to the nipple line and vertically from the angle of Louis to the xiphoid process. (From Maron BJ, et al.,[87] reproduced with permission of Journal of Cardiovascular Electrophysiology.)

nerable phase of repolarization, ventricular fibrillation resulted instantaneously and reproducibly.[88] Conversely, when the precordium was struck during depolarization (on the QRS complex), transient complete heart block often occurred.

Furthermore, in the swine model, softer-than-standard safety baseballs reduced the risk of ventricular fibrillation,[88] suggesting that prevention of sudden death from commotio cordis during certain youth sporting activities could be achieved through the modification of athletic equipment. Chest protection and padding may be appropriate for selected cir-

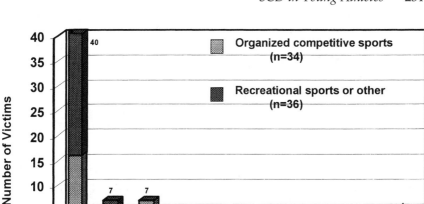

Figure 7. Sports participation at the time of blunt chest impact-induced sudden cardiac arrest (commotio cordis), shown separately for competitive and recreational athletic activities. (From Maron BJ, et al.,[87] reproduced with permission of Journal of Cardiovascular Electrophysiology.)

cumstances or sports such as in ice hockey, karate, or youth baseball. However, the low event rate for commotio cordis is an obstacle to documenting the effectiveness of any protective intervention. Indeed, it is probably not possible to achieve absolute protection and "zero risk" from all adverse eventualities of athletic participation while at the same time preserving the integrity of the competition.[61]

Commotio cordis events are not uniformly fatal and approximately 10% of reported victims are known to have survived, usually when afforded reasonably prompt cardiopulmonary resuscitation and defibrillation.[90] With enhanced public awareness of this syndrome, emergency measures are more likely to be promptly implemented on the athletic field, possibly avoiding many future deaths.

The frequency that commotio cordis occurs is unknown, but the phenomenon is undoubtedly uncommon. On the other hand, because systematic and comprehensive identification of cases is exceedingly difficult, it is reasonable to assume that such events are underreported. Nevertheless, the issue of prevalence should not detract from the significance of commotio cordis as a newly appreciated risk of the athletic field or its recognition as a true clinical event. Indeed, blunt chest impact-induced cardiac arrest has been so poorly understood in the lay community that some such events have been regarded as criminal acts, rather than physiologically based catastrophes and accidents.[87]

Therefore, the commotio cordis syndrome accounts for an important subset of sudden deaths during sports activities occurring in the absence of cardiovascular disease. The mechanical energy of chest impact over the precordium is almost instantaneously converted into a devastating electrophysiological event in which ventricular fibrillation is caused when 3 criteria are fulfilled: (1) chest impact located directly over the heart, usually of relatively low energy;[86,87] (2) precise timing of the blow to a narrow 15-ms segment of the cardiac cycle during repolarization, vulnerable to potentially lethal ventricular arrhythmias, just prior to the T wave peak,[88] and apparently by activation of the $K^+_{ATP}$ channel;[89] and (3) a narrow, compliant chest wall, typical of young children.

> *Death should stay away from young men's games. Death belongs in musty hospital rooms, sickbeds. It should not impinge its terrible presence on the celebrations of youth, reap its frightful harvest in fields where cheers ring and bands play and banners wave.*
> Jim Murray

> To An Athlete Dying Young
> *The time you won your town the race*
> *We chaired you through the marketplace;*
> *Man and boy stood cheering by,*
> *And home we brought you shoulder high.*
>
> *Today, the road all runners come,*
> *Shoulder-high we bring you home,*
> *And set you at your threshold down,*
> *Townsman of a stiller town.*
> Alfred Edward Housmann, 1895

## References

1. Maron BJ. Sudden death in young athletes: lessons from the Hank Gathers affair. N Engl J Med 1993; 329:55–57.
2. Burke AP, Farb V, Virmani R, et al. Sports-related and non-sports-related sudden cardiac death in young adults. Am Heart J 1991; 121:568–575.
3. Maron BJ, Shirani J, Poliac LC, et al. Sudden death in young competitive athletes: clinical, demographic and pathological profiles. JAMA 1996; 276:199–204.
4. van Camp SP, Bloor CM, Mueller FO, et al. Nontraumatic sports death in high school and college athletes. Med Sci Sports Exer 1995; 27:641–647.
5. Maron BJ, Roberts WC, McAllister HA, et al. Sudden death in young athletes. Circulation 1980; 62:218–229.

6. Corrado D, Thiene G, Nava A, et al. Sudden death in young competitive athletes: clinicopathologic correlations in 22 cases. Am J Med 1990; 89:588–596.
7. Thiene G, Nava A, Corrado D, et al. Right ventricular cardiomyopathy and sudden death in young people. N Engl J Med 1988; 318:129–133.
8. Tsung SH, Huang TY, Chang HH. Sudden death in young athletes. Arch Pathol Lab Med 1982; 106:168–170.
9. James TN, Froggatt P, Marshall TK. Sudden death in young athletes. Ann Intern Med 1967; 67:1013–1021.
10. Furlanello F, Bettini R, Cozzi F, et al. Ventricular arrhythmias and sudden death in athletes. Ann N Y Acad Sci 1984; 427:253–279.
11. Maron BJ, Epstein SE, Roberts WC. Causes of sudden death in competitive athletes. J Am Coll Cardiol 1986; 7:204–214.
12. Drory Y, Turetz Y, Hiss Y, et al. Sudden unexpected death in persons <40 years of age. Am J Cardiol 1991; 68:1388–1392.
13. Topaz O, Edwards JE. Pathologic features of sudden death in children, adolescents and young adults. Chest 1985; 87:476–482.
14. Liberthson RR. Sudden death from cardiac causes in children and young adults. N Engl J Med 1996; 334:1039–1044.
15. Thompson PD, Stern MP, Williams P, et al. Death during jogging or running: a study of 18 cases. JAMA 1979; 242:1265–1267.
16. Thompson PD, Funk EJ, Carleton RA, et al. Incidence of death during jogging in Rhode Island from 1975 through 1980. JAMA 1982; 247:2535–2538.
17. Waller BF, Roberts WC. Sudden death while running in conditioned runners aged 40 years or over. Am J Cardiol 1980; 45:1292–1300.
18. Virmani R, Robinowitz M, McAllister HA Jr. Nontraumatic death in joggers: a series of 30 patients at autopsy. Am J Med 1982; 72:874–882.
19. Maron BJ, Mitchell JH. Revised eligibility recommendations for competitive athletes with cardiovascular abnormalities. (Introduction to Bethesda Conference #26). J Am Coll Cardiol 1994; 24:848–850.
20. Maron BJ, Poliac L, Kaplan JA, et al. Blunt impact to the chest leading to sudden death from cardiac arrest during sports activities. N Engl J Med 1995; 333:337–342.
21. Maron BJ, Garson A. Arrhythmias and sudden cardiac death in elite athletes. Cardiol Rev (D Zipes, ed), 1994; 2(1):26–32.
22. Maron BJ, Thompson PD, Puffer JC, et al. Cardiovascular preparticipation screening of competitive athletes. Circulation 1996; 94:850–856.
23. Maron BJ, Mitchell JH. 26th Bethesda Conference. Recommendations for determining eligibility for competition in athletes with cardiovascular abnormalities. J Am Coll Cardiol 1994; 24:845–899.
24. Wigle ED, Sasson Z, Henderson MA, et al. Hypertrophic cardiomyopathy: the importance of the site and extent of hypertrophy—a review. Prog Cardiovasc Dis 1985; 28:1–83.
25. Maron BJ, Bonow RO, Cannon RO, et al. Hypertrophic cardiomyopathy: interrelation of clinical manifestations, pathophysiology, and therapy. N Engl J Med 1987; 316:780–789 and 844–852.
26. Louie EK, Edwards LC. Hypertrophic cardiomyopathy. Prog Cardiovasc Dis 1994; 36:275–308.
27. Spirito P, Seidman CE, McKenna WJ, et al. The management of hypertrophic cardiomyopathy. N Engl J Med 1997; 336:775–785.
28. Klues HG, Schiffers A, Maron BJ. Phenotypic spectrum and patterns of left ventricular hypertrophy in hypertrophic cardiomyopathy: morphologic observa-

tions and significance as assessed by two-dimensional echocardiography in 600 patients. J Am Coll Cardiol 1995; 26:1699–1708.

29. Maron BJ. Hypertrophic cardiomyopathy. Lancet 1997; 3350:127–133.

30. Maron BJ, Moller JH, Seidman CE, et al. Impact of laboratory molecular diagnosis on contemporary diagnostic criteria for genetically transmitted cardiovascular diseases: hypertrophic cardiomyopathy, long-QT syndrome, and Marfan syndrome. Circulation 1998; 98:1460–1471.

31. Thierfelder L, Watkins H, MacRae C,et al. α-Tropomyosin and cardiac troponin T mutations cause familial hypertrophic cardiomyopathy: a disease of the sarcomere. Cell 1994; 77:701–712.

32. Niimura H, Bachinski LL, Sangwatanaroj S, et al. Mutations in the gene for human cardiac myosin-binding protein C and late-onset familial hypertrophic cardiomyopathy. N Engl J Med 1998; 338:1248–1257.

33. Schwartz K, Carrier L, Guicheney P, et al. Molecular basis of familial cardiomyopathies. Circulation 1995; 91:532–540.

34. Marian AJ, Roberts R. Recent advances in the molecular genetics of hypertrophic cardiomyopathy. Circulation 1995; 91:532–540.

35. Maron BJ, Gardin JM, Flack JM, et al. Asssessment of the prevalence of hypertrophic cardiomyopathy in a general population of young adults: echocardiographic analysis of 4111 subjects in the CARDIA Study. Circulation 1995; 92:785–789.

36. Maron BJ, Shen WK, Link MS, et al. Efficacy of the implantable cardioverter-defibrillator for the prevention of sudden death in hypertrophic cardiomyopathy (abstract). Circulation (in press).

37. Maron BJ, Pelliccia A, Spirito P. Cardiac disease in young trained athletes: insights into methods for distinguishing athlete's heart from structural heart disease with particular emphasis on hypertrophic cardiomyopathy. Circulation 1995; 91:1596–1601.

38. Maron BJ, Isner JM, McKenna WJ. Hypertrophic cardiomyopathy, myocarditis and other myopericardial diseases, and mitral valve prolapse. Task Force 3. In: Maron BJ, Mitchell JH (eds). 26th Bethesda Conference. Recommendations for Determining Eligibility for Competition in Athletes with Cardiovascular Abnormalities. J Am Coll Cardiol 1994; 24:880–885.

39. Cheitlin MD, De Castro CM, McAllister HA. Sudden death as a complication of anomalous left coronary origin from the anterior sinus of Valsalva: a not-so-minor congenital anomaly. Circulation 1974:50:780–787.

40. Roberts WC. Congenital coronary arterial anomalies unassociated with major anomalies of the heart or great vessels. In: Adult Congenital Heart Disease. FA Davis Co., Philadelphia,1987, p 583.

41. Basso C, Maron BJ, Corrado D, et al. Clinical profile of congenital coronary artery anomalies with origin from the wrong aortic sinus leading to sudden death in young competitive athletes. In press.

42. Gaither NS, Rogan KM, Stajduhar K, et al. Anomalous origin and course of coronary arteries in adults: identification and improved imaging utilizing transesophageal echocardiography. Am Heart J 1991; 122:69–75.

43. Maron BJ, Leon BJ, Swain JA. Prospective identification by two-dimensional echocardiography of anomalous origin of the left main coronary artery from the right sinus of Valsalva. Am J Cardiol 1991; 68:140–142.

44. Jureidini SB, Eaton C, Williams J, Nouri S, Appleton RS. Transthoracic two-dimensional and color flow echocardiographic diagnosis of aberrant left coronary artery. Am Heart J 1994; 127:438–440.

45. Bharati S, Lev M. Congenital abnormalities of the conduction system in sudden death in young adults. J Am Coll Cardiol 1986; 8:1096–1104.
46. Thiene G, Pennelli N, Rossi L. Cardiac conduction system abnormalities as a possible cause of sudden death in young athletes. Human Pathol 1983; 14:706–709.
47. Benson DW, Benditt DG, Anderson RW, et al. Cardiac arrest in young, ostensibly healthy patients: clinical, hemodynamic and electrophysiologic findings. Am J Cardiol 1983; 52:65–69.
48. Vincent GM, Timothy KW, Leppert M, et al. The spectrum of symptoms and QT intervals in carriers of the gene for the long-QT syndrome. N Engl J Med 1992; 327:846–852.
49. Moss AJ, Schwartz PJ, Crampton RS, et al. The long QT syndrome: prospective longitudinal study of 328 families. Circulation 1991; 84:1136–1144.
50. Roden DM, Lazzara R, Rosen M, et al. Mutiple mechanisms in the long-QT syndrome: current knowledge, gaps, and future directions. Circulation 1996; 94:1996–2012.
51. McKenna WJ, Thiene G, Nava A, et al. Diagnosis of arrhythmogenic right ventricular dysplasia/cardiomyopathy. Br Heart J 1994; 71:215–218.
52. Kark JA, Posey DM, Schumacher HR, et al. Sickle-cell as a risk factor for sudden death in physical training. N Engl J Med 1987; 317:781–787.
53. Virmani R, Robinowitz M, Smialek JE. Cardiovascular effects of cocaine: an autopsy study of 40 patients. Am Heart J 1988; 115:1068–1076.
54. Isner JM, Estes NAM III, Thompson PD, et al. Acute cardiac events temporally related to cocaine abuse. N Engl J Med 1986; 315:1438–1443.
55. Kloner RA, Hale S, Alkekr K, et al. The effects of acute and chronic cocaine use on the heart. Circulation 1992; 85:407–419.
56. Kaplan NM, Deveraux RB, Miller HS Jr. Systemic hypertension. Task Force 4. In: Maron BJ, Mitchell JH (eds). 26th Bethesda Conference. Recommendations for Determining Eligibility for Competition in Athletes with Cardiovascular Abnormalities. J Am Coll Cardiol 1994; 24:885–888.
57. Maron BJ, Poliac LC, Roberts WO. Risk for sudden cardiac death associated with marathon running. J Am Coll Cardiol 1996; 28:428–431.
58. Kerber RE, Becker LB, Bourland JD, et al. Automatic external defibrillators for public access defibrillation: recommendations for specifying and reporting arrhythmia analysis, algorithm performance, incorporating new waveforms, and enhancing safety. Circulation 1997; 95:1677–1682.
59. Maron BJ, Gohman TE, Aeppli D. Prevalence of sudden cardiac death during competitive sports activities in Minnesota high school athletes. J Am Coll Cardiol 1998; 32:1881–1884.
60. Pelliccia A, Maron BJ. Preparticipation cardiovascular evaluation of the competitive athlete: perspectives from the 30-year Italian experience. Am J Cardiol 1995; 75:827–831.
61. Maron BJ, Brown RW, McGrew CA, et al. Ethical, legal and practical considerations affecting medical decision-making in competitive athletes. In: Maron BJ, Mitchell JH, eds. 26th Bethesda Conference. Recommendations for Determining Eligibility for Competition in Athletes with Cardiovascular Abnormalities. J Am Coll Cardiol 1994; 24:854–860.
62. Mitten MJ, Maron BJ. Legal considerations that affect medical eligibility for competitive athletes with cardiovascular abnormalities and acceptance of Bethesda Conference recommendations. J Am Coll Cardiol 1994; 24:861–863.
63. Mitten MJ. Team physicians and competitive athletes: allocating legal responsibility for athletic injuries. U Pitt L Rev 1993; 55:129–169.

64. Maron BJ, Mitten MJ, Quandt EK, et al. Competitive athletes with cardiovascular disease: the case of Nicholas Knapp. N Engl J Med 1998; 339:1632–1635.
65. Glover DW, Maron BJ. Profile of preparticipation cardiovascular screening for high school athletes. JAMA 1998; 179:1817–1819.
66. Corrado D, Basso C, Schiavon M, et al. Screening for hypertrophic cardiomyopathy in young athletes. N Engl J Med 1998; 339:364–369.
67. Maron BJ, Epstein SE. Hypertrophic cardiomyopathy: a discussion of nomenclature. Am J Cardiol 1979; 43:1242–1244.
68. Ricci C, Longo R, Pagnan L, et al. Magnetic resonance imaging in right ventricular dysplasia. Am J Cardiol 1992; 70:1589–1595.
69. Weidenbener EJ, Krauss MD, Waller BF, et al. Incorporation of screening echocardiography in the preparticipation exam. Clin J Sport Med 1995; 5:86–89.
70. Feinstein RA, Colvin E, Oh MK. Echocardiographic screening as part of a preparticipation examination. Clin J Sport Med 1993; 3:149–152.
71. Risser WL, Hoffman HM, Gordon BG Jr, et al. A cost-benefit analysis of preparticipation sports examination of adolescent athletes. J School Health 1985; 55:270–273.
72. Murry PM, Cantwell JD, Heith DL, et al. The role of limited echocardiography in screening athletes. Am J Cardiol 1995; 76:849–850.
73. Lewis JF, Maron BJ, Diggs JA, et al. Preparticipation echocardiographic screening for cardiovascular disease in a large, predominantly black population of collegiate athletes. Am J Cardiol 1989; 64:1029–1033.
74. Huston TP, Puffer JC, Rodney McW. The athlete heart syndrome. N Engl J Med 1985; 4:24–32.
75. Maron BJ. Structural features of the athlete heart as defined by echocardiography. J Am Coll Cardiol 1986; 7:190–203.
76. Pelliccia A, Maron BJ, Spataro A, et al. The upper limit of physiologic cardiac hypertrophy in highly trained elite athletes. N Engl J Med 1991; 324:295–301.
77. Pelliccia A, Maron BJ, Culasso F, et al. Athlete's heart in women: echocardiographic characterization of highly trained elite female athletes. JAMA 1996; 276:211–215.
78. Pelliccia A, Cullasso F, Di Paolo F, et al. Physiologic left ventricular cavity dilatation in elite athletes. Ann Intern Med 1999; 130:23–31.
79. Maron BJ, Spirito P, Wesley YE, et al. Development and progression of left ventricular hypertrophy in children with hypertrophic cardiomyopathy. N Engl J Med 1986; 315:610–614.
80. Maron BJ, Bodison SA, Wesley YE, et al. Results of screening a large group of intercollegiate competitive athletes for cardiovascular disease. J Am Coll Cardiol 1987; 10:1214–1221.
81. Maron BJ, Wolfson JK, Ciró E, et al. Relation of electrocardiographic abnormalities and patterns of left ventricular hypertrophy identified by two-dimensional echocardiography in patients with hypertrophic cardiomyopathy. Am J Cardiol 1983; 51:189–194.
82. Pelliccia A, Cullasso F, Di Paolo FM, et al. Clinical significance of abnormal electrocardiographic patterns in elite athletes: the impact of gender and cardiac morphologic adaptations to training (abstract). Circulation 1996; 94:I-326.
83. Zehender M, Meinertz T, Keul J, et al. ECG variants and cardiac arrhythmias in athletes: clinical relevance and prognostic importance. Am Heart J 1990; 119:1378–1391.
84. Fuller CM, McNulty CM, Spring DA, et al. Prospective screening of 5,615 high school athletes for risk of sudden cardiac death. Med Sci Sports Exerc 1997; 29:1131–1138.

85. Maron BJ, Poliac LC, Mathenge R. Hypertrophic cardiomyopathy as an important cause of sudden cardiac death on the athletic field in African-American athletes (abstract). J Am Coll Cardiol 1997; 29(Suppl A):462A.
86. Maron BJ, Poliac L, Kaplan JA, et al. Blunt impact to the chest leading to sudden death from cardiac arrest during sports activities. N Engl J Med 1995; 333:337–342.
87. Maron BJ, Link MS, Wang PJ, et al. Clinical profile of commotio cordis: an under-appreciated cause of sudden death in the young during sports and other activities. J Cardiovasc Electrophysiol 1999:10:114–120.
88. Link MS, Wang PJ, Pandian NG, et al. An experimental model of sudden death due to low-energy chest-wall impact (commotio cordis). N Engl J Med 1998; 338:1805–1811.
89. Link MS, Wang PJ, VanderBrink BA, et al. Selective activation of the $K^+_{ATP}$ is a mechanism by which sudden death is produced by low energy chest wall impact (commotio cordis). Circulation 1999; 100:413–418.
90. Maron BJ, Strasburger JF, Kugler JD, et al. Survival following blunt chest impact-induced cardiac arrest during sports activities in young athletes. Am J Cardiol 1997; 79:840–841.

# 16

# Idiopathic Ventricular Fibrillation

*Silvia G. Priori, MD, PhD, and*
*Lia Crotti, MD*

## Introduction

Ventricular tachyarrhythmias are the leading cause of sudden unexpected cardiac death. More than 90% of these deaths occur in patients with structural heart disease such as coronary artery disease, cardiomyopathies, and valvular abnormalities.[1]

Recently, attention has been focused on sudden arrhythmic death occurring in individuals with an apparently normal heart. These subjects are very often young, active, and otherwise healthy. Data collected from a large series of victims of cardiac arrest show that ventricular fibrillation in the absence of structural heart disease may be more common than previously recognized, occurring in 1% of survivors of cardiac arrest and in up to 8% of victims of sudden death.[2,3]

Idiopathic ventricular fibrillation is the term that is most frequently used to describe the occurrence of ventricular fibrillation in the intact heart. This term best acknowledges the inability to identify a causal relationship between the clinical circumstance and the arrhythmia, yet does not exclude the existence of "predisposing" and "precipitating" factors.[4]

The first problem concerning idiopathic ventricular fibrillation (IVF) is the definition of this entity. Idiopathic ventricular fibrillation is a diagnosis of exclusion. It is therefore of major importance to define the criteria on which the diagnosis is based, and more specifically, to determine which clinical diagnoses need to be ruled out before an IVF diagnosis is advocated. A consensus document has been prepared by a panel convened by the Working Group of Arrhythmias of the European Society of Cardiology[4] to define the clinical examinations that should be performed before a survivor of cardiac arrest is labeled as affected by IVF. A summary of these recommendations is outlined below.

From: Aliot E, Clementy J, Prystowsky EN (editors). *Fighting Sudden Cardiac Death: A Worldwide Challenge.* ©Futura Publishing Company, Armonk, NY, 2000.

# Criteria for Diagnosis of Idiopathic Ventricular Fibrillation

The clinical evaluations that should be performed in individuals with documented ventricular fibrillation to exclude with an appropriate level of confidence the presence of a structural heart disease are:

1. Collection of clinical history with attention devoted to recording of pharmacological treatment as well as the use of "recreational " drugs.
2. Blood biochemistry: cardiac enzymes; thyroid function tests; serum alcohol level; sedimentation rate; inflammatory indexes; glucose; serum electrolytes; white blood cell count.
3. Electrocardiography (12-lead ECG, 24-hour ambulatory ECG recording, exercise stress test).
4. 2D-echocardiography.
5. Coronary angiography.
6. Left and right ventricular cineangiography.
7. Electrophysiological study with assessment of atrioventricular conduction.

Ventricular biopsy is not considered a mandatory examination; however, it is recommended when it may be targeted to specific regions of the ventricles where "dubious" morphologic or kinetic abnormalities have been suspected.

The role of programmed electrical stimulation in subjects with an apparently "intact" heart is controversial and, therefore, despite the fact that most electrophysiologists would include it in the series of investigations of a survivor of cardiac arrest, the authors of the document[4] have decided to consider programmed electrical stimulation an elective procedure. The role of drug testing in the setting of programmed electrical stimulation will be discussed in a later chapter.

It is important to acknowledge that despite having IVF, patients have by definition a structurally intact heart, but this does not imply that their heart is free from any "abnormality"; it simply means that their heart is free from abnormalities associated with increased susceptibility to ventricular tachyarrhythmias. Therefore, the presence of common abnormalities such as mitral valve prolapse not associated with hemodynamic consequences or QT prolongation may well be acceptable within the diagnosis of IVF.

Although these criteria will help render the diagnosis of IVF more uniformly, clinical difficulties are far from being solved. For example, the interpretation of "minimal cardiac abnormalities" is one of the most debated issues for the diagnosis of IVF. In addition to nonspecific biopsy findings, the significance of minor hemodynamic abnormalities, borderline right and left ventricular indexes, and subtle wall motion abnormalities have an unclear meaning in survivors of IVF. The interpretation of these findings is difficult mainly because the incidence of these abnormalities in the general population is unknown.

In recent years the contribution of molecular genetics to clinical cardiology has focused the attention toward a novel class of arrhythmogenic diseases characterized by normal cardiac morphology and normal cardiac function. This cluster of diseases called "ion channel diseases"[5] includes the different genetic variants of the long QT syndrome[6] and the recently described Brugada syndrome.[7]

A novel question arises of whether ion channel diseases should be included in the diagnosis of IVF.

A few years ago nobody would have considered including long QT syndrome in IVF; however, today it is accepted by many that the diagnosis of Brugada syndrome equals that of IVF. Since long QT syndrome and Brugada syndrome are, at least in one form, allelic variants of the same genetic abnormality (*SCN5A* defects), it seems reasonable that the 2 disorders are both considered separate from IVF.

Most of the controversy arose as a consequence of the paper by Chen et al.[8] describing the identification of mutations in the cardiac sodium channel gene in some families with diagnosis of Brugada syndrome. It is now time to put things into perspective.

In analogy to the long QT syndrome that is characterized by QT interval prolongation, Brugada syndrome is also characterized by a typical ECG pattern (right bundle branch block and ST segment elevation in leads $V_1$ to $V_3$). Even if in most cases the typical ECG pattern can be clearly identified, "concealed" forms of the long QT syndrome and Brugada syndrome have been reported.[9,10] If cardiac arrest occurs in a patient with a subclinical form of long QT syndrome or Brugada syndrome, that patient is likely to be diagnosed as having IVF because no structural heart disease will be identified. Nevertheless, this is by no means an appropriate diagnosis. It is our opinion that *diagnosis of long QT syndrome and of Brugada syndrome should be carefully searched for and excluded in survivors of IVF.* This should be done by repeated ECG recordings at rest and during stress, by 12-lead Holter monitoring, and, in case of Brugada syndrome, by a provocative test with sodium channel blockers. Since both diseases may remain undiagnosed despite careful clinical evaluation, it will be only through the widespread availability of genetic testing with much higher sensitivity and specificity than is presently available that exclusion of long QT syndrome and Brugada syndrome will be possible in the vast majority of IVF survivors.

After having discussed the definition of IVF, it is time to move to the most pressing clinical problem for the cardiologist, i.e., how to manage survivors of IVF. These individuals are often young and active subjects, anxious to resume a normal life and to be informed about their long-term prognosis and treatment.[11,12]

Physicians are thus faced with some key questions that influence therapeutic decisions: What is the risk of recurrence in IVF survivors? What are the acute and long-term responses to "pharmacological" versus "device" treatment? How often does ventricular fibrillation represent the first clinical sign of a structural disease that will become manifest years later?

The Working Group on Arrhythmias of the European Society of Cardiology recognized the clinical relevance of these questions and in 1992 established a prospective long-term registry of cardiac arrest in the normal heart, with the goal of addressing this problem.[13] This international database is called Unexplained Cardiac Arrest Registry of Europe (UCARE) and has already enrolled more than 200 patients who survived IVF episodes. The data available in UCARE represent the world's largest experience on IVF. These data provide preliminary answers needed to define the optimal long-term management of IVF patients.

## What Is the Risk of Recurrence of Cardiac Arrest?

Five years after cardiac arrest, IVF patients have a 30% chance of recurrence of cardiac arrest.[14] This means that the majority of patients (70%) remain free of symptoms at follow-up, so it would be extremely important to devise risk stratification protocols leading to the identification of those patients at higher risk of recurrence. Unfortunately, at present, no predictors of poor outcome are available; as a consequence, UCARE investigators recommend an implantable cardioverter-defibrillator (ICD) for all IVF survivors in order to protect the 30% that will experience recurrence. Despite advocating "aggressive" treatment (ICD implantation) for IVF survivors, we should not forget when counseling the patients that in the majority of them, a lethal event will not recur. Obviously this is not satisfactory and new strategies for risk stratification have to be devised.

Peeters et al.[15] proposed that 62-lead body surface QRST integral maps could help in the identification of patients at higher risk. In 17 patients with a first episode of IVF, 29% had a normal dipolar map, 24% had a dipolar map with an abnormally large negative area on the right side of the thorax, and 47% had a nondipolar map. All subjects of a healthy control group had a normal dipolar QRST integral map. A recurrent arrhythmic event occurred in 7 patients (41%), all of whom had an abnormal QRST integral map.

Schaefers et al.[16] studied cardiac radioactive iodine-labeled meta-iodobenzylguanidine (I-123-MIBG) uptake in 45 patients with idiopathic right ventricular outflow tract tachycardia (RVO-VT), 25 patients with idiopathic left ventricular tachycardia (ILVT), 15 patients with IVF, and 10 control patients. I-123-MIBG cardiac imaging is used to evaluate presynaptic norepinephrine reuptake in different parts of the heart since MIBG is a norepinephrine analog. Locally reduced I-123-MIBG uptake was found in 27 of 45 RVO-VT patients (60%), 5 of 15 ILVT patients (33%), and 17 of 25 IVF patients (68%). In conclusion, patients with RVO-VT and IVF show significantly reduced I-123-MIBG uptake in the posterior left ventricular wall compared with control patients. The determination of impaired cardiac sympathetic innervation assessed by MIBG activity may be useful for patients at risk for sudden cardiac death.

So far none of these parameters has been tested and confirmed in other laboratories, so their clinical applicability is still limited.

# What Are the Acute and Long-Term Responses to Drug Versus Device Treatment?

According to UCARE investigators, prevention of recurrence with antiarrhythmic agents and beta-blockers has failed.[17] A different view comes from the Israeli studies led by Belhassen and Viskin,[18] who reported a limited but positive experience with the use of sodium channel blockers in 15 patients. This result is not confirmed by the UCARE Registry: 9% of the patients were treated with sodium channel blockers and this group had a 30% recurrence rate with 2 sudden deaths. Long-term follow-up of 6 IVF patients in whom programmed electrical stimulation had predicted suppression of inducibility with sodium channel blockers showed a recurrence rate of 100%.[19]

Thus, according to the UCARE experience, IVF survivors do not benefit from antiarrhythmic therapy and should be considered as candidates for an implantable defibrillator.[17]

# How Often Does Ventricular Fibrillation Represent the First Clinical Sign of a Structural Disease that Will Become Manifest Years Later?

This is one of the most interesting speculative questions concerning IVF. Since the early description of IVF cases, clinicians have handled the frustration of being unable to make a diagnosis by expecting development of an "overt heart disease" at follow-up.

The possibility of a lethal arrhythmia developing at the site of the initial degeneration of the cardiac muscle due to a preclinical form of structural heart disease seemed a plausible possibility to the UCARE investigators who included, as part of the follow-up visit, a thorough clinical evaluation in order to detect signs of developing heart disease. A diagnosis of "structural heart disease" became apparent at follow-up in only 4% of the patients. Silent ischemia was identified in 4 patients (in 2 cases because of positive ergonovine tests, in 1 case because of an episode of chest pain during exercise, and in 1 case because of spontaneous coronary spasm during angiography); dilated cardiomyopathy was diagnosed in 2 patients after a follow-up of 104 and 69 months, respectively, and in 1 patient arrhythmogenic right ventricular dysplasia was diagnosed.

The paucity of patients in whom structural heart disease is identified at follow-up suggests that the cause for development of ventricular tachyarrhythmias remains elusive in most individuals originally diagnosed as having IVF.

## On the Mechanism of IVF

Patients with IVF are individuals with a morphologically "normal" heart that revealed electrical instability at least once.

What can be the cause of this electrical instability? According to UCARE investigators, 70% of patients remain free of symptoms at follow-up.

The evidence that most of the IVF survivors will not experience a second event may suggest that transient factors could represent the trigger for the episode of cardiac arrest in these patients. *Electrolyte imbalance or viral infections* may be among the "silent" and "transitory" factors leading to IVF. It is most likely that if the presence of such a transient abnormality is missed immediately after resuscitation of the patient, it will remain undetected in the future; therefore, these individuals will remain labeled as survivors of "idiopathic VF."

On the contrary, in the 30% of patients that experience a recurrence, it is most likely that a "permanent" abnormality causing electrical instability does exist.

How can we reconcile the concept of "heart disease" with the absence of "structural" defects? As anticipated in a previous section of this chapter, genetic diseases in "nonpenetrant" variants may represent a group of diseases underlying IVF. Diseases such as hypertrophic cardiomyopathy or long QT syndrome are best recognized in their most typical forms associated with clearly distinguishable clinical manifestations. However, one of the most interesting contributions of molecular genetics to clinical cardiology is the unequivocal demonstration of an unexpected variable manifestation of the clinical phenotype of genetic defects. This variability, called in genetic terms "incomplete penetrance,"[9] is in some families so pronounced that individuals with the same genetic defect may have a wide range of clinical manifestations.

Preliminary data have confirmed that among survivors of cardiac arrest, there are "forme fruste" of "long QT syndrome" (SG Priori, unpublished data) and of Brugada syndrome (SG Priori and T Giovannini, unpublished data); the quantification of the percentage is presently limited by the lack of knowledge about the genes implicated in both diseases.

## The Link Between IVF and SUDS

Whether IVF and sudden and unexpected death syndrome (SUDS) endemic to Japan and Southeast Asia[20] are part of the same clinical entity has been debated for some time. A major confounding factor for the classification of the various forms of SUDS has been the description of the manifestations preceding death such as nightmares, contractions, screaming, and moaning, probably rooted in traditional medicine and superstition more than in contemporary clinical medicine. Another striking factor that has contributed to maintaining SUDS separate from IVF is the much higher prevalence of SUDS in eastern countries as compared to IVF in western countries. Recently, Nademanee et al.[20] identified elevation of ST segment in the right chest leads (Brugada syndrome) in the majority of SUDS patients from Thailand; 63% of the victims of either aborted sudden death or syncope (or seizure) had a dynamic pattern of ST segment elevation in precordial leads $V_1$ to $V_3$, often accompanied by apparent conduction block in the right ventricle.[20] We are not aware of genetic analysis performed in SUDS victims; therefore, if we accept the evidence that "incomplete penetrance" is a feature of the Brugada syndrome, this number is likely to be an underestimation of the total number of SUDS cases caused by the Brugada syndrome. It will be very important to perform population genetic studies in order to understand why these genetic defects are so common in Eastern countries.

## The Future of IVF

Since the term IVF acknowledges our inability to identify the substrate for the development of a lethal arrhythmic episode, it is our hope that in the future, the number of survivors of cardiac arrest labeled as IVF will decrease. The identification of "hidden" diseases accounting for the 30% of cases that will experience a recurrence is certainly the most important step toward better management for IVF patients.

When molecular diagnosis will reach a sensitivity close to 100% in the detection of genetic diseases, it will be possible to define whether inherited abnormalities account for the patients who experience recurrences of cardiac arrest. This hypothesis appears very appealing and, if confirmed, will allow targeting the use of defibrillators to the higher risk subgroups.

## References

1. Myerburg RJ, Castellanos A. Cardiac arrest and sudden cardiac death. In: Braunwald E (ed). Heart Disease. A Textbook of Cardiovascular Medicine. 4th ed. W.B. Saunders Co., Philadelphia, 1992:756–789.
2. Poole JE, Bardy GH. Sudden cardiac death. In: Zipes DP, Jalife J (eds). Cardiac Electrophysiology: From Cell to Bedside, 2nd ed. W.B. Saunders Co., Philadelphia, 1995, pp 812–832.
3. Bowker TJ, Wood DA, Davies MJ, Shepard MN, Cary NRB, et al. A national survey of sudden unexpected cardiac or unexplained death in adults (SUDS). Heart 1996; 75(5):80.
4. Bardy GH, Bigger JT Jr, Borggrefe M, Camm AJ, Cobb LA, et al., for the Working Group on Arrhythmias of the European Society of Cardiology. Consensus statement. Survivors of out-of-hospital cardiac arrest with apparently normal heart: need for definition and standardized clinical evaluation. Circulation 1997; 95:265–272.
5. Schwartz PJ, Locati EH, Napolitano C, Priori SG. The long QT syndrome. In: Zipes DP, Jalife J (eds). Cardiac Electrophysiology: From Cell to Bedside, 2nd ed. W.B. Saunders Co., Philadelphia, 1995, pp 788–811.
6. Priori SG, Barhanin J, Hauer RNW, Haverkamp W, Habo JJ, et al. Genetic and molecular basis of cardiac arrhythmias: impact on clinical management. Parts I and II. Circulation 1999; 99:518–528; Eur Heart J 1999; 20:174–195.
7. Brugada J, Brugada R, Brugada P. Right bundle-branch block and ST segment elevation in leads $V_1$ through $V_3$: a marker for sudden death in patients without demonstrable structural heart disease. Circulation 1998; 97:457–460.
8. Chen Q, Kirsch GE, Zhang D, Brugada R, Brugada J, et al. Genetic basis and molecular mechanism for idiopathic ventricular fibrillation. Nature 1998; 392:293–294.
9. Priori SG, Napolitano C, Schwartz PJ. Low penetrance in the long QT syndrome: clinical impact. Circulation 1999; 99:529–533.
10. Priori SG, Napolitano C, Terreni L, Crotti L, Bloise R, et al. Incomplete penetrance and variable response to sodium channel blockade in Brugada's syndrome (abstract). Eur Heart J 1999; 20(Suppl):465.
11. Martini B, Nava A, Thiene G, Buja GF, Canciani B, et al.. Ventricular fibrillation without apparent heart disease: description of six cases. Am Heart J 1989; 118:1203–1209.
12. Myerburg RJ, Kessler KM, Castellanos A. Sudden cardiac death: epidemiology, transient risk, and intervention assessment. Ann Intern Med 1993; 119:1187–1197.
13. Priori SG, Borggrefe M, Camm AJ, Hauer RNW, Klein H, et al. Unexplained cardiac arrest: the need for a prospective registry. Eur Heart J 1992; 13:1445–1446.
14. Priori SG, Paganini V. Idiopathic ventricular fibrillation: epidemiology, pathophysiology, primary prevention, immediate evaluation and management, long-term evaluation and management, experimental and theoretical developments. Cardiac Electrophysiol Rev 1997; 1:244–247.
15. Peeters HAP, Sippensgroenewegen A, Wever EFD, Potse M, Danieels MCG, et al. Electrocardiographic identification of abnormal ventricular depolarization

and repolarization in patients with idiopathic ventricular fibrillation. J Am Coll Cardiol 1998; 31:1406–1413.

16. Schaefers M, Wichter T, Lerch H, Matheja P, Kuwert T, et al. Cardiac 123I-MIBG uptake in idiopathic ventricular tachycardia and fibrillation. J Nucl Med 1999; 40:1–5.

17. Priori SG, Borggrefe M, Camm AJ, Hauer RNW, Klein H, et al., on behalf of UCARE. Role of the implantable defibrillator in patients with idiopathic ventricular fibrillation: data from the UCARE international registry. PACE 1995; 18(4, Part II):799.

18. Belhassen B, Viskin S. Idiopathic ventricular tachycardia and fibrillation. J Cardiovasc Electrophysiol 1993; 4:356–368.

19. Tsai CF, Chen SA, Tsai CT, Chiang CE, Ding YA, et al. Idiopathic ventricular fibrillation: clinical, electrophysiologic characteristics and long-term outcomes. Int J Cardiol 1998; 64:47–55.

20. Nademanee K. Sudden unexplained death syndrome in Southeast Asia. Am J Cardiol 1997; 79:10–11.

# IV

## *Arrhythmogenic Right Ventricular Dysplasia*

# 17

# Why Patients with Arrhythmogenic Right Ventricular Dysplasia Die Suddenly

G. Fontaine, MD, PhD, P. Fornes, MD, PhD,
Z. Mallat, MD, F. Fontaliran, MD, and
R. Frank, MD

## Introduction

Sudden death is the most frightening and spectacular symptom of arrhythmogenic right ventricular dysplasia (ARVD). It is always a familial and a social tragedy because it is observed most frequently in adolescents or young adults. The diagnosis is generally overlooked by routine autopsy. ARVD, which was originally considered as a rare condition, is now of rising interest among doctors who are involved in the investigation of sudden unexpected deaths, such as medical examiners.[1]

According to some researchers, and at least in the Veneto region of Italy, the disease strikes 1 out of 5,000 individuals, but only a small percentage of them die suddenly.[2] Most of the victims experience ventricular arrhythmias with QRS complexes showing a left bundle branch block pattern. Others may experience supraventricular or atrial arrhythmias.[3] However, sudden death can be the first manifestation of the disease.

Nevertheless, as also observed in ischemic heart disease, ventricular arrhythmias in ARVD are in fact an epiphenomenon. Therefore, it could be suspected that these patients have a similar basic histological substrate and that a large percentage of them go unrecognized, because they are free of symptomatic cardiac arrhythmias and have a preserved cardiac function.

The prevalence of sudden death in ARVD patients treated empirically has been estimated at 2% per year. However, few publications have re-

From: Aliot E, Clementy J, Prystowsky EN (editors). *Fighting Sudden Cardiac Death: A Worldwide Challenge.* ©Futura Publishing Company, Armonk, NY, 2000.

ported the prevalence of the arrhythmogenic substrate of right ventricular dysplasia in the general population.[4]

The purpose of this chapter is to examine possible factors that may explain sudden cardiac death in ARVD, and to put them into perspective with the basic structure of this new category of cardiomyopathy.

## The Classic Understanding of ARVD

ARVD was originally identified by its cardiac arrhythmias. A young patient who died suddenly and unexpectedly with a documented episode of ventricular fibrillation was diagnosed as having ARVD at autopsy.[5] This disease was demonstrated to lead to sudden death. A prospective study performed in the Veneto region has demonstrated that among 60 adults who died suddenly under the age of 35, 12 had a "cardiomyopathy of the right ventricle."[6] However, such a high prevalence of the disease has not been found elsewhere. Nevertheless, pathological findings in these cases seemed to be in agreement with the previous description of ARVD.

Therefore, a link seemed to exist between the frequency of cardiac arrhythmias (isolated extrasystoles to ventricular tachycardia) and the risk of ventricular fibrillation, the lethal event, in patients with dissociation of myocardial fibers by adipose tissue in the right ventricle.

After the classic description of right ventricular dysplasia was made by Marcus et al. in 1982,[7] this new entity was more clearly identified even though it was previously reported as a form of partial Uhl's anomaly.[8] Since then, it has become of interest as a mechanism of cardiac arrhythmia during recent decades. It was also the time of successful therapeutic results obtained with antiarrhythmic drugs, pacemakers, and defibrillators, used alone or in combination. ARVD has multiple, but nonspecific, clinical features. Nevertheless, diagnosis can be made by a thorough analysis of clinical data. Criteria for the diagnosis of ARVD, including major and minor structural and functional signs, have been proposed by experts under the auspices of the Scientific Council of Cardiomyopathies of the International Society and Federation of Cardiology (ISFC) now called the World Heart Federation (WHF) and the Working Group on Myocardial and Pericardial Diseases of the European Society of Cardiology.[9]

Another way to evaluate the incidence of the disease in the population at large is the identification of its histological characteristics observed in patients who died suddenly and/or had a typical clinical presentation of ARVD. When histological criteria have been defined, it is possible to use them for recognition of this condition in the general population of people who died of various causes.

The most important pathological trait of the disease, which was originally observed at the time of surgery, was a generally dilated right ventricle covered by an exceedingly large amount of fat. This ventricle had also abnormal contractions. When the right ventricle was cut by a "simple ventriculotomy" at the site of origin of ventricular tachycardia identified by epicardial mapping during ventricular tachycardia, it was clear that most of the free wall had a dramatic decrease in muscular component, which remained only in the subendocardial layers. This was particularly visible in the infundibulum, the apex, and under the tricuspid valve, the so-called triangle of dysplasia.[7] The most important part of the overall wall was thicker than normal and occupied by fatty tissue (Figure 1). The ventricular myocardium seemed to remain in the subendocardial layers only. However, microscopically, fat was not uniform but intermingled with strands of fibromyocytic bundles. It was therefore possible to surmise that most of the fat, which seemed to cover an apparently atrophic endocardium, was in fact the result of an abnormal replacement of myocardium by adipose tissue.

In addition, it was later reported that in many specimens it was possible to recognize the original border of epicardium, which may or may not have been covered by normal epicardial fat. This epicardial fat was similar to that observed in other areas of the myocardium, such as the AV

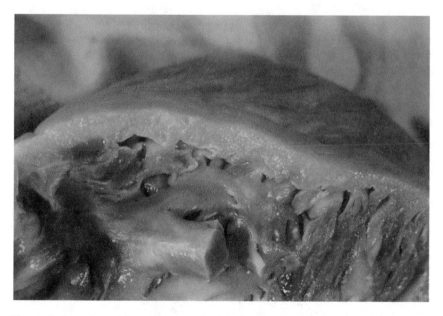

Figure 1. A section of the anterior wall of the right ventricle along the border of the right interventricular septum. Almost the whole myocardial wall has been replaced by fat, which appears thicker than normal with only a few myocardial cells remaining in the endocardium. In contrast, the physiological trabeculations are hypertrophied. The moderator band appears devoid of fatty infiltration. These features explain certain images obtained by contrast angiography of the right ventricle. (Courtesy of Pr JP Fauchier, Tours, France.)

groove, the interventricular groove, or fat surrounding the coronary vessels. Therefore, the structure of ARVD seems to be the consequence of a dysontogenetic phenomenon, leading to the transdifferentiation of cardiomyoblasts into adipoblasts.[10] In addition, the concept that the disease progresses from the epicardium toward the endocardium was deduced from gross pathology or histological findings in the most advanced forms of the disease, in which the epicardial layers were replaced by fat. In 11 out of 12 cases that we have recently studied, disease was found to begin inside the mediomural layers and to progress preferentially toward the epicardium rather than toward the endocrdium.

## Minimal Prerequisite for Cardiac Arrhythmias

We recently examined the heart from a spontaneously aborted 27-week-old fetus who was arrhythmogenic in utero. It was dissociated by distaff-like clusters of adipocytes following the general orientation of myocardial fibers[11] (Figure 2). In this specimen, fibrosis was minimal and there

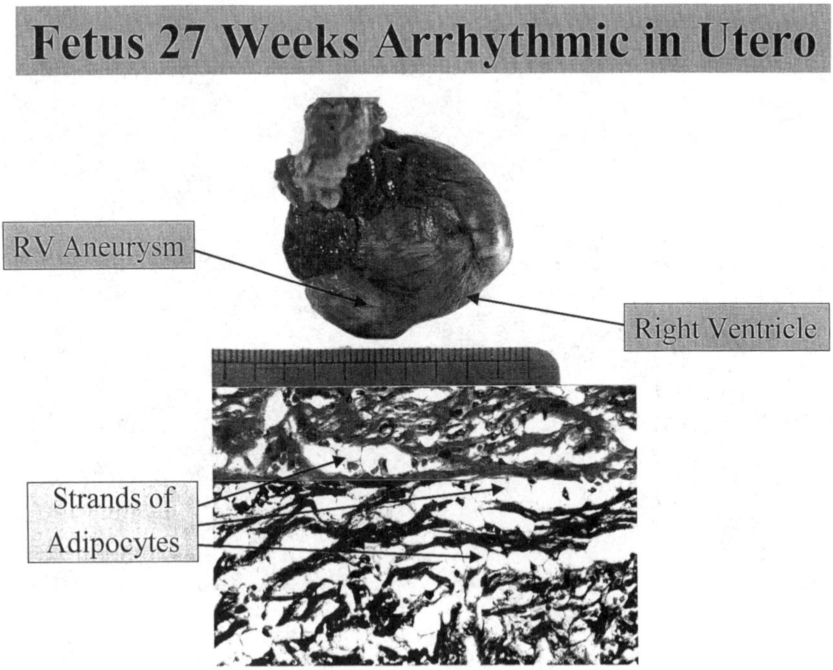

Figure 2. Right ventricular myocardium of a 27-week-old fetus, arrhythmic in utero, showing dissociation of myocardium by strands of adipose tissue in the absence of colliding vacuoles. (Same specimen as presented in Circulation[11]; used with persmission.)

was no acute inflammation. Exceptional lymphocytes were observed. It was concluded that dissociation of myocardial fibers by layers of adipose tissue could have been responsible for a possible reentry phenomenon producing ventricular arrhythmias. Such arrhythmias may cause sudden death.

Histological slides provide only bidimensional information on pathological structure. Nevertheless, examination of serial sections demonstrates that apparently isolated strands of cardiomyocytes are in fact part of a continuous layer of cardiomyocytes. This concept is particularly important since this kind of geometric structure could be the background of a drifting vortex tachycardia.

## Genesis of Drifting Vortex Ventricular Tachycardia

A patient with ARVD died suddenly at night with a Holter recording showing a torsades de pointes-like ventricular tachycardia preceded by isolated extrasystoles during a period of relative slowdown of the sinus rhythm. Histology demonstrated the presence of foliated epicardial layers in the right ventricular myocardium on both its anterior and diaphragmatic aspects, with persistence of a thin layer of flat and compact endocardium 0.8 mm in thickness[12-14] (Figure 3). It was interesting to make a parallel between this structure and the laboratory model developed to induce torsades de pointes-like ventricular tachycardia, studied by optical mapping.[15] Therefore, our case was probably the first clinical illustration of this interesting phenomenon of a reentrant mechanism drifting inside the myocardium when a small continuous layer of cardiomyocytes was present.

A similar phenomenon is likely to have occurred in a 32-year-old patient who died suddenly after several episodes of syncope. This patient was diagnosed by Dr. Pedro Brugada as having the Brugada syndrome,[16] characterized by ST segment elevation in leads $V_1$ to $V_3$. The histological material of this case was referred to us by Dr. Pedro Brugada. The right ventricular free wall was divided into 2 layers: epicardial and endocardial. Between these 2 layers, a line of adipocytes was observed and the adjacent myocardium was bordered by a thin rim of fibrosis (Figure 4). This fibroadipose tissue, which had different orientations, separated the epicardial from endocardial layers of myocardium that had different orientations. This suggests that adipose tissue and fibrosis were the result of differently oriented mechanical forces, acting on an already diseased myocardium. However, these 2 layers were interconnected in some areas, where the genetically determined sodium and potassium channel disorders could have occurred.[17] When the conduction between these 2 layers is interrupted, the epicardial layers become isolated. This may ex-

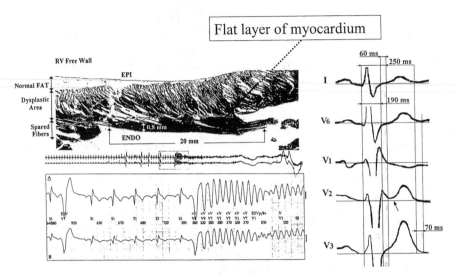

Figure 3. Onset of sudden death at night in a patient with ARVD. Holter recording demonstrated polymorphic, torsades de pointes-like ventricular tachycardia preceded by 4 isolated extrasystoles during a relative slowdown of the sinus rhythm. Histology of the right ventricular free wall showed foliated epicardial myocardial fibers. A small endocardial layer of compact myocardium could have been the background for a drifting vortex ventricular tachycardia leading to cardiac desynchronization. In the same patient, the tracing recorded a few days before the catastrophe showed saddle-back ST segment elevation in lead $V_2$, "more than complete bundle branch block pattern," and QT dispersion. (Modified from Fontaine G, et al.[13,14])

plain both ST segment elevation in leads $V_1$ to $V_3$ and the isolation of a thin endocardial structure. This structure could be, as suggested by the previous case, the background for polymorphic torsades de pointes-like ventricular tachycardia.[18] The improper connection between this thin layer and adjacent myocardium, due to a major reduction of the safety margin for the propagation of activation, results in activation of the adjacent septum, leading in that particular case to the torsades de pointes-like ventricular tachycardia. A drifting vortex ventricular tachycardia could end spontaneously, but can also transmit erratic activation to the left ventricle, leading to desynchronization of fibers, ventricular fibrillation, and sudden death.

Therefore, the abnormal ST segment elevation in the Brugada syndrome seemed to be related to the loss of electrical forces in the subepicardial layers. It is noteworthy that the previous case that had foliated epicardial layers also showed a "saddleback" ST segment elevation in lead $V_2$ (Figure 3).

# BRUGADA SYNDROME
# PATHOLOGY in one PATIENT

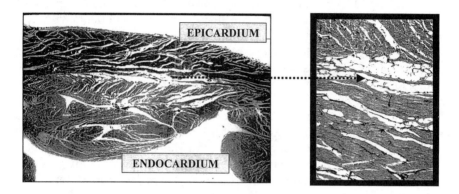

EPICARDIUM

ENDOCARDIUM

Two myocardial layers separated by adipocytes and fibrosis

Figure 4. A patient with Brugada syndrome who died suddenly after several episodes of syncope. At low magnification, the epicardial as opposed to endocardial layers shows fibers with different orientation. Adipocytes and a thin rim of fibrosis separated them. This was more clearly visible at higher magnification (HE, G×20, G×400).

## The Histological Structure of ARVD
## Prevalence in the General Population

To assess the prevalence of the disease in the general population, one may consider a control group of right ventricular biopsy samples of people who died of various causes and look for the specific histological structure of the right ventricular free wall. We published in 1991 a study of 143 patients who had biopsy samples taken from the anterior aspect of the right ventricle in a systematic examination of the heart at autopsy.[4] The samples were taken from the middle of the anterior aspect of the right ventricle, halfway between the apex and the base. From this material, we selected 140 patients who had a dominant right coronary artery with no or nonsignificant stenosis. In addition, we excluded elderly obese women who usually have an exceedingly large amount of fat surrounding the heart. From this study, it appeared that only a small percentage of cases, approximately

40%, had a normal right ventricular free wall, i.e., compact myocardium without strands of adipose tissue. This normal feature was similar to that found in most laboratory animals such as rat, mouse, hamster, chicken, rabbit, goat, dog, pig, cow, and monkey.[19] The remaining 60% of patients had various degrees of fat dissociating myocardial fibers in the right ventricular free wall. In the most extensive form, the histological feature was similar to that of patients with ARVD except that there was no fibrosis.

In our study, the 140 patients were used as controls and compared to a group of ARVD patients. Our conclusion was that in patients with dysplasia, histology should demonstrate not only the presence of cardiomyocytic bundles inside fat but also collagen tissue bordering or embedding these bundles. This feature seemed to be a necessary prerequisite for the diagnosis of ARVD, and constituted histological criteria for the typical form of the disease.[4]

However, in this work, the mean age of patients including 75 females and 65 males was quite high (69.3 ± 13; range 27–88). All patients were hospitalized in our cardiology department. This could have created a bias in the selection of cases. To overcome this criticism, a later study was performed involving 82 patients (52 females and 30 males) from different departments in a general hospital, who died of various causes. These cases were also selected on the basis of the same previous criteria. They were younger (48.2 ± 12.2 ; range 17–68).

The same pathologist (FF) examined the histological material (Figure 5). The same percentage of cases, 37%, as in our previous study had a compact myocardium (group I).

Groups II to IV were composed of patients who had a moderate to important amount of fat dissociating myocardial fibers. In group IV, the amount of fat in the most severe cases was similar to that found in ARVD patients.

In this study, we defined group V by the presence of fibrosis bordering myocytic bundles (fibromyocytic bundles), suggesting a quiescent form of right ventricular dysplasia. This group accounted for 3.7% of patients who died of noncardiac causes, and is likely to represent the incidence of right ventricular dysplasia in the population at large. Because 1 out of 5,000 individuals in the general population was reported to have ARVD in the Veneto region, one may estimate that less than 0.5% of right ventricular dysplasia patients are prone to develop arrhythmias. However, the reason that explains why several members of the same family die suddenly, suggesting a stronger severity of the disease, is unknown.[20]

## Substrate Remodeling

The anatomic arrhythmogenic substrate of ARVD consists of fat, fibrosis, and apparently normal cardiomyocytes. Additional multiple fac-

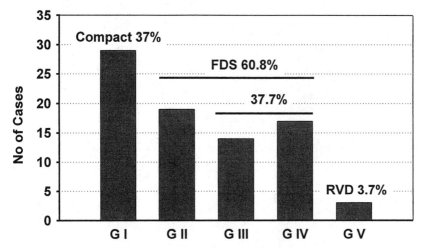

Figure 5. Histological features of right ventricular myocardium obtained in a control group of 140 patients who died of various causes. Fat dissociating myocardial fibers (FDS) without fibrosis was observed in 60% of the cases. A later study performed on 82 patients who died of various causes in a general hospital showed the presence of fat dissociation in the same percentage as the previous study, but 3.7% had also fibrosis bordering myocardial fibers, suggesting a quiescent form of right ventricular dysplasia (RVD). GI to GV: see text, page 258.

tors are likely to be superimposed. Among these factors, inflammation has been found to be involved in 2 out of 3 cases.[21] Identification of superimposed inflammation as a determinant of arrhythmogenicity has been one of the most important steps in the understanding of the disease mechanism. This concept was suggested by the observations that some patients had a stable or slowly progressing disease, whereas others had a rapidly progressing left ventricular dysfunction and developed congestive heart failure that could become irreversible in a few years or months.[22]

In some of these patients, analysis of biopsy samples taken at the time of surgery showed inflammatory infiltrates (Figure 6). Some had fever several weeks before the major event. Others had severe chest pain mimicking myocardial infarction except that the CK-MB was not significantly increased. The hearts of some of these ARVD patients who died suddenly showed exceedingly large amounts of fibrosis. Fibrosis was present in both ventricles and might have explained the progressive left ventricular dysfunction despite no evidence of fatty replacement of left ventricular myocardial fibers.

## ACUTE INFLAMMATION in a ARVD PATIENT

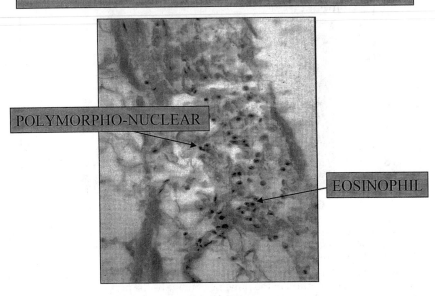

**Figure 6.** Acute inflammation in a patient who had acute chest pain, suggesting hyperacute myocardial infarction and ventricular tachycardia of right ventricular origin, and who had successful antiarrhythmic surgery. Histology showed typical signs of acute myocarditis with eosinophils, polymorphonuclears, and macrophages.

However, these signs, suggesting myocarditis, could present various clinical features:

- *Acute,* or even superacute features, leading to fulminant heart failure in which the systematic study of the right ventricle showed the presence of typical dysplasia with hyaline fibrosis that cannot be the result of the acute event.[22] Inflammatory infiltrates consist of neutrophils, eosinophils and lymphocytes.
- *Chronic,* when fibrosis is associated with inflammatory infiltrates consisting mostly of lymphocytes and plasmocytes. In case of healing, these cells progressively disappear, leaving only fibrosis.[1]
- *Chronic active,* when lymphocytes and plasmocytes predominate with scarce neutrophils still present.[23] This latter form progresses more rapidly toward cardiac insufficiency, mimicking a late stage of idiopathic dilated cardiomyopathy.[24,25]

In all cases, the infective agent leading to the creation of the arrhythmogenic substrate has destroyed some cardiomyocytes. The electrophysiological properties have been modified in such a way that the previously nonarrhythmogenic structures became arrhythmogenic. This is the consequence of modification of critical electrophysiological parameters, including speed of conduction, refractory period, and connection of abnormal to normal tissue.

The cause of inflammation is of interest. Few reports have mentioned the presence of enteroviruses, especially coxsackie B.[26] However, other agents could also play a role, independently or in association with the enterovirus. The role of hepatitis C has not been determined in ARVD.[27] The role of apoptosis at any stage of the disease might be considered independently or in association with inflammation.[28,29] We have reported that the importance of apoptosis was directly related to the severity of inflammation.[29]

Finally, the role of fibrosis that is correlated to (and not the cause of) late potential development may be an important indirect determinant of arrhythmia and sudden death.[30]

Hoffman et al. have recently demonstrated that activation of neutrophils and eosinophils produces early afterdepolarization[31] and reperfusion arrhythmia. This finding establishes for the first time a direct link between inflammation and electrophysiological phenomena. Triggering of arrhythmias by acute inflammation was suggested in Naxos disease, in which patients have a stepwise pattern of the disease progression, associated with the occurrence of cardiac arrhythmias.

# Conclusion

Sudden death in ARVD is a rare event, contrasting with the frequent histological background of ARVD in the whole population. However, the reason for the occurrence of several sudden deaths in certain families is unknown.

In addition to the basic electrophysiological complex structure of ARVD involving fat and fibrosis interspersed with cardiomyocytes favoring reentrant tachycardia, new mechanisms of sudden death have been recently identified:

- Dissociation of myocardial fibers by fat without fibrosis in exceptional cases.
- Thin endocardial layer leading to drifting vortex ventricular tachycardia. This may also explain sudden death at night in the Brugada syndrome.

262 • Fighting Sudden Cardiac Death: A Worldwide Challenge

- Remodeling of the arrhythmia substrate by a superimposed inflammation with multiple clinical presentations.
- Acute inflammation leading to early afterdepolarization triggering arrhythmogenicity.

## References

1. Lecomte D, Fornes P, Fouret P, Nicolas G. Isolated myocardial fibrosis as a cause of sudden cardiac death and its possible relation to myocarditis. J Forensic Sci 1993; 38:617–621.
2. Thiene G, Gambino A, Corrado D, Nava A. The pathological spectrum underlying sudden death in athletes: new trends in arrhythmias 1985; 3:323–331.
3. Tonet J, Castro Miranda R, Iwa T, Poulain F, et al. Frequency of supraventricular tachyarrhythmias in arrhythmogenic right ventricular dysplasia. Am J Cardiol 1991; 67:1153.
4. Fontaliran F, Fontaine G, Fillette F, Aouate P, Chomette G, et al. Frontieres nosologiques de la dysplasie arythmogene: variations quantitatives du tissu adipeux ventriculaire droit normal. Arch Mal Coeur 1991; 84:33–38.
5. Olsson SB, Edvardsson N, Emanuelsson H, Enestrom S. A case of arrhythmogenic right ventricular dysplasia with ventricular fibrillation. Clin Cardiol 1982; 5:591–596.
6. Thiene G, Nava A, Corrado D, Rossi L, Pennelli N. Right ventricular cardiomyopathy and sudden death in young people. N Engl J Med 1988; 318:129–133.
7. Marcus FI, Fontaine G, Guiraudon G, Frank R, Laurenceau JL, et al. Right ventricular dysplasia: a report of 24 cases. Circulation 1982; 65:384–399.
8. Froment R, Perrin A, Loire R, Dalloz CL. Ventricule droit papyrace du jeune adulte par dystrophie congenitale: a propos de 2 cas anatomo-cliniques et de 3 cas cliniques. Arch Mal Coeur 1968; 61:477–503.
9. McKenna WJ, Thiene G, Nava A, Fontaliran F, Blomstrom-Lundqvist C, et al. Diagnosis of arrhythmogenic right ventricular dysplasia/cardiomyopathy. Br Heart J 1994; 71:215–218.
10. Hu E, Tontonoz P, Spiegelman BM. Transdifferentiation of myoblasts by the adipogenic transcription factors PPAR gamma and C/EBP alpha. Proc Natl Acad Sci USA 1995; 92:9856–9860.
11. Fontaine G, Fontaliran F, Frank R. Arrhythmogenic right ventricular cardiomyopathies: clinical forms and main differential diagnoses (editorial). Circulation 1998; 97:1532–1535.
12. Aouate P, Fontaliran F, Fontaine G, Frank R, Benassar A, et al. Holter et mort subite: interet dans un cas de dysplasie ventriculaire droite arythmogene. Arch Mal Coeur 1993; 86:363–367.
13. Fontaine G, Aouate P, Fontaliran F. Repolarization and the genesis of cardiac arrhythmias: role of body surface mapping (editorial). Circulation 1997; 12:2600–2602.
14. Fontaine G, Aouate P, Fontaliran F. Dysplasie ventriculaire droite arythmogene, torsades de pointes et mort subite: nouveaux concepts. Ann Cardiol Angiol 1997; 46:531–538.
15. Davidenko JM. Spiral wave activity: a possible common mechanism for polymorphic and monomorphic ventricular tachycardias. J Cardiovasc Electrophysiol 1993;4:730–746.

16. Brugada P, Brugada J. Right bundle branch block, persistent ST segment elevation and sudden cardiac death: a distinct clinical and electrocardiographic syndrome. J Am Coll Cardiol 1992;20:1391–1396.

17. Chen Q, Kirsch GE, Zhang D, Brugada R, Brugada J, et al. Genetic basis and molecular mechanism for idiopathic ventricular fibrillation. Nature 1998; 392:293–296.

18. Yan GX, Antzelevitch C. Induction of torsades de pointes in an isolated arterially perfused canine left ventricular wedge preparation: role of intramural reentry (abstract). Circulation 1996; 94(Suppl I):712.

19. Fontaine G, Fontaliran F, Zenati O, Guzman CE, Rigoulet J, et al. Fat in the heart: a feature unique to the human species? Observational reflections on an unsolved problem. Acta Cardiol 1999; 54:189–194.

20. Nava A, Thiene G, Canciani B, Scognamiglio R, Daliento L, et al. Familial occurrence of right ventricular dysplasia: a study involving nine families. J Am Coll Cardiol 1988; 12: 1222–1228.

21. Basso C, Thiene G, Corrado D, Angelini A, Nava A, et al. Arrhythmogenic right ventricular cardiomyopathy: dysplasia, dystrophy or myocarditis? Circulation 1996; 94: 983–991.

22. Fontaine G, Brestescher C, Fontaliran F, Himbert C, Tonet J, et al. Modalites evolutives de la dysplasie ventriculaire droite arythmogene: a propos de 4 observations. Arch Mal Coeur 1995; 88: 973–980.

23. Girard F, Fontaine G, Fontaliran F, Zenati O, Gajdos P. Catastrophic global heart failure in a case of nonarrhythmogenic right ventricular dysplasia. Heart Vessels 1997; 12:152–154.

24. Nemec J, Edwards BS, Osborn MJ, Edwards WD. Arrhythmogenic right ventricular dysplasia masquerading as dilated cardiomyopathy. Am J Cardiol 1999; 84:237–239.

25. Pinamonti B, Pagnan L, Bussani R, Ricci C, Silvestri F, et al. Right ventricular dysplasia with biventricular involvement. Circulation 1998; 98:1943–1945.

26. Heim A, Grumbach I, Hake S, Muller G, Pring-Akerblom P, et al. Enterovirus heart disease of adults: a persistent, limited organ infection in the presence of neutralizing antibodies. J Med Virol 1997; 53:196–204.

27. Matsumori A, Matoba Y, Nishio R, Shioi T, Ono K, et al. Detection of hepatitis C virus RNA from the hearts of patients with hypertrophic cardiomyopathy. Biochem Biophys Res Comm 1996; 222:678–682.

28. James TN. Normal and abnormal consequences of apoptosis in the human heart: from postnatal morphogenesis to paroxysmal arrhythmias. Circulation 1994; 90:556–573.

29. Mallat Z, Tedgui A, Fontaliran F, Frank R, Durigon M, et al. Evidence of apoptosis in arrhythmogenic right ventricular dysplasia. N Engl J Med 1996; 335:1190–1196.

30. Valente M, Calabrese F, Angelini A, Basso C, Thiene G. In vivo evidence of apoptosis in arrhythmogenic right ventricular cardiomyopathy. Am J Pathol 1998; 152:479–484.

31. Hoffman BF, Feinmark SJ, Guo SD. Electrophysiologic effects of interactions between activated canine neutrophils and cardiac myocytes. J Cardiovasc Electrophysiol 1997; 8:679–687.

# 18

# Arrhythmogenic Right Ventricular Cardiomyopathy/Dysplasia:

## A Genetic or an Acquired Disease?

Domenico Corrado, MD,
Cristina Basso, MD, PhD,
Marialuisa Valente, MD, and
Gaetano Thiene, MD

## Introduction

Arrhythmogenic right ventricular (RV) cardiomyopathy/dysplasia (ARVC/D) is a heart muscle disease of unknown etiology, often familial, that is characterized pathologically by fibrofatty replacement of the RV myocardium and clinically by ventricular arrhythmias of RV origin that may lead to sudden death, mostly in young people and in athletes.[1-7] Although several theories have been advanced, the etiopathogenesis of ARVC/D is still unknown. The different terminologies—dysplasia versus cardiomyopathy—proposed for this entity reflect different viewpoints about the etiopathogenesis—congenital versus acquired—of the lack of the RV myocardium.[1-9]

The term "dysplasia" was originally used to describe an entity that was considered to be the result of a developmental defect of the RV myocardium.[1,8,9] According to this etiopathogenetic view, ARVC/D should be regarded as a congenital heart disease present at birth. A better understanding of clinical manifestations and morphological findings of ARVC/D does not support the theory of a congenital absence of the myo-

This study was supported by the Veneto Region, Venice, and by the National Council for Research, Rome, Italy.
From: Aliot E, Clementy J, Prystowsky EN (editors). *Fighting Sudden Cardiac Death: A Worldwide Challenge.* ©Futura Publishing Company, Armonk, NY, 2000.

cardium, but is in keeping with a nonischemic, ongoing atrophy of the RV myocardium that becomes symptomatic in adolescents and young adults.[2–5,10] On the basis of its nature of progressive heart muscle disease of unknown etiology, characterized by a most likely genetically determined myocyte loss with fibrofatty substitution, ARVC/D has been more appropriately included among the cardiomyopathies in the recent classification proposed by the Task Force of the World Health Organization/International Society and Federation of Cardiology.[11]

## Clinical Manifestations and Natural History

The distinctive clinical manifestation of ARVC/D consists of ventricular arrhythmias with left bundle branch morphology, ranging from isolated premature ventricular beats to sustained ventricular tachycardia or ventricular fibrillation.[1–6,12] Other clinical features include global and/or regional dysfunction and structural alterations of the right ventricle or both ventricles, and ECG depolarization/repolarization changes mostly localized to right precordial leads.[1–3,13] There is definitive clinicopathological evidence that ARVC/D is a progressive heart muscle disease. Clinicopathological investigations and long-term follow-up data from clinical studies indicate that ARVC/D with time may lead to more diffuse RV changes and left ventricular (LV) involvement, culminating in heart failure.[4,14–16] Recently, a multicenter clinicopathological investigation was carried out to further define the anatomoclinical profile of ARVC/D, with special reference to disease progression and LV involvement.[5] By examining 42 affected whole hearts, including those removed at transplant, and correlating pathological findings with the patient's clinical history, the study demonstrated that at least in this subgroup, representing an extreme of the disease spectrum, ARVC/D can no longer be regarded as an isolated disease of the right ventricle. Macroscopic or histological involvement of the left ventricle was found in 76% of hearts with ARVC/D. It was age-dependent, was more common in patients with long-standing clinical history, and was progressive as evaluated by serial echocardiographic examinations. Moreover, LV lesions were associated with clinical arrhythmic events, more severe cardiomegaly, inflammatory infiltrates, and heart failure (Table 1). Therefore, the natural history of ARVC/D is a function of both the electrical instability of diseased ventricular myocardium, which can precipitate "arrhythmic" cardiac arrest any time during the disease course, and the progressive myocardial loss that results in right or biventricular dysfunction and heart failure. The following clinicopathological phases can be considered[17]: (1) "concealed disease" characterized by subtle RV structural changes, with or without minor ventricular arrhythmias, during which sudden death may be the first manifestation of the disease,

## Table 1

## Clinical Characteristics and Morphologic Findings in ARVC Patients with or without Left Ventricular Involvement

|  | (Isolated RV Involvement) Group A n= 10 pts | (Histologic LV Involvement) Group B n= 15 pts | (Gross LV Involvement) Group C n= 17 pts |
|---|---|---|---|
| Age (years) | 20±8.8 | 25±9.7 | 39±15*§ |
| Familial history for ARVC and/or SD | 3 (30%) | 8 (53%) | 6 (35%) |
| Athletes | 2 (20%) | 7 (46%) | 4 (23%) |
| Disease duration (yrs) | 1.2±2.1 | 3.4±2.2 | 9.3±7.3*§ |
| Asymptomatic | 7 (70%) | 3 (20%)* | 2 (13%)* |
| Syncope | 3 (30%) | 5 (33%) | 3 (18%) |
| Inverted T waves: |  |  |  |
| -right precordial leads ($V_1$–$V_4$) | 2/2 (100%) | 11/12 (92%) | 14/14 (100%) |
| -lateral leads ($V_5$,$V_6$) | 0/2 | 1/12 (10%) | 9/14 (71%)§ |
| Ventricular arrhythmias | 2 (20%) | 11 (73%)* | 14 (82%)* |
| "Normal" echo | 2/2 (100%) | 5/9 (55%) | 0/11*§ |
| PM implantation | 0 | 0 | 5 (29%) |
| Heart failure | 0 | 0 | 8 (47%)*§ |
| Heart weight (g) | 328±40 | 380±95 | 500±150*§ |
| Significant RV wall thinning (≤2 mm) | 2 (20%) | 13 (87%)* | 12 (71%)* |
| RV aneurysms | 3 (30%) | 10 (66%) | 7 (41%) |
| Inflammatory infiltrates | 3 (30%) | 11 (73%)* | 15 (88%)* |

Comparison between ARVD/C patients with and without left ventricular involvement with respect to a series of clinical and morphological variables. Patients are classified into 3 groups according to the presence and severity of left ventricular involvement: (1) Group A = patients with isolated right ventricular involvement; (2) Group B = patients with right ventricular and istologic left ventricular involvement only; (3) Group C = patients with right ventricular and macroscopic left ventricular involvement (see text for details).
RV = right ventricular; LV = left ventricular; ARVD = arrhythmogenic RV dysplasia.
* = p < .05 vs. group A.
§ = p < .05 vs. group B.
From Corrado et al.[5] with permission.

mostly in young people and athletes; (2) "overt electrical disorder" in which severe RV arrhythmias and impending cardiac arrest are associated with overt RV functional and structural abnormalities; (3) "RV failure" due to the progression and extension of the RV muscle disease that provokes global RV dysfunction; (4) final stage of "biventricular pump failure" due to significant LV involvement. At this stage, ARVC/D mimics a biventricular dilated cardiomyopathy leading to congestive heart failure and thromboembolic complications.[4,5]

# Pathological Features of RV Dysplasia/Cardiomyopathy

The most striking morphological feature of ARVC/D is the diffuse or segmental loss of the myocardium of the RV free wall and its replacement by fibrofatty tissue, which is frequently transmural and accounts for aneurysmal dilations of the diaphragmatic, apical, and infundibular regions (so called "triangle of dysplasia") in nearly 50% of the cases in the autopsy series.[1-5,18] The wavefront of the pathological process progresses from the subepicardium to the endocardium, so that residual myocardium is confined to the inner subendocardial layer and to the trabeculae of the RV, whereas islands of surviving myocardiual cells are scattered throughout the fibrofatty tissue.[2-5] Patchy acute myocarditis with myocyte death and round cell (mostly lymphocytes) inflammatory infiltrates is present nearly in two-thirdsof the cases.[4,5]

Two morphological variants of ARVC/D have been reported.[2,4] The *fatty* form is exclusively confined to the right ventricle, which predominantly involves the apical and infundibular regions. It is characterized by partial or almost complete substitution of the myocardium by fatty tissue without wall thickness decrease (4–5 mm). There is evidence of myocardial degeneration and death in about half of the cases, in the absence of significant fibrous tissue and inflammatory infiltrates. The left ventricle and the interventricular septum are typically spared.

In the *fibrofatty* variant, the adipose infiltration is associated with significant replacement-type fibrosis, thinning of the RV wall (<3 mm), aneurysmal dilatation, and inflammatory infiltrates. There is usually involvement of the diaphragmatic wall underneath the posterior leaflet of the tricuspid valve, the left ventricle, and, more rarely, the ventricular septum may be involved to a lesser extent.

## Genetics

A familial history of ARVC/D has been demonstrated in 30–50% of cases.[19-26] The most common pattern of inheritance is autosomal dominant, although an autosomal recessive pattern has also been reported. Linkage analysis has located the genetic abnormality on chromosomes 1, 2, 3, and 14 for the dominant form[20-24] and on chromosome 17 for the recessive form of the disease (Table 2).[25] This latter variant is characterized by associated epidermal abnormalities such as palmoplantar keratosis and woolly hair (so-called Naxos disease), more severe signs of the disease, and higher penetrance in family members (90%). Although 6 ARVC/D loci have been identified so far, the involved genes and the molecular defect

Table 2

Genetic Basis for Arrhythmogenic Right Ventricular
Dysplasia/Cardiomyopathy

| Reference | Inheritance | Chromosome | Locus |
|-----------|-------------|------------|-------|
| Rampazzo et al. (20) | Autosomal dominant | 14 | q23–q24 |
| Rampazzo et al. (21) | Autosomal dominant | 1 | q42–q43 |
| Severini et al. (22) | Autosomal dominant | 14 | q12–q22 |
| Rampazzo et al. (23) | Autosomal dominant | 2 | q32.1–q32.2 |
| Ahamad et al (24) | Autosomic dominant | 3 | p23 |
| Coonar et al. (25) | Autosomal recessive | 17 | q21 |

causing the disease are still unknown.[3] Genes encoding for actinin and keratine have been considered potential candidates for the dominant and recessive variant of ARVC/D, respectively.[20,25] It is noteworthy that in the Padua experience, about 50% of the ARVC/D families undergoing clinical and genetic screening did not show linkage with any of the known chromosomal loci.[26] Therefore, further genetic heterogeneity can be postulated. Although a preclinical diagnosis of ARVC/D by DNA characterization is warranted, at the present time a genetic test is not currently available.

## Etiopathogenetic Hypotheses

All the hypotheses advanced to explain the progressive loss of the RV myocardium are not in conflict with the well-established genetic background of ARVC/D.[27,28]

### Dystrophy

According to the dystrophic theory, the disappearance of the RV myocardium is caused by a genetically determined dystrophy leading to myocyte death as the result of some metabolic or ultrastructural defects.[4] The concept of a progressive muscle atrophy linked to a genetic abnormality, as observed in patients with Duchenne's or Becker's skeletal muscle dystrophies, is supported by the frequent familial occurrence of ARVC/D[19] and the recent discovery of the aforementioned genetic defects.[20,25] Duchenne's or Becker's diseases may share with ARVC/D the histopathological finding of muscular atrophy with fatty infiltration (so-called "pseudohypertrophy"). Mutations of genes encoding for the molecules such as merosin, DAGs, and dystrophin, which are involved in the connection of the cytoskeleton with the extracellular matrix via transmembrane glycoproteins, may induce severe muscle damage and result in a muscular dystrophy.[20,28] It is noteworthy that segments of actinin molecule, which has been implicated in the pathogenesis of ARVC/D, show a structural homology with parts of dystrophin.[20] Nevertheless, no skeletal muscular involvement was detected in patients with ARVC/D.

Why the dystrophic process in ARVC/D is confined to the right ventricle remains unexplained.

## Inflammation

The frequent histopathological finding of inflammatory infiltrates associated with myocardial degeneration and necrosis suggests a myocarditis.[2,4,5,29,30] Accordingly, the loss of the RV myocardium would be regarded as a consequence of an inflammatory myocardial "injury" with myocyte death due to an infectious and/or immune reaction, and the fibrofatty replacement would be considered as a "repair" process in the setting of chronic myocarditis.[4] The familial occurrence of ARVC/D is not in contrast with the inflammatory hypothesis since a genetically determined vulnerability of the RV myocardium to viral infection has been shown in experimental studies in animals. Matsumori and Kavai obtained a selective RV perimyocarditis in BALB/c mice after coxsackievirus infection that later resulted in the development of ventricular aneurysms.[31] Of note, this experimental RV pericardiomyocarditis could explain the peculiar subepicardial involvement of the RV wall in ARVC/D.

In human hearts, an enteroviral infection was recently ruled out by means of PCR and RT-PCR techniques that never detected entoviral genome particles either in hearts obtained at the time of cardiac transplantation or in endomyocardial biopsy samples from ARVC/D patients.[32] Likewise, the hypothesis of a humoral autoimmunity was also ruled out by the finding of similar frequency of circulating organ antibodies, either cardiac-specific or skeletal muscle cross-reactive, in ARVC/D patients and controls.[32] Whether a cell-mediated immunity plays a pathogenetic role, like that observed in some experimental models of lymphocytic myocarditis, remains to be assessed by further investigations.

## Apoptosis

Apoptosis (or programmed cell death) is a genetically mediated process that allows individual cells to be deleted from tissues.[33] Apoptosis has a homeostatic function to counterbalance mitosis in the normal turnover of cells and a remodeling function during embryogenesis. It has been shown to be involved in a series of physiological and pathological biological processes such as morphogenesis, autoimmune reaction, and growth and regression of malignancy. Recently it was advanced that apoptosis may account for the progressive disappearance of the RV myocardium in the setting of the physiological postnatal involution of the right ventricle as well as of the pathological myocardial atrophy with fibrofatty substitution that is observed in ARVC/D.[34,35] This is not in conflict with the genetic background of ARVC/D, since the apoptotic process is regulated by the expression of genes such as *bcl-2*, which is a major apoptosis-suppressing gene, and *p53* and *c-myc*, which are apoptosis-promoting genes.[36–38] Cells undergoing apoptosis show distinctive morphological features, mostly consisting of compaction and margination of nuclear chromatin, nuclear and cytoplasmatic aggregation, and fragmentation into apoptotic bodies that are phagocytosed by macrophages.[33] TUNEL is a recently developed technique that identifies apoptosis in paraffin sections by in situ end-labeling of DNA fragmentation into regular nucleosome-sized units.[39] Using the TUNEL method, apoptosis has been demonstrated by James et al. in an infant with Uhl's anomaly and complete AV block,[40] and by Mallat et al. in a series of postmortem hearts with ARVC/D.[34] In vivo evidence of apoptosis in ARVC/D has been provided by Valente et al. by examining endomyocardial biopsies from 20 ARVC/D patients; apoptotic myocytes were found in 35% of the cases with a mean apoptotic index (calculated as percentage of positive nuclei in sections stained with TUNEL) of $24.4 \pm 9.8$.[35] Moreover, apoptosis was significantly related to an "acute" clinical presentation with angina, pyrexia, ST segment elevation, and rise of ESR or CPK.[35] These findings might reflect a cause-effect relationship among an acute viral infection, autoimmune reaction or other inflammatory process, and apoptosis. Recent studies have demonstrated that apoptosis may be induced in the setting of a myocardial inflammation by cytotoxic T lymphocytes and antibody-dependent cytotoxic cells.[41] Therefore, the frequent finding of focal lymphocytic myocarditis in hearts with ARVC/D is not in contrast with the apoptotic theory.

# Conclusions

There is clear-cut evidence that ARVC/D is an acquired, nonischemic atrophy of the RV myocardium. A dynamic injury/repair process accounts for the progressive loss of the myocardium and its fibrofatty replacement. Myocyte death may be the result of a genetically determined myocardial dystrophy due to some metabolic or ultrastructural defect (dystrophic theory), a chronic myocarditis caused by an infection and/or immune myocardial reaction (inflammation theory), or a programmed cell death (apoptosis) in the setting of an enhanced postnatal involution of the right ventricle (apoptotic theory). All of the above fit with the frequent familial occurrence and the well-established genetic background of ARVC/D.

## References

1. Marcus FI, Fontaine G, Guiraudon G, et al. Right ventricular dysplasia: a report of 24 adult cases. Circulation 1982; 65:384–398.
2. Thiene G, Nava A, Corrado D, Rossi L, Pennelli N. Right ventricular cardiomyopathy and sudden death in young people. N Engl J Med 1988; 318:129–133.
3. Nava A, Rossi L, Thiene G (eds): Arrhythmogenic Right Ventricular Cardiomyopathy-Dysplasia. Elsevier, Amsterdam, 1997.
4. Basso C, Thiene G, Corrado D, Angelini A, Nava A, et al. Arrhythmogenic right ventricular cardiomyopathy: dysplasia, dystrophy, or myocarditis? Circulation 1996; 94:983–991.
5. Corrado D, Basso C, Thiene G, et al. Spectrum of clinicopathologic manifestations of arrhythmogenic right ventricular cardiomyopathy/dysplasia: a multicenter study. J Am Coll Cardiol 1997; 30:1512–1520.
6. Corrado D, Thiene G, Nava A, Rossi L, Pennelli N. Sudden death in young competitive athletes: clinicopathologic correlation in 22 cases. Am J Med 1990; 89:588–596.
7. Corrado D, Basso C, Schiavon M, Thiene G. Screening for hypertrophic cardiomyopathy in young athletes. N Engl J Med 1998; 339:364–369.
8. Fontaine G, Guiraudon G, Frank R, Tereau Y, Fillette F, et al. Dysplasie ventriculaire droite arythmogène et maladie de Uhl. Arch Mal Coeur 1982; 4:361–372.
9. Gerlis LM, Schmidt-Ott C, Ho SY, Anderson RH. Dysplastic conditions of the right ventricular myocardium: Uhl's anomaly vs arrhythmogenic right ventricular dysplasia. Br Heart J 1993; 69:142–150.
10. Daliento L, Turrini P, Nava A, Rizzoli G, Angelini A, et al. Arrhythmogenic right ventricular cardiomyopathy in young versus adult patients: similarities and differences. J Am Coll Cardiol 1995; 25:655–664.
11. Richardson P, McKenna WJ, Bristow M, Maisch B, Mautner B, et al. Report of the 1995 WHO/ISFC Task Force on the definition and classification of cardiomyopathies. Circulation 1996; 93:841–842.
12. Fontaine G, Frank R, Fontaliran F, Lascault G, Tonet J. Right ventricular tachycardias. In: Parmley WW, Chatteryce K (eds). Cardiology. JB Lippincott Co., New York, 1992, pp 1–17.
13. McKenna WJ, Thiene G, Nava A, et al. Diagnosis of arrhythmogenic right ventricular dysplasia/cardiomyopathy. Br Heart J 1994; 71:215–218.
14. Blomström-Lundqvist C, Sabel CG, Olsson SB. A long-term follow-up of 15 patients with arrhythmogenic right ventricular dysplasia. Br Heart J 1987; 58:477–488.
15. Marcus FI, Fontaine GH, Frank R, Gallagher JJ, Reiter MJ. Long-term follow-up in patients with arrhythmogenic right ventricular disease. Eur Heart J 1989; 10 (Suppl D):61–67.
16. Pinamonti B, Sinagra G, Salvi A, et al. Left ventricular involvement in right ventricular dysplasia. Am Heart J 1992; 123:711–724.
17. Thiene G, Nava A, Angelini A, Daliento L, Scognamiglio R, et al. Anatomoclinical aspects of arrhythmogenic right ventricular cardiomyopathy. In:

Baroldi G, Camerini F, Goodwin JF (eds). Advances in Cardiomyopathy. Springer Verlag, Berlin, 1990, pp 397–408.

18. Burke AP, Farb A, Tashko G, Virmani R. Arrhythmogenic right ventricular cardiomyopathy and fatty replacement of the right ventricular myocardium: are they different diseases? Circulation 1998; 97:1571–1580.
19. Nava A, Thiene G, Canciani B, Scognamiglio R, Daliento L, et al. Familial occurrence of right ventricular dysplasia: a study involving nine families. J Am Coll Cardiol 1988; 12:1222–1228.
20. Rampazzo A, Nava A, Danieli GA, Buja GF, Daliento L, et al. The gene for arrhythmogenic right ventricular cardiomyopathy maps to chromosome 14q23–q24. Hum Mol Genet 1994; 3:959–962.
21. Rampazzo A, Nava A, Erne P, Eberhard M, Vian E, et al. A new locus for arrhythmogenic right ventricular cardiomyopathy (ARVD2) maps to chromosome 1q42-q43. Hum Mol Genet 1995; 4:2151–2154.
22. Severini GA, Krajinovic M, Pinamonti B, Sinagra G, Fioretti P, et al. A new locus for arrhythmogenic right ventricular dysplasia on the long arm of chromosome 14. Genomics 1996; 31:193–200.
23. Rampazzo A, Nava A, Miorin M, Fonderico P, Pope B, et al. A new locus for arrhythmogenic right ventricular cardiomyopathy (ARVD4) maps to chromosome 2q32. Genomics 1997; 45:259–263.
24. Ahmad F, Li D, Karibe A, Gonzales O, Tapscott T, et al. Localization of a gene responsible for arrhythmogenic right ventricular dysplasia to chromosome 3p23. Circulation 1998; 98:2791–2795.
25. Coonar AS, Protonotarius N, Tsatsopoulou A, Needham EWA, Houlston RS, et al. Gene for arrhythmogenic right ventricular cardiomyopathy with diffuse nonepidermolytic palmoplantar keratoderma and woolly hair (Naxos disease) maps to 17q21. Circulation 1998; 97:2049–2058.
26. Nava A, Bauce B, Villanova C, Rampazzo A, Muriago M, et al. Arrhythmogenic right ventricular cardiomyopathy: long-term follow-up of 37 families (abstract). J Am Coll Cardiol 1999; 33:497A.
27. Thiene G, Basso C, Danieli GA, Rampazzo A, Corrado D, et al. Arrhythmogenic right ventricular cardiomyopathy: a still underrecognized clinical entity. TCM 1997; 7:84–90.
28. Danieli GA, Nava A, Rampazzo A. A first insight into molecular genetics. In: Nava A, Rossi L, Thiene G (eds). Arrhythmogenic Right Ventricular Cardiomyopathy-Dysplasia. Elsevier, Amsterdam, 1997, pp 166–173.
29. Thiene G, Corrado D, Nava A, Rossi L, Poletti A, et al. Right ventricular cardiomyopathy: is there evidence of an inflammatory etiology? Eur Heart J 1991; 12:22–25.
30. Lobo FV, Heggtveit HA, Butany J, Silver MD, Edwards JE. Right ventricular dysplasia: morphological findings in 13 cases. Can J Cardiol 1992; 8: 261–268.
31. Matsumori A, Kawai C. Coxsackievirus B3 perimyocarditis in BALB/c mice: experimental model of chronic perimyocarditis in the right ventricle. J Pathol 1980; 131:97–106.
32. Valente M, Calabrese F, Angelini A, Caforio A, Basso C, et al. Pathobiology. In: Nava A, Rossi L, Thiene G (eds). Arrhythmogenic Right Ventricular Cardiomyopathy/Dysplasia. Elsevier, Amsterdam,1997, pp 147–158.
33. Kerr JFR, Wyllie AH, Currie AR. Apoptosis: a basic biological phenomenon with wide-ranging implications in tissue kinetics. Br J Cancer 1972,26:239–257.
34. Mallat Z, Tedgui A, Fontaliran F, Frank R, Durigon M, et al. Evidence of apoptosis in arrhythmogenic right ventricular dysplasia. N Engl J Med 1996; 335:1190–1196.

35. Valente M, Calabrese F, Thiene G, Angelini A, Basso C, et al. In vivo evidence of apoptosis in arrhythmogenic right ventricular cardiomyopathy. Am J Pathol 1998; 152:479–484.
36. Misao J, Hayakawa Y, Ohno M, Nato S, Fujwara T, et al. Expression of bcl-protein, an inhibitor of apoptosis, in ventricular myocytes of human hearts with myocardial infarction. Circulation 1996; 94:1506–1512.
37. Kajstura J, Mansukhani M, Cheng W, Reiss K, Krajewski S, et al. Programmed cell death and expression of the protooncogene bcl-2 in myocytes during postnatal maturation of the heart. Exp Cell Res 1995; 219:110–121.
38. Olivetti G, Abbi R, Quaini F, Kajstura J, Cheng W, et al. Apoptosis in the failing human heart. N Engl J Med 1997; 336:1131–1141.
39. Gavrieli Y, Sherman Y, Ben- Sasson SA. Identification of programmed cell death in situ via specific labelling of nuclear DNA fragmentation. J Cell Biol 1992; 119: 493–501.
40. James TM, Nichols MM, Sapire DW, Di Patre, PL, Lopez SM. Complete heart block and fatal right ventricular failure in an infant. Circulation 1996; 93:1588–1600.
41. Nagata S. Apoptosis mediated by the Fas system. Prog Mol Subcell Biol 1996; 16:87–103.

# 19

# Therapies for Prevention of Sudden Cardiac Death in Arrhythmogenic Right Ventricular Cardiomyopathy

*Thomas Wichter, MD,*
*Martin Borggrefe, MD,*
*Dirk Böcker, MD, and*
*Günter Breithardt, MD*

## Introduction

In recent years, arrhythmogenic right ventricular cardiomyopathy/dysplasia (ARVCD) has been recognized as a major cause of ventricular tachyarrhythmias and sudden death in young patients and in athletes with apparently normal hearts.

ARVCD is characterized by localized or diffuse degeneration and atrophy of predominantly right ventricular myocardium with subsequent replacement by fatty and fibrous tissue.[1-4] These structural abnormalities progress from the epicardium toward the endocardium and are predominantly located in the right ventricular outflow tract, apex, and subtricuspid area of the right ventricular free wall ("triangle of dysplasia"),[5] whereas the interventricular septum and the left ventricular myocardium are usually spared. As a result of these pathomorphologic alterations, ventricular tachyarrhythmias and regional or global right (and left) ventricular dysfunction are major clinical findings and manifestations of ARVCD.

The prognosis of ARVCD is determined mainly by ventricular tachyarrhythmias and sudden cardiac death. In a young population of sudden death victims below the age of 35 years, the proportion of ARVCD as the underlying disease has been estimated at 15% to 25%.[4,6-8] This corresponds with a 20% to 25% mortality rate after 10 years on empiric (uncontrolled)

From: Aliot E, Clementy J, Prystowsky EN (editors). *Fighting Sudden Cardiac Death: A Worldwide Challenge.* ©Futura Publishing Company, Armonk, NY, 2000.

antiarrhythmic drug therapy.[9–12] Therefore, ARVCD cannot be considered a benign disease but requires an individualized, tailored, and effective treatment to prevent sudden cardiac death.

## Clinical Presentation

ARVCD usually manifests with ventricular tachycardia (VT) of left bundle branch block configuration (hallmark) in apparently healthy adolescents or young adults. In the majority of cases, the age at the time of first manifestation ranges between 15 and 35 years. In contrast, a first manifestation of ARVCD during early childhood or beyond the age of 60 years is unusual. Males are more frequently affected than females and usually present with more extensive forms or manifestations of the disease.[5,13–15]

In the majority of patients, ARVCD manifests with the sporadic occurrence of monomorphic VT. Others present with frequent premature ventricular beats, repetitive ventricular runs, or nonsustained VT. Associated symptoms range from palpitations and paroxysmal tachycardia to dizziness, syncope, and sudden cardiac arrest. Despite the fact that even rapid ventricular tachyarrhythmias may be well tolerated due to the normal left ventricular function, there is a potential risk of sudden cardiac death in untreated patients. In a minority of cases, resuscitation from cardiac arrest or sudden death may be the first manifestation of ARVCD. The disease has been recognized as an important underlying cause of unexpected sudden death in young patients and in athletes.[4,8]

Patients with ARVCD are usually not limited in their exercise capacity and may participate in sports activities without complaints. Not infrequently, they are even competitive athletes. This is of special interest and importance, because in patients with ARVCD, ventricular arrhythmias and cardiac arrest often occur during or immediately after physical exercise or competitive sports, particularly during the early phase of the disease. Therefore, particular attention should be directed toward recognizing ARVCD during the medical screening of athletes. With increasing age and more advanced stages of the disease, this exercise dependence diminishes and the arrhythmias more frequently occur at rest.

Cardiomegaly, left ventricular involvement, or clinical signs and symptoms of heart failure are unusual in early stages of ARVCD and are rarely a primary manifestation of the disease. They almost exclusively occur in patients with a long history and advanced stages of ARVCD.[16]

# Data on Treatment and Prognosis in ARVCD

## Data on Epidemiology

The proportion of ARVCD as the underlying disease in cases of sudden and unexpected cardiac death is unknown. Provided a detailed postmortem investigation of the right ventricle is performed by an experienced pathologist looking for the typical morphological signs of ARVCD, the proportion of ARVCD among sudden death victims below the age of 35 years has been reported at 15% and 25%.[4,6–8] However, since these conditions are frequently not fulfilled or postmortem investigations are not performed at all, the true frequency of ARVCD among sudden deaths is probably underestimated. Therefore, the assessment of the prevalence and also the prognosis of ARVCD remains difficult.

## Data on Treatment

Concerning the treatment of patients with ARVCD, the available data are also limited. Multicenter reports or controlled randomized studies have not been published so far. International registries were recently initiated but are just beginning to enroll patients. The available data to date, therefore, refer to (mostly retrospective) analyses of the treatment results in single centers with limited numbers of patients. Only a few groups have published prospective data on the long-term outcome of ARVCD patients on different treatment modalities.[15,17–23] Furthermore, the comparability of patient cohorts from different centers is limited due to discrepancies in patient selection (i.e., referral bias, treatment strategies) and application of diagnostic criteria.

# Management of Asymptomatic Patients and Family Members

## Asymptomatic Patients

Asymptomatic patients with ARVCD without a history of tachycardia, syncope, or cardiac arrest, without documented complex or sustained ventricular tachyarrhythmias, and without signs or symptoms of heart failure do not require specific antiarrhythmic or otherwise cardiac treatment. However, they should be followed by regular noninvasive cardiac investigations for the early recognition of ventricular arrhythmias and the potential progression of the disease with worsening of global or regional myocardial dysfunction. These follow-up visits should include a detailed interview concerning the interim occurrence of arrhythmic symptoms or events, ECG at rest, exercise tests, Holter monitoring, and cardiac imaging by echocardiography and/or magnetic resonance imaging. Patients with ARVCD should be advised against participation in competitive sports since this appears to be associated with an increased risk of sudden cardiac death.[4,6,7]

## Family Members

Family members of patients with ARVCD should visit a cardiologist experienced with the disease at regular intervals (3–5 years or with onset of symptoms). Twelve-lead surface ECG and echocardiography represent essential baseline diagnostic investigations that should be completed by exercise testing, Holter monitoring, and signal-averaged ECG whenever possible and suitable. If these investigations show signs suspicious of ARVCD or if complex ventricular arrhythmias are documented or syncope occurs, more detailed investigations should be performed to establish the diagnosis, to stratify the risk, and to develop an individualized treatment strategy. This extended diagnostic work-up should include supplemental cardiac imaging (cine-ventriculography, magnetic resonance imaging, radionuclide imaging, possibly endomyocardial biopsy) as well as electrophysiological investigations (invasive electrophysiological study, isoproterenol provocation). Criteria for the diagnosis of ARVCD were proposed and published by an international study group on ARVCD.[24]

Affected but asymptomatic family members of ARVCD patients should be followed up and investigated closely by experienced cardiologists familiar with the disease. In general, there is no indication for prophylactic antiarrhythmic therapy in these patients. However, in selected cases with familial ARVCD and frequent occurrence of sudden cardiac deaths within a family, an empiric treatment with beta blockers or amiodarone, or even the implantation of an implantable cardioverter-defibrillator (ICD) on a prophylactic basis may be discussed. However, it should be emphasized that at the present time, this approach is an individual borderline decision supported by only a few reports in single cases, and not an established treatment indication with evidence for general benefit.

## Treatment of Heart Failure

Symptomatic heart failure requiring treatment is present in only 10–20% of patients with ARVCD.[14,16] In ARVCD patients, heart failure usually occurs in advanced stages of the disease with a long history of preceding arrhythmias. In addition to a progressive dilatation and global dysfunction of the right ventricle, these patients frequently show signs of left ventricular involvement and therefore exhibit clinical signs and symptoms of biventricular heart failure.

There is no causal treatment option for heart failure in ARVCD. Pharmacological therapy of heart failure follows conventional guidelines and includes vasodilators, diuretics, beta blockers, and digitalis. In rare and selected patients with ARVCD and severe progressive heart failure intractable by pharmacological treatment, heart transplantation has been successfully performed by our group and others.[1] The implantation of a uni- or biventricular mechanical assist device may be considered as a bridging procedure in selected patients awaiting urgent transplantation and has been performed in 1 of our patients.

## Treatment of Arrhythmias

Recent studies indicate that ARVCD underlyies approximately 20% of sudden and unexpected cardiac deaths in a young population below the age of 35 years.[4,6–8] This corresponds well with studies reporting on 10-year mortality rates of up to 20% on empiric (uncontrolled) antiarrhythmic drug therapy.[9–12] Therefore, ARVCD should not be considered a benign disease and there is wide agreement on the need for antiarrhythmic therapy to reduce symptoms and to improve prognosis by the prevention of serious arrhythmic events and (most importantly) sudden cardiac death. However, to date, risk stratification for the identification of ARVCD patients at high risk for sudden cardiac death is still unsatisfactory and requires significant further improvement.

## General Considerations

*Sports Activities*

Patients with ARVCD should not participate in competitive sports, since this appears to be associated with an increased incidence of life-threatening ventricular arrhythmias and sudden cardiac death in ARVCD.[4,6–7] Therefore, preparticipation medical screening of athletes should pay particular attention not only to hypertrophic cardiomyopathy as a major cause of sudden death in athletes, but also to ARVCD, which has been identified as another important and frequent disease underlying unexpected sudden cardiac death on the athletic field.[25–27]

*Monitoring of Drug Effects*

If a patient is on antiarrhythmic drug treatment, 12-lead surface ECG should be performed at regular intervals with particular attention to the QRS width (Class I drugs) and the QT interval (Class III drugs). In addition, electrolyte disturbances (hypokalemia) should be avoided and potential drug interactions (QT prolongation) should be noticed to prevent proarrhythmic drug effects.

## Follow-Up Visits

To assess the long-term course of ARVCD and the long-term efficacy of antiarrhythmic treatment, follow-up visits should be scheduled at regular intervals by cardiologists with experience in evaluating the disease. To optimize compliance, the patients should be motivated to continue with the prescribed antiarrhythmic medication without changes in dosage to prevent arrhythmia recurrence. To achieve this goal, detailed information about the patient concerning the underlying disease and the individual treatment strategy may be helpful.

# Antiarrhythmic Drug Therapy

## Symptomatic Extrasystoles

In patients with ARVCD, premature ventricular beats, couplets, or short ventricular runs are not associated with an increased risk of sudden cardiac death and therefore do not require specific antiarrhythmic treatment, provided there is no history of syncope or cardiac arrest. In many cases, reassurance of the patient by detailed information on the harmlessness of these arrhythmias results in an improvement of symptoms so that drug therapy can be avoided. However, if a patient still suffers severe symptoms from palpitations, treatment with conventional beta blockers or with verapamil may be considered. Beta blockers appear to be more effective in patients with exercise-provocable ventricular arrhythmias, whereas verapamil may be successful in those cases with predominant occurrence of arrhythmias at rest and suppression during exercise. Because of their potential for adverse effects (in particular proarrhythmia), the use of specific antiarrhythmic drugs should be restricted to selected cases with severe symptoms from palpitations that cannot be controlled by reassurance, beta blockers, or verapamil.

## Ventricular Tachyarrhythmias

In patients with ARVCD and documented VT, antiarrhythmic treatment is considered to be indicated to prevent recurrent VT with serious symptoms and complications, to reduce emergency hospital admissions, and most importantly to prevent sudden cardiac death. Reports of prospective randomized studies or multicenter trials for the assessment of antiarrhythmic drug efficacy in ARVCD are not available.

The largest experience on the acute and long-term efficacy of antiarrhythmic drug therapy in ARVCD was published by Wichter et al.[18] and includes 147 patients in their latest published series.[19] In 63% of patients, serial testing identified an effective antiarrhythmic drug that completely suppressed the clinical arrhythmia during acute testing. Multivariate analysis identified extensive right ventricular dysfunction (advanced stage of ARVCD) and the inducibility of VT during programmed electrical stimulation as independent predictors of drug refractoriness. In another 15% of patients, the clinical arrhythmia was rendered more diffucult to induce or was sufficiently suppressed and a partial drug efficacy was assumed.[19]

The efficacy rates of different antiarrhythmic drugs in 191 ARVCD patients investigated at our institution are depicted in Figure 1. Sotalol in a dosage of 320 mg to 480 mg/day (up to 640 mg/day in selected cases) was identified as the most effective drug in this study, reaching a 68% overall efficacy rate.[18,19] A combination of amiodarone with beta blockers has a similar antiarrhythmic profile (Class III activity plus beta blockade) and was reported with comparable efficacy rates by French authors.[28] However, treatment with amiodarone alone or in combination with Class I antiarrhythmic drugs resulted in less favorable efficacy rates when com-

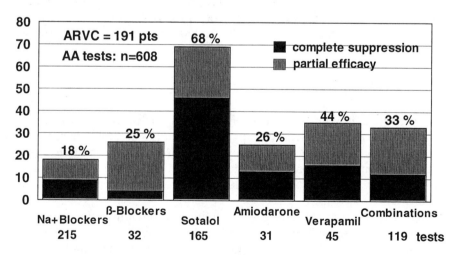

Figure 1. Efficacy rates of different antiarrhythmic drugs for treatment of VT in ARVCD (n=191 patients, n=608 tests). Sotalol in a dosage of 320–480 mg/day showed the highest efficacy rates. Amiodarone mono-treatment was less effective than sotalol and does not appear to be an alternative. Verapamil was tested only in patients with nonreentrant VT and may be an alternative therapy only in VT underlying triggered activity or abnormal automaticity. See text for details.

pared with sotalol.[18,19] Therefore, and because of the high incidence of serious side effects during long-term treatment with amiodarone in a young patient cohort, amiodarone does not appear to be advantageous. For these reasons, treatment with sotolol should be attempted or alternative treatment modalities considered prior to the initiation of amiodarone therapy.

Class I antiarrhythmic drugs proved efficacious to suppress the clinical arrhythmia in only a minority (18%) of patients with ARVCD, although some patients received several different Class I drugs.[18,19] Similar results were reported by other groups.[17,28]

In a small subset of patients with ARVCD and triggered activity of the underlying arrhythmia mechanism, verapamil and beta blockers demonstrated efficacy rates of 44% and 25% of patients treated.[18,19] In this selected small patient subgroup, these agents may therefore constitute an alternative treatment option with a low risk of adverse effects. However, to suppress reentrant ventricular arrhythmias, which are present in the majority of cases with ARVCD, verapamil and beta blockers are usually not effective.

Studies with long-term follow-up showed that patients in whom drug efficacy was monitored by serial electrophysiological study (inducible VT) or Holter monitoring combined with exercise testing (noninducible VT) provided better long-term outcome when compared with empiric drug treatment.[17,19,28] Sudden cardiac death and VT recurrences predominantly occurred in patients without successful suppression of arrhythmias at discharge, those with significant progression of ARVCD, or those with inappropriate dosage and/or intake of the tested antiarrhythmic drug (noncompliance).[19]

## Treatment Monitoring

Adequate monitoring of drug efficacy is a prerequisite for pharmacological antiarrhythmic drug therapy. Empiric antiarrhythmic drug treatment without evidence for appropriate suppression of the clinical arrhythmia cannot be recommended due to a high recurrence rate of VT and a significant mortality from sudden cardiac death during long-term follow-up.[9-12]

Due to the high spontaneous variability and sometimes only sporadic occurrence of arrhythmias in ARVCD, antiarrhythmic drug efficacy should be monitored by serial programmed electrical stimulation whenever feasible. The available data suggest that this approach offers best results with respect to long-term survival and freedom of VT recurrences. The requirement of reproducible inducibility of the clinical VT at baseline EP study is fulfilled in the majority of patients with ARVCD and sustained monomorphic VT.

However, in patients with only nonsustained VT, ventricular runs, or frequent premature ventricular beats, sustained monomorphic VT is less frequently inducible by programmed stimulation. Because these arrhythmias are frequently provocable by catecholamines, the clinical arrhythmia may be reproducibly provoked by exercise tests, intravenous catecholamines (i.e., isoproterenol), or programmed stimulation during catecholamine infusion.[18,29] In such patients with ARVCD, these tests may be used to monitor antiarrhythmic drug efficacy or nonpharmacological treatment.

In patients with ARVCD and frequent ventricular arrhythmias, Holter monitoring may be of additional help to assess and monitor the efficacy of antiarrhythmic treatment. In particular, this approach is useful for those patients in whom the clinical arrhythmia cannot be induced or provoked by programmed ventricular stimulation, or by exercise or catecholamines. However, due to the variability in the occurrence of spontaneous arrhythmias in these patients, the assessment of drug efficacy on the basis of Holter monitoring alone is unsafe and should therefore be restricted to patients at low risk of sudden cardiac death.

## Catheter Ablation

In patients with ARVCD, the arrhythmogenic substrate is represented by progressive atrophy predominantly of right ventricular myocardium with subsequent replacement by fatty and fibrous tissue.[1-4] The presence of surviving myocytes interspersed within fat and fibrosis results in areas of slow conduction predisposing to reentrant arrhythmias.[3,20] The anatomic substrate is comparable to that in patients with VT after myocardial infarction in whom viable myocardium is interspersed within fibrotic scar tissue at the border zone of the infarcted area.

### Endocardial Catheter Mapping

Endocardial catheter mapping using pacing interventions (resetting, entrainment) demonstrated that reentrant mechanisms underlie VT in the majority of ARVCD patients.[20,22,30,31] However, in patients with localized or concealed forms of ARVCD, triggered activity due to delayed afterdepolarizations and abnormal automaticity were also discussed as potential VT mechanisms.[20,32]

Our group[20,33] and others[22,30,31,34-36] showed that mapping criteria developed for catheter ablation of VT in patients after myocardial infarction[37-39] can also be applied in patients with ARVCD. In particular, activation mapping, mid-diastolic potentials, and entrainment mapping are helpful techniques for the localization of the critical site for energy delivery.[36,37,39] Pace mapping, which has been widely used for targeting ablation sites in patients with idiopathic VT, may be helpful in patients with localized or concealed ARVCD and VT underlying a mechanism of triggered activity or abnormal automaticity.

Detailed endocardial mapping studies by Aizawa et al.,[30] Yamabe et al.,[31] and Ellison et al.[36] in patients with typical manifestations of ARVCD demonstrated an entrainment of reentrant VT and thereby confirmed the presence of an area of slow conduction. Stark et al.[35] also showed entrainment and ablated the clinical VT in a patient with ARVCD by targeting radiofrequency (RF) energy delivery to an area of the tricuspid annulus acting as one of the barriers of an isthmus of slow conduction. Ellison et al.[36] mapped 19 VTs in 5 patients with ARVCD using activation and entrainment mapping. The reentrant circuit sites were clustered predominantly around the tricuspid annulus and in the right ventricular outflow tract.

## Results of Catheter Ablation in ARVCD (Table 1)

The published data on catheter ablation of VT in ARVCD show that acute success can be achieved in 60–80% of patients. However, during

Table 1

Catheter Ablation of Ventricular Tachycardia in ARVCD

| | Patients [n] | Energy | Acute Success | Procedure-Related Death | Follow-up [months] | VT-Recurrence |
|---|---|---|---|---|---|---|
| Fontaine[23] | 23 | DC | 83% | 9% | 71 | NI |
| Haissaguerre[58] | 7 | DC | 60% | 29% | 32 | NI |
| Leclercq[59] | 11 | DC | 72% | 0% | 32 | NI |
| Shoda[34] | 11 | DC | 91% | 0% | 17 | 50% |
| Trappe[60] | 12 | DC | 85% | 0% | 35 | 58% |
| Asso[61] | 6 | RF | 66% | 0% | 18 | 17%* |
| Ellison[36] | 5 | RF | 20% | 0% | 17 | 0%** |
| Gonska[62] | 32 | RF | 78% | 0% | NI | NI |
| Weiss[63] | 6 | RF | 75% | 0% | 21 | 50% |
| Wichter[20] | 30 | RF | 73% | 0% | 52 | 60% |

ARVCD = arrhythmogenic right ventricular cardiomyopathy/dysplasia; DC = direct current; RF = radiofrequency current; NI = no information.
*But 50% of patients on prophylactic antiarrhythmic drug treatment or ICD implantation.
**But 4 of 5 patients remained on antiarrhythmic drugs (n=2 amiodarone) or received an ICD. (n=1)

long-term follow-up of 3–5 years, the recurrence rates are as high as 50–70%.[20] In the early reports, catheter ablation was performed using direct current energy (DC), which was later replaced by RF current, which is still the technique most widely used today.

In 1984, Puech et al.[32] first reported the successful DC catheter ablation of drug-refractory catecholamine-sensitive VT in a patient with ARVCD. Fontaine et al.[22] studied the acute results and follow-up of DC catheter ablation in ARVCD and reported 2 procedure-related deaths during the initial phase and learning curve of DC ablation. In their latest series,[23] they report on 23 patients with an overall acute clinical success rate of 83%. Complete suppression of the clinical arrhythmia was achieved in 44% of patients; in another 39%, partial success was attained. To achieve these results, a second ablation session was necessary in 14, and a third in 3 of the 23 patients. The incidence of VT recurrences during follow-up was not reported in this study. In the latest series,[23] the authors also reported on their results with RF catheter ablation in 8 patients with ARVCD, which were, however, less favorable.

Ellison et al.[36] reported their results of entrainment mapping and RF catheter ablation of 19 VTs in 5 patients with ARVCD. VT terminated at 13 sites or 22% of RF applications. Eight of the 19 VTs were rendered noninducible and another 3 were modified. No procedure-related complications were observed. However, only 1 patient with VTs originating from the right ventricular outflow tract has remained free of VT during postprocedural EP testing and follow-up. The remaining 4 patients with VT still inducible after ablation were treated by amiodarone or ICD implantation.[36]

In our own experience with catheter ablation in 30 patients with ARVCD,[20,33] RF energy was used in the majority of cases and showed favorable acute results with complete suppression of drug-refractory VT in 22 patients (73%). However, the long-term results were less satisfactory with 2 sudden deaths (6.7%) and 18 patients suffering from VT recurrence (n=16) or syncope (n=2) during a follow-up period of 52 ± 37 months. Event-free survival was 63% after 1 year, 43% after 3 years, and 32% after 5 years, respectively[20] (Figure 2). The majority of early VT relapses (<1 year) after catheter ablation was due to the clinical arrhythmia and preferentially occurred in patients with unsuccessful ablation. In contrast, the majority of late VT recurrences (>1 year) showed a different QRS morphology when compared with the target VT.

Similar results were reported by Shoda et al.,[34] who achieved acute success in 10 of their 11 ARVCD patients (91%) using DC catheter ablation. However, 5 of them (50%) suffered VT relapses during follow-up of 15 ± 4 months after the intervention. In all cases, the QRS morphology of the recurrent VT was different from the clinical target VT during ablation.

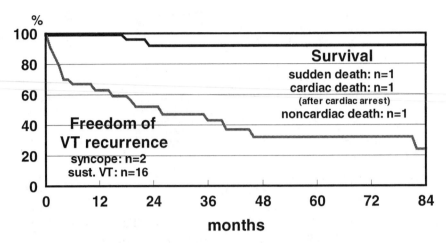

Figure 2. Long-term results after catheter ablation of VT in 30 patients with ARVCD (follow-up: 56 ± 32 months). Despite a rate of 73% acute success, the event-free survival was as low as 63% after 1 year, 43% after 3 years, and 32% after 5 years. The majority of late VT recurrences (>1 year) were due to new VT morphologies (new arrhythmogenic foci) during the progressive long-term course of ARVCD.

These observations suggest that the development of new arrhythmogenic substrates in different or neighboring areas may occur during the progressive long-term course of ARVCD and may be responsible for VT recurrences and sudden cardiac deaths occurring late after initially successful catheter ablation. This hypothesis also explains the discrepancy between the favorable acute results and the unsatisfactory long-term efficacy of catheter ablation for the treatment of VT in ARVCD.

## Limitations of Catheter Ablation in ARVCD

Successful catheter ablation of VT in patients with ARVCD offers the potential for long-term prevention of the targeted VT. This has been demonstrated by high success rates of catheter ablation in patients with a single site of VT origin and localized manifestation of ARVCD and in patients with a single or dominant form of drug-refractory frequent or incessant VT. However, additional antiarrhythmic drug therapy and/or repeated ablation sessions are frequently necessary to prevent recurrences of the clinical (targeted) or newly developed VT.

The progressive nature of ARVCD as the underlying myocardial disease constitutes the major relevant limitation for catheter ablation of VT in ARVCD. Discharge after successful catheter ablation bears a risk of potentially life-threatening or fatal VT recurrences from new arrhythmogenic foci developed during follow-up (2 late deaths in our series). On the other hand, it has not been shown to date that prophylactic antiarrhythmic drug therapy in ARVCD or other entities improves the long-term prognosis in this situation. Therefore, several authors have recommended restricting catheter ablation of VT in ARVCD to those patients with localized forms of the disease and only a single site of VT origin and/or combining catheter ablation with the implantation of a cardioverter-defibrillator (ICD) to prevent sudden cardiac deaths and VT recurrences during the progressive long-term course of ARVCD.[15,20,34]

Due to insufficient mapping conditions, not all patients with ARVCD and monomorphic VT are suitable candidates for catheter ablation. In addition to the problem of accurately localizing the critical parts of the reentrant circuit that are responsible for the induction and maintenance of VT, several features may limit the feasibility and success of catheter ablation in ARVCD. These include intramural, epicardial, or multiple sites of VT origin, a large arrhythmogenic area, and hemodynamically or electrically unstable VT. To be successful, the VT targeted by catheter ablation not only must be mappable, but also requires a critical portion of a reentrant pathway sufficiently small and with adequate electrode stability, wall contact, and tissue heat transfer so that the lesion induced by the RF current can interrupt and prevent VT.

## Current Indications for Catheter Ablation in ARVCD

In selected patients with ARVCD and drug-refractory VT, RF catheter ablation represents a therapeutic alternative. However, the technical limitations and the acute and long-term results indicate a palliative rather than a curative claim for this treatment modality in ARVCD. Nevertheless, in specific situations, catheter ablation may be a favored treatment option. These may include a single site of origin of a well-tolerated VT in a patient with localized ARVCD and, in particular, frequent or incessant VT refractory to drugs, or frequent VT episodes after ICD implantation.[20] In the latter situations, catheter ablation may even be the only available treatment option.

## Antitachycardia Surgery

During map-guided antitachycardia surgery in patients with drug-refractory VT and without demonstrable structural heart disease, Fontaine and co-workers in 1977–78 were the first to recognize and report ARVCD as a unique entity entitled "right ventricular dysplasia."[40]

*Surgical Techniques*

Different surgical techniques have been developed and applied for the treatment of VT in patients with ARVCD. Localized arrhythmogenic foci were usually treated by circumscribed surgical interventions including simple ventriculotomy, local excision, and endomyocardial circumcision of the arrhythmogenic zone in the area of earliest electrical activation.[41,42] In the border zone of the arrhythmogenic substrate, these interventions were sometimes combined with cryoablation.[41] In contrast to these techniques that are targeted to the arrhythmogenic substrate, partial or total disconnection of the right ventricular free wall [43,44] results in an electrical isolation of the right ventricular wall with its arrhythmogenic foci. The aim is to limit VT to the isolated right ventricle and to prevent expansion of VT to the left ventricle and thereby the systemic circulation.

*Results of Antitachycardia Surgery in ARVCD (Table 2)*

Various groups have reported favorable acute and long-term results of localized surgical interventions targeting the clinical VT in ARVCD. However, similar to catheter ablation, there is a risk of VT recurrence from new arrhythmogenic foci developing during the long-term progressive course of ARVCD. In patients with left ventricular involvement of ARVCD, long-term results of antitachycardia surgery appear to be unsatisfactory because the prognosis in these patients is determined mainly by VT recurrences of left ventricular origin or biventricular heart failure.[42]

A total disconnection of the right ventricular free wall has been per-

### Table 2
### Antitachycardia Surgery in ARVCD

| | Patients [n] | Localized vs. Diconnection | Follow-up [months] | Postop. Heart Failure | VT- Recurrence | Death at Follow-up |
|---|---|---|---|---|---|---|
| Cox[43] | 4 | 2/2 | 39 | 50% | 25% | 0% |
| Fontaine[41] | 12 | 12/0 | 36 | 9% | 33% | 17% |
| Guiraudon[44] | 20 | 12/8 | 38 | 20% | 30% | 15% |
| Lawrie[45] | 2 | 0/2 | 22 | 0% | 50% | 50% |
| Misaki[42] | 8 | 8/0 | 60 | 25% | 13% | 25% |
| Nimkhedkar[46] | 10 | 1/9 | 24 | 90% | 20% | 0% |

ARVCD = arrhythmogenic right ventricular cardiomyopathy/dysplasia.
Localized = circumscribed ventriculotomy, excision or endomyocardial circumcision.
Disconnection = total disconnection of the right ventricular free wall.

formed in selected ARVCD patients with multiple sites of VT origin and diffuse right ventricular involvement of ARVCD. The surgical technique was first described by Guiraudon et al.[44] followed by a few other groups.[43,46] All authors report a relevant proportion of postoperative right heart failure that was intractable and sometimes lethal. On the other hand, right ventricular function recovered in some patients during long-term follow-up after surgery.[46]

## Current Indications for Antitachycardia Surgery in ARVCD

Since localized surgical interventions bear a similar risk of VT recurrence due to new arrhythmogenic foci during the progressive long-term course of ARVCD, and the total disconnection of the right ventricular free wall is associated with a high incidence of postoperative right heart failure, antitachycardia surgery for VT in ARVCD has been abandoned by most groups.

# Implantable Cardioverter-Defibrillator

During recent years, the marked reduction of morbidity and mortality of ICD implantation and the tremendous progress in the technical development of ICDs have expanded the indications for ICD therapy.[21,47,50] Technical improvements include the introduction of purely transvenous ICD systems, antitachycardia pacing algorithms, biphasic shock waves (reduction of defibrillation threshold), sophisticated detection algorithms for ventricular tachyarrhythmias (multiple zones, QRS width, sudden onset, rate stability, dual chamber detection, and others), and improved battery longevity.

# Results of ICD Therapy in ARVCD

Similar to patients with coronary artery disease and remote myocardial infarction,[49–54] ICD therapy may also improve long-term prognosis in a high-risk subgroup of patients with ARVCD. Prospective randomized studies comparing ICD therapy with conventional antiarrhythmic drug therapy or with catheter ablation are not available for ARVCD patients. Prior to our own studies,[21,47,55] no results were published in relevant patient cohorts and information was limited to a few case reports.

After previous preliminary reports,[47,55] we recently reported the results of transvenous ICD implantation in 30 patients with ARVCD.[21] During long-term follow-up of 34 ± 19 months, no perioperative or sudden deaths were observed. One patient died from intractable biventricular heart failure 34 months after ICD implantation. Recurrent ventricular tachyarrhythmias were treated by cardioversion (n=15) and/or antitachycardia pacing (n=14) in 20 of 30 patients (67%). The majority of episodes were terminated by overdrive pacing. Event-free survival rates were 41% after 1 year, 36% after 2 years, and 27% after 3 years, respectively. The projected benefit on survival by ICD therapy, calculated by the difference between total mortality and the incidence of fast VT (>240 bpm),[53,54] was 29% after 1 year, 40% after 2 years, and 52% after 3 years, respectively[21] (Figure 3). These calculations assume that VT recurrences >240 bpm would have been fatal without ICD intervention, but also that all VT relapses <240 bpm would have been survived. Despite the limited data available, these data strongly suggest the benefits of ICD therapy in selected high-risk subgroups of ARVCD.

Comparable data were recently published by Link et al.,[48] who reported the results of ICD therapy in 12 patients with ARVCD. During follow-up of 13 ± 10 months, 1 patient died suddenly and 7 patients (58%) experienced appropriate ICD therapies for VT recurrences. In 5 patients, additional antiarrhythmic drug therapy with sotalol was considered indicated to reduce frequent VT relapses and subsequent ICD therapies.

## Complications of ICD Therapy in ARVCD

In our experience of ICD therapy in 30 patients with ARVCD,[21] there is a low risk of procedure-related complications. In particular, we have not

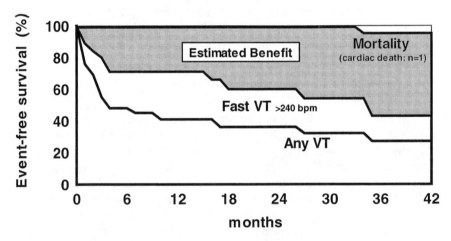

Figure 3. Long-term results after ICD implantation in 30 patients with ARVCD (follow-up: 34 ± 19 months). Three months after ICD implantation, there is a 50% recurrence rate of VT. The projected benefit on survival (shaded area), calculated by the difference between total mortality and fast VT (>240 bpm), was 29% after 1 year, 40% after 2 years, and 52% after 3 years, respectively.

observed ventricular perforations. Perioperative mortality, infections, lead-related complications, inappropriate ICD therapies, and other adverse events were also not increased and not different from other patient cohorts.[56] These results were confirmed by the study of Link et al.,[48] who observed no complications of ICD therapy in their 12 patients with ARVCD. However, due to the structural abnormalities of the right ventricular myocardium in patients with ARVCD, meticulous attention has to be paid to the placement of the right ventricular defibrillation leads during lead implantation, in order to achieve satisfactory acute and long-term pacing and sensing results.[21,47] In single cases, progression of myocardial atrophy and subsequent replacement by fat and fibrosis at the site of lead implantation may result in a loss of sensing function of the right ventricular defibrillation lead and may require the additional implantation of a pace/sense lead.[21]

### Current Status and Indications of ICD Therapy in ARVCD

The limited data available to date indicate that the majority of patients with ARVCD receive appropriate ICD therapies within the first year after ICD implantation.[21,47–58] These ICD therapies were probably life-saving in a relevant proportion of patients because of the high rate of VT recurrences. Therefore, it may be assumed that ICD therapy improves the long-term prognosis and survival in a selected high-risk population of patients with ARVCD and an otherwise normal life expectancy.[21]

In patients with ARVCD, indications for ICD implantation currently include episodes of survived cardiac arrest and high-risk patients with drug-refractory VT unsuitable for catheter ablation (extensive ARVCD, large or multiple arrhythmogenic foci, insufficient mapping conditions).

## Prognosis and Risk Stratification

Different studies reported a 10-year overall mortality of 5–25% according to the treatment strategy applied. The best results concerning long-term survival (Figure 4) were achieved by individualized treatment strategies, including serial drug testing monitored by repeated EP study and ICD implantation in selected high-risk patients with ARVCD.[17,19] (Figures 5, 6).

Patients with ARVCD and effective antiarrhythmic medication monitored by serial electrophysiological testing were reported to have a favorable long-term prognosis provided there was adequate dosage and intake of the tested and prescribed medication (compliance) and exclusion of significant progression of the underlying disease.[17,19] In this context, it is im-

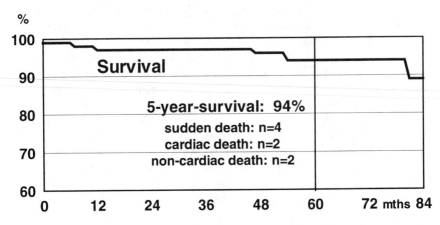

**Figure 4.** Long-term survival of 148 patients with ARVCD followed-up at our institution (follow-up: 54 ± 39 months). Tailored treatment of ventricular tachyarrhythmias was mainly guided according to the strategy depicted in Figure 6. The overall survival rate after discharge was 94% at 5 years of follow-up.[19]

portant to stress the importance of long-term follow-up of patients with follow-up visits at regular intervals not only to detect a progressive course of ARVCD but also to improve and optimize patient compliance. ARVCD patients without effective antiarrhythmic drug therapy frequently experience VT recurrences and mortality rates of up to 25% after 10 years or 2.5% per

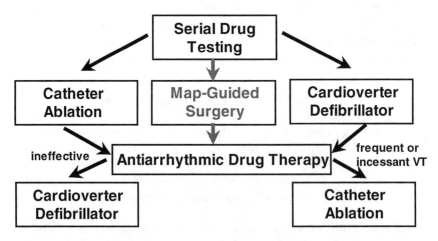

**Figure 5.** Stepwise treatment for VT in patients with ARVCD. Antitachycardia surgery has been abandoned by most groups because of improvement in catheter ablation techniques and the introduction of transvenous ICD systems. See text for details.

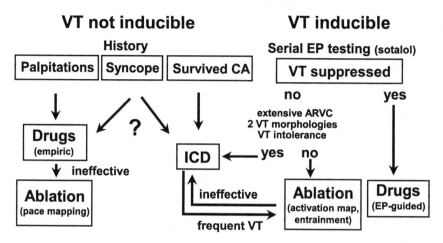

Figure 6. Strategy for the treatment of VTs in patients with ARVCD (proposal based on results at our institution). See text for details. EP-Testing = antiarrhythmic drug testing guided by electrophysiological study; CA = cardiac arrest.

year were reported on empiric antiarrhythmic drug therapy.[9–12] These data probably correspond with the natural history of ARVCD; however, the rate of sudden death as a primary manifestation of the disease is not taken into account.

Multivariate analyses identified several independent predictors of arrhythmic events during long-term follow-up of patients with ARVCD.[19,57] These include a severe enlargement and dysfunction of the right ventricle, left ventricular involvement, the inducibility of ventricular tachyarrhythmias during EP study, late potentials in the signal-averaged ECG, and a history of syncope or cardiac arrest. Future improvement of risk stratification is required to identify patients at high risk of sudden cardiac death and to optimize the proposed treatment strategies for patients with ARVCD outlined below.

## Treatment Strategies to Prevent Sudden Cardiac Death

Patients with ARVCD and asymptomatic ventricular runs or premature ventricular beats require no specific antiarrhythmic treatment, provided there is no history of cardiac arrest or syncope due to arrhythmias. If such arrhythmias are symptomatic, treatment with beta blockers or verapamil should be considered and specific antiarrhythmic drugs should be avoided wherever possible because of potential (proarrhythmic) side effects.

In asymptomatic patients with a family history of sudden cardiac death due to ARVCD, prophylactic treatment may be considered. However, there is no evidence that empiric antiarrhythmic treatment with beta blockers, sotalol, amiodarone, or other agents is effective to prevent serious arrhythmic events and sudden cardiac death. Therefore, the implantation of an ICD system on a prophylactic basis has been discussed and performed in selected ARVCD patients with a malignant family history for the primary prevention of cardiac arrest and sudden death. This approach, however, is still controversial and requires an individual decision based on the specific constellation of risks rather than a general recommendation as long as sufficient data are lacking.

Patients with nonsustained and sustained VT should undergo a detailed diagnostic work-up and invasive electrophysiological study to stratify the risk and to assess the inducibility of the clinical ventricular arrhythmia, both having a major impact on the subsequent treatment strategy (Figures 5, 6). In patients with inducible VT during programmed ventricular stimulation, the efficacy of subsequent drug therapy should be monitored by repeated electrophysiological study of medication, because this approach yields the most successful long-term results.

Antiarrhythmic drug therapy with sotalol (320–480 mg/day) yielded the highest efficacy rates in retrospective studies on drug efficacy for VT in ARVCD.[18,19] However, although there is no doubt that antiarrhythmic treatment reduces VT recurrences, there is no proof from prospective or randomized studies that it is also effective in the prevention of sudden death. Nevertheless, in our experience, mortality rates during long-term follow-up were low in those patients with ARVCD who were on electrophysiological study-guided and effective antiarrhythmic drug therapy (preferably sotalol).

In cases of drug-refractoriness, localized ARVCD, and a single morphology of a hemodynamically well-tolerated VT, catheter ablation may be considered as an alternative option and may lead to good acute results. However, recurrences were frequently observed during follow-up.[20,34] However, in selected cases of drug-refractory frequent or incessant VT, catheter ablation may be the only treatment option available with a palliative claim.

In patients with ARVCD and well-tolerated episodes of monomorphic VT but no reproducible VT induction during electrophysiological study, monitoring of drug efficacy may be performed by repeated exercise tests, catecholamine provocation, or Holter monitoring, provided there is no history of life-threatening arrhythmias or cardiac arrest in the patient or his family.[15]

For those patients who survived cardiac arrest or potentially life-threatening VT, the implantation of a transvenous ICD system should be considered as the treatment of choice to prevent recurrent cardiac arrest or sudden death. Also, in patients with drug-refractory VT and advanced stages of ARVCD, or multiple sites of VT origin, the implantation of an ICD may be the most appropriate therapeutic alternative to date to prevent life-threatening VT recurrences and sudden cardiac death.[21,47]

## References

1. Basso C, Thiene G, Corrado D, et al. Arrhythmogenic right ventricular cardiomyopathy: dysplasia, dystrophy, or myocarditis? Circulation 1996; 94:983–991.
2. Corrado D, Basso C, Thiene G, et al. Spectrum of clinicopathologic manifestations of arrhythmogenic right ventricular cardiomyopathy/dysplasia: a multicenter study. J Am Coll Cardiol 1997; 30:1512–1520.
3. Fontaine G, Fontaliran F, Linares-Cruz E, et al. The arrhythmogenic right ventricle. In: Iwa T, Fontaine G (eds). Cardiac Arrhythmias: Recent Progress in Investigation and Management. Elsevier Science Publishers BV, New York, 1988, pp 189–202.
4. Thiene G, Nava A, Corrado D, et al. Right ventricular cardiomyopathy and sudden death in young people. N Engl J Med 1988; 318:129–133.
5. Marcus FI, Fontaine GH, Guiraudon G, et al. Right ventricular dysplasia: a report of 24 cases. Circulation 1982; 65:384–398.
6. Corrado D, Basso C, Thiene G. Pathological findings in victims of sport-related sudden cardiac death. Sports Exerc Inj 1996; 2:78–86.
7. Corrado D, Thiene G, Nava A, et al. Exercise-related sudden death in the young. Eur Heart J 1993; 14(Suppl):368A.
8. Shen WK, Edwards WD, Hammill SC, Gersh BJ. Is right ventricular dysplasia a specific finding in the cause of sudden death in young subjects? Eur Heart J 1994; 15(Suppl):363.
9. Blomström-Lundqvist C, Sabel KG, Olsson SB. A long-term follow-up of 15 patients with arrhythmogenic right ventricular dysplasia. Br Heart J 1987; 58:477–488.
10. Canu G, Atallah G, Claudel JP, et al. Prognostic et évolution à long terme de la dysplasie arythmogène du ventricule droit. Arch Mal Coeur 1993; 86:41–48.
11. Leclercq JF, Coumel P, Denjoy I, et al. Long-term follow-up after sustained monomorphic ventricular tachycardia: causes, pump failure, and empiric antiarrhythmic therapy that modify survival. Am Heart J 1991; 121:1685–1692.
12. Marcus FI, Fontaine GH, Frank R, et al. Long-term follow-up in patients with arrhythmogenic right ventricular disease. Eur Heart J 1989; 10(Suppl D):68–73.
13. Marcus FI, Fontaine G. Arrhythmogenic right ventricular dysplasia/cardiomyopathy: a review. PACE 1995; 18:1298–1314.
14. Wichter T, Borggrefe M, Breithardt G. Arrhythmogene rechtsventrikuläre kardiomyopathie: ätiologie, diagnostik und therapie. Med Klin 1998; 93:268–277.
15. Wichter T, Borggrefe M, Breithardt G. How to diagnose and manage right ventricular cardiomyopathy today. In: Raviele A (ed). Cardiac Arrhythmias 1997. Springer-Verlag, Milan, 1998, pp 313–322.
16. Pinamonti B, Singara G, Salvi A, et al. Left ventricular involvement in right ventricular dysplasia. Am Heart J 1992; 123:711–724.

17. Berder V, Vauthier M, Mabo P, et al. Characteristics and outcome in arrhythmogenic right ventricular dysplasia. Am J Cardiol 1995; 75:411–415.
18. Wichter T, Borggrefe M, Haverkamp W, et al. Efficacy of antiarrhythmic drugs in patients with arrhythmogenic right ventricular disease: results in patients with inducible and noninducible ventricular tachycardia. Circulation 1992; 86:29–37.
19. Wichter T, Haverkamp W, Martinez-Rubio A, Borggrefe M. Long-term prognosis and risk-stratification of arrhythmogenic right ventricular dysplasia/cardiomyopathy. Circulation 1995; 92(Suppl I):I-97.
20. Wichter T, Hindricks G, Kottkamp H, et al. Catheter ablation of ventricular tachycardia. In: Nava A, Rossi L, Thiene G (eds). Arrhythmogenic Right Ventricular Cardiomyopathy/Dysplasia. Elsevier Science Publishers BV, Amsterdam, 1997, pp 376–391.
21. Wichter T, Böcker D, Borggrefe M, et al. Cardioverter-defibrillator therapy. In: Nava A, Rossi L, Thiene G (eds). Arrhythmogenic Right Ventricular Cardiomyopathy/Dysplasia. Elsevier Science Publishers BV, Amsterdam,1997, pp 364–375.
22. Fontaine G, Frank R, Rougier I, et al. Electrode catheter ablation of resistant ventricular tachycardia in arrhythmogenic right ventricular dysplasia: experience of 15 patients with a mean follow-up of 45 months. Heart Vessels 1990; 5:172–187.
23. Fontaine G, Frank R, Gallais Y, et al. Fulguration et radiofrequence dans la tachycardie ventriculaire. Arch Mal Coeur 1994; 87:1589–1607.
24. McKenna WJ, Thiene G, Nava A, et al., on behalf of the Task Force of The Working Group Myocardial and Pericardial Disease of the European Society of Cardiology and of the Scientific Council on Cardiomyopathies of the International Society and Federation of Cardiology. Diagnosis of arrhythmogenic right ventricular dysplasia/cardiomyopathy. Br Heart J 1994; 71:215–218.
25. Maron BJ, Thompson PD, Puffer JC, et al. Cardiovascular preparticipation screening of competitive athletes: a statement for health professionals from the Sudden Death Committee (Clinical Cardiology) and Congenital Cardiac Defects Committee (Cardiovascular Disease in the Young), American Heart Association. Circulation 1996; 94:850–856.
26. Furlanello F, Bertoldi A, Dallago M, et al. Cardiac arrest and sudden death in competitive athletes with arrhythmogenic right ventricular dysplasia. PACE 1998; 21:331–335.
27. Corrado D, Basso C, Schiavon M, Thiene G. Screening for hypertrophic cardiomyopathy in young athletes. N Engl J Med 1998; 339:364–369.
28. Tonet J, Frank R, Fontaine G, Grosgogeat Y. Efficacité de l'association de faibles doses de bêta-bloquants à l'amiodarone dans le traitement des tachycardies ventriculares réfractaires. Arch Mal Coeur 1989; 82:1511–1517.
29. Haissaguerre M, Chavernac P, Le Metayer P, et al. Valeur complementaire du test à l'isoprénaline et de l'ECG à haute amplification dans le diagnostic de la dysplasie arythmogène du ventricule droit. Ann Cardiol Angiol 1992; 41:425–432.
30. Aizawa Y, Funazaki T, Takahashi M, et al. Entrainment of ventricular tachycardia in arrhythmogenic right ventricular tachycardia. PACE 1991; 14:1606–1613.
31. Yamabe H, Okumura K, Tsuchiya T, Yasue H. Demonstration of entrainment and presence of slow conduction during ventricular tachycardia in arrhythmogenic right ventricular dysplasia. PACE 1994; 17:172–178.
32. Puech P, Gallay P, Grolleau R, Koliopoulos N. Traitement par electrofulgura-

tion endocavitaire d'une tachycardie ventriculaire récidivante par dysplasie ventriculaire droite. Arch Mal Coeur 1984; 77:826–834.

33. Haverkamp W, Borggrefe M, Chen X, et al. Radiofrequency catheter ablation in patients with sustained ventricular tachycardia and arrhythmogenic right ventricular disease. Circulation 1993; 88(Suppl):I-353.

34. Shoda M, Kasanuki H, Ohnishi S, Umemura J. Recurrence of new ventricular tachycardia after successful catheter ablation in patients with arrhythmogenic right ventricular dysplasia. Circulation 1992; 86(Suppl I):I-580.

35. Stark SI, Arthur A, Lesh MD. Radiofrequency catheter ablation of ventricular tachycardia in right ventricular cardiomyopathy: use of concealed entrainment to identify the slow conduction isthmus bounded by an aneurysm and the tricuspid annulus. J Cardiovasc Electrophysiol 1996; 7:967–971.

36. Ellison KE, Friedman PL, Ganz LI, Stevenson WG. Entrainment mapping and radiofrequency catheter ablation of ventricular tachycardia in right ventricular dysplasia. J Am Coll Cardiol 1998; 32:724–728.

37. Borggrefe M, Chen X, Hindricks G, et al. Catheter ablation of ventricular tachycardia in patients with coronary artery disease. In: Zipes DP, Jalife J (eds). Cardiac Electrophysiology: From Cell to Bedside (2nd edition). WB Saunders Company, Philadelphia, 1995, pp 1502–1517.

38. Morady F, Harvey M, Kalbfleisch SJ, et al. Radiofrequency catheter ablation of ventricular tachycardia in patients with coronary artery disease. Circulation 1993; 87:363–372.

39. Stevenson WG, Khan H, Sager P, et al. Identification of reentry circuit sites during catheter mapping and radiofrequency ablation of ventricular tachycardia late after myocardial infarction. Circulation 1993; 88:1647–1670.

40. Fontaine G, Guiraudon G, Frank R, et al. Stimulation studies and epicardial mapping in ventricular tachycardia: study of mechanism and selection for surgery. In: Kulbertus HE (ed). Reentrant Arrhythmias. MTP, Lancaster, 1977, pp 334–350.

41. Fontaine G, Guiraudon G, Frank R, et al. Surgical management of ventricular tachycardia unrelated to myocardial ischemia or infarction. Am J Cardiol 1982; 49:397–410.

42. Misaki T, Watanabe G, Iwa T, et al. Surgical treatment of arrhythmogenic right ventricular dysplasia: long-term outcome. Ann Thorac Surg 1994; 58:1380–1385.

43. Cox JL, Bardy GH, Damiano RJ Jr, et al. Right ventricular isolation procedures for nonischemic ventricular tachycardia. J Thorac Cardiovasc Surg 1985; 90:212–224.

44. Guiraudon G, Klein GJ, Gulamhusein SS, et al. Total disconnection of the right ventricular free wall: surgical treatment of right ventricular tachycardia associated with right ventricular dysplasia. Circulation 1983; 67:463–470.

45. Lawrie GM, Pacifico A, Kaushik R. Results of direct surgical ablation of ventricular tachycardia not due to ischemic heart disease. Ann Surg 1989; 209:716–727.

46. Nimkhedkar K, Hilton CJ, Furniss SS, et al. Surgery for ventricular tachycardia associated with right ventricular dysplasia: disarticulation of right ventricle in 9 of 10 cases. J Am Coll Cardiol 1992; 19:1079–1084.

47. Breithardt G, Wichter T, Haverkamp W, et al. Implantable cardioverter defibrillator therapy in patients with arrhythmogenic right ventricular cardiomyopathy, long QT syndrome, or no structural heart disease. Am Heart J 1994; 127(Suppl):1151–1158.

48. Link MS, Wang PJ, Haugh CJ, et al. Arrhythmogenic right ventricular dyspla-

sia: clinical results with implantable cardioverter-defibrillators. J Interven Cardiac Electrophysiol 1997; 1:41–48.
49. Böcker D, Haverkamp W, Block M, et al. Comparison of d,l-sotalol and implantable defibrillators for treatment of sustained ventricular tachycardia or fibrillation in patients with coronary artery disease. Circulation 1996; 94:151–157.
50. Moss AJ, Hall WJ, Cannom DS, et al., for the MADIT Investigators. Improved survival with an implanted defibrillator in patients with coronary artery disease at high risk of ventricular arrhythmia. N Engl J Med 1996; 335:1933–1940.
51. Nisam S, Breithardt G. Mortality trials with implantable defibrillators. Am J Cardiol 1997; 79:468–471.
52. The Antiarrhythmics Versus Implantable Defibrillators (AVID) Investigators. A comparison of antiarrhythmic drug therapy with implantable defibrillators in patients resuscitated from near-fatal ventricular arrhythmias. N Engl J Med 1997; 337:1576–1583.
53. Böcker D, Bänsch D, Heinecke A, et al. Potential benefit from ICD therapy in patients with and without heart failure. Circulation. 1998; 98:1636–1643.
54. Böcker D, Block M, Isbruch F, et al. Do patients with an implantable defibrillator live longer? J Am Coll Cardiol 1993; 21:1638–1644.
55. Wichter T, Block M, Böcker D, et al. Arrhythmogenic right ventricular disease: implantable cardioverter defibrillator therapy in a subgroup of patients at high risk of sudden death. Eur Heart J 1992; 13(Suppl):151.
56. Block M, Hammel D, Bänsch D, et al. Prevention of ICD complications. In: Allessie M, Fromer M (eds). Atrial and Ventricular Fibrillation—Mechanisms and Device Therapy. Futura Publishing Company, Armonk, NY, 1996, pp 291–309.
57. Peters S, Reil GH. Risk factors of cardiac arrest in arrhythmogenic right ventricular dysplasia. Eur Heart J 1995; 16:77–80.
58. Haissaguerre M, Warin JF, Lemêtayer P, et al. Fulguration of ventricular tachycardia using high cumulative energy: results in thirty-one patients with a mean follow-up of twenty-seven months. PACE 1989; 12:245–251.
59. Leclercq JF, Chouty F, Cauchemez B, et al. Results of electrical fulguration in arrhythmogenic right ventricular disease. Am J Cardiol 1988; 62:220–224.
60. Trappe HJ, Brugada P, Talajic M, et al. Prognosis of patients with ventricular tachycardia and ventricular fibrillation: role of the underlying etiology. J Am Coll Cardiol 1988; 12:166–174.
61. Asso A, Farré J, Zayas R, et al. Radiofrequency catheter ablation of ventricular tachycardia in patients with arrhythmogenic right ventricular dysplasia. J Am Coll Cardiol 1995; 25(Suppl):315A.
62. Gonska BD, Raab J, Cao K. Catheter ablation of ventricular tachycardia in patients with arrhythmogenic right ventricular disease. Eur Heart J 1996; 17(Suppl):206.
63. Weiss C, Cappato R, Willems S, et al. Impact of underlying heart disease on long-term outcome following catheter ablation of ventricular tachycardia. J Am Coll Cardiol 1996; 27(Suppl):76A.

# V

# Sudden Cardiac Death and Repolarization

# 20

# The Long QT Syndrome:

# From Genotype to Phenotype

*Peter J. Schwartz, MD*

## Introduction

There are not many examples in clinical cardiology of relatively uncommon diseases which, within a few years, become the focus of massive and multidisciplinary research resulting in a flood of articles in scientific journals and of presentations at scientific meetings as is currently happening with the long QT syndrome (LQTS).

The objective of this brief chapter is not that of reviewing its main clinical features, which have been carefully described over the years,[1-4] or of reporting in detail the impressive acquisitions of knowledge related to the genes involved in the disease[3,5,6]; instead, the focus is on the rationale and preliminary data related to the unfolding saga of genotype-phenotype correlation.

It is essential to keep in mind a few basic facts. All genes for LQTS identified so far encode ion channels involved in the control of ventricular repolarization. The "expression" techniques available coupled with in situ mutagenesis[7] make it possible, once a specific mutation has been identified, to reproduce of the electrophysiological characteristics of the mutated protein and to appreciate the consequences on the action potential. The resulting understanding may guide the exploration of novel therapeutic approaches, either mutation- or gene-specific, and may help in designing genotype-phenotype studies.[8] The latter may in turn contribute to more accurate diagnosis, risk stratification, and therapeutic management.

Thus far, 6 loci have been related to LQTS and 5 genes have been identified. Two of them, *minK* and *Mirp1*, responsible respectively for LQT5 and LQT6, are rare. The most common forms, responsible respectively for LQT1, LQT2, and LQT3, depend on mutations on *KvLQT1*—encoding the $I_{Ks}$ current, on *HERG*—encoding the $I_{Kr}$ current, and on *SCN5A*—encoding the Na$^+$ current. The data available for genotype-phenotype correlation studies on adequate numbers are limited to LQT1, LQT2, and LQT3.

From: Aliot E, Clementy J, Prystowsky EN (editors). *Fighting Sudden Cardiac Death: A Worldwide Challenge.* ©Futura Publishing Company, Armonk, NY, 2000.

So far, genotype-phenotype studies have focused on a few selected areas and they will be succinctly described here because, for the most part, they have not yet been published other than in abstract form.

## Genotype and ECG

Moss et al.[9] were the first to call attention to the fact that different genotypes appeared to correlate with rather specific electrocardiographic patterns. LQT1 patients tend to have smooth, broad-based T waves whereas LQT2 patients frequently have low amplitude and notched T waves; LQT3 patients have a more distinctive pattern characterized by a late onset of the T wave. Additional, and relatively specific, patterns have been identified.[10] Unfortunately, these morphological differences are not always so well defined; there is some degree of overlap, and in some families extreme heterogeneity of T wave morphology may be observed. Therefore, the ECG morphology may be useful in suggesting to look first for mutations on a certain gene, thus saving time for the molecular diagnosis. On the other hand, it does not represent a valid surrogate for actual genotyping and it should not be used to make a molecular diagnosis.

## Genotype and Drug-Induced QT Shortening

The realization[11–14] that some of the mutations on $SCN5A$, the sodium channel gene, produce a delayed inactivation of the $Na^+$ current and result in the persistence of a small inward current—responsible for the QT prolongation—provided the rationale for the first attempt to shorten the QT interval as a gene-specific therapy.[8] We used the $Na^+$ channel blocker mexiletine to verify the possibility of achieving, in selected patients, a degree of QT shortening that might be expected to reduce the risk of life-threatening arrhythmias. Our data, based on approximately 40 genotyped patients, show that among LQT3 patients, mexiletine shortens the QT interval by an average of 90 ms whereas among LQT1 and LQT2 patients the change averages only 20–30 ms. These preliminary data suggest that mexiletine, which can be considered as a relatively safe drug in LQTS patients independently of their mutations, may contribute to clinical management by shortening the QT interval of some LQT3 patients.

Recent and partially unpublished data suggest that flecainide—another $Na^+$ channel blocker—may be particularly effective in patients with delayed inactivation of the $Na^+$ current because the drug inhibits preferentially late $Na^+$ openings, thereby reducing the late current with little effect on the early current.[15] A clinical counterpart may already exist, because Moss and associates[16] have observed a striking degree of QT shortening in some patients with the ΔKPQ mutation (the most common among those producing delayed inactivation of the $Na^+$ current). Adequate comparative data are not yet available, but it may very well be that flecainide is more effective than mexiletine in these patients.

A few words of caution may be necessary. Although it is reasonable to expect that QT shortening will reduce the risk of arrhythmic events, this has not yet been proven. Thus, drugs that may effectively shorten the QT interval cannot substitute for therapies of proven efficacy, such as antiadrenergic interventions; they might be used in conjunction with the established therapies with the reasonable hope of further reducing the arrhythmic risk. Some patients with *SCN5A* mutations appear to have both QT prolongation and the Brugada syndrome[17]; the use of flecainide in these patients may unmask a previously unrecognized Brugada syndrome with devastating consequences. Very appropriately, Moss and associates limit the use of flecainide to patients with the ΔKPQ mutation. However, one would expect flecainide to have similar efficacy in the other mutations producing delayed inactivation of the $Na^+$ current.[12]

While the therapeutic trials with $Na^+$ channel blockers, mexiletine, flecainide, or others, merit careful attention because of the exciting concept of gene-specific therapy, it is also important to remember that the number of families with mutations producing a delayed inward $Na^+$ current constitutes a very small minority. LQT3 patients appear to represent less than 5% of all LQTS patients and half of them have mutations producing different electrophysiological consequences. In this sense, $Na^+$ channel blockers represent, in my opinion, more a "mutation-specific" than a "gene-specific" therapy.

Another approach, based on the realization that $K^+$ current (impaired by *HERG* mutations) is activated by higher levels of $K^+$ plasma concentration, has been based on the understanding that quantitatively reduced $I_{Kr}$ function leads to prolongation of repolarization, and $I_{Kr}$ conductance is heightened by increased extracellular $K^+$.[18] $I_{Kr}$ conductance can be stimulated toward a quantitatively normal current magnitude by an increase in serum $K^+$ in LQT2 patients both during acute[19] and chronic $K^+$ therapy. While this approach was designed specifically to counteract the genetic defect in LQT2, it may provide a means of normalizing repolarization duration in patients with LQTS due to any cause. A current limitation is represented by the difficulty in achieving persistent increases in serum $K^+$ levels by chronic administration.[20]

## Genotype and Tachycardia-Induced QT Shortening

In 1995 we realized that exercise-induced heart rate changes could produce differential degrees of QT shortening according to genotype.[8]

These preliminary observations have been extended and can be summarized as follows. Compared to 50 healthy controls, there is a tendency among LQT1 patients for a lesser degree of QT shortening for each 100 ms of RR shortening; despite a significant overlap, several of 30 LQT1 patients had only a minimal degree of QT shortening. This is in agreement with what could be expected of patients with an impairment in the $I_{Ks}$ current. This important repolarizing current is indeed activated by increases in heart rate and by catecholamine release.

LQT2 patients do not differ from the control population. By contrast, the behavior of LQT3 patients is strikingly different: during heart rate increases they shorten their QT interval much more than controls. A possible explanation for this unexpected finding has been provided by an experimental study attempting to reproduce the defects of *SCN5A* and of *HERG* at the cellular level.[21] By exposing guinea pig ventricular myocytes to anthopleurin, a toxin that interferes with the inactivation of $I_{Na}$, and to dofetilide, a selective blocker of $I_{Kr}$, we obtained marked prolongation of the action potential. This mimicked the alterations thought to be present in LQT3 and in LQT2 patients, respectively. The behavior of LQT3 patients closely mimicked that of myocytes pretreated with anthopleurin, which during fast pacing shortened action potential duration more than control and more than dofetilide-pretreated cells. With rapid rates $Na^+$ accumulates in the cell, lowering the $Na^+$ gradient across the membrane and, consequently, the magnitude of $I_{Na}$. The effect of such a reduction would be negligible during the rising phase of the action potential, when $I_{Na}$ is of overwhelming magnitude. However, the $I_{Na}$ contribution of the mutant channels is of much smaller magnitude—being due to delayed inactivation of $I_{Na}$[11-14]—and could be significantly affected by such changes. It is indeed important to remember that this current operates at a critical time, when the action potential is determined by a very delicate balance of small currents.[5,6] It is, therefore, conceivable that a reduction of $I_{Na}$ during this phase—as it can result from faster heart rates—can shorten action potential duration and, hence, the QT interval. The obvious implication of these findings is that LQT3 patients may be at relatively lower risk during physical exercise, when the progressive heart rate increase may allow appropriate QT shortening. These patients may also be less likely to be protected by beta-blockers that would produce an excessively slow heart rate and would prevent an adequate heart rate increase during exercise.

## Genotype and Triggers for Life-Threatening Cardiac Events

The differential effects of heart rate increases on the duration of the QT interval and the surprising preliminary observations on apparently different precipitating factors for cardiac events among LQT2 and LQT3 patients[8] have prompted a large collaborative study among several investigators in order to assess whether or not different genotypes were associated with different risk factors for cardiac events.[22]

The most recent data, based on over 750 genotyped and symptomatic LQTS patients, indicate the existence of amazing differences. In summary, LQT1 patients are at particularly high risk during exercise (69% of the events) and at very low risk (4% of the events) while at rest or during sleep; the remaining 27% of the events occur during emotional arousal. An almost opposite pattern is present among LQT3 patients who have 52% of their episodes at rest or during sleep without any known arousal and in only 19% of cases during exercise. LQT2 patients do not appear to have a preferential trigger, but they also have a surprisingly low incidence of events (16%) during exercise.

Many different conclusions and inferences can be drawn from these data. Here only 2 will be mentioned: 1 concerning management and 1 concerning mechanisms.

It is clear that almost all arrhythmic episodes among LQT1 patients occur under conditions of augmented sympathetic activity. It would be logical to expect a high degree of protection for these patients by the use of antiadrenergic interventions, particularly beta blockers. The data available from several groups with direct clinical experience and adequate follow-up on large numbers of genotyped LQT1 patients (such as the groups in Paris, in Salt Lake City, and in Pavia) fully support this view.

At first glance it is difficult to comprehend why patients with mutations so different (i.e., affecting $I_{Na}$ and $I_{Kr}$) should share the striking feature of a relatively low risk during exercise, a condition resulting in a major elevation in catecholamines. As a matter of fact, a very sensible explanation does exist. What LQT2 and LQT3 have in common is that they both have a perfectly functional $I_{Ks}$ current. $I_{Ks}$, being activated by catecholamines and by increases in heart rate, plays a major role in the QT adaptation during exercise by accelerating repolarization. Thus, at variance with LQT1 patients, most of whom have an impaired ability to shorten their QT interval during exercise and are indeed at high risk for life-threatening arrhythmias in this condition, LQT2 and LQT3 patients can appropriately adapt their QT interval to progressive shortening in the cardiac cycle, thus escaping some of the risk involved in exercise.

# Conclusion

The study of genotype-phenotype correlation is currently offering interesting paradigms that foster our knowledge and might also provide useful clues for a more targeted clinical approach, whether it is gene-specific or mutation-specific. However, as often happens in life, it seems that the dark side of the moon hides the most exciting secrets, namely, those LQTS patients in whom there is no correlation between genotype and phenotype.

## References

1. Schwartz PJ. Idiopathic long QT syndrome: progress and questions. Am Heart J 1985; 109:399–411.
2. Schwartz PJ. The long QT syndrome. In: Camm AJ (ed). Clinical Approaches to Tachyarrhythmias series. Futura Publishing Co, Armonk, NY, 1997, pp 1–108.
3. Schwartz PJ, Priori SG, Napolitano C. Long QT syndrome. In: Zipes DP, Jalife J (eds). Cardiac Electrophysiology: From Cell to Bedside, 3rd edition. WB Saunders Co., Philadelphia (In press).
4. Zareba W, Moss AJ, Schwartz PJ, Vincent GM, Robinson JL, et al., for the International Long-QT Syndrome Registry Research Group. Influence of the genotype on the clinical course of the long QT syndrome. N Engl J Med 1998; 339:960–965.
5. Roden DM, Lazzara R, Rosen MR, Schwartz PJ, Towbin JA, et al., for the SADS Foundation Task Force on LQTS. Multiple mechanisms in the long-QT syndrome: current knowledge, gaps, and future directions. Circulation 1996; 94:1996–2012.
6. Priori SG, Barhanin J, Hauer RNW, Haverkamp W, Jongsma HJ, et al. Genetic and molecular basis of cardiac arrhythmias: impact on clinical management. Parts I and II. Circulation 1999; 99:518–528; Part III. Circulation 1999; 99:674–681; and Eur Heart J 1999; 20:174–195.
7. Chien KR (ed). Molecular Basis Of Cardiovascular Disease. WB Saunders Co., Philadelphia, 1999.
8. Schwartz PJ, Priori SG, Locati EH, Napolitano C, Cantù F, et al. QT syndrome patients with mutations on the SCN5A and HERG genes have differential responses to $Na^+$ channel blockade and to increases in heart rate: implications for gene-specific therapy. Circulation 1995; 92:3381–3386.
9. Moss AJ, Zareba W, Benhorin J, Locati EH, Hall WJ, et al. ECG T-wave patterns in genetically distinct forms of the hereditary long QT syndrome. Circulation 1995; 92:2929–2934.
10. Zhang L, Timothy KW, Fox J, Moss AJ, Schwartz PJ, et al. Genotypes of long QT syndrome patients with non-specific ST-T wave patterns can be recognized by family ECG characteristics (abstract). PACE 1998; 21:859.
11. Bennett PB, Yazawa K, Makita N, George AL Jr. Molecular mechanism for an inherited cardiac arrhythmia. Nature 1995; 376:683–685.
12. Dumaine R, Wang Q, Keating MT, Hartmann HA, Schwartz PJ, et al. Multiple mechanisms of $Na^+$ channel-linked long-QT syndrome. Circ Res 1996; 78:916–924.
13. An RH, Bangalore R, Rosero SZ, Kass RS. Lidocaine block of LQT-3 mutant human $Na^+$ channels. Circ Res 1996; 79:103–108.
14. An RH, Wang XL, Kerem B, Benhorin J, Medina A, et al. Novel LQT-3 mutation affects $Na^+$ channel activity through interactions between $\alpha$- and $\beta_1$-subunits. Circ Res 1998; 83:141–146.
15. Nagatomo T, Kyle JW, Tonkovich GS, January CT, Makielski JC. The open channel blocker flecainide preferentially inhibits persistent Na current in the ΔKPQ mutant in the LQT3 syndrome. Circulation 1997; 96:I-121.

16. Moss et al., in preparation.
17. Postma AV, Alshinawi C, van der Berg MP, Viersma JW, van Langen IM, et al. A single *SCN5A* mutation causing both long-QT and Brugada's syndrome (abstract). Eur Heart J 1999; 20(Suppl):465.
18. Sanguinetti MC, Jiang C, Curran ME, Keating MT. A mechanistic link between an inherited and an acquired cardiac arrhythmia: HERG encodes the $I_{Kr}$ potassium channel. Cell 1995; 81:299–307.
19. Compton SJ, Lux RL, Ramsey MR, Strelich KT, Sanguinetti MC, et al. Genetically defined therapy of inherited long QT syndrome: correction of abnormal repolarization by potassium. Circulation 1996; 94:1018–1022.
20. Tan HL, Alings M, Van Olden RW, Wilde AA. Long-term (subacute) potassium treatment in congenital HERG-related long QT syndrome (LQTS2). J Cardiovasc Electrophysiol 1999; 10:229–233.
21. Priori SG, Napolitano C, Cantù F, Brown AM, Schwartz PJ. Differential response to $Na^+$ channel blockade, β-adrenergic stimulation, and rapid pacing in a cellular model mimicking the *SCN5A* and *HERG* defects present in the long QT syndrome. Circ Res 1996; 78:1009–1015.
22. Schwartz PJ, Priori SG, Spazzolini C, Moss AJ, Vincent GM, et al. Gene-specific triggers for life-threatening arrhythmias in the long QT syndrome. (In preparation)

# 21

# Congenital Long QT Syndrome:

## Therapeutic Considerations Based on the International LQTS Registry

*Arthur J. Moss, MD, and*
*Wojciech Zareba, MD, PhD*

## Introduction

The long QT syndrome (LQTS) is a familial disorder in which affected family members have prolonged ventricular repolarization on the ECG and a propensity to syncope, polymorphous ventricular tachycardia (torsades de pointes), and sudden cardiac death.[1] Approximately 10,000 persons in the United States are affected with this disorder. Four specific mutant cardiac ion channel genes have been identified (KvLQT1, *HERG*, *SCN5A*, and KCNE1), and each encodes an abnormal channel protein, resulting in altered ion channel kinetics.[2-5]

Early attempts at therapy for LQTS date back to the mid-1960s when diphenylhydantoin and phenobarbital were used because of the presumed similarity of arrhythmic "seizure" episodes to classic epilepsy, with the thought being that electrical discharge from the brain was responsible for sudden cardiac arrhythmic events in LQTS. In 1969, surgical therapy with left cervicothoracic sympathetic ganglionectomy (LCTSG) was used in 1 patient with recurrent syncope that was due to documented runs of transient polymorphic ventricular tachycardia, and the success of this therapy was reported in 1970 after 2 years of follow-up.[6] This therapy was based on animal

Supported in part by a General Clinical Research Center (GCRC) Grant, 5M01-RR00044 from the National Center for Research Resources, and by Research Grants HL-33843, HL-51618, and HL-58731, all from the NIH, Bethesda, Maryland.

From: Aliot E, Clementy J, Prystowsky EN (editors). *Fighting Sudden Cardiac Death: A Worldwide Challenge.* ©Futura Publishing Company, Armonk, NY, 2000.

studies in which left stellate ganglion stimulation produced QT prolongation,[7] and only later was it appreciated that the antiadrenergic effects of the left-sided cardiac sympathectomy contributed to the therapeutic efficacy. Shortly thereafter, beta-blocker therapy was used in treatment of LQTS, with the rationale based on the fact that a majority of syncopal episodes and sudden death occurred in the setting of acute arousal situations. The subsequent results with beta blockers in the treatment of LQTS appeared quite favorable,[8] but this conclusion was based on retrospective historical comparisons of cardiac event rates before beta-blocker therapy became available.

Other forms of therapy for LQTS have included pacemakers,[9,10] implanted cardioverter-defibrillators (ICDs),[11–13] and more recently, pharmacological therapy tailored to the specific dysfunctional genetic channelopathy.[14–18] The purpose of this chapter is to focus on 5 therapies for LQTS based on experience from the International LQTS Registry that has actively enrolled and followed over 800 LQTS families and more than 5,500 family members during the past 20 years.

# Left Cervicothoracic Sympathectic Ganglionectomy (LCTSG)

Following the initial case report of LCTSG for LQTS in 1970,[7] this technique was subsequently applied to LQTS patients with recurrent syncope and aborted cardiac arrest refractory to beta-blocker therapy. In 1984, Bhandari et al. reported only limited success with this approach in 10 patients with a mean follow-up of 3 years,[19] but questions have been raised about the adequacy of the sympathetic ganglionectomy in that study. In 1991, Schwartz et al. evaluated the efficacy of LCTSG in 85 LQTS patients, mostly from the LQTS registry but also including the 10 patients reported by Bhandari, during an average follow-up of almost 6 years per patient (Figure 1).[20] The LCTSG surgery was performed during a 21-year period from 1969 to 1990. The mean age of the population at surgery was 20 years, and LCTSG was followed by a significant decrease in the number of patients with cardiac events (99% to 45%), in the average number of cardiac events per patient (from $22\pm32$ to $1\pm3$), and in the number of patients with 5 or more cardiac events (from 71% to 10%). There were 7 sudden deaths (8%) after LCTSG, and the 5-year survival rate was 94%. These findings indicate that LCTSG can reduce the rate of recurrent syncope, but sudden death continues to occur at an unacceptably high rate.

In 1995, Ouriel and Moss reported their experience with LCTSG in 6 patients with refractory LQTS who underwent surgery over a 3.5-year period between 1990 and 1993, with median follow-up of 1.3 years.[21] The frequency of symptomatic episodes decreased from 7.1 events per year before

## INCIDENCE PER YEAR

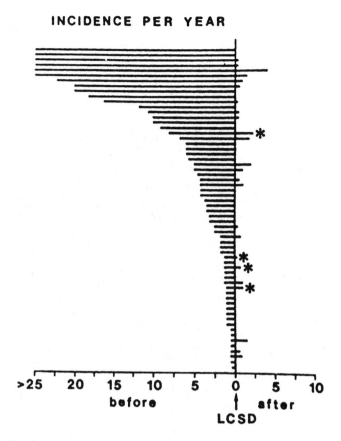

Figure 1. Cardiac event rates before and after left cardiac sympathetic denervation (LCSD) in 62 LQTS patients. * = sudden death. (Adapted from Schwartz et al.[20] Reproduced with permission from Circulation. Copyright ©1991 Lippincott Williams & Wilkins. All rights reserved).

LCTSG to 0.1 events per year after operation. All but 1 patient remained asymptomatic during follow-up. The youngest patient with a very severe form of LQTS was operated on at 1 month of age and died suddenly 10 months after the procedure.

The optimal technique for LCTSG involves a nonthoracotomy, supraclavicular approach to the left stellate ganglion with removal of the lower half of the stellate ganglion and the second and third thoracic ganglia. The surgical technique in experienced hands is not difficult, but removal of the second and third thoracic ganglia is essential.[21]

The overall experience with LCTSG suggests that this surgical technique is associated with some clinical benefit in patients with LQTS. This procedure may be useful in symptomatic patients refractory to beta-blocker therapy, in high-risk patients with contraindications to beta blockers, and in very high-risk patients who are too small for an ICD.

## Pacemakers

Syncope and cardiac arrest in LQTS are due primarily to malignant ventricular tachyarrhythmias, and these arrhythmias can be exacerbated by sinus bradycardia, which frequently occurs in this syndrome. Profound sinus bradycardia may develop with full-dose beta-blocker therapy. In addition, abnormalities of atrioventricular conduction may occur in infants with severe forms of LQTS, resulting in 2:1 conduction block.[22] Regardless of the etiology of the bradycardia, a slow heart rate and/or long beat-to-beat pauses can augment the heterogeneity of ventricular repolarization in patients with QT prolongation and can contribute to ventricular afterpotentials that are thought to be responsible for the initiation of torsades de pointes. In 1987, Eldar et al. reported their clinical experience with permanent cardiac pacing in 8 LQTS patients with refractory symptoms.[9] With atrial or ventricular pacing at 70 to 85 beats/min combined with beta-blocker therapy, there was elimination of recurrent syncope during a mean follow-up of 35 months. In 1992, this same group reported their expanded experience with combined pacing (atrial, ventricular, or dual chamber pacing) and beta-blocker therapy in 21 LQTS patients during a 45-month follow-up.[23] Most patients did very well, but pacemaker problems and discontinuance of beta-blocker therapy were associated with recurrent events. Overall, pacemaker therapy provided excellent adjunctive therapy to beta blockers for symptomatic LQTS patients, especially those with primary or beta blocker-related bradycardia.

In 1991, Moss et al. reported the efficacy of permanent pacing in the management of 30 high-risk LQTS patients from the International LQTS Registry.[10] Most of the patients were female (87%), the average age at implantation was 19 years, 67% of the patients had a resting heart rate less than 60 beats/min, 57% were receiving antiadrenergic therapy for LQTS, and the mean baseline QTc was 550 ms. Cardiac event rates were significantly reduced with the addition of pacing (Figure 2), and 21 of the 30 patients experienced no cardiac events during an average pacemaker follow-up of 49 months. Eight patients experienced recurrent arrhythmic events after pacemaker implantation. Augmentation of the heart rate was associated with significant reduction in the QT interval but minimal change in the QTc interval.

The above-referenced studies substantiated the usefulness of pacemaker therapy in selected LQTS patients. Although permanent cardiac pacing reduces the rate of recurrent syncopal events in high-risk LQTS pa-

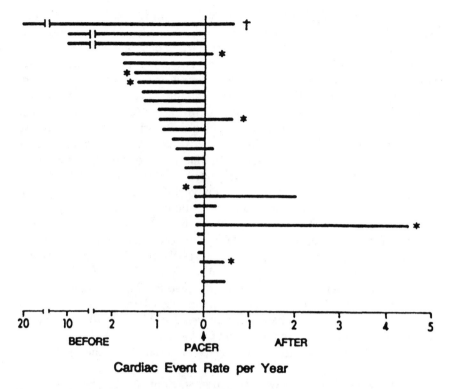

BEFORE   PACER   AFTER

Cardiac Event Rate per Year

Figure 2. Cardiac event rates before and after implantation of a permanent pacemaker in 30 LQTS patients. * = left cervicothoracic sympathetic ganglionectomy; [†] = cardiac death; (From Moss et al.[10] Reproduced with permission from Circulation. Copyright c1991 Lippincott Williams & Wilkins. All rights reserved).

tients, it does not provide complete protection against recurrent syncope or sudden cardiac death. It should be emphasized that beta-blocker therapy should always be continued in patients treated with pacemakers.

## Beta Blockers

Although beta blockers are routinely prescribed in LQTS and the rationale for their use is quite reasonable, there has never been a randomized, double-blind, placebo-controlled trial to evaluate the safety and efficacy of this treatment in this disorder. Recently, Moss et al. carried out a detailed study of all LQTS patients from the International Registry who were treated with beta blockers. An abstract of this investigation was reported at the Scientific Sessions of the American College of Cardiology in March 1999,[24] and has been published.[25]

A total of 869 LQTS patients from the International Registry have been treated with beta blockers. The effectiveness of beta blockers was analyzed during matched periods before and after starting beta blockers, and by survivorship methods to determine factors associated with cardiac events while on prescribed beta blockers. After initiation of beta blockers, there was a significant (P<0.001) reduction in the rate of cardiac events in both probands and affected family members during 5-year matched periods. On-therapy survivorship analyses revealed that patients who had cardiac symptoms before beta blockers (n=598) had a hazard ratio of 5.8 for recurrent cardiac events (syncope, aborted cardiac arrest, or death) during beta-blocker therapy compared with asymptomatic patients (P<0.001). Of note, 32% of these symptomatic patients will have another cardiac event within 5 years while on prescribed beta blockers. Patients with a history of aborted cardiac arrest before starting beta blockers (n=113) have a hazard ratio of 12.9 for aborted cardiac arrest or death while on prescribed beta blockers compared with asymptomatic patients (P<0.001); 14% of these patients will have another arrest (aborted or fatal) within 5 years (Figure 3).

Beta-blocker analyses were also performed in 69 LQT1, 42 LQT2, and 28 LQT3 genotyped patients. Beta-blocker therapy had minimal effects on QTc in all 3 genotypes, but beta blockers were associated with a significant reduction in events and event rates in LQT1 and LQT2 patients. There was no evident effect of beta blockers on events in the small number of patients with LQT3.

Among the 33 patients who died after starting beta blockers, 76% had a known prescription for beta blockers at last contact before death. Females made up 67% of the deaths, and the mean baseline QTc value among the fatal cases (530±60 ms) was only slightly longer than in the overall study population (510±50 ms). Among those who died, beta blockers were started mostly before adolescence (mean age 9 years), with death on average 5 years later (mean age 14 years).

The appropriate or optimal dose of beta blockers for treatment of LQTS is not known. We evaluated the relationship among 3 different prescribed dose ranges of propranolol (=1.5 [n=80], 1.6–2.5 [n=75], and >2.5 [n=73] mg/kg body weight/day) and recurrent cardiac events. To our surprise, there were similar and significant reductions in the cardiac event rates at the 3 propranolol dose ranges. We also observed sudden death events over a spectrum of beta-blocker doses from low levels to full therapeutic doses.

These findings from the International LQTS Registry indicate that beta-blocker therapy reduces the syncopal event rate but is not entirely effective in preventing arrhythmic sudden death in LQTS. LQTS patients with aborted cardiac arrest prior to beta-blocker therapy have a very high likelihood of experiencing recurrent aborted cardiac arrest or death de-

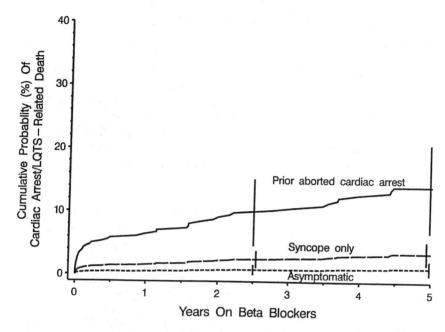

**Figure 3.** Estimated cumulative probability of experiencing aborted cardiac arrest or death while receiving beta-blocker therapy in LQTS patients who were asymptomatic (dotted line), had only syncope (dashed line), or had experienced aborted cardiac arrest (solid line) before beta blockers. Vertical lines are 95% confidence intervals. The risk curves are for LQTS patients who were started on beta blockers at 10 years of age or older. Time periods off therapy for more than 2 days are excluded. (From Moss et al.[25] Reproduced with permission from Circulation. Copyright ©1999 Lippincott Williams & Wilkins. All rights reserved).

spite beta-blocker therapy, and ICD therapy in combination with beta blockers is most reasonable and appropriate for the prevention of sudden cardiac death in this very high-risk subset.

## Implanted Cardioverter-Defibrillator

We have only recently examined the International LQTS Registry data regarding experience with ICDs in this disorder, and a presentation of the preliminary findings was made at the XI[th] World Symposium on Cardiac Pacing and Electrophysiology in Berlin in June 1999. We know from the beta-blocker study described above that sudden death can occur in LQTS, even in patients on full therapeutic doses of beta blockers.

From the Registry, a total of 88 patients were identified with an ICD, with various reasons for implanting the device. Forty-eight percent had an aborted cardiac arrest, and most of the remaining patients had documented long runs of life-threatening torsades de pointes. A few patients were asymptomatic with long QTc and came from families with a high frequency of sudden cardiac death as the first clinical event. The average age at ICD implantation was 23±10 years with a mean QTc of 520±60 ms. During an average follow-up of 2.5 years per patient (range 0.1 to 9.0 years), there were no deaths. Eighty-two percent of the patients were receiving beta-blocker therapy before and 89% after implantation of the device. Four patients had aborted cardiac arrest events after the ICD was implanted. Findings from device interrogation in 1 patient with aborted cardiac arrest are shown in Figure 4.

ICD therapy is not without its potential problems. Until more definitive treatment becomes available, ICD implantation should be considered life-long therapy. As with pacemakers, skin erosion at the battery implantation site, wound infection, and lead fracture are potential complications, but the rate of these problems continues to diminish with smaller units and more experience. If the lead is not positioned properly, malsensing may result in inappropriate shock delivery. On occasion, LQTS patients may develop arrhythmic storm and experience a burst of shocks for termination of torsades de pointes and/or ventricular fibrillation. Supplementary intravenous beta blockers and augmentation of the pacing rate of the defibrillator unit will usually provide stabilization, but it may take 24 to 48 hours of aggressive therapy. Such situations tax the therapeutic skill of the cardiologist and the emotional reserve of the patient. It is clear that after ICD implantation, maximal beta-blocker therapy should be maintained to minimize the frequency of subsequent arrhythmic events.

# Pharmacological Therapy Tailored to the Genetic Channelopathy

With the identification of mutation-related disordered ion channel kinetics involving the LQTS KvLQT1, *HERG*, and *SCN5A* genes, the potential for tailored pharmacological therapy to correct specific ion channel defects has become a reality. The potassium channel defects associated with LQT1 (KvLQT1) and LQT2 (*HERG*) mutations result in a loss of function whereas the LQT3 (*SCN5A*) mutation is associated with a gain in function. In 1995, Schwartz et al.[14] demonstrated that a single oral dose of mexiletine (acute loading with 6–8 mg/kg) administered to 6 LQT3 patients with the ΔKPQ deletion produced significant shortening of the QT interval within 4 hours, with QTc diminishing from 535±32 to 445±31 msec (P<0.005). Mexiletine had minimal, if any, effect on the QTc in LQT2 pa-

# LQTS: ICD

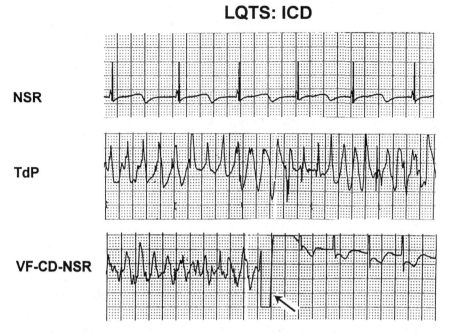

NSR

TdP

VF-CD-NSR

**Figure 4.** Interrogated intracardiac electrograms that were retrieved from an ICD following an episode of aborted cardiac arrest in a 12-year-old male with LQTS (*HERG* mutation). The ICD had been implanted 3 months earlier following external resuscitation from ventricular fibrillation. Top panel: normal sinus rhythm (NSR) with QTc 660 ms. Middle panel: torsades de pointes-pattern of polymorphic ventricular tachycardia (TdP) that coincided with acute loss of consciousness. Bottom panel: termination of ventricular fibrillation (VF) with discharge of the implanted cardioverter-defibrillator (CD) at the arrow, with return to normal sinus rhythm (NSR) 600 ms after the defibrillator discharge. The rhythm strips are sequential but not continuous. The patient regained full consciousness within 1 minute after internal ventricular defibrillation, and there was no neurological deficit. The subject was receiving the beta blocker nadolol, 60 mg twice daily, at the time of this episode. (From Moss et al.[13] Reproduced with permission from The New England Journal of Medicine. Copyright © 1999 Massachusetts Medical Society. All rights reserved.)

tients with the *HERG* mutation. In 1996, Compton et al.[16] reported that an acute increase in serum potassium with intravenous potassium loading and oral spironolactone improves abnormalities of repolarization duration, T-wave morphology, QT/RR slope, and QT dispersion in patients with LQT2-*HERG* mutations. However, a recent report by Tan et al.[26] indicates that a long-lasting rise of serum potassium is only partially achievable because in the presence of normal renal function, potassium homeostasis limits the amount of serum potassium increase.

The Rochester component of the International LQTS Registry has had limited but interesting experience with pharmacological therapy tailored to a specific genetic channelopathy. In 1997, Rosero et al.[15] reported the effects of sodium channel blocker therapy in 2 LQT3 Registry family members with the mutant SCN5A-ΔKPQ deletion. In each of the 2 affected carriers, intravenous infusion of lidocaine (40 μg/kg/min for 90 min), and separately, the oral administration of the tocainide (400 mg q8h for 48 hours) were associated with 15–18% shortening of the QTc and near normalization of the morphology of the repolarization T wave. Chronic administration of tocainide to one of the symptomatic LQT3 carriers for over 12 months has been associated with persistent shortening of the QTc and improvement in the configuration of the T wave without arrhythmias or syncope.

Oral mexiletine was administered to 2 Rochester-based LQT3-ΔKPQ patients in a dose-response protocol to full therapeutic doses of the drug with therapy extending for at least a week at each dose. Mexiletine in this protocol had negligible effects on the QTc interval or the morphology of the repolarization T wave.

Subsequent oral administration of the potent sodium channel blocker flecainide (100 mg q12h for 3 days) to the 2 Rochester-based patients who were previously unresponsive to mexiletine was associated with dramatic normalization of both the QTc interval and the configuration of the T wave (Figure 5). Three additional patients from the Registry with the LQT3-ΔKPQ mutation have also been studied with oral flecainide with similar results, including shortening of the QTc from 543 ms to 443 ms and full normalization of the morphology of the T wave and the ST interval. This preliminary experience with flecainide in these 5 LQT3-ΔKPQ patients[18] is the background for a recently funded research grant from the National Institutes of Health (USA) for a long-term, randomized, double-blind, placebo-controlled trial to evaluate the safety and efficacy of oral flecainide in 30 LQT3-ΔKPQ patients enrolled in the International LQTS Registry.

The Israeli component of the International LQTS Registry (Dr. J. Benhorin and associates) has also studied oral flecainide (100 mg q12h) in 8 adult LQT3 patients with the D1790G mutation, and a report of their 1-year experience with this therapy is in press.[17] Flecainide was well tolerated and was associated with marked and sustained shortening of the QTc interval during long-term follow-up without any evident adverse effects.

These preliminary studies from the International LQTS Registry indicate that the sodium channel blocker flecainide may be useful in genotype-identified LQT3 patients with the ΔKPQ or D1790G SCN5A mutations. Flecainide should not be considered as a treatment option in any of the other forms of LQTS.

## BASELINE    FLECAINIDE

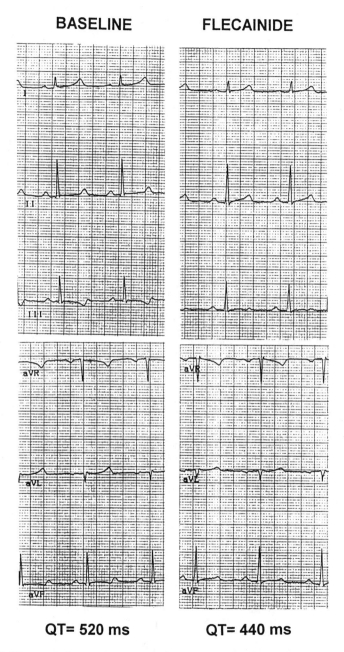

QT= 520 ms        QT= 440 ms

Figure 5. Electrocardiographic tracings of 6 limb leads before and after 2 days of oral flecainide 100 mg every 12 hours in a 31-year-old male with LQT3-ΔKPQ mutation. The QTc was 520 ms before flecainide (left panel) and was reduced to 440 ms after flecainide (flecainide blood level 0.2 mg/L) (right panel), with normalization of the T-wave morphology.

## Conclusions

Based on the experience of the International LQTS Registry, 5 different types of therapy for LQTS have been presented. Beta blockers effectively reduce the frequency of recurrent syncope in patients with the more common LQT1 and LQT2 forms of this disorder, with uncertain benefit in the less frequent LQT3 genotype. Sudden cardiac death can occur in patients taking beta blockers. Pacemakers, left cervicothoracic sympathetic ganglionectomy, and ICDs are useful adjunctive therapies, in addition to beta blockers, in carefully selected, high-risk patients. ICDs should be implanted in all LQTS patients who experience an aborted cardiac arrest. Pharmacological therapy tailored for specific genetic channelopathies is very promising, although the experience to date is quite limited.

## *References*

1. Moss AJ, Schwartz PJ, Crampton RS, Tzivoni D, Locati EH, et al. The long QT syndrome: prospective longitudinal study of 328 families. Circulation 1991; 84:1136–1144.
2. Wang Q, Curran ME, Splawski I, Burn TC, Millholland JM, et al. Positional cloning of a novel potassium channel gene: KVLQT1 mutations cause cardiac arrhythmias. Nature Genetics 1996; 12:17–23.
3. Curran ME, Splawski I, Timothy KW, Vincent GM, Green ED, et al. A molecular basis for cardiac arrhythmia: HERG mutations cause long QT syndrome. Cell 1995; 80:795–803.
4. Wang Q, Shen J, Splawski I, Atkinson D, Li Z, et al. SCN5A mutations associated with an inherited cardiac arrhythmia, long QT syndrome. Cell 1995; 80:805–811.
5. Splawski I, Tristani-Firouzi M, Lehmann MH, Sanguinetti MC, et al. Mutations in the hminK gene cause long QT syndrome and suppress $I_{Ks}$. Nature Genetics 1997; 17:338–340.
6. Moss AJ, McDonald J. Unilateral cervicothoracic sympathetic ganglionectomy for the treatment of the long QT interval syndrome. N Engl J Med 1970; 285:903–904.
7. Yanowitz P. Preston JB, Abildskov AJ. Functional distribution of right and left stellate innervation of the ventricles. Circ Res 1966; 18:416–428.
8. Schwartz PJ, Locati E. Idiopathic long QT syndrome: pathogenic mechanisms and therapy. Eur Heart J 1985; 6(Suppl D):103–114.
9. Eldar M, Griffin JC, Abbott JA, Benditt D, Bhandari A, et al. Permanent cardiac pacing in patients with the long QT syndrome. J Am Coll Cardiol 1987; 10:600–607.
10. Moss AJ, Liu JE, Gottlieb S, Locati E, Schwartz PJ, et al. Efficacy of permanent pacing in the management of high-risk patients with long QT syndrome. Circulation 1991; 84:1524–1529.
11. Groh WJ, Silka MJ, Oliver RP, Halperin BD, McAnulty JH, et al. Use of implantable cardioverter-defibrillator in the congenital long QT syndrome. Am J Cardiol 1996; 78:703–706.
12. Priori SG, Zareba WJ, Napolitano C, Locati EH, Robinson JL, et al. The im-

plantable cardioverter defibrillator (ICD) in the long QT syndrome: data from the international registry. PACE 1996; 19(2):556.

13. Moss AJ, Daubert JP. Internal ventricular defibrillation. N Engl J Med (in press).
14. Schwartz PJ, Priori SG, Locati EH, Napolitano C, Cantu F, et al. Long QT syndrome patients with mutations of the SCN5A and HERG genes have differential responses to Na$^+$ channel blockade and to increases in heart rate: implications for gene-specific therapy. Circulation. 1995; 92:3381–3386.
15. Rosero SZ, Zareba W, Robinson JL, Moss AJ. Gene-specific therapy for long QT syndrome: QT shortening with lidocaine and tocainide in patients with mutation of the sodium channel gene. Ann Noninvas Electrocardiol 1997; 2:274–278.
16. Compton SJ, Lux RL, Ramsey MR, Strelich KR, Sanguinetti MC, et al. Genetically defined therapy of inherited long-QT syndrome: correction of abnormal repolarization by potassium. Circulation 1996; 94:1018–1022.
17. Benhorin J, Taub R, Goldmit M, Kerem B, Kass RS, et al. Effects of flecainide in patients with a new SCN5A mutation: mutation-specific therapy for long QT syndrome? Circulation (in press).
18. Windle JR, Geletka RC, Adkins DL, Moss AJ. Normalization of ventricular repolarization with flecainide in LQT3 form (SCN5A:ΔKPQ mutation) of long QT syndrome. Circulation (abstract in press).
19. Bhandari A, Scheinman MM, Morady F, Svinarich J, Mason J, et al. Efficacy of left sympathectomy in the treatment of patients with the long QT syndrome. Circulation 1984; 70:1018–1023.
20. Schwartz PJ, Locati E, Moss AJ, Crampton RS, Trazzi R, et al. Left cardiac sympathetic denervation in the therapy of the congenital long QT syndrome: a worldwide report. Circulation 1991; 84:503–511.
21. Ouriel K, Moss AJ. Long QT syndrome: an indication for cervicothoracic sympathectomy. Cardiovasc Surg 1995; 3:475–478.
22. Scott WA, Dick MD II. Two:one atrioventricular block in infants with congenital long QT syndrome. Am J Cardiol 1987; 60:1409–1410.
23. Eldar M, Griffin JC, Van Hare GF, Witherell C, Bhandari A, et al. Combined use of beta-adrenergic blocking agents and long-term cardiac pacing in patients with the long QT syndrome. J Am Coll Cardiol 1992; 20:830–837.
24. Moss AJ, Zareba W, Hall WJ, Robinson JL, Benhorin J, et al. Efficacy and limitations of beta-blocker therapy in long QT syndrome. J Am Coll Cardiol 1999; 33:138A.
25. Moss AJ, Zareba W, Hall WJ, Schwartz PJ, Crampton RS, et al. Effectiveness and limitations of beta-blocker therapy in congenital long QT syndrome. Circulation 2000; 101:616–623.
26. Tan HL, Alings M, van Olden RW, Wilde AAM. Long-term (subacute) potassium treatment in congenital HERG-related long QT syndrome (LQTS2). J Cardiovasc Electrophysiol 1999; 10:229–233.

# 22

# Brugada Syndrome:

## From Genetics to Clinical Management

*Pedro Brugada, MD, PhD,*
*Josep Brugada, MD, PhD,*
*Ramon Brugada, MD,*
*Jeffrey Towbin MD, and*
*Charles Antzelevitch, PhD*

## Background

Sudden cardiac death is responsible for 25% of all causes of natural death and has epidemic (and pandemic) proportions. Many advances have been made on the understanding of the mechanisms leading to sudden cardiac death. However, the diversity of its causes makes prevention very difficult. The more exactly the cause of a disease is known, and the better the pathophysiological mechanisms are understood, the easier it becomes to design effective diagnostic, preventive, and therapeutic strategies.

A few years ago a new disease, now known as Brugada syndrome, was described. This disease causes sudden cardiac death in apparently healthy individuals with an otherwise structurally normal heart. Six years after the initial description of the disease, we showed that it is genetically determined, transmitted with an autosomal dominant pattern and caused by mutations in the gene encoding for the human cardiac sodium channel *SCN5A*. At least 6 different mutations are known at present that encompass the whole spectrum of possible genetic mistakes (insertion, deletion, missense, and nonsense mutations). Both males and females may carry the disease; however, some genetic modifiers seem to make males more prone to manifesting the phenotype. Rapid polymorphic ventricular arrhythmias caused by phase 2 reentry result in episodes of syncope when self-

From: Aliot E, Clementy J, Prystowsky EN (editors). *Fighting Sudden Cardiac Death: A Worldwide Challenge.* ©Futura Publishing Company, Armonk, NY, 2000.

terminating and in (aborted) sudden death when long lasting. The disease is ubiquitous but more prevalent in some areas, such as South Asia where it causes up to 1 sudden death per 1,000 inhabitants per year. The electrocardiogram during sinus rhythm is the most important clue to the phenotypic diagnosis of the disease. It shows a right bundle branch block-like morphology with a peculiar elevation of the ST segment in leads $V_1$ to $V_3$. However, the ST segment elevation as well as the apparent conduction disturbances may disappear spontaneously over time. The intravenous administration of a sodium channel blocker may unmask the abnormal electrocardiogram in affected individuals. Symptomatic patients with this disease are best managed by the implantation of a cardioverter-defibrillator. Many questions still remain on how to manage asymptomatic carriers of the disease, but present data support an aggressive approach with electrophysiological investigation and the prophylactic implantation of a defibrillator in inducible individuals. The Brugada syndrome is an excellent example of the value of a multidisciplinary approach to disease. Without this approach it could never have been possible to move so fast from genetics to clinical management.

# Introduction

Sudden cardiac death is responsible for one quarter of all deaths from natural causes. Understanding the exact mechanisms causing sudden cardiac death may have a major impact on general morbidity and mortality. An acute ischemic episode in patients with underlying coronary artery disease still remains the major cause of sudden cardiac death. However, there exist many other causes of sudden cardiac death unrelated to coronary artery disease. Particularly in individuals less than 50 years of age, most sudden deaths are caused by diseases different from arteriosclerotic heart disease.

In 1992 we described a new syndrome that is caused by inheritable mutations in the gene encoding for the human cardiac sodium channel *SCN5A*. Carriers of one of the mutations may experience sudden cardiac death because of rapid ventricular arrhythmias.

The description of this disease renewed scientific interest in the causes of sudden cardiac death not related to coronary artery disease, including the long QT syndrome and hypertrophic and idiopathic congestive cardiomyopathy.

# Definition

The syndrome of right bundle branch block, ST segment elevation from $V_1$ to $V_3$, and sudden cardiac death (Brugada syndrome) is a clinical electrocardiographic diagnosis based on syncopal or sudden death episodes in patients with a structurally normal heart with a characteristic electrocardiographic pattern:[1] ST segment elevation in the right precordial leads $V_1$ to $V_3$ with a morphology of the QRS complex resembling a right bundle branch block (Figure 1). This pattern of right bundle branch block is not present in all patients, and has also been considered an elevation of the J point instead of a true conduction disturbance.[2,3] The episodes of syncope and (aborted) sudden death are caused by rapid polymorphic ventricular arrhythmias similar to the ones shown in Figure 2. Figure 2 is an exceptional example, however, of initiation of polymorphic ventricular tachycardia after a short-long sequence in a patient with Brugada syn-

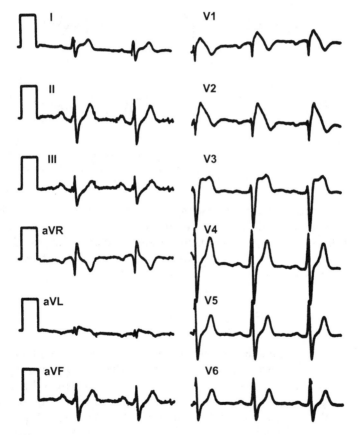

**Figure 1.** Typical electrocardiogram at 25 mm/sec paper speed in a patient with Brugada syndrome. Note the ST segment elevation from $V_1$ to $V_3$ with a pattern resembling a right bundle branch block. There is also a negative T wave from $V_1$ to $V_3$ and a slightly prolonged PR interval, which is the result of a prolonged H-V interval.

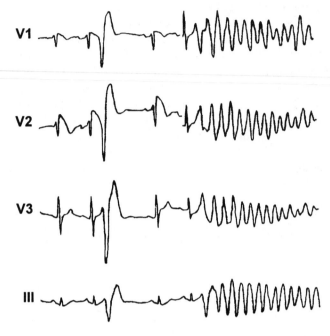

Figure 2. Spontaneous initiation of a polymorphic ventricular tachycardia in a patient with Brugada syndrome. Note the typical electrocardiogram in leads $V_1$ to $V_3$.

drome. Short-long sequences are a very common initiation of torsades de pointes in patients with long QT syndrome,[4] but are exceptional in Brugada syndrome. In Brugada syndrome, there is no preceding acceleration of the sinus rate before the arrhythmias as happens in cathecolamine-dependent torsades de pointes.[5]

## Etiology and Genetics

This disease is genetically determined. We have shown that mutations in the gene *SCN5A* encoding for the human cardiac sodium channel cause the disease, which is transmitted with an autosomal dominant pattern of inheritance.[6] Both genders may be affected, but some genetic modifiers seem to make males more prone to manifest the phenotype (typical electrocardiogram and ventricular arrhythmias). In some areas, such as South Asia,[7] only males seem to manifest the phenotype. The first 3 mutations that we described included a missense mutation (T1620M), a 2 base pair insertion, and a 1 base deletion. The missense mutation is temperature-dependent when expressed in frog oocytes and results in loss of function of the sodium channel (unpublished observations). The mutation resulting from a 2 base insertion has unknown physiological effects so far. The 1 base deletion results in a stop codon whereby no sodium channels are expressed in the mutant xenopus oocytes resulting in a total loss of function. The other 3 mutations resulting in Brugada syndrome have been reported at international meetings by other groups. These mutations also affect the sodium channel and result in loss of function. So far, no full report is available on any of these 3 mutations. Also, no full report is available at the time of writing this manuscript on a mutation in the sodium channel causing Brugada syndrome and long QT syndrome in the same family. The electrophysiological effects of this mutation have not been presented, but it is very difficult to understand how a single mutation may result in effects that are theoretically incompatible. The long QT syndrome results from a gain of function in the sodium channel (leakage current) while the Brugada syndrome results from a loss of function. We will have to wait for the full report to get sound explanations about this apparent paradox.

## Incidence and Distribution

The disease is ubiquitous. Cases have been identified all over the world. It seems, however, that the disease clusters, something that is not surprising for a genetically determined, autosomal dominant disease. In Laos, it may cause up to 1 sudden death per 1,000 inhabitants per year. This prevalence is similar to the overall prevalence of sudden death in Western countries. Brugada syndrome may be overall the cause of 4–12% of all sudden deaths. When apparently healthy individuals below age 50 are taken into account, Brugada syndrome is the cause of about 50% of all sudden deaths.

The prevalence of the disease is difficult to study because the electrocardiogram may be completely normal at certain moments. Fortunately, sodium channel blockers such as ajmaline, flecainide, pilsicainide, or procainamide may be given intravenously to unmask the abnormal electrocardiogram (Figure 3). Although false negative tests may occur with these drugs (Silvia Priori, unpublished observations) false positive tests have been not reported so far. Thus, any individual showing an electrocardiogram typical of Brugada syndrome, either spontaneously or after the administration of a sodium channel blocker, must be considered affected by the disease.

## Electrophysiological Mechanisms

The electrophysiological mechanisms of Brugada syndrome have been the subject of intensive investigation.[8] The ventricular arrhythmias

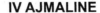

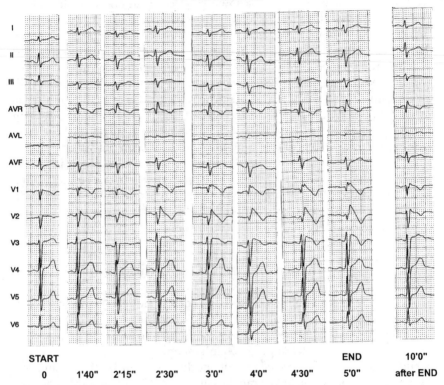

Figure 3. A patient with Brugada syndrome and a normal electrocardiogram in whom the abnormal electrocardiogram is unmasked by the intravenous administration of 50 mg ajmaline over a 5-min period. Note the progressive elevation of the ST segment in leads $V_1$ to $V_3$ induced by the drug, with practically full normalization of the electrocardiogram 10 min after end of the injection.

result from phase 2 reentry between epicardial and endocardial layers. This reentry phenomenon occurs because of a voltage gradient between epicardium and endocardium (Figure 4). The voltage gradient is the result of a dominant transient outward potassium current ($I_{to}$) unopposed by a sodium channel that has lost function because of the mutation. These electrophysiological mechanisms explain very nicely why sodium channel blockers worsen the electrocardiographic manifestations of the disease, while calcium channel enhancers and sodium channel enhancers such as isoproterenol improve the electrocardiographic manifestations of the disease. Also, several cases are known at present of patients with Brugada syndrome with electrical storms (multiple episodes of ventricular fibrillation within 1 day) who have been controlled by the acute intravenous ad-

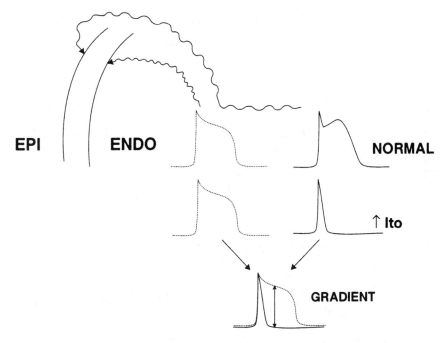

**EPI**  **ENDO**  **NORMAL**

↑ **Ito**

**GRADIENT**

**Figure 4.** Electrophysiological mechanisms involved in Brugada syndrome. See text for details. EPI = epicardium; ENDO = endocardium; Ito = transient outward potassium current.

ministration of isoproterenol. Belhassen and co-workers showed a beneficial effect of low-dose quinidine in patients with so-called idiopathic ventricular fibrillation.[9] At that time they did not know exactly how many of their patients were affected by what we now know as Brugada syndrome. However, low-dose quinidine is a blocker of $I_{to}$, explaining the beneficial effect on Brugada syndrome.

## Prognosis and Treatment

The poor prognosis of Brugada syndrome when left untreated has been confirmed from our series,[10] and also from the studies by other authors, including Nademanee, and other large series from Japan (unpublished observations). Figure 5 shows that at 4 years of follow-up, about 40% of patients with previous episodes of syncope or sudden death (symptomatic patients) will develop a new episode of ventricular fibrillation or will die suddenly during follow-up. Unfortunately, this figure also shows that the same percentage of individuals who were found to have the disease but were asymptomatic at the time of diagnosis (asympto-

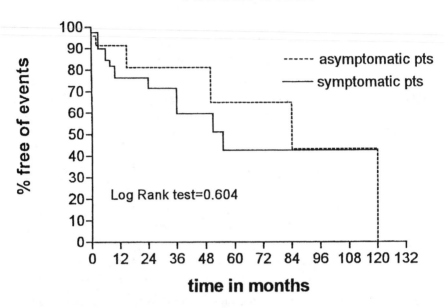

**Figure 5.** Actuarial curves for freedom of recurrent ventricular fibrillation or sudden death in symptomatic and asymptomatic individuals with proven Brugada syndrome. Both symptomatic and asymptomatic individuals have a high incidence of events during follow-up. (Used with permission from Brugada J, et al.[10])

matic patients) will develop their first episode of ventricular fibrillation or sudden death within the same time period. Thus, symptomatic as well as asymptomatic individuals need protection against sudden cardiac death. Figure 6 shows that only the implantable cardioverter-defibrillator gives 100% protection against sudden cardiac death. Patients receiving antiarrhythmic drugs (quinidine not included) or no treatment have a poor prognosis.

## Conclusions

The Brugada syndrome is a fascinating disease which, like the long QT syndrome, has opened new approaches to prevention, diagnosis, and treatment of patients at risk of sudden arrhythmic death. Notwithstanding the still remaining limitations in our knowledge, the Brugada syndrome is another example of the power of a multi-disciplinary approach to disease.

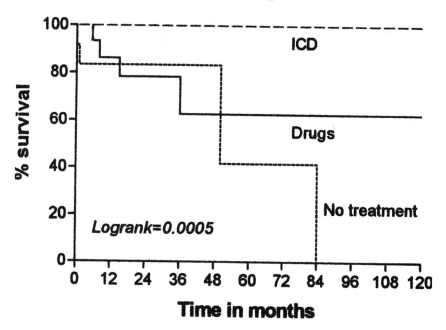

**Figure 6.** Survival of patients with Brugada syndrome according to treatment. Only patients receiving an implantable cardioverter-defibrillator have a 100% survival (in spite of a 40% recurrence rate of ventricular fibrillation during follow-up). (Used with permission from Brugada J, et al.[10])

Without this approach, advances in the understanding of the pathophysiological mechanisms of this disease could not have been made

## References

1. Brugada P, Brugada J. Right bundle branch block, persistent ST segment elevation and sudden cardiac death: a distinct clinical and electrocardiographic syndrome. J Am Coll Cardiol 1992; 20:1391–1396.
2. Bjerregaard P, Gussak I, Kotar SL, et al. Recurrent syncope in a patient with prominent J wave. Am Heart J 1994; 127:1426–1430.
3. Yan GX, Antzelevitch C. Cellular basis for the electrocardiographic J wave. Circulation 1996; 93:372–379.
4. Priori SG, Diehl L, Schwartz PJ. Torsades de pointes. In: Podrid PJ, Kowey PR (eds). Cardiac Arrhythmia. Williams & Wilkins, Baltimore, MD, 1995, pp 951–963.
5. El-Sherif N. Polymorphic ventricular tachycardia. In: Podrid PJ, Kowey PR

(eds). Cardiac Arrhythmia. Williams & Wilkins, Baltimore, MD, 1995, pp 936–950.
6. Chen Q, Kirsch GE, Zhang D, et al. Genetic basis and molecular mechanisms for idiopathic ventricular fibrillation. Nature 1998; 392:293–296.
7. Nademanee K, Veerakul G, Nimmannit S, et al. Arrhythmogenic marker for the sudden unexplained death syndrome in Thai men. Circulation 1997; 96:2595–2600.
8. Antzelevitch C. The Brugada syndrome. J Cardiovasc Electrophysiol 1998; 9:513–516.
9. Belhassen B, Shapira I, Shoshani D, et al. Idiopathic ventricular fibrillation: inducibility and beneficial effects of class I antiarrhythmic agents. Circulation 1987; 75:809–816.
10. Brugada J, Brugada R, Brugada P. Right bundle branch block and ST segment elevation in leads $V_1$–$V_3$: a marker for sudden death in patients with no demonstrable structural heart disease. Circulation 1998; 97:457–460.

# VI

## Heart Failure

# 23

# Are There Specific Risk Markers of Sudden Cardiac Death in Heart Failure Patients?

*J. Y. Le Heuzey, MD,*
*X. Copie, MD,*
*O. Piot, MD, T. Lavergne, MD,*
*S. Digeos-Hasnier, MD,*
*and L. Guize, MD*

## Introduction

Sudden cardiac death is frequent in heart failure patients. About 50% of heart failure patients will die of sudden cardiac death. The title of this chapter may be understood in different ways and raises some questions. The first question is: "Are there markers of sudden death that are specific in heart failure patients?" In fact, no; all of the studies that have been made, especially in postinfarction patients, included patients with normal and with abnormal ejection fraction. The second question is: "Are markers of sudden cardiac death specific in heart failure patients?" The specificity of all the markers usually analyzed is rather high, but their positive predictive value is low, even if their negative predictive value is high. The positive predictive value is low because in most of the series the events are rare. Finally, the most relevant question is: "Are there markers of cardiac death that are specific to sudden death in heart failure patients?" Indeed, the most interesting challenge is to be able to define what patients need an implantable cardioverter-defibrillator (ICD). To be able to answer to this question, we need specific markers of sudden cardiac death that are able to differentiate between death from progressive pump failure and death due to arrhythmias.

From: Aliot E, Clementy J, Prystowsky EN (editors). *Fighting Sudden Cardiac Death: A Worldwide Challenge.* ©Futura Publishing Company, Armonk, NY, 2000.

# Risk Markers

Several markers have been proposed to stratify the risk of sudden death. Numerous publications have demonstrated the interest in predicting cardiac mortality of markers such as the cardiothoracic ratio, the peak $VO_2$, left ventricular end-diastolic volume, sodium, potassium, creatinine, ejection fraction, baroreflex sensitivity, heart rate, presence of couplets and nonsustained ventricular tachycardias, heart rate variability, late potentials, and programmed ventricular stimulation. "New" markers have been recently proposed, such as the QT interval (analysis of length, dispersion, and dynamicity), T wave alternans, and heart rate turbulence after ventricular premature beats.

## "Classic" Markers

It is well known that ejection fraction, even if it is a hemodynamic parameter, is able to predict sudden death. There is a clear correlation between the level of the ejection fraction, the total mortality rate, and the mortality rate by sudden cardiac death.[1]

By Holter monitoring,[2] it is possible to analyze the presence of couplets and nonsustained ventricular tachycardias. Couplets and nonsustained ventricular tachycardias are markers of cardiac death; but it is not currently known if these markers are independent factors or if they are related to ventricular dysfunction. There is no clear evidence that these markers are specific of sudden death.

The late potentials have a high negative predictive value but a low positive predictive value. Furthermore, the high prevalence of bundle branch blocks in heart failure patients is a major problem in the interpretation of this marker in these patients. Late potentials could be predictive of sustained spontaneous or inducible ventricular tachycardias, but no clear demonstration about the prediction of sudden death has been reported in the literature.[3]

Concerning programmed ventricular stimulation, there is no specificity of the induction of polymorphic ventricular tachycardia or ventricular fibrillation.[4] The induction of monomorphic ventricular tachycardia is observed in about 40% of ischemic patients and in 10% of patients with idiopathic dilated cardiomyopathies. There is a high risk of sudden death if the patient has inducible ventricular tachycardias and if this patient remains inducible after antiarrhythmic treatment. Finally, it is well known that programmed ventricular stimulation has a lower predictive value in idiopathic dilated cardiomyopathy compared to ischemic patients.

Heart rate variability may be of great interest in risk stratification in heart failure patients. It has been demonstrated that heart rate variability is decreased in congestive heart failure patients, using time domain analysis[5] or frequency domain analysis.[6] In the UK-heart study,[7] the authors demonstrated a reduction in the standard deviation of normal-to-normal beats, which identifies patients at high risk of death. Nevertheless, this marker seems to be a better predictor of death due to progressive heart failure than other conventional clinical measurements. Therefore, in this study, heart rate variability is not a specific marker of sudden cardiac death when compared to total cardiac mortality.

In the work of Brouwer,[8] a nonlinear analysis was performed. In multivariate analysis, abnormal Poincaré plots (obtained by plotting each RR interval by the preceding one) still had independent prognostic value, both for all-cause cardiac mortality and for sudden cardiac death. Poincaré plots may be also of great interest in analyzing the effects of drugs. It has been demonstrated in the CIBIS I trial[9] that beta blockers were able to increase the area of the Poincaré plots after 1 month of treatment. The data obtained by Poincaré plots are additional to those obtained by time and frequency domain analyses.[10] In the same patients, the shape of Poincaré diagrams remained the same, but the measurement of the area showed an increase during beta blocker treatment (Figure 1).

There is a controversy concerning the significance of low heart rate variability in terms of ventricular arrhythmia occurrence. Fei[11] considers that depressed heart rate variability, in congestive heart failure patients, is related principally to the degree of left ventricular impairment and is independent of etiology and the presence of ventricular arrhythmias. On the contrary, in the study of Fauchier,[12] a decreased heart rate variability is an independent predictor of arrhythmic events and sudden death in idiopathic dilated cardiomyopathy, whether or not the mechanism of sudden death is ventricular tachyarrhythmia. This last study clearly shows that heart rate variability can be a good predictor of sudden cardiac death, but it is also a predictor of total cardiac mortality; and thus it is not possible to think that heart rate variability is really a specific marker of sudden death.

In fact, in these different studies, it is very difficult to separate predictors of sudden death and predictors of progressive heart failure death. In the UK-heart study,[13] Brooksby et al. demonstrated that the best predictors of sudden cardiac death, in multivariate analysis, are cardiothoracic ratio, left ventricular end-diastolic diameter, and potassium. The best predictors of progressive heart failure death are creatinine, sodium, cardiothoracic ratio, and couplets. These results show that some markers may be predictors of both sudden death and progressive heart failure death, so none is really specific for sudden cardiac death.

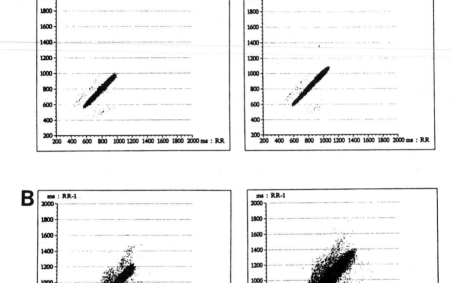

Figure 1. Poincaré diagram in congestive heart failure patients from the CIBIS I study. In panel A, Poincaré diagrams at control and after 1 month of treatment in the placebo group. In panel B, Poincaré diagrams at control and after 1 month of treatment with bisoprolol. The surface of the Poincaré diagram is increased by beta-blocker therapy.

## "New" Markers

New markers have been proposed in recent years, including analysis of QT interval, T wave alternans, and heart rate turbulence.

Concerning QT, it is possible to analyze QT length, QT dispersion, and QT dynamicity. QT length is known to have a good predictive value in ischemic patients,[14] but the demonstration of its value in congestive heart failure has not been clearly made. In the UK-heart study,[13] including 554 patients with 421 days of follow-up, the authors did not find any predictive value of QT length.

For QT dispersion there are also contradictory results. There is no predictive value reported by Fei[11] when QT dispersion has a predictive value of arrhythmias and also in Fu's report on sudden death occurrence.[15] In the work of Galinier,[16] there is a predictive value for sudden death in idiopathic dilated cardiomyopathy, but not in ischemic cardiomyopathy.

QT dynamicity seems to be a better approach. Alterations in heart failure patients have been demonstrated.[17] In heart failure patients, the RR/QT relationship is more abrupt. This finding has also been noted by Fauchier,[18] but the prognostic value concerned the occurrence of cardiac events (cardiac death and heart transplantation).

Other new markers may be proposed in the risk stratification of congestive heart failure patients. For the moment, these markers have been tested in postmyocardial infarction patients, but no large study has been performed in congestive heart failure patients. Electrical alternans affecting the ST segment and T wave are common among patients at increased risk for ventricular arrhythmias.[19] Subtle electrical alternans on the electrocardiogram may serve as a noninvasive marker of vulnerability to ventricular arrhythmias. Rosenbaum reported a good correlation between T wave alternans and results of electrophysiological testing in relation to arrhythmia survival in a series of 66 patients.[19] It is likely that the validity of this marker will be tested in large-scale studies in congestive heart failure patients.

The same observation can be made for heart rate turbulence proposed by Schmidt et al.[20] The absence of heart rate turbulence after ventricular premature beats is a very potent postinfarction risk stratifier that is independent of other known risk factors and is stronger than other presently available risk predictors. It is necessary to test the validity of this marker in a series of congestive heart failure patients. In Holter recordings obtained from MPIP[21] and EMIAT,[22] the authors found that a turbulence slope lower that 2.5 ms per RR interval could be a factor of bad prognosis, but the demonstration of this bad outcome concerns only total mortality.

## Definition of Sudden Cardiac Death

In fact, the main problem is that it is very difficult, in clinical trials concerning congestive heart failure patients, to have an exact definition of sudden cardiac death. Sudden cardiac death describes the unexpected natural death from a cardiac cause with a short time period, generally less than 1 hour from the onset of symptoms in a person without any prior condition that would appear fatal.[23] But in fact it is difficult to know, in congestive heart failure patients, if the death is cardiac or noncardiac, if it is sudden or nonsudden, and if it is arrhythmic or nonarrhythmic. It is even difficult to know the definition of sudden death in the different publications trying to evaluate the predictive value of the different markers.

If the definition of sudden death is not precise, the results of the predictive values that are calculated in the different publications remain debatable. Pratt[24]observed that in some similar trials, for example, SOLVD Rx and V-HeFT I, the ratio of sudden death varies from 22% in the first study to 61% in the second one.

Even the definition of cardiac death[25] may be difficult to obtain as demonstrated by the paper of Kürkciyan,[26] dealing with the accuracy and impact of presumed cause in patients with cardiac arrests. They demonstrated that causes of cardiac arrests are not as easily recognized as anticipated, especially when the initial rhythm is different from ventricular fibrillation. These data have been obtained by retrospective analysis of the primarily presumed cause of cardiac death as determined by the emergency room physician on admission in all patients admitted to the emergency department of an urban tertiary care hospital. The presumed causes were compared to the diagnosis made after an autopsy. The sensitivity of a cardiac presumed cause of cardiac arrest is high, 94.8%, but the specificity is low, 76.5%.

# Conclusion

Several markers are good predictors of total cardiac mortality in heart failure patients, but their negative predictive value is better than their positive predictive value.

Even if some markers are more predictive of sudden death than others, on multivariate analysis, there is no formal marker for the risk of sudden death in heart failure patients. Nevertheless, the combination of different markers allows a better prediction.

The fact that there is no formal marker for the risk of sudden death is due to the diversity of heart failure etiologies, the complexity of arrhythmia mechanisms, and the difficulties in defining and identifying sudden death.

## References

1. Cohn JN, Johnson GR, Shabetai R, et al. Ejection fraction, peak exercise oxygen consumption, cardiothoracic ratio, ventricular arrhythmias and plasma norepinephrine are determinants of prognosis in heart failure. Circulation 1993; 97(VI):5–9.
2. Podrid BJ, Fogel RI, Tordjman Fuchs T. Ventricular arrhythmia in congestive heart failure. Am J Cardiol 1992; 69:82G-96G.
3. Galinier M, Albenque JP, Aschar N, et al. Prognostic value of late potentials in patients with congestive heart failure. Eur Heart J 1996; 17:264–271.
4. Dennis AR, Richards DA, Cody DV, et al. Prognostic significance of ventricular tachycardia and fibrillation induced at programmed stimulation and delayed potentials detected by the signal averaged electrocardiogram of survivors of acute myocardial infarction. Circulation 1968; 74:741–745.

5. Casolo G, Balli E, Taddei T, Amumasi J, Gori C. Decreased spontaneous heart rate variability in congestive heart failure. Am J Cardiol 1989; 64:1162–1167.
6. Saul JP, Arai Y, Berger RD, Lilly LS, Colucci WS, et al. Assessment of autonomic regulation in chronic congestive heart failure by heart rate spectral analysis. Am J Cardiol 1988; 61:1292–1299.
7. Nolan J, Batin PD, Andrews R, et al. Prospective study of heart rate variability and mortality in chronic heart failure: results of the United Kingdom Heart Failure Evaluation and Assessment of Risk Trial (UK-Heart). Circulation 1998; 98:1510–1516.
8. Brouwer J, Van Veldhuisen DJ, Man In't Veld AJ, et al. Prognostic value of heart rate variability during long-term follow-up in patients with mild to moderate heart failure. J Am Coll Cardiol 1996; 28:1183–1189.
9. Copie X, Pousset F, Lechat P, Jaillon P, Guize L, et al. Effects of beta blockade with bisoprolol on heart rate variability in advanced heart failure: analysis of scatterplots of RR intervals at selected heart rate. Am Heart J 1996; 132:369–375.
10. Pousset F, Copie X, Lechat P, et al. Effects of bisoprolol on heart rate variability in heart failure. Am J Cardiol 1996; 77:612–617.
11. Fei L, Keeling BJ, Gille JS, et al. Heart rate variability and its relation to ventricular arrhythmias in congestive heart failure. Br Heart J 1994; 71:322–328.
12. Fauchier L, Babuty D, Cosnay P, Fauchier JP, et al. Prognostic value of heart rate variability for sudden death and major arrhythmic events in patients with idiopathic dilated cardiomyopathy. J Am Coll Cardiol 1999; 33:1203–1207.
13. Brooksby P, Batin PD, Nolan J, et al. The relationship between QT intervals and mortality in ambulant patients with chronic heart failure: the United Kingdom heart failure evaluation and assessment of risk trial (UK-Heart).    Eur Heart J 1999; 20:1335–1341.
14. Schwartz PJ, Wolf S. QT interval prolongation as predictor of sudden death in patients with myocardial infarction. Circulation 1978; 57:1074–1077.
15. Fu GS, Meissner A, Simon R. Repolarisation dispersion and sudden cardiac death in patients with impaired left ventricular function. Eur Heart J 1997; 18:281–289.
16. Galinier M, Vialette JC, Fourcade J, et al. QT interval dispersion as a predictor of arrhythmic events in congestive heart failure: importance of etiology. Eur Heart J 1998; 19:1054–1062.
17. Maison Blanche P, Catuli D, Fayn J, Coumel P. QT interval, heart rate and ventricular arrhythmias. In: Moss AJ, Stern S (eds). Noninvasive Electrocardiology: Clinical Aspects of Holter Monitoring. WB Saunders, London, 1995, pp 383–404.
18. Fauchier L, Babuty D, Poret P, Autret ML, Fauchier JP, et al.
Heart rate variability and risk stratification for major arrhythmic events in idiopathic dilated cardiomyopathy (abstract). Eur Heart J 1999; 20(Suppl):8.
19. Rosenbaum DS, Jackson LE, Smith JM, Garan H, Ruskin J, et al.
Electrical alternans and vulnerability to ventricular arrhythmias. N Engl J Med 1994; 330:235–241.
20. Schmidt G, Malik M, Barthel P, et al. Heart rate turbulence after ventricular premature beats as a predictor of mortality after acute myocardial infarction. Lancet 1999; 353:1390–1416.
21. Multicenter Post-Infarction Research Group. Risk stratification and survival after myocardial infarction. N Engl J Med 1983; 309:331–336.
22. Julian DG, Camm AJ, Frangin G, et al. Randomized trial of effects of amiodarone and mortality in patients with left ventricular dysfunction after recent myocardial infarction: EMIAT. Lancet 1997; 349:667–674.

23. Zipes DP, Wellens HJJ. Sudden cardiac death. Circulation 1998; 98:2334–2351.
24. Pratt CG, Greenway PS, Schoenfeld MH, Ibben ML, Reiffel JA. Exploration of the precision of classifying sudden cardiac death: implications for the interpretation of clinical trials. Circulation 1996; 93:519–524.
25. Narang R, Cleland JFG, Erhardt L. Mode of death in chronic heart failure: a request and proposition for more accurate classifications. Eur Heart J 1996; 17:1390–1403.
26. Kürkciyan I, Meron G, Behringer W, et al. Accuracy and impact of presumed cause of death in patients with cardiac arrest. Circulation 1998; 98:766–771.

# 24

# Sudden Cardiac Death in Idiopathic Dilated Cardiomyopathy

Pierre Cosnay, MD, Laurent Fauchier, MD,
Dominique Babuty, MD, PhD,
Danielle Casset-Senon, PhD,
David Tena-Carbi, MD,
Jean-Christophe Charniot, MD,
Philippe Poret, MD, and
Jean-Paul Fauchier, MD

## Introduction

Dilated cardiomyopathy is a genetically and clinically heterogeneous disease that can affect newborns, children, adolescents, adults, and the elderly population.[1] This common disease has an annual incidence of 7.5 cases per 100,000 persons[2] and is a syndrome of impaired systolic function characterized by hemodynamic, neurohormonal, and electrical derangements. As expected, many deaths are secondary to progressive pump failure in patients (in whom heart transplantation can be performed), but a large proportion of patients die suddenly,[3] most secondary to ventricular arrhythmia and a smaller proportion due to bradyarrhythmia. The mechanism of these rhythm disturbances could be different at each stage, and the prognostic significance of ventricular arrhythmias remains poorly understood. Our lack of knowledge of the electrophysiological and associated biochemical alterations in the failing heart is due do the limited number of experimental animal preparations of idiopathic dilated cardiomyopathy (IDC) that demonstrate spontaneously occurring arrhythmia as well as the limited access to myopathic human ventricular tissue.[4] Transgenic mice models of dilated idiopathic cardiomyopathy and heart failure could be useful in the future to understand the mechanism of sudden death in this disease.[5]

From: Aliot E, Clementy J, Prystowsky EN (editors). *Fighting Sudden Cardiac Death: A Worldwide Challenge.* ©Futura Publishing Company, Armonk, NY, 2000.

## Pathogenesis of Ventricular Arrhythmias

### Experimental Studies

Alterations in ventricular mechanics produce electrophysiological changes (mechanical electrical feedback) that may increase vulnerability to sustained ventricular arrhythmias because the acute stretch of the ventricle produces a shortening of the action potential and early afterdepolarization.[6] Stretching of myocytes accompanying ventricular dilation and high filling pressures opens the membrane mechanical channels that are nonselective for the sodium and potassium ions.[7] In the cardiomyopathic Syrian hamster, during the development of cardiac dilation, a reduction of $i_{to1}$ may contribute to changes in the shape of the action potential.[8] A reduction in $i_{to1}$ density has also been associated with canine cardiomyopathy similar to that seen in Duchenne's muscular dystrophy in humans.[9] At the stage of cardiac failure in the cardiomyopathic Syrian hamster, the sarcoplasmic reticulum function can be altered, and $Na^+/Ca^{2+}$ exchanger activated at resting membrane potential delivering a small inward depolarizing current.[10] In another genetically determined cardiomyopathic Syrian hamster that develops a progressive and fatal congestive heart failure, $i_{CaT}$ had a high density, suggesting a contribution of $i_{CaT}$ to the pathogenesis overload and to the arrhythmogenic activity in this cardiomyopathy.[11]

### Structural, Humoral, Electrophysiological and Genetic Factors in Human Idiopathic Dilated Cardiomyopathy

#### Structural Factors

In IDC, areas of fibrosis that contribute to the slow conduction necessary for reentry have been found, as well as pulmonary emboli, a potential cause of electromechanical dissociation on autopsy findings.[12] The compensatory ventricular hypertrophy improving survival[13] has not been evaluated in specific relation to sudden death.

#### Humoral Factors

Myocardium from failing hearts is more sensitive to changes in extracellular environment and response with a greater propensity toward developing afterdepolarizations and triggered activity. Automaticity arising from a normal maximal diastolic potential is observed in 50% of failing human hearts but only after exposure to an extracellular environment containing low potassium, low magnesium, and high norepinephrine levels.[14]

High sympathetic tone, manifested by elevated plasma norepinephrine levels, reduced myocardial norepinephrine content and decreased myocardial beta receptor density;[15] abnormalities of the autonomic nervous system and renin angiotensine aldosterone axis appear to promote the occurrence of ventricular arrhythmias. Modulation of calcium flux by alpha and beta adrenergic stimulation may also impact significantly on the development of arrhythmias in the failing heart.

## Electrophysiological Factors

A significant prolongation of the action potential with delayed repolarization has been observed in the end-stage heart failure caused by IDC.[16] This lengthening can result from either an increase in inward currents or a decrease in outward currents, or both.[17] In IDC, there is a prolonged diastolic $Ca^{2+}$ transient resulting from a diminished capacity to restore low resting $Ca^{2+}$ levels,[18,19] but no significant $i_{CaT}$ has been detected in ventricular cells isolated from humans.[20] Dilatation of the left ventricle in combination with a low ejection fraction predisposes to stretch that can induce early afterdepolarization, delayed afterdepolarization, and triggered activity, depending on the timing of applied stretch in this disease. In human IDC, epicardial reentrant wavefronts and transmural scroll waves were present during ventricular fibrillation.[21]

Increased fibrosis provides a site for conduction block, leading to the continuous generation of reentry.[21] Mapping of the epicardial surface in hearts of patients with IDC has demonstrated slowing conduction velocity, either longitudinal or transverse to fiber orientation, during induced ectopic beats. The presence of conduction block during pacing or associated with induced ectopic beats suggests that reentry could potentially underlie the degree of interstitial fibrosis at the sites of focal activation but were spatially distant from the sites initiating ventricular tachycardia.[22]

## Genetic Factors

In some cases, genetic studies have shown cardiomyopathy with conduction defects[1] but no study has demonstrated a strong relation between genetic factors and sudden death in IDC.

## Mechanisms of Sudden Death in Idiopathic Dilated Cardiomyopathy

Spontaneous and induced ventricular arrhythmias in patients with end-stage IDC can arise in the subendocardium or subepicardium by a focal mechanism.[23] Interestingly, macroreentry within the bundle branches, a relatively uncommon mechanism of ventricular tachycardia in coronary artery disease, has been observed frequently in nonischemic cardiomyopathy.[24] The relative incidences of arrhythmogenic or nonarrhythmogenic mechanisms of sudden death are ventricular tachycardia (Figure 1) and ventricular fibrillation in 50% and bradycardia and

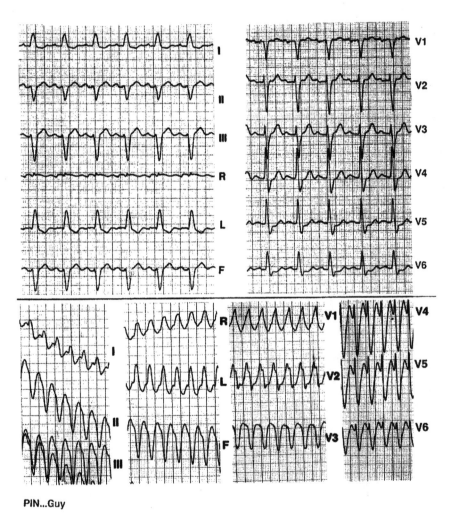

PIN...Guy

Figure 1. Electrocardiograms of a patient with an idiopathic dilated cardiomyopathy, who had died suddenly. Top: Sinus rhythm with left bundle branch block and left QRS axis. Bottom: Spontaneous monomorphic ventricular tachycardia with right bundle branch block and left QRS axis.

electromechanical dissociation in the remaining 50% in the end stage of IDC.[25]

## Clinical Findings

Many patients with IDC die suddenly and unexpectedly, and this creates an important clinical problem, especially in patients who are awaiting a heart transplantation. The mechanism underlying sudden death could be different at each stage of the New York Heart Association (NYHA) classification. In stages I and II, ventricular tachyarrhythmias could play a major part in unexpected sudden death in patients with stable hemodynamic status. In stages III and IV, ventricular arrhythmias indicate only the degree of ventricular dysfunction, and sudden death may follow bradyarrhythmias and electromechanical dissociation. Some clinical factors have to be considered in the determination of patients who are at increased risk for sudden death. Familial disease is probably a predictor of adverse prognosis. The familial form of IDC is the more malignant form; it occurs at an earlier age and progresses more rapidly than the nonfamilial idiopathic dilated form.[26] The natural history of IDC in children is not well characterized, but there is a persistent risk of late sudden death in children whose echocardiographic dimensions remain abnormal.[27] In the adult population, age is not a clear predictor of adverse prognosis; however, Fuster reported an increased mortality rate for those over age 55.[28] The relation between NYHA functional class and risk of sudden death is controversial. The cumulative mortality rate from sudden death for the Class III group was significantly higher than that for the functional Class I and II groups in Stewart's study,[29] but neither Hoffman[30] nor Romeo[31] found a significant correlation between NYHA functional class and risk of sudden death. In contrast, syncope is a significant prognostic finding.[32,33] The actuarial risk of sudden death at 1 year for patients with a history of syncope is high. Syncope may identify a patient who is at high risk for arrhythmias or who has impaired ability to maintain adequate cerebral perfusion in response to physiological stresses.

Concerning the left and right ventricular function and hemodynamic parameters, some results have been observed in IDC patients; those with spontaneous nonsustained ventricular tachycardia had lower left ejection fractions and increased left ventricular end-diastolic pressures.[34,35] The right ventricular function is a parameter of great interest because sudden death was associated with more severe right ventricular dysfunction.[31] Significant right ventricular dilation in IDC increased the mortality over 4 years nearly 3-fold, and created more rapid deterioration of left ventricular function than did a less significant initial right ventricular dilation (Figure 2).

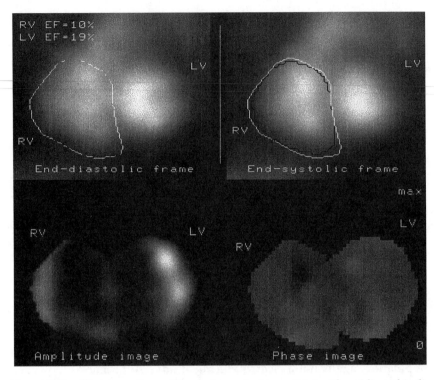

**Figure 2.** Equilibrium radionuclide angiography in a patient with an idiopathic dilated cardiomyopathy who had died suddenly. Top: End-diastolic and end-systole frames in the left anterior oblique view, showing a biventricular enlargement, low left and right ventricular ejection fractions (respectively, 19% and 10%), and diffuse biventricular hypokinesia. Bottom: Amplitude image (Fourier), revealing a small contraction amplitude, only in the right ventricular free wall and in the left ventricular lateral wall. Phase image shows a biventricular heterogeneity of the activation-contraction mapping.

In summary, with the exception of syncope and severe right ventricular dysfunction, historical and physical findings yield few clues for the clinician as to which patients are at increased risk for sudden death.

## Electrocardiogram Findings

No significant association between intraventricular conduction delay and risk of sudden death has been demonstrated.[30,31] In contrast, in a study of 94 patients followed prospectively for 49 ± 37 months, the presence of first or second degree AV block was found to be an independent risk factor of sudden death in patients with IDC.[36]

Concerning atrial fibrillation, some studies show that this arrhythmia is associated with an increased risk of sudden death[30,31] or that it has no influence on sudden death.[12,37]

# Noninvasive Tests

Spontaneous ventricular ectopy is a very common finding in patients with IDC, but the prognostic significance of Holter monitoring remains controversial. Therefore, other noninvasive methods (late ventricular potentials, QT dispersion) have been developed.

## Holter Monitoring

### Ventricular Ectopy Activity

In IDC, the ventricular ectopic activity is extremely high and remains asymptomatic. Most patients have complex ventricular ectopy, and approximately one half of them have at least 1 episode of nonsustained ventricular tachycardia recorded in a 24-hour period that was a sensitive but not a specific marker of sudden death. Some studies have found a relationship between premature ventricular contractions and sudden death,[29,31] but in contrast, other studies[34,38] have not established a correlation between ventricular tachyarrhythmias and sudden death in IDC. A left ventricular ejection fraction lower than 40% together with a nonsustained ventricular tachycardia was associated with a high risk of sudden death in this disease.[39]

### Heart Rate Variability

In a study of 71 patients with IDC and shorter follow-up (15 ± 5 months), Hoffman[40] has not found a significant relation between heart rate variability and major arrhythmic events (sustained ventricular tachycardia, sustained ventricular fibrillation, and sudden death). In contrast, Fauchier,[41] in a study concerning 116 patients with IDC with a mean follow-up of 53 ± 39 months has found that heart rate variability is predictive of major arrhythmic events and sudden cardiac death, whether or not the mechanism of sudden death is ventricular tachyarrhythmia (Figure 3).

### QT Dispersion

In 107 patients with IDC, arrhythmic events occurred in 12 patients during 13 ± 7 months of follow-up. QTc dispersion and adjusted QTc dis-

GLOBAL RESULTS

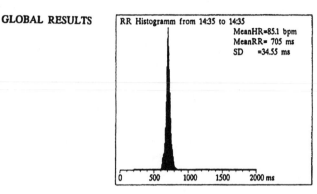

| | H.R. | PNN50 | PNN30 | rMSSD | Var.Index | ASDNN/5 | SDANN/5 | SD |
|---|---|---|---|---|---|---|---|---|
| 24H | 85.1 bpm | 0.35 % | 3.44 % | 11.85 ms | 1.04 % | 13.73 ms | 31.40 ms | 34.55 ms |

Figure 3. An example of heart rate variability in a patient with an idiopathic dilated cardiomyopathy; the standard deviation of the RR histogram is very low. This patient had died suddenly a few months after this Holter recording.

person were not significantly different between patients with and those without arrhythmic events.[42] During follow-up, the QT dispersion usefulness for the arrhythmia risk prediction was limited by a large overlap of QT dispersion between patients with and without arrhythmic events.[42] In another study of 135 patients with congestive heart failure secondary to IDC, QT dispersion was not a predictor for arrhythmic events or death.[43]

## Other Methods

Methods such as decreased baroreflex sensitivity and T wave alternans have to be studied for noninvasive arrhythmia risk stratification. These parameters are being evaluated in a study of Grimm et al., beginning in 1998 with a follow-up of 5 years.[44]

### Signal-Averaged Electrocardiogram

In a different series of IDC, the prevalence of late ventricular potentials was between 25% and 30%.[45-48] The presence of left bundle branch block on the surface electrocardiogram is relatively frequent in IDC. The detection of late ventricular potentials is not very accurate in this situation, and spectral analysis does not improve the ventricular tachycardia prediction in patients with a conduction defect,[47] but predicts the development of progressive heart failure and in some cases of sudden death.[49] In the study of Poll et al.,[45] 14% of patients with nonsustained ventricular tachycardia had late ventricular potentials versus 83% in patients with sustained ventricular tachycardia. In our series of IDC (Figure 4), we detected 21% of late ventricular potentials in patients without ventricular tachycardia, 43% in patients with nonsustained ventricular tachycardia, and 67% in patients with sustained ventricular tachycardia.[46] Concerning the predictive value of late ventricular potentials for cardiac death in IDC, Turitto et al.[50] found that the 2-year actuarial survival rate free of arrhythmic events was similar in patients with and without abnormal findings on signal-averaged electrocardiogram or induced ventricular tachycardia. In this study, the normal findings on the signal-averaged electrocardiogram as well as the failure to induce ventricular tachycardia was not always associated with a benign outcome. In contrast, Mancini[51] showed that an abnormal signal-averaged electrocardiogram was a marker for future ventricular tachycardia or death. Some patients with spontaneous sustained ventricular tachycardia were free of late ventricular potentials in IDC because mechanisms other than reentry are possible to explain the arrhythmogenicity of this disease.[52]

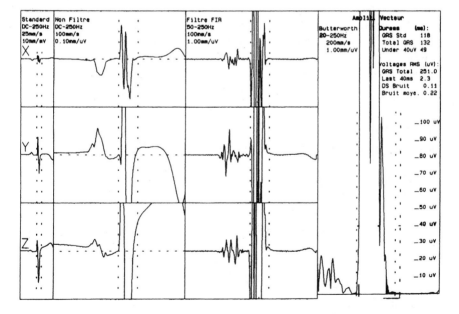

Figure 4. Presence of late ventricular potentials in a patient with an idiopathic dilated cardiomyopathy. This patient, who is alive 3 years after the diagnosis, also has episodes of spontaneous ventricular tachycardia.

## Programmed Ventricular Stimulation

### Inducible Ventricular Arrhythmias in Patients with Spontaneous Ventricular Arrhythmias

Poll and co-workers,[53] using up to 3 stimuli, were able to induce monomorphic sustained ventricular tachycardia in all patients in whom this arrhythmia occurred spontaneously. In contrast, monomorphic sustained ventricular tachycardia was inducible in only 1 of 14 patients with ventricular fibrillation and in 2 of 20 patients with nonsustained ventricular tachycardia. In a large study by Chen et al.[54] of IDC with documented sustained ventricular tachycardia (n = 63) or ventricular fibrillation (n = 39), there was no relationship between documented and inducible ventricular tachyarrhythmias, and programmed ventricular stimulation seems not to be useful in this group of patients.

### Programmed Ventricular Stimulation for Arrhythmia Risk Stratification in Patients with IDC and without History of Symptomatic Ventricular Arrhythmia

Das and co-workers[55] found inducible monomorphic sustained tachycardia in only 1 of 24 patients with IDC who had no history of symptomatic ventricular tachyarrhythmia. In another study,[56] programmed ventricular stimulation did not appear to be helpful for arrhythmia risk stratification in patients with IDC with a left ventricular ejection fraction (35% and spontaneous nonsustained ventricular tachycardia.

### Programmed Ventricular Stimulation and Correlation with Impairment of Left Ventricular Function

In the study of Das,[55] there was no correlation between hemodynamic variables and inducibility of polymorphic ventricular tachycardia or ventricular fibrillation. For Meinertz and co-workers,[57] there was no correlation between electrically induced polymorphic ventricular arrhythmias and the degree of impairment of the left ventricular function.

### Prognostic Value of Programmed Ventricular Stimulation

In the study of Brembilla-Perrot et al.,[32] inducible ventricular tachycardia in patients with IDC was associated with a poor prognosis. In other studies,[53,54] sudden cardiac death was not predicted by the response to programmed stimulation and was unrelated to arrhythmia initiation. Electrophysiological testing also has limitations for guiding therapy in patients with ventricular tachyarrhythmias and IDC.[53]

# Therapy

Current therapeutic options, including neurohormonal blockade, antiarrhythmic drugs, and implantable cardioverter-defibrillators, are discussed.

## Medical Treatment

Patients with a lower cardiac left ejection fraction and increased left ventricular end-diastolic pressures often have spontaneous nonsustained ventricular tachycardia. Sudden death is also associated with a more severe ventricular dysfunction. Many of the agents such as digitalis or diuretics used to treat congestive heart failure in IDC may exacerbate ventricular arrhythmias. Only angiotensin-converting enzyme inhibitors and beta-blocking agents can improve morbidity and mortality. First, we consider the place of the neurohormonal blockade agents.

### Angiotensin-Converting Enzyme Inhibitors

These drugs can improve parasympathetic activity, which may be protective against fatal ventricular arrhythmias and have a positive effect in the prevention of arrhythmias related to the electrolyte and catecholamine disturbances. In the Veterans Trial II,[58] enalapril therapy was associated with a significantly decreased incidence of sudden death compared with the treatment with isosorbide dinitrate and hydralazine.

### Beta-Blocking Agents

The rationale for using beta blockers in congestive heart failure secondary to IDC is based on the hypothesis that the disease is worsened by abnormal activity of the sympathetic nervous system.[15] Three large prospective studies with carvedilol,[59] metoprolol,[60] and bisoprolol[61] have demonstrated a beneficial effect concerning cardiac mortality and sudden death in congestive heart failure. An antiarrhythmic effect was documented with carvedilol in the treatment of ventricular tachycardia in a patient with IDC.[62] In the MERIT HF study group,[60] there were fewer sudden deaths in the metoprolol group than in the placebo group. The decrease in sudden death (41%) was similar to that in the CIBIS II study[61] with bisoprolol (44%). The decreased incidence of sudden death in these studies suggests an antifibrillatory effect of metoprolol and bisoprolol, but the studies were not designed for a separate analysis of patients with IDC.

## Antiarrhythmic Drugs

No study reported to date has shown a benefit connected with the use of any of the non-amiodarone antiarrhythmic agents in the prevention of sudden cardiac death. Proarrhythmic effects occur more commonly in patients with congestive heart failure.

However, in a study by Rae and colleagues,[63] success during serial drug testing is associated with a good follow-up in patients with IDC and noninducible arrhythmias, but this situation is uncommon.[53] With amiodarone treatment, the results are better, but it is difficult to analyze the different studies. In the GESICA study,[64] both sudden death and death due to progressive heart failure were reduced in all analyzed subgroups, including the presence or absence of nonsustained ventricular tachycardia, but many of the patients had Chagas' disease and non-IDC. In the STAT-CHF study,[65] the subgroup with IDC appeared to have a better prognosis. Some uncontrolled studies suggest that amiodarone may have some benefit in the primary prevention of sudden death. Prospective studies are needed for confirmation. In a study by Castelli,[66] in unselected patients with IDC, cardiovascular mortality did not differ between those with nonsustained ventricular tachycardia on chronic amiodarone treatment and those without nonsustained ventricular tachycardia who have not undergone antiarrhythmic therapy; the disappearance of nonsustained ventricular tachycardia during amiodarone treatment was not predictive of a reduced rate in sudden death, so that the potential effect of the drug does not appear to be related to the suppression of nonsustained ventricular tachycardia at Holter monitoring.

The preceding results indicate that many patients without inducible tachycardia during baseline study or without suppressed inducibility on drugs have a poor outcome. Therefore, nonpharmacological therapy must be considered for these patients.[67] Mapping directed surgery is presumably not appropriate because of the diffuse myocardial disease. Catheter ablation may be tried in patients with monomorphic tachycardia (for example, bundle branch reentry). Since antiarrhythmic drug therapy was of limited value, implantation of a cardiac defibrillator may improve the prognosis of these high-risk patients. In New York Heart Association stages I and II, ventricular tachyarrhythmias could play a major part in unexpected sudden death of patients whose stable hemodynamic status suggested a more prolonged survival. The value of an implantable cardioverter-defibrillator would seem to be proved in this group of patients at least as a secondary prevention. When heart failure symptoms are severe despite medical therapy, the prevention of sudden death remains important especially when transplantation is planned. If we consider the significant role of ventricular arrhythmias in sudden cardiac death, it would seem logical that the implantable cardioverter-defibrillator would improve survival rates. The data of Fazio et al.[68] suggest a survival benefit with implantable cardioverter-defibrillator in 40 consecutive patients with cardiac arrest, syncope or near syncope. Grimm and Marchlinski[69] reported 49 patients with IDC presenting with cardiac arrest (82%), syncope (12%), and ventricular tachycardia without syncope (6%); they were followed for 28 ± 28 months after cardioverter-defibrillator implants according to the intention to treat. The majority of patients received appropriate shocks during follow-up, and the sudden death rate was low with implantable cardioverter-defibrillators in these data. Thus, in a selected population with IDC, for example, with unexplained syncope,[70] the majority of patients received appropriate shocks during follow-up and the sudden death rate with active implantable cardioverter-defibrillator was low. Borggrefe et al.[71] feel that implantation of a cardioverter-defibrillator should be considered in most of patients with IDC.

Prospective implantable cardioverter-defibrillator trials are focusing on IDC:

- The German Cardiomyopathy Trial (CAT) enrolls patients with advanced dilated cardiomyopathy and no symptomatic ventricular arrhythmias. The investigators decided to evaluate the study hypotheses of a yearly mortality of 12% for sudden cardiac death after analyzing the results from the first 100 patients.[72]
- In the Definite study, the treatment with implantable cardioverter-defibrillators was compared with beta blockers in nonischemic cardiomyopathy and symptomatic heart failure with nonsustained ventricular tachycardia or premature ventricular complex.[73]

In end-stage failure, heart transplantation may be the ultimate treatment. In some cases, when heart transplantation is not possible, alternative therapy combining dynamic cardiomyoplasty with internal defibrillation is a new approach for treatment of advanced cardiomyopathy.[68]

## Conclusion

Many sudden cardiac deaths occur in IDC. Spontaneous ventricular ectopy is a very common finding, but the prognostic significance remains controversial. Late ventricular potentials, heart rate variability, and QT dispersion are used to stratify the long-term prognosis. Concerning the predictive value of programmed electrical stimulation, this method failed to identify some patients with a high risk of sustained ventricular arrhythmias or sudden death. Preliminary data for the use of the implantable cardioverter-defibrillator appear to be promising.

## References

1. Priori SG, Barhanin J, Hauer RN, et al. Genetic and molecular basis of cardiac arrhythmias: impact on clinical management. Eur Heart J 1999; 20:174–195.
2. Tamburro P, Wilber D. Sudden death in idiopathic dilated cardiomyopathy. Am Heart J 1992; 124:1035–1045.
3. Wu AH, Das SK. Sudden death in dilated cardiomyopathy. Clin Cardiol 1999; 22:267–272.
4. Pogwizd SM, Corr PB. Biochemical and electrophysiological alterations underlying ventricular arrhythmias in the failing heart. Eur Heart J 1994; 15:145–154.
5. Christensen G, Wang Y, Chien K. Physiological assessment of complex cardiac phenotypes in genetically engineered mice. Am J Physiol 1997; 272:H2513-H2524.
6. Lab MJ. Contraction-excitation feedback in myocardium. Circ Res 1982; 50:757–766.
7. Hansen DE, Craig CS, Hondeghem LM. Stretch-induced arrhythmias in the isolated canine ventricle: evidence for the importance of mechanoelectrical feedback. Circulation 1990; 81:1094–1105.
8. Thuringer D, Coulombe A, Deroubaix E, et al. Depressed transient outward current density in ventricular myocytes from cardiomyopathic Syrian hamsters of different ages. J Mol Cell Cardiol 1996; 28:387–401.
9. Pacioretty LM, Cooper BJ, Gilmour RF. Reduction of the transient outward potassium current in canine X-linked muscular dystrophy. Circulation 1994; 90:1350–1356.
10. Hatem SN, Sham JSK, Morad M. $Na^+$–$Ca^{2+}$ exchange activity is enhanced in cardiomyopathic Syrian hamster. Circ Res 1994; 74:253–261.
11. Sen L, Smith TW. T-type $Ca^{2+}$ channels are abnormal in genetically determined cardiomyopathic hamster hearts. Circ Res 1994; 75:149–155.
12. Roberts WC, Siegel RJ, McManus BM. Idiopathic dilated cardiomyopathy: analysis of 152 necroscopy patients. Am J Cardiol 1987; 60:1340–1355.
13. Benjamin IJ, Shuster EH, Bulkley BH. Cardiac hypertrophy in idiopathic dilated congestive cardiomyopathy: a clinicopathologic study. Circulation 1981; 64:442–447.
14. Vermeulen JT. Mechanisms of arrhythmias in heart failure. J Cardiovasc Electrophysiol 1998; 9:208–221.
15. Cohn JN, Levine TB, Olivari MT. Plasma norepinephrine as a guide to prognosis in patients with congestive heart failure. N Engl J Med 1984; 311:819–823.
16. Beuckelmann DJ, Näbauer M, Erdmann E. Alterations of $K^+$ currents in isolated human ventricular myocytes from patients with terminal heart failure. Circ Res 1993; 73:379–385.
17. Richard S, Leclercq F, Lemaire S, et al. $Ca^{2+}$ currents in compensated hypertrophy and heart failure. Cardiovasc Res 1998; 37:300–311.
18. Pieske B, Kretshmann B, Meyer M, et al. Alterations in intracellular calcium handling associated with the inverse force-frequency relation in human dilated cardiomyopathy. Circulation 1995; 92:1169–1178.

19. Beuckelmann DL, Näbauer M, Erdmann E. Intracellular calcium handling in isolated human ventricular myocytes from patients with terminal heart failure. Circulation 1992; 85:1046–1055.
20. Coraboeuf E, Nargeot J. Electrophysiology of human cardiac cells. Cardiovasc Res 1993; 27:1713–1725.
21. Wu TJ, Ong JJC, Hwang C, et al. Characteristics of wave fronts during ventricular fibrillation in human hearts with dilated cardiomyopathy: role of increased fibrosis in the generation of reentry. J Am Coll Cardiol 1998; 32:187–196.
22. Anderson KP, Walker R, Urie P, et al. Myocardial electrical propagation in patients with idiopathic dilated cardiomyopathy. J Clin Invest 1993; 92:122–140.
23. Pogwizd SM, McKenzie JP, Cain ME. Mechanisms underlying spontaneous and induced ventricular arrhythmias in patients with idiopathic dilated cardiomyopathy. Circulation 1998; 98:2404–2014.
24. Caceres J, Jazayeri M, McKinnie J, et al. Sustained bundle branch reentry as a mechanism of clinical tachycardia. Circulation 1989; 79:256–270.
25. Luu M, Stevenson WG, Stevenson LW, et al. Diverse mechanisms of unexpected cardiac arrest in advanced heart failure. Circulation 1989; 80:1675–1680.
26. Csanady M, Hogye M, Kallai A, et al. Familial dilated cardiomyopathy: a worse prognosis compared with sporadic forms. Br Heart J 1995:171–173.
27. Burch M, Siddiqi SA, Celermajer DS, et al. Dilated cardiomyopathy in children: determinants of outcome. Br Heart J 1994; 72:246–250.
28. Fuster V, Gersh B, Giuliani ER, et al. The natural history of idiopathic dilated cardiomyopathy. Am J Cardiol 1981; 47:525–531.
29. Stewart RA, Mc Kenna WJ, Oakley CM. Good prognosis for dilated cardiomyopathy without severe heart failure or arrhythmia. QJ Med 1990; 74:309–318.
30. Hoffmann T, Meinertz T, Kasper W, et al. Mode of death in idiopathic dilated cardiomyopathy: a multivariate analysis of prognostic determinants. Am Heart J 1988; 116:1455–1463.
31. Romeo F, Pelliccia F, Cianfrocca C, et al. Predictors of sudden death in idiopathic dilated cardiomyopathy. Am J Cardiol 1989; 63:138–140.
32. Brembilla-Perrot B, Donetti J, Terrier de la Chaise A, et al. Diagnostic value of ventricular stimulation in patients with idiopathic dilated cardiomyopathy. Am Heart J 1991; 121:1124–1131.
33. Tchou PJ, Krebs AC, Sra J, et al. Syncope: a warning sign in idiopathic dilated cardiomyopathy patients. J Am Coll Cardiol 1991; 17:196A.
34. Von Olshausen K, Schafer A, Mehmel HC, et al. Ventricular arrhythmias in idiopathic dilated cardiomyopathy. Br Heart J 1984; 51:195–201.
35. Sun JP, James KB, Yang XS, et al. Comparison of mortality rates and progression of left ventricular dysfunction in patients with idiopathic dilated cardiomyopathy and dilated versus nondilated right ventricular cavities. Am J Cardiol 1997; 80:1583–1587.
36. Schoeller R, Andresen D, Büttner P, et al. First or second degree atrioventricular block as a risk factor in idiopathic dilated cardiomyopathy. Am J Cardiol 1993; 71:720–726.
37. Likoff MJ, Chandler SL, Kay HR. Clinical determinants of mortality in chronic congestive heart failure secondary to idiopathic dilated or to ischemic cardiomyopathy. Am J Cardiol 1987; 59:634–638.
38. Huang SK, Messer JV, Denes P. Significance of ventricular tachycardia in idiopathic dilated cardiomyopathy: observations in 35 patients. Am J Cardiol 1983; 51:507–512.
39. Meinertz T, Hofmann T, Kasper W, et al. Significance of ventricular arrhythmias in idiopathic dilated cardiomyopathy. Am J Cardiol 1984; 53:902–907.

40. Hoffmann J, Grimm W, Menz V, et al. Heart rate variability and major arrhythmic events in patients with idiopathic dilated cardiomyopathy. PACE 1996; 19 (II):1841–1844.
41. Fauchier L, Babuty D, Cosnay P, et al. Prognostic value of heart rate variability for sudden death and major arrhythmic events in patients with idiopathic dilated cardiomyopathy. J Am Coll Cardiol 1999; 5:1203–1207.
42. Grimm W, Steder U, Menz V, et al. QT dispersion and arrhythmic events in idiopathic dilated cardiomyopathy. Am J Cardiol 1996; 78:458–461.
43. Fei L, Goldman JH, Prasad K, et al. QT dispersion and RR variations on 12-lead ECGs in patients with congestive heart failure secondary to idiopathic dilated cardiomyopathy. Eur Heart J 1996; 17:258–263.
44. Grimm W, Glaveris C, Hoffmann J, et al. Noninvasive arrhythmia risk stratification in idiopathic dilated cardiomyopathy: design and first results of the Marburg cardiomyopathy study. PACE 1998; 21:2551–2556.
45. Poll DS, Marchlinski FE, Buxton AE, et al. Sustained ventricular tachycardia in patients with idiopathic dilated cardiomyopathy: electrophysiologic testing and lack of response to antiarrhythmic drug therapy. Circulation 1984; 70:451–456.
46. Fauchier JP, Cosnay P, Babuty D, et al. Etude du potentiel arythmogène des myocardiopathies:les myocardiopathies dilatées. Arch Mal Coeur 1991; 84:95–103.
47. Turitto G, Ahuja RK, Bekheit S, et al. Incidence and prediction of induced ventricular tachyarrhythmias in idiopathic dilated cardiomyopathy. Am J Cardiol 1994; 73:770–773.
48. Galinier M, Albenque JP, Afchar N, et al. Prognostic value of late potentials in patients with congestive heart failure. Eur Heart J 1996; 17:264–271.
49. Yi G, Keeling PJ, Goldman JH, et al. Prognostic significance of spectral turbulence analysis of the signal-averaged electrocardiogram in patients with idiopathic dilated cardiomyopathy. Am J Cardiol 1995; 75:494–497.
50. Turitto G, Ahuja RK, Caref EB, et al. Risk stratification for arrhythmic events in patients with nonischemic dilated cardiomyopathy and nonsustained ventricular tachycardia: role of programmed ventricular stimulation and the signal-averaged electrocardiogram. J Am Coll Cardiol 1994; 24:1523–1528.
51. Mancini IDC, Wong KL, Simson MB. Prognostic value of an abnormal signal-averaged electrocardiogram in patients with nonischemic congestive cardiomyopathy. Circulation 1993; 87:1083–1092.
52. Winters SL, Goldman DS, Banas JS. Prognosis impact of late potentials in nonischemic dilated cardiomyopathy. Circulation 1993; 87:1405–1407.
53. Poll DS, Marchlinski FE, Buxton AE, et al. Usefulness of programmed stimulation in idiopathic dilated cardiomyopathy. Am J Cardiol 1986; 58:992–997.
54. Chen X, Shenasa M, Borggrefe M, et al. Role of programmed ventricular stimulation in patients with idiopathic dilated cardiomyopathy and documented sustained ventricular tachyarrhythmias: inducibility and prognostic value in 102 patients. Eur Heart J 1994; 15:76–82.
55. Das SK, Morady F, DiCarlo L, et al. Prognostic usefulness of programmed ventricular stimulation in idiopathic dilated cardiomyopathy without symptomatic ventricular arrhythmias. Am J Cardiol 1986; 58:998–1000.
56. Grimm W, Hoffmann J, Menz V, et al. Programmed ventricular stimulation for arrhythmia risk prediction in patients with idiopathic dilated cardiomyopathy and nonsustained ventricular tachycardia. J Am Coll Cardiol 1998; 32:739–745.
57. Meinertz T, Treese N, Kasper W, et al. Determinants of prognosis in idiopathic

dilated cardiomyopathy as determined by programmed electrical stimulation. Am J Cardiol 1985; 56:337–341.

58. Cohn JN, Johnson G, Ziesche, et al. A comparison of enalapril with hydralazine-isosorbide dinitrate in the treatment of chronic congestive heart failure (V-HeFT II). N Engl J Med 1991; 325:303–310.

59. Packer M, Bristow MR, Cohn J et al for the US Carvedilol Heart Failure Study Group. The effect of carvedilol on morbidity and mortality in patients with chronic heart failure. N Engl J Med 1996; 334:1349–1355.

60. Effect of metoprolol CR/XL in chronic heart failure: metoprolol CR/XL randomised intervention trial in congestive heart failure (MERIT-HF). Lancet 1999; 353:2001–2007.

61. The Cardiac Insufficiency Bisoprolol Study II (CIBIS II). Lancet 1999; 353:9–13.

62. Wright DJ, Cooke GA, Tan LB. Intractable recurrent ventricular tachycardia in dilated cardiomyopathy controlled by a vasodilating β blocker. Heart 1997; 77:581–582.

63. Rae AP, Spielman SR, Kutalek SP, et al. Electrophysiologic assessment of antiarrhythmic drug efficacy for ventricular tachyarrhythmias associated with dilated cardiomyopathy. Am J Cardiol 1987; 59:291–295.

64. Doval HC, Nul DR, Grancelli HO et al for the GESICA Group. Randomized trial of low dose amiodarone in severe congestive heart failure. Lancet 1994; 344:493–498.

65. Singh SN, Fletcher RD, Gross-Fischer S, et al. Amiodarone in patients with congestive heart failure and asymptomatic ventricular arrhythmia. N Engl J Med 1995; 333:77–82.

66. Castelli G, Ciaccheri M, Cecchi F, et al. Nonsustained ventricular tachycardia as a predictor for sudden death in patients with idiopathic dilated cardiomyopathy: the role of amiodarone treatment. G Ital Cardiol 1999; 29:514–523.

67. Brachmann J, Hilbel T, Grünig E, et al. Ventricular arrhythmias in dilated cardiomyopathy. PACE 1997; 20:2714–2718.

68. Fazio G, Veltri EP, Tomaselli G, et al. Long-term follow-up of patients with nonischemic dilated cardiomyopathy and ventricular tachyarrhythmias treated with implantable cardioverter defibrillators. PACE 1991; 14:1905–1910.

69. Grimm W, Marchlinski FE. Shock occurrence and survival in 49 patients with idiopathic dilated cardiomyopathy and implantable cardioverter-defibrillators. Eur Heart J 1995; 16:218–222.

70. Knight BP, Goyal R, Pelosi F, et al. Outcome of patients with nonischemic dilated cardiomyopathy and unexplained syncope treated with an implantable defibrillator. J Am Coll Cardiol 1999; 33:1964–1970.

71. Borggrefe M, Chen X, Martinez-Rubio A, et al. The role of implantable cardioverter defibrillators in dilated cardiomyopathy. Am Heart J 1994; 127:1145–1150.

72. The Cardiomyopathy Trial Investigators. The Cardiomyopathy Trial. PACE 1993; 16:576–581.

73. Nisam S, Mower M. ICD trials: an extraordinary means of determining patient risk? PACE 1998; 21:1341–1346.

# 25

# Mechanisms of Sudden Death in Hypertrophic Cardiomyopathy:

## Implications for Risk Stratification

*Paul Sorajja, MD, Perry M. Elliott, MD, and William J. McKenna, MD*

## Introduction

Population studies using 2-D echocardiography have reported the prevalence of hypertrophic cardiomyopathy (HCM) to be between 0.2% and 0.5%.[1-4] Although the majority of these persons live without cardiac morbidity, a subset of these patients die suddenly. Studies from referral institutions report an incidence of sudden death of ~4% in adolescents and young adults and 1–2% in adults.[5-7] Although the propensity for sudden death has been noted since early descriptions of HCM, the identification of those at high risk still remains an important challenge in clinical management. This need for stratification has spurred a wealth of investigations into the mechanisms responsible for sudden death in HCM. These studies have pointed to the presence of a susceptible myocardial substrate as well as hemodynamic triggers that, when identified, can aid in the recognition of the HCM patient at increased risk for sudden death.

## Pathogenesis of Sudden Death

Sudden death in HCM has been attributed to multiple pathogenic mechanisms (Figure 1). These abnormalities either have been found or have long been suspected in HCM patients, although the role of each fac-

From: Aliot E, Clementy J, Prystowsky EN (editors). *Fighting Sudden Cardiac Death: A Worldwide Challenge.* ©Futura Publishing Company, Armonk, NY, 2000.

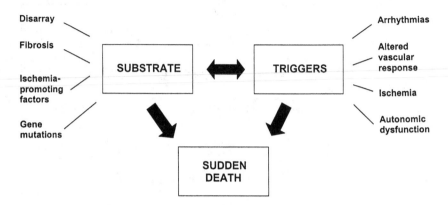

Figure 1. Scheme of mechanisms of sudden death in HCM. An abnormal myocardial substrate and the presence of either hemodynamic or ischemic triggers have been implicated in the pathogenesis of sudden death in HCM. Either component may act singly or in combination with other factors to lead to sudden death. Ischemia-promoting factors include reduced arteriole density and coronary arteries that have decreased lumen size and impaired reserve.

tor in sudden death has been the subject of controversy. Myocyte hypertrophy and disarray, myocardial fibrosis, and ischemia-promoting factors, all as a direct or indirect consequence of disease-causing gene mutations, contribute to an abnormal myocardial substrate. This substrate may be primarily responsible for sudden death or act in a secondary manner in response to an external provocative measure, such as an unfavorable hemodynamic alteration. Evidence for the latter contention comes from investigations that have shown that autonomic dysfunction, abnormal vascular responses, myocardial ischemia, and syncope are common in HCM and confer an increased risk of sudden death.

VF is the final common pathway for sudden death in HCM, although its antecedent events have been difficult to ascertain due to the rarity of monitored cases. Conclusions on mechanisms of sudden death in HCM, therefore, have relied on either anecdotal reports or inferences from investigations of persons deemed to be at high risk for sudden death (e.g., those patients with prior cardiac arrest or syncope). Although a diurnal variation in the occurrence of sudden death due to HCM has been suggested,[8] sudden death in these patients commonly takes place without regard to the presence of symptoms or functional limitation, and, in near-equal proportions, during periods of rest and periods of moderate to severe physical exertion (Figure 2).[9] This heterogeneity has suggested that the relative importance of the substrate and corresponding hemodynamic triggers varies among individuals.

Several natural history observations illustrate this likelihood. In the majority of patients, the ARG403GLN β-myosin heavy chain mutation confers an adverse prognosis with up to 50% of persons succumbing to disease-

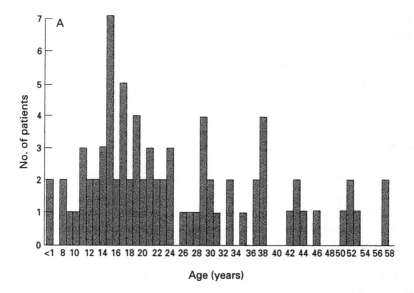

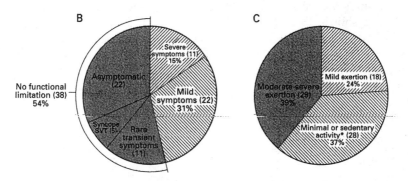

Figure 2. Clinical profile of patients with HCM and sudden death. A: Age distribution of 78 patients who died suddenly or experienced cardiac arrest. B: Functional state prior to sudden death or cardiac arrest. C: Activity at time of death or cardiac arrest. *Includes 4 patients who died during sleep. SVT = supraventricular tachycardia. (Reproduced with permission from Maron et al.[5,73])

related death by 50 years of age.[10] Nonetheless, other families who harbor other mutations may have normal or near-normal survival.[10] Clinical heterogeneity has also been observed within single families. Mutations in the cardiac troponin T (cTnT) gene are ominous with a mortality rate that equals or exceeds that of the ARG403GLN β-myosin heavy chain mutation in severity. In a family with the Intron 15 $G_1 \rightarrow A$ cTnT mutation, 10 disease-related deaths (9 sudden deaths) had taken place before 25 years of age yet 8 family members with the same mutation had survived into the seventh or eighth decade of life.[11] Furthermore, in studies of survivors of cardiac arrest due to HCM, approximately two-thirds of those who had not received antiarrhythmic medical therapy (i.e., amiodarone) are alive after 5 years of follow-up.[12] Although the risk of sudden death is high in this subset of patients, the absence of a recurrence of terminal ventricular arrhythmias in the remaining patients points to the possibility that determinants of sudden death in HCM may even vary within an individual over time.

## Case Reports of Monitored Sudden Death

In 1988, Nicod and co-workers published their report of a 30-year-old man with HCM who died suddenly during ambulatory monitoring.[13] Clinical evaluation had revealed asymmetric left ventricular hypertrophy (maximum left ventricular wall thickness, MLVWT, 28 mm) and symptoms consisting of slight dyspnea on exertion. The initial ambulatory electrocardiogram (ECG) had documented only rare multiform premature ventricular contractions. A second ambulatory ECG, performed during subsequent follow-up, recorded the terminal events of this patient. While walking at a beach, sinus tachycardia with marked ST segment depression was noted, followed shortly thereafter (within 10 min), by polymorphic ventricular tachycardia (VT) and VF. A prominent artifact was present on the recordings, which suggested that syncope, in addition to myocardial ischemia, may have preceded the death of this patient.[14,15] Sinus tachycardia and myocardial ischemia, which led to VF, were also observed in a 7-year-old girl.[16] These events happened during a syncopal episode from which she was resuscitated. Profound hypotension during rapid atrial pacing (> 130 bpm) was later demonstrated in this patient. Similarly, sinus tachycardia and myocardial ischemia occurred prior to the death of a 63-year-old man with HCM.[17] In a 27-year-old man with obstructive HCM, VF was precipitated during exercise at a heart rate of 136 bpm.[18] His history was significant for nonsustained VT on ambulatory ECG monitoring, symptoms of dyspnea, chest pain, and syncope, and prior cardiac arrest on 1 occasion. Prior to the exercise study, he had been prescribed amiodarone at 600 mg/day, which had suppressed his VT on later ambulatory ECG recordings.

Three other reports have cited arrhythmias as the primary event leading to sudden death in HCM. The first case involved a 32-year-old man who was in a hospital after resuscitation from cardiac arrest. While standing, spontaneous polymorphic VT occurred without antecedent symptoms and degenerated into VF.[16] The second case involved a patient who had been diagnosed at birth with HCM and arthrogryposis multiplex congenita.[19] Nonsustained VT had been noted prior to and after surgical myotomy, which was performed at 16 years of age for exercise intolerance. Fifty days after surgery, she died while sleeping. The ambulatory ECG recorded a single premature ventricular complex followed by polymorphic VT and VF. Intermittent, asymptomatic bradycardia and third-degree atrioventricular block had been noted postoperatively, but these events were absent near the time of her death. The third case was a 48-year-old woman with atrial fibrillation and symptoms of paroxysmal nocturnal dyspnea and angina.[20] In addition to verapamil and oxprenolol, she had been taking amiodarone at 200 mg/day that was later reduced to 100 mg/day due to keratopathy. While standing in a shop, a ventricular couplet preceded 12 beats of atrial fibrillation, followed by polymorphic VT and VF. Resuscitative measures by an ambulance team were unsuccessful for this patient.

## Abnormal Myocardial Substrate

The importance of the abnormal myocardial substrate in the genesis of sudden death in HCM has been noted since the early investigation of Teare.[21] In his report of 8 HCM patients who died suddenly, postmortem examinations revealed a "bizarre arrangement of muscle bundles" and "considerable fibrosis" in the hearts of these patients.

Myocyte disarray is now considered to be the pathological hallmark of HCM. Marked variation in myocyte width and length, and the disorderly arrangement of these cells are characteristic of HCM, with > 95% of these patients exhibiting disarray in postmortem examinations.[22] Disarray has been observed in other cardiac disorders and in normal hearts, but it occurs to a much greater degree in HCM (> 5% of total myocardium) than in other conditions (< 1% of total myocardium).[23] Nonhomogeneous electrical conduction resulting from the structural/functional abnormalities of disarray likely provides the setting for microreentry pathways that may degenerate into terminal arrhythmias. Of note, multiple premature sudden deaths have been observed in HCM patients who harbored prominent disarray without ventricular hypertrophy.[24] Moreover, disarray is commonly associated with replacement and/or diffuse interstitial myocardial fibrosis that may involve the ventricular septum, free wall, and, occasionally, the papillary muscles.[25,26] Other features also are observed in HCM and are likely to contribute to the susceptibility of the myocardial substrate. These abnormalities include myocardial bridging, coronary arteries with narrow lumens (external diameter < 1,500 mm), impaired coronary reserve, diminished arteriolar density, and altered loading conditions (resting or latent left ventricular outflow tract obstruction).[27–30]

Through modern molecular techniques, the concept of an altered myocardial substrate in HCM has been extended beyond histopathological features to include the underlying gene mutations present in these patients. Within the past decade, mutations in 8 sarcomeric genes have been found to be responsible for HCM. The affected proteins are β-myosin heavy chain (β-MHC), cTnT, myosin-binding protein C (MyBP-C), actin, α-tropomyosin, cardiac troponin I, and the essential and regulatory myosin light chains (Figure 3).[31–34] Importantly, the natural history of

HCM is influenced by the particular sarcomeric protein affected, as well as by the specific changes within the protein encoded by the mutation. Disease due to mutations in the aforementioned β-MHC gene is characteristically heterogeneous. Some mutations (ARG403GLN, ARG719TRP, ARG453CYS) have a mean age of death in the fourth decade of life, other mutations (VAL606MET, LEU908VAL, GLY256GLU) are associated with near-normal survival, and still others confer an intermediate prognosis (Figure 4) .[10,35–39] The typical features of HCM caused by cTnT mutations are mild ventricular hypertrophy (maximum LV wall thickness, MLVWT = 15–20 mm) and a high risk of sudden death. In 112 persons with cTnT mutations, 39 sudden deaths and an additional 11 disease-related deaths were observed.[11] The mean MLVWT of this entire study population was 16 mm. MyBP-C mutations have age-related penetrance and confer an adverse prognosis once disease expression occurs.[40] Most commonly, HCM due to MyBP-C manifests after the age of 40 years, highlighting the importance of continued family screening of HCM in older populations.[40] Early investigations of HCM-related α-tropomyosin disease have suggested a favorable prognosis.[41] The true proportion of disease due to the remaining sarcomeric mutations is uncertain. These mutations have yet to be evaluated systematically, and, therefore, conclusions on their associated risk of sudden death have not been made.

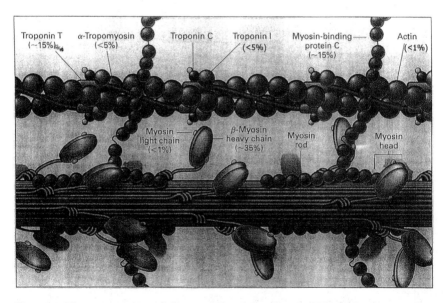

Figure 3. The sarcomere and disease-related proteins in HCM. Numbers within parentheses indicate estimated frequencies with which mutations in the corresponding gene cause hypertrophic cardiomyopathy. (Modified with permission from Seidman and Seidman.[74])

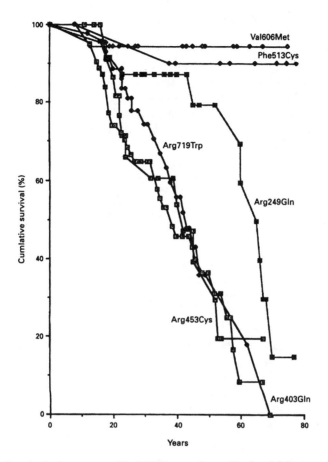

Figure 4. Survival of persons with -MCH mutations. Kaplan-Meier survival plots for persons harboring the corresponding -MHC mutations are shown, illustrating differing survival rates for different -MCH mutations. The VAL606MET -MHC mutation carries a more favorable prognosis than the ARG249GLN, ARG453CYS, and ARG403GLN -MHC mutations. (Reproduced with permission from Watkins et al.[6])

## Quantitative Importance of the Substrate

The importance of the abnormal myocardial substrate has been demonstrated through paced electrogram fractionation, a novel electrophysiological technique developed by Saumarez and co-workers.[42] This technique is based on the hypothesis that variations in myocyte size and shape in HCM (i.e., disarray) lead to an increased number of conduction paths and velocities in accordance with their effective refractory period (Figure 5). During extrastimulation, fast-conducting pathways are blocked, revealing slower conducting pathways that are detected in electrogram transitions recorded at multiple ventricular sites. Using a computer-controlled pacing sequence, an extrastimulus is placed every third beat and the $S_1S_2$ coupling interval is decreased in 1-ms steps until the effective ventricular refractory period is reached. A plot of the latency of the transitions against the coupling interval (Figure 6) is then used to determine 2 variables: (1) the $S_1S_2$ coupling interval at which latency begins to increase by more than a 75 ms/20 ms decrease in $S_1S_2$ coupling interval; and (2) the change in width of the electrogram between an $S_1S_2$ coupling interval of 350 ms and the ventricular effective refractory period.

Saumarez and co-workers used paced electrogram fractionation of the right ventricle to examine 37 patients with HCM, 4 of whom had spontaneous VF.[42] A spectrum of electrophysiological abnormalities was observed in the study population, with greater dispersion of intraventricular conduction in those patients with clinical risk factors. A higher coupling interval at which latency begins to increase and a larger electrogram du-

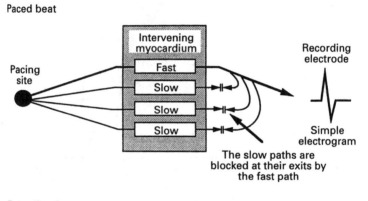

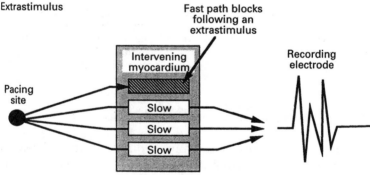

Figure 5. Intraventricular conduction model that is the basis of electrogram fractionation technique. Premature stimulation leads to a refractory state in fast conducting pathways, allowing slow pathways to be exposed and recorded on an electrogram. (Reproduced with permission from Saumarez.[75])

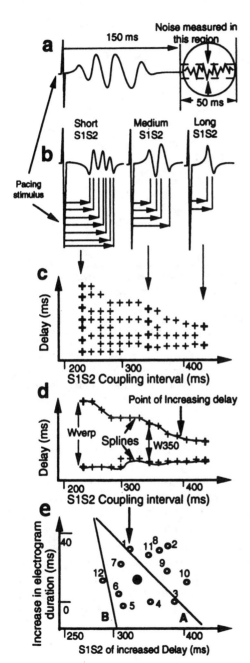

Figure 6. Electrogram analysis. Noise from the portion of the electrogram between 150 and 200 ms after the pacing stimulus is used to set the detection threshold for fractionated potentials (a). The latency of each potential in relation to the pacing stimulus is determined (b). Each latency is plotted against the $S_1S_2$ interval to create the intraventricular conduction curve (c). Cubic splines are fitted to the upper and lower bounds of the curve, which is used to the change in electrogram width between an S of 350 ms and the ventricular effective refractory period. The $S_1S_2$ interval at which the latency begins to increase by greater than 75 ms/20 ms $S_1S_2$ also is determined through differentiation of the cubic spline (d). Results for all curves are plotted and averaged to obtain a single observation (•) for each patient (e). (Reproduced with permission from Saumarez et al.[43])

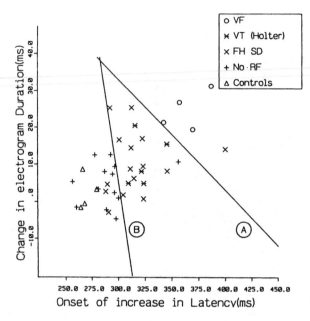

Figure 7. Differentiation of HCM patients according to risk profile by electrogram fractionation. Each point is the mean of observations for each individual patient. Line A is the discriminant line that separates survivors of cardiac arrest from the remainder; line B is the discriminant line that separates those patients with a history of cardiac arrest, nonsustained VT on ambulatory ECG monitoring, and a family history of sudden death from patients without these risk factors. These data point to variations in the susceptible myocardial substrate within HCM patients. (Reproduced with permission from Saumarez et al.[42])

ration discriminated patients with VF (high risk) from patients with either VT on an ambulatory ECG, a family history of HCM and sudden death, or syncope (medium risk) from patients without these risk factors (low risk) (Figure 7). These results suggest that delays in ventricular activation in HCM may be at least partly due to diseased myocardial regions, and that the quantitative presence of these regions influences the propensity of the myocardial substrate to mechanisms of sudden death. A subsequent investigation of 64 other HCM patients by Saumarez and co-workers validated their initial investigation.[43] These conclusions also are supported by the aforementioned observations of sudden death in HCM patients without ventricular hypertrophy but with prominent disarray on autopsy.[24]

## Triggers for Sudden Death

Potential triggers for sudden death in HCM include supraventricular and ventricular arrhythmias, abnormal vascular responses, autonomic dysfunction, myocardial ischemia, and conduction disease involving the sinoatrial node, atrioventricular node, and the His-Purkinje system.[44] Although these events are common in other cardiac disorders, their effects may be magnified in HCM by the presence of diastolic impairment, underlying myocardial ischemia, myocyte disarray, and myocardial fibrosis, all of which can reduce the threshold for ventricular arrhythmias.

## Arrhythmia

Polymorphic VT/VF represents the terminal arrhythmia in HCM, with sustained monomorphic VT being rare. Sustained monomorphic VT in HCM is usually associated with aneurysms,[45] which may arise from midcavity systolic obliteration and the resultant high apical intracavitary pressures.

Nonsustained VT, defined as bursts of 3 or more consecutive ventricular extrasystoles at a heart rate greater than 120 bpm, occurs in ~25% of HCM patients on ambulatory ECG recordings.[46] Nonsustained VT in HCM more commonly appears after 25 years of age, although its appearance in children and adolescents is more ominous. Early studies conducted at tertiary centers demonstrated that the presence of VT signifies an increased risk of sudden death with an annual mortality rate of 8%.[47,48] More recent reports from unselected nonreferral-based populations, however, have suggested that isolated, nonrepetitive episodes may carry a lower risk, particularly if these episodes occur asymptomatically.[49,50]

Suppression or reduction in the frequency of nonsustained VT has been associated with improvement in prognosis. McKenna and co-workers first demonstrated this effect through the use of amiodarone in low doses (200–300 mg/day).[51,52] Twenty-one consecutive HCM patients with VT were treated with amiodarone and compared to the previous 24 consecutive HCM patients with VT who received therapy with conventional antiarrhythmics (mainly beta blockers, disopyramide, mexiletine, or quinidine). During a 3-year follow-up, none of the patients who had been treated with amiodarone died, while death occurred in 5 of the patients in the conventional therapy group (Figure 8). Cecchi and co-workers, in a separate investigation, noted similar survival (<1%) between patients without VT and patients with multiple repetitive episodes of VT who were treated with amiodarone (220 mg/day).[53]

Supraventricular tachyarrhythmias are evident in 15–20% of adolescents and adults with HCM.[7] In addition to the associated embolic risk, these electrical disturbances carry significant morbidity due to the tachycardia-related impairment of ventricular filling, which may be exaggerated in HCM because of preexisting diastolic dysfunction. Several reports have documented cardiovascular deterioration following the onset of such rhythms, particularly in the presence of accessory ventricular pathways.[54,55] Supraventricular arrhythmias may be more common in patients who die of

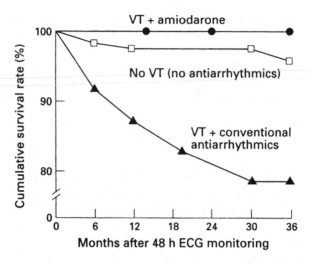

Figure 8. Cumulative survival rate for patients with nonsustained ventricular tachycardia treated with amiodarone (●), patients with nonsustained ventricular tachycardia treated with conventional antiarrhythmics (▲), and patients without nonsustained VT (□). (Reproduced with permission from McKenna et al.[38])

sudden death (33%) than in those who do not (10–18%).[5,48] This difference, however, has not been found to be statistically significant, possibly due to other modifying factors (e.g., propensity for hemodynamic collapse).

## Abnormal Vascular Response

In approximately one-third of HCM patients, the blood pressure fails to rise appropriately and remain sustained during exercise.[56] This abnormality occurs despite a proper rise in cardiac output and is due to an exaggerated fall in systemic vascular resistance. Inappropriate vasodilation of nonexercising vascular beds has been documented, suggesting that the abnormal response is due to premature withdrawal of sympathetic tone and is possibly related to ventricular mechanoreceptor activation.[57] The presence of heightened mechanoreceptor sensitivity may explain the poor tolerance of supraventricular tachyarrhythmias in some patients. We have observed the tolerance of fast atrial fibrillation in patients with severe hypertrophy and a normal vascular response to exercise, but prompt clinical deterioration from slow atrial fibrillation in patients with mild hypertrophy and an abnormal vascular response.

A prospective study of 161 consecutive HCM patients with an abnormal vascular response to exercise demonstrated the prognostic significance of this clinical risk factor.[58] These patients (mean age, 27 years; range, 8–40 years) underwent maximal, symptom-limited treadmill exercise off cardioactive medications and were followed for a mean of 44 months. An abnormal vascular response was defined as a fall in systolic blood pressure >20 mm Hg during exercise or the failure of the systolic blood pressure to rise >20 mm Hg by peak exercise. Of note, lethal arrhythmias related to exercise were not found in any of the study patients. For the end-point of sudden death, the presence of an abnormal vascular response had a sensitivity of 75%, a specificity of 66%, a positive predictive accuracy of 15%, and a negative predictive accuracy of 97%. Patients with an abnormal vascular response had reduced survival with ~75% being alive after 60 months (Figure 9). In contrast, ~95% of those with normal vascular response were alive over the same time period. The association of an adverse prognosis with an abnormal vascular response to exercise has also been found in patients with myocardial ischemia and aortic stenosis, supporting the role of hemodynamic instability in mechanisms of sudden death.[59,60] Furthermore, because nonsustained VT is relatively infrequent in young patients with HCM (~10%), several authors have concluded that such instability may predominate over primary arrhythmias as the mechanism of sudden death in these patients.[61]

## Myocardial Ischemia

Patients with HCM are prone to myocardial ischemia due to inherent imbalances in myocardial oxygen supply and demand, which may trigger sudden death through the promotion of nonhomogeneous conduction and repolarization abnormalities. Postmorten studies have shown abnormally small intramural arteries in areas of extensive myocardial fibrosis,[62,63] suggesting another mechanism by which myocardial ischemia may lead to lethal arrhythmias in HCM. ST segment depression, despite a normal coronary angiogram, occurs in 25% of these patients during ambulatory ECG monitoring and in 40% during exercise testing.[64,65]

Several anecdotal reports have observed ST segment depression in association with sinus tachycardia to immediately precede sudden death in HCM.[13,16,17] These reports constitute a significant proportion of the published cases of monitored sudden death. The significance of myocardial ischemia in HCM has been examined most commonly with stress (dipyridamole or exercise) thallium-201 nuclear scanning. Reversible thallium defects are evident in 25–40% of HCM patients.[66,67] Those HCM patients with positive stress thallium studies are more likely to have nonsustianed VT on an ambulatory ECG, syncope, and a history of prior cardiac arrest.[61] Follow-up data also point to an association between reversible thallium defects and "soft" cardiac events, such as supraventricular arrhythmias, cardiac dilatation, conduction abnormalities, and further symptoms of angina or syncope.[68]

Nonetheless, the role of myocardial ischemia in sudden death due to

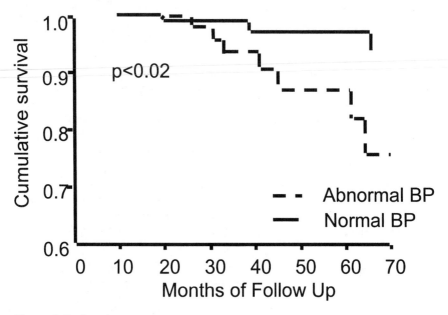

Figure 9. Reduced survival in patients with an abnormal blood pressure (BP) response to exercise. Solid line indicates patients with a normal BP response; dotted line indicates patients with an abnormal ABPR. (Reproduced with permission from Sadoul et al.[58])

HCM may be only in concert with other mechanisms. Fixed and reversible thallium defects do not appear to be related directly to cardiac mortality in HCM, although the studies conducted thus far may have been confounded by the use of amiodarone in high-risk patients during follow-up.[69] Discontinuation of amiodarone for the purposes of such a study may not be possible for ethical reasons. Of note, the treatment of HCM patients with anti-ischemic drugs (i.e., beta blockers and calcium channel blockers) has also not been shown to improve prognosis in HCM.

## Autonomic Dysfunction

Imbalance of sympathovagal tone carries an increased risk of sudden death and overall mortality for patients with heart failure and/or recent myocardial infarction.[70–72] A proportion of patients with HCM also exhibit autonomic derangements, which, among other mechanisms, may lead to death through the precipitation of hypotension, myocardial ischemia, and ventriuclar arrhythmias.

Thomson and co-workers recently investigated 29 patients with HCM (7 with syncope) for evidence of autonomic dysfunction.[73] In this study, forearm vascular resistance (FVR) was examined during the application of lower body negative pressure. The authors observed a lower mean increase in FVR in HCM patients (2.3 U) than in controls (12.3 U), and a fall in FVR in those HCM patients with a history of syncope (mean fall, 4.9 U). These results, which are similar to the observations of vasodilation of nonexercising vascular beds, suggest paradoxical activation of ventricular mechanoreceptors in response to the unloading of central filling pressures. Similarly, other studies have demonstrated reflex hypotension during head-up tilt (with isoproterenol augmentation) in syncopal HCM patients,[74] although the sensitivity and specificity of this test has been challenged.[75]

Diminished heart rate variability during short-term (deep breathing and Valsalva maneuvers)[76] and long-term (24-hour ambulatory ECG) assessment also has been noted.[77–79] Some investigations have suggested that blunted heart rate variability may be more common in HCM patients with outflow tract obstruction,[77] symptoms of dyspnea or chest pain, and supraventricular arrhythmias or nonsustained VT.[79] Although an increased risk of sudden death may be inferred with these observations, the prognostic value of heart rate variability itself has not been demonstrated.[79] This lack of correlation may be due to the prolonged periods of time used in its measurement. Events of importance in mechanisms of sudden death in HCM may occur sporadically and not be reflected through these assessments.

## Risk Stratification

The most important challenge in the management of HCM is the identification of those persons at risk of sudden death. The inheritable fashion of the disorder and the relative ease with which HCM patients can be identified (i.e., electrocardiography and echocardiography) warrants the cardiac screening of at least all first-degree relatives of these patients. The goals of such screening are (1) to identify afflicted individuals; (2) to perform risk stratification in order to reassure those patients with a favorable prognosis; and (3) to be able to intervene therapeutically once risk stratification has identified those patients at increased risk.

Established risk factors for sudden death in HCM include prior cardiac arrest, nonsustained VT on an ambulatory ECG, abnormal vascular response to exercise, positive family history for sudden death due to HCM, massive left ventricular hypertrophy, and recurrent, unexplained syncope.[31] Youth at clinical presentation also is a proposed risk factor, although its use requires the differentiation of those patients who present on their own accord (e.g., due to symptoms) from those patients who are being seen due to aggressive family screening. The association of certain sarcomeric mutations with an adverse prognosis also carries potential for risk stratification. The considerable time and technical expertise required for genotype analysis, however, currently limits its use to the confines of research institutions. Moreover, each of the other risk factors for sudden death in HCM can be obtained through simple, noninvasive means, facilitating their broad application to the HCM patient population. Due to the clinical heterogeneity of HCM, the positive predictive power of each factor alone is relatively low, but their presence in combination helps to recognize those patients at increased risk. Perhaps more importantly, their collective absence of suggests a benign prognosis.

The use of programmed ventricular stimulation for risk assessment in HCM has been proposed. In protocols using 3 or more premature ventricular stimuli to either the left or the right ventricle, approximately 40% of HCM patients have either sustained polymorphic VT or VF.[80–83] These inducible arrhythmias are more common in patients with a history of cardiac arrest or syncope, and may be associated with reduced survival. Nonetheless, several reservations about the utility of programmed ventricular stimulation do exist. Nearly three-fourths of HCM patients require at least 3 premature ventricular stimuli to demonstrate the presence of a sustained ventricular arrhythmia. These aggressive protocols can lead to a disproportionate number of false positive tests, as this compromise has been demonstrated in other cardiac disorders. Because of the reduced sensitivity of less aggressive protocols and the considerable loss of specificity with more aggressive techniques, electrophysiology studies do not add to the knowledge gained from current noninvasive, risk-stratification studies. Furthermore, the inducible arrhythmias in about three-fourths of HCM patients are polymorphic VT and VF rather than sustained monomorphic VT. The presence of sustained monomorphic VT may be more related to sudden death risk than other inducible ventricular arrhythmias. Of further concern is the safety of programmed ventricular stimulation in patients with HCM. These patients often demonstrate hemodynamic collapse during a ventricular arrhythmia and can be difficult to resuscitate due to the inherent properties of the myocardial substrate. The questionable utility of programmed ventricular stimulation in HCM patients, therefore, currently restricts its application in risk stratification.

Because the presence of 2 or more risk factors confers an annual mortality rate of 2–4%, the current policy at this institution is that their presence warrants consideration of either low-dose amiodarone therapy or the placement of an implantable cardioverter-defibrillator (ICD). This approach is based on evidence from several investigations that have pointed to the therapeutic effect and safety of low-dose amiodarone, particularly in HCM patients who have multiple or prolonged episodes of nonsustained VT, and recent studies that have documented successful resuscitation from out-of-hospital cardiac arrest by ICDs in HCM.[12,83,84] Amiodarone not only promotes electrical stability of the myocardium, but also has beneficial negative inotropic and coronary vasodilatory properties.[85,86] Although early studies highlighted the potential toxicity of amiodarone, evidence from large observational trials has concluded that severe side effects of amiodarone are rare and not associated with increased mortality.[87] Furthermore, the efficacy of low-dose amiodarone also has been established for the treatment of supraventricular tachyarrhythmias, which are common in HCM.[88,89] Nonetheless, it is clear failures do occur in HCM with both amiodarone[18,20,90] and ICDs (Prof. Borggrefe, personal communication). Anecdotal evidence suggests that these failures commonly occur in patients with disease due to mutations in the cardiac troponin T gene. Furthermore, ICDs are limited by their costs and their invasiveness, which may not be desirable to some patients. ICDs also carry social stigmata that may also have occupational implications. Evaluations of further follow-up after ICD placement should clarify its utility in HCM.

Risk stratification in HCM does have inherent limitations. HCM is a clinically heterogeneous disorder, in which sudden death likely occurs due to multiple mechanisms. This heterogeneity poses problems for the broad application of conventional risk factors. Criticism directed at approaches to risk stratification in HCM has also raised the issue of the referral bias of the institutions where these risk factors have been delineated. Increased cardiac screening of proband relatives and other community-based populations (e.g., athletes) have found higher prevalence rates of HCM than previously thought, and that many of these affected persons are asymptomatic and otherwise would have gone undiagnosed. The preclinical diagnosis of a number of otherwise healthy individuals through molecular studies also points to this likelihood. Risk stratification in HCM, nonetheless, currently relies on data from tertiary referral due to the requirement for large databases of affected patients in the evaluation of potential risk factors. Data from current cardiac screening programs are becoming available, and these should help in risk assessment across all populations of HCM patients.

## Conclusions

Multiple mechanisms are likely to be responsible for the pathogenesis of sudden death in HCM. Current evidence points to the importance of an altered myocardial substrate and the propensity for hemodynamic collapse in the events leading to sudden death. Useful noninvasive measures for risk assessment include clinical history, ambulatory ECG monitoring, echocardiography, and exercise testing. Genotype analysis also represents a future area of risk stratification. The combined use of the established clinical risk factors aids in the recognition of those patients at increased risk for sudden death, while their collective absence points to a favorable prognosis.

## References

1. Maron BJ, Peterson EE, Maron MS, et al. Prevalence of hypertrophic cardiomyopathy in an outpatient population referred for echocardiographic study. Am J Cardiol 1994; 73:577–580.

378 • Fighting Sudden Cardiac Death: A Worldwide Challenge

2. Codd MB, Sugrue DD, Gersh BJ, et al. Epidemiology of idiopathic dilated and hypertrophic cardiomyopathy: a population based study in Olmstead County, Minnesota, 1975–84. Circulation 1989; 80:564–572.
3. Maron BJ, Gardin JM, Flack JM, et al. Prevalence of hypertrophic cardiomyopathy in a population of young adults: echocardiographic analysis of 4111 subjects in the CARDIA study: Coronary Artery Risk Development in Young Adults. Circulation 1995; 92:785–789.
4. Savage DD, Castelli WP, Abbott RD, et al. Hypertrophic cardiomyopathy and its markers in the general population: the great masquerader revisited: The Framingham Study. J Cardiovasc Ultrason 1983; 2:41–47.
5. McKenna WJ, Deanfield J, Faruqui A, et al. Prognosis in hypertrophic cardiomyopathy: role of age and clinical, electrocardiographic and hemodynamic features. Am J Cardiol 1981; 47:532–538.
6. McKenna WJ, Deanfield JE. Hypertrophic cardiomyopathy: an important cause of sudden death. Arch Dis Child 1984; 59:971–975.
7. McKenna WJ, Franklin RCG, Nihoyannopoulos P, et al. Arrhythmia and prognosis in infants, children and adolescents with hypertrophic cardiomyopathy. J Am Coll Cardiol 1988; 11:147–153.
8. Maron BJ, Kogan J, Proschan MA, et al. Circadian variability in the occurrence of sudden cardiac death in patients with hypertrophic cardiomyopathy. J Am Coll Cardiol 1994; 23:1405–1409.
9. Maron BJ, Roberts WC, Epstein SE. Sudden death in hypertrophic cardiomyopathy: a profile of 78 patients. Circulation 1982; 65: 1388–1394.
10. Watkins H, Rosenzweig A, Hwang DS, et al. Characteristics and prognostic implications of myosin missense mutations in familial hypertrophic cardiomyopathy. N Engl J Med 1992; 326:1108–1114.
11. Watkins H, McKenna WJ, Thierfelder L, et al. Mutations in the genes for cardiac troponin T and α-tropomyosin in hypertrophic cardiomyopathy. N Engl J Med 1995; 332:1058–1064.
12. Elliott PM, Sharma A, Varnava A, et al. Survival after cardiac arrest or sustained ventricular tachycardia in patients with hypertrophic cardiomyopathy. J Am Coll Cardiol 1999; 33:1590–1595.
13. Nicod P, Polikar R, Peterson KL. Hypertrophic cardiomyopathy and sudden death. N Engl J Med 1988; 318:1255–1257.
14. Bernstein SB, Shandling AH. Hypertrophic cardiomyopathy and sudden death. N Engl J Med 1988; 319:1091.
15. Losordo DW, Kosowsky BD. Hypertrophic cardiomyopathy and sudden death. N Engl J Med 1988; 319:1091.
16. Fananapazir L, Epstein SE. Hemodynamic and electrophysiologic evaluation of patients with hypertrophic cardiomyopathy surviving cardiac arrest. Am J Cardiol 1991; 67:280–287.
17. Sato M, Takenaka K, Yamashita T, et al. Sudden death during Holter electrocardiographic monitoring in a patient with hypertrophic cardiomyopathy. J Cardiol 1998; 31:297–303.
18. Mercereau D, Kubac G, Klinke WP. Failure of amiodarone to prevent ventricular fibrillation (sudden death) in hypertrophic cardiomyopathy. Can J Cardiol 1989; 5:77–80.
19. Gardin LL, Nanton MA, Hanna BD. Ambulatory monitoring of the sudden death of an adolescent with hypertrophic cardiomyopathy. Can J Cardiol 1994; 10:548–550.
20. Gilligan DM, Missouris CG, Boyd MJ, et al. Sudden death due to ventricular tachycardia during amiodarone therapy in familial hypertrophic cardiomyopathy. Am J Cardiol 1991; 68:971–973.

21. Teare D. Asymmetrical hypertrophy of the heart in young adults. Br Heart J 1958; 20:1–8.
22. Davies MJ. The current status of myocardial disarray in hypertrophic cardiomyopathy. Br Heart J 1984; 51:361–374.
23. Maron BJ. Hypertrophic cardiomyopathy. Curr Probl Cardiol 1993; 18:639.
24. McKenna WJ, Stewart JT, Nihoyannopoulos P, et al. Hypertrophic cardiomyopathy without hypertrophy: two families with myocardial disarray in the absence of increased myocardial mass. Br Heart J 1990; 63:287–290.
25. Maron BJ, Epstein SE, Roberts WC. Hypertrophic cardiomyopathy and transmural infarction without significant atherosclerosis of the extramural coronary arteries. Am J Cardiol 1979; 43:1086–1102.
26. Factor SM, Butany J, Sole MJ, et al. Pathological fibrosis and matrix connective tissue in the subaortic myocardium of patients with hypertrophic cardiomyopathy. J Am Coll Cardiol 1991; 17:1343–1351.
27. Schwartzkopff B, Mundhenke M, Strauer BE. Alterations of the architecture of subendocardial arterioles in patients with hypertrophic cardiomyopathy and impaired coronary vasodilator reserve: a possible cause for myocardial ischemia. J Am Coll Cardiol 1998; 31:1089–1096.
28. Tanaka M, Fujiwara H, Onodera T, et al. Quantitative analysis of narowing of intramyocardial small arteries in normal hearts, hypertensive hearts, and hearts with hypertrophic cardiomyopathy. Circulation 1987; 75:1130–1139.
29. Yetman AT, McCrindle BW, MacDonald C, et al. Myocardial bridging in children with hypertrophic cardiomyopathy: a risk factor for sudden death. N Engl J Med 1998: 339:1201–1209.
30. Maron BJ, Bonow RO, Cannon RO III, et al. Hypertrophic cardiomyopathy: interrelations of clinical manifestations, pathophysiology, and therapy. N Engl J Med 1987; 316:780–789, 844–852.
31. Spirito P, Seidman CE, McKenna WJ, et al. The management of hypertrophic cardiomyopathy. N Engl J Med 1997; 336:775–785.
32. Mogensen J, Klausen IC, Pedersen AK, et al. α-Cardiac actin is a novel disease gene in familial hypertrophic cardiomyopathy. J Clin Invest 1999; 103:R39–R43.
33. Poetter K, Jiang H, Hassanzadeh S, et al. Mutations in either the essential or regulatory light chains of myosin are associated with a rare myopathy in human heart and skeletal muscles. Nature Genet 1996; 13:63–69.
34. Kimura A, Harada H, Park J-E, et al. Mutations in the cardiac troponin I gene associated with hypertrophic cardiomyopathy. Nature Genet 1997; 16:379–382.
35. Epstein ND, Cohn GM, Cyran F, et al. Differences in clinical expression of hypertrophic cardiomyopathy associated with two distinct mutations in the β-myosin heavy chain gene. Circulation 1992; 86:345–352.
36. Marian AJ, Mares A Jr, Kelly DP, et al. Sudden cardiac death in hypertrophic cardiomyopathy: variability in phenotypic expression of β-myosin heavy chain mutations. Europ Heart J 1995; 16:368–376.
37. Anan R, Greve G, Thierfelder L, et al. Prognostic implications of novel β cardiac myosin heavy chain gene mutations that cause familial hypertrophic cardiomyopathy. J Clin Invest 1994; 93:280–285.
38. Charron P, Dubourg O, Desnos M, et al. Genotype-phenotype correlations in familial hypertrophic cardiomyopathy: a comparison between mutations in the cardiac protein-C and the beta-myosin heavy chain genes. Europ Heart J 1998; 19:139–145.
39. Fananazapir L, Epstein ND. Genotype-phenotype correlations in hypertrophic cardiomyopathy. Circulation 1994; 89:22–32.
40. Nimura H, Bachinski LL, Sangwatanaroj S, et al. Mutations in the gene for car-

diac myosin-binding protein C and late-onset familial hypertrophic cardiomy-opathy. N Engl J Med 1998; 338:1248–1257.

41. Coviello DA, Maron BJ, Spirito P, et al. Clinical features of hypertrophic car-diomyopathy caused by mutation of a "hot spot" in the alpha-tropomyosin gene. J Am Coll Cardiol 1997; 29:635–640.

42. Saumarez RC, Camm AJ, Panagos A, et al. Ventricular fibrillation in hyper-trophic cardiomyopathy is associated with increased fractionation of paced right ventricular electrograms. Circulation 1992; 86:467–474.

43. Saumarez RC, Slade AKB, Grace AA, et al. The significance of paced electro-gram fractionation in hypertrophic cardiomyopathy: a prospective study. Cir-culation 1995; 91:2762–2768.

44. Maron BJ, Fananapazir L. Sudden cardiac death in hypertrophic cardiomy-opathy. Circulation 1992; 85:(Suppl I):57–63.

45. Mantica M, Della Bella P, Arean V. Hypertrophic cardiomyopathy with apical aneurysm: a case of catheter and surgical therapy of sustained monomorphic ventricular tachycardia. Heart 1997; 77:481–483.

46. McKenna WJ, Chetty S, Oakley CM, et al. Arrhythmia in hypertrophic car-diomyopathy: exercise and 48-hour ambulatory electrocardiographic assessment with and without beta adrenergic blocking therapy. Am J Cardiol 1980; 45:1–5.

47. Maron BJ, Savage DD, Wolfson JK, et al. Prognostic significance of 24-hour am-bulatory electrocardiographic monitoring in patients with hypertrophic car-diomyopathy: a prospective study. Am J Cardiol 1981; 48:252–257.

48. McKenna WJ, England D, Doi YL, et al. Arrhythmia in hypertrophic car-diomyopathy I: influence on prognosis. Br Heart J 1981; 46:168–172.

49. Spirito P, Rapezzi C, Autore C, et al. Prognosis of asymptomatic patients with hypertrophic cardiomyopathy and nonsustained ventricular tachycardia. Cir-culation 1994; 90:2743–2747.

50. Cecchi F, Olivotto I, Montereggi A, et al. Prognostic value of non-sustained ven-tricular tachycardia and the potential role of amiodarone treatment in hyper-trophic cardiomyopathy: assessment in an unselected non-referral based pa-tient population. Heart 1998; 79:331–336.

51. McKenna WJ, Harris L, Rowland E, et al. Amiodarone for long-term manage-ment of patients with hypertrophic cardiomyopathy. Am J Cardiol 1984; 54:802–810.

52. McKenna J, Oakley CM, Krikler DM, et al. Improved survival with amiodarone in patients with hypertrophic cardiomyopathy and ventricular tachycardia. Br Heart J 1985; 53:412–416.

53. Cecchi F, Olivotto I, Montereggi A, et al. Prognostic value of non-sustained ventricular tachycardia and the potential role of amiodarone treatment in hy-pertrophic cardiomyopathy: assessment in an unselected non-referral based patient population. Heart 1998; 79:331–336.

54. Madariaga I, Carmona JR, Mateas FR, et al. Supraventricular arrhythmia as the cause of sudden death in hypertrophic cardiomyopathy. Eur Heart J 1994; 15:134–137.

55. Favale S, Di Biase M, Rizzo U, et al. Ventricular fibrillation induced by trans-esophageal atrial pacing in hypertrophic cardiomyopathy. Eur Heart J 1987; 8:912–916.

56. Frenneaux MP, Counihan PJ, Caforio ALP, et al. Abnormal blood pressure re-sponse during exercise in hypertrophic cardiomyopathy. Circulation 1990; 82:1995–2002.

57. Counihan PJ, Frenneaux MP, Webb DJ, et al. Abnormal vascular responses to supine exercise in hypertrophic cardiomyopathy. Circulation 1991; 84:686–696.

Hypertrophic Cardiomyopathy and Sudden Death • 381

58. Sadoul N, Prasad K, Elliott PM, et al. Prospective assessment of blood pressure response as a marker of risk of sudden death in hypertrophic cardiomyopathy. Circulation 1997; 96:2987–2991.
59. Lele SS, Scalia G, Thomson HL, et al. Mechanism of exercise hypotension in patients with ischemic heart disease: role of neurocardiogenically medicated vasodilation. Circulation 1994; 90:2701–2709.
60. Mark AL, Kioschos JM, Abboud FM, et al. Abnormal vascular responses in patients with aortic stenosis. J Clin Invest 1973; 52:1385–1394.
61. Dilsizian V, Bonow RO, Epstein SE, et al. Myocardial ischemia detected by thallium scintigraphy is frequently related to cardiac arrest and syncope in young patients with hypertrophic cardiomyopathy. J Am Coll Cardiol 1993; 22:796–804.
62. Maron BJ, Wolfson JK, Epstein SE, et al. Intramural ("small vessel") coronary artery disease in hypertrophic cardiomyopathy. J Am Coll Cardiol 1986; 8:545.
63. Tanaka M, Fujiwara H, Onodera T, et al. Quantitative analysis of narrowings of intramyocardial small arteries in normal hearts, hypertensive hearts, and hearts with hypertrophic cardiomyopathy. Circulation 1987; 75:1130–1139.
64. Elliott PM, Kaski JC, Prasad K, et al. Chest pain during daily life in patients with hypertrophic cardiomyopathy: an ambulatory electrocardiographic study. Eur Heart J 1996; 17:1056–1064.
65. Cannon RO, Dilsizian V, O'Gara P, et al. Myocardial metabolic, hemodynamic, and electrocardiographic significance of reversible thallium-201 abnormalities in hypertrophic cardiomyopathy. Circulation 1991; 83:1660–1667.
66. Pitcher D, Wainwright R, Maisey M, et al. Assessment of chest pain in hypertrophic cardiomyopathy using exercise thallium-201 myocardial scintigraphy. Br Heart J 1980; 44:650–665.
67. Von Dohlen TW, Prisant LM, Frank MJ. Significance of positive or negative thallium-201 scintigraphy in hypertrophic cardiomyopathy. Am J Cardiol 1989; 64:498–503.
68. Lazzeroni E, Picano E, Morozzi L, et al. Dipyridamole-induced ischemia as a prognostic marker of future adverse cardiac events in adult patients with hypertrophic cardiomyopathy. Circulation 1997; 96:4268–4272.
69. Yamada M, Elliott PM, Kaski JC, et al. Dipyridamole stress thallium-201 perfusion abnormalities in patients with hypertrophic cardiomyopathy. Relationship to clinical presentation and outcome. Eur Heart J 1998; 19:500–07.
70. Farrel TG, Bashir Y, Cripps T, et al. Risk stratification for arrhythmic events in postinfarction patients based on heart rate variability, ambulatory electrocardiographic variables and the signal-averaged electrocardiogram. J Am Coll Cardiol 1991; 18:687–97.
71. Kleiger RE, Miller JP, Bigger JT, et al. Decreased heart rate variability and its association with increased mortality after acute myocardial infarction. Am J Cardiol 1987; 59:256–62.
72. Stein PK, Bosner MS, Kleiger RE, et al. Heart rate variability: a measure of cardiac autonomic tone. Am Heart J 1994; 127:1376–81.
73. Thomson HL, Thurgood-Morris J, Atherton J, et al. Reduced cardiopulmonary baroreflex sensitivity in patients with hypertrophic cardiomyopathy. J Am Coll Cardiol 1998; 31:1377–1382.
74. Gilligan DM, Nihoyannopoulos P, Chan WL, et al. Investigation of a hemodynamic basis for syncope in hypertrophic cardiomyopathy: use of a head-up tilt test. Circulation 1992; 85:2140–2148.
75. Sneddon JF, Slade A, Seo H, et al. Assessment of the diagnostic value of head-up tilt testing in the evaluation of syncope in hypertrophic cardiomyopathy. Am J Cardiol 1994; 73:601–604.

76. Gilligan DM, Chan WL, Sbarouni E, et al. Autonomic function in hypertrophic cardiomyopathy. Br Heart J 1993; 69:525–629.
77. Limbruno U, Strata G, Zucchi R, et al. Altered autonomic cardiac control in hypertrophic cardiomyopathy: role of outflow tract obstruction and myocardial hypertrophy. Eur Heart J 1998; 19:146–153.
78. Tanabe T, Iwamoto T, Fusegawa Y, et al. Alterations of sympathovagal balance in patients with hypertrophic and dilated cardiomyopathies assessed by spectral analysis of RR interval variability. Eur Heart J 1995; 16:799–807.
79. Counihan PJ, Fei L, Bashir Y, et al. Assessment of heart rate variability in hypertrophic cardiomyopathy: association with clinical and prognostic features. Circulation 1993; 88(Part 1):1682–1690.
80. Kuck K-H, Kunze K-P, Schluter M, et al. Programmed electrical stimulation in hypertrophic cardiomyopathy: results in patients with and without cardiac arrest or syncope. Eur Heart J 1988; 9:177–185.
81. Watson RM, Schwartz JL, Maron BJ, et al. Inducible polymorphic ventricular tachycardia and ventricular fibrillation in a subgroup of patients with hypertrophic cardiomyopathy at high risk for sudden death. J Am Coll Cardiol 1987; 10:761–774.
82. Fananapazir L, Chang AC, Epstein SE, et al. Prognostic determinants in hypertrophic cardiomyopathy: prognostic evaluation of a therapeutic strategy based on clinical, Holter, hemodynamic, and electrophysiological findings. Circulation 1992; 86:730–740.
83. Zhu DWX, Sun H, Hill R, et al. The value of electrophysiology study and prophylactic implantation of cardioverter defibrillator in patients with hypertrophic cardiomyopathy. PACE 1998; 21:299–302.
84. Primo J, Geelen P, Brugada J, et al. Hypertrophic cardiomyopathy: role of the implantable cardioverter-defibrillator. J Am Coll Cardiol 1998; 31:1081–1085.
85. Singh BN, Vaughan Williams EM. The effect of amiodarone, a new anti-anginal drug on cardiac muscle. Br J Pharmacol 1970; 39:657–667.
86. Meyer BJ, Amann FN. Additional antianginal efficacy of amiodarone in patients with limiting angina pectoris. Am Heart J 1993; 125:996–1001.
87. Podrid PJ. Amiodarone: reevaluation of an old drug. Ann Int Med 1995; 122:689–700.
88. Nolan PE Jr, Nappi J, Pollak PT. Clinical efficacy of amiodarone. Pharmacotherapy 1998; 18(6 Pt 2):127S–137S.
89. Singh B. Antiarrhythmic actions of amiodarone: a profile of a paradoxical agent. 1996; 78:41–53.
90. Fananapazir L, Leon MB, Bonow RO, et al. Sudden death during empiric amiodarone therapy in symptomatic hypertrophic cardiomyopathy. Am J Cardiol 1991; 67:169–174.
91. Maron BJ, Cecchi F, McKenna WJ. Risk factors and stratification for sudden cardiac death in patients with hypertrophic cardiomyopathy. Br Heart J 1994; 72(Suppl):S13–S18.
92. Seidman CE, Seidman JG. Gene mutations that cause familial hypertrophic cardiomyopathy. In: Haber E (ed). Molecular Cardiovascular Medicine. Scientific American, NY, 1995, pp 193–209.
93. Saumarez RC. Electrophysiological investigation of patients with hypertrophic cardiomyopathy: evidence that slowed intraventricular conduction is associated with an increased risk of sudden death. Br Heart J 1994; 72(Suppl):S19–23.

# 26

# Prevention of Sudden Cardiac Death in Hypertrophic Cardiomyopathies

*Riccardo Cappato, MD*

## Introduction

Hypertrophic cardiomyopathy (HCM) is a clinical syndrome characterized by ventricular hypertrophy in the absence of an obvious cause and hyperdynamic ventricular function.[1] In the usual case, myocardial stiffness is increased and results in abnormal diastolic relaxation.[2] This abnormality in diastolic relaxation produces increased left ventricular end-diastolic pressure with resulting pulmonary congestion and dyspnea, the most common clinical findings in patients with HCM. Mechanical obstruction to intracardiac flow may occur in about 25% of patients secondary to asymmetric hypertrophy, with the left ventricular septal wall being thicker than the left ventricular free wall, and abnormal systolic anterior motion of the mitral valve against the hypertrophied septum.[1,3]

Although the cause of hypertrophic cardiomyopathy remains unknown, recent data suggest the presence of a link between specific features of HCM and abnormal myocardial calcium kinetics.[1,4] In particular, an increased number of calcium channels associated with abnormal transmembrane calcium fluxes would result in increased intracellular calcium concentrations;[5,6] this in turn may produce hypertrophy and disarray in an as yet undefined process.

HCM appears to be genetically transmitted in about half of the patients as an autosomal dominant trait with identified diseased loci in at least 4 different chromosomes (chromosomes 1,11,14,15).[7,8] The cause of HCM in the remainder of patients is unknown.

Distinction of HCM from a variety of conditions presenting similar gross morphological features may sometimes be difficult; among them are

From: Aliot E, Clementy J, Prystowsky EN (editors). *Fighting Sudden Cardiac Death: A Worldwide Challenge.* ©Futura Publishing Company, Armonk, NY, 2000.

the athlete's heart, myocardial hypertrophy secondary to systemic hypertension or aortic stenosis, hyperparathyroidism, infants of diabetic mothers, neurofibromatosis, generalized lipodystrophy, lentiginosis, pheocrocytoma, Friedrich's ataxia, and Noonan's syndrome.[9,10]

The overall prevalence of HCM in the general population is between 0.02% and 0.2%;[11-13] in most patients, symptoms are absent or mild and clinical deterioration is usually slow, with the percentage of severely symptomatic patients increasing with age.[14] The annual mortality is about 3% in adults seen in large referral centers[15] but probably is closer to 1% when all patients with HCM are included.[16-18] The risk of sudden death is higher in children,[19] and HCM accounts for about one-third of fatal cases in younger competitive athletes in the United States.[20-22]

A variety of conditions may precipitate death in HCM, including myocardial ischemia, congestive heart failure, bradyarrhythmias, tachyarrhythmias (supraventricular and ventricular), and mechanical obstruction to left ventricular cardiac flow. Although peripheral cardiovascular collapse may occur in response to each condition, it may play a primary role in precipitating death in subgroups of patients. Effort-related death mainly accounts for death in younger HCM patients and occurs as a consequence of severe myocardial ischemia, sustained ventricular arrhythmias, and mechanical obstruction to left ventricular cardiac flow. In contrast, death in adult patients occurs as a consequence of late left ventricular dilation observed during long-term follow-up in a minority of patients (10–15%) and leading to congestive heart failure.[1,23] In summary, although death in HCM is a rare event, it may not infrequently occur as the first clinical symptom. In addition, death in HCM is mostly sudden in younger affected individuals, and competitive athletes unaware of their underlying condition likely represent the category at highest risk.

# How to Prevent Sudden Death in Patients with Hypertrophic Cardiomyopathy

The low prevalence of HCM, the low incidence of death among affected patients, and the different potential causes of death make it difficult to provide evidence-based criteria for effective prevention of sudden death in the individual case. In symptomatic patients, prior studies have shown that loss of consciousness is the only independent clinical predictor of future events during follow-up[24] and that mortality rates in this subgroup are still very low (about 9% after 5 years from the index event). Despite this observation, risk assessment in patients with HCM may reasonably be afforded by subdividing affected patients into 2 groups: (1) asymptomatic or mildly symptomatic patients; and (2) patients with symptoms of impaired consiousness. The first group also includes those individuals who are unaware of their disease and in whom identification of an underlying HCM is achieved during an occasional check-up.

## Asymptomatic or Mildly Symptomatic Patients

Because of the high prevalence of HCM among young competitive athletes dying suddenly during effort,[20-22] identification of the underlying disease at preparticipation screening and disqualification of affected individuals from further intense physical activity may substantially reduce their risk of sudden death during follow-up. This hypothesis was tested in a recent study by Corrado et al.[13] Based on a national program for systematic preparticipation screening of all young competitive athletes established in Italy approximately 20 years ago, the authors investigated the impact that disqualification of identified HCM patients had on their future risk of sudden death in the Veneto region. During the investigated time, the incidence of sudden death was 1.6 per 100,000 per year among competitive athletes and 0.75 per 100,000 among nonathletes 35 years of age or less (relative risk among athletes 2.1; confidence interval, 1.5 to 2.9). Out of 33,735 competitive athletes undergoing preparticipation screening, 22 were identified with HCM and disqualified from further physical activity. During the follow-up time, the prevalence of HCM among young nonathletes who died suddenly was similar in this study (7.3%) and in another population-based study performed by Burke et al.[21] in the United States (3%). In contrast, the prevalence of HCM among athletes who died suddenly was at 2%, which is markedly lower in the Italian study than it was at 24% in the American study. These data suggest that disqualification from further physical activity of identified patients with asymptomatic or mildly symptomatic HCM may substantially reduce the risk of sudden death during follow-up and indicate that a search for HCM should be mandatory in young people involved in competitive sport disciplines.

## Patients with Symptoms of Impaired Consciousness

In one of the largest collectives of HCM patients investigated prospectively, cardiac arrest, syncope, and presyncope were the strongest predictors of future cardiac events during long-term follow-up.[24] In patients with these symptoms at the time of referral for diagnostic and therapeutic assessment, the 5-year overall survival free of cardiac events (i.e., sudden death, cardiac arrest, or syncope) was more than 95% in patients without symptoms of impaired consciousness, about 90% in those with presyncope, about 75% in those with syncope, and less than 30% in patients surviving a cardiac arrest episode.[24] According to multivariate analysis, only 2 out of 31 investigated parameters were significant independent predictors of future cardiac events: (1) a history of cardiac arrest or syncope ($\beta$, 2.9); and (2) the inducibility of a sustained ventricular arrhythmia at programmed electrical stimulation ($\beta$, 3.5). In these subgroups of patients, the risk of future cardiac events was increased if they presented nonsustained ventricular tachycardia during 24-hour Holter monitoring.

Treatment of patients at increased risk of sudden death varies, depending on the cause leading to loss of consiousness. In a study by Fananapazir et al.[25] on cardiac arrest survivors with HCM, potential causes were found in all 30 patients and were multiple in 43%. Ventricular electrical instability, as defined by the presence of nonsustained ventricular tachycardia at Holter monitoring and/or sustained ventricular arrhythmia at programmed electrical stimulation, was found in 70% of patients; other causes included mechanical obstruction of the left ventricular outflow tract in 30%, bradyarrhythmias in 17%, myocardial ischemia associated with hypotension in 17%, and atrial tachycardia leading to hypotension in 13%. During 18 ± 19 months follow-up, 4 patients (13%) died suddenly, of which 3 had shown ventricular electrical instability and 1 had atrial tachycardia and hypotension. Of note, none of the victims with ventricular electrical instability had received an implantable cardioverter-defibrillator and no therapy was initiated in the 1 victim with atrial tachycardia. No deaths were reported in another 17 patients with ventricular electrical instability who underwent implantable cardioverter-defibrillator therapy and in another 3 patients with atrial tachycardia and hypotension who received effective antiarrhythmic drug treatment or radiofrequency current ablation. The use of amiodarone in these patients is controversial[26-30] and should be avoided in patients in whom, compared to baseline, a sustained ventricular arrhythmia is more easily or only inducible after drug loading.[31] Although not controlled, these data suggest that survivors of cardiac arrest with HCM should receive an implantable defibrillator unless correctable causes are found and effectively removed. This is further supported by data obtained in large collectives of patients with sustained ventricular arrhythmias and hemodynamic impairment.[32]

## Summary

HCM is a rare disease and affected individuals present with an overall low risk of death during long-term follow-up. In HCM patients, sudden death accounts for a variable percentage of all deaths and tends to decrease with older age; in particular, strenuous physical activity by young athletes may precipitate sudden death by different mechanisms. Identification of HCM by means of routine preparticipation screening is highly recommended and becomes mandatory for competitive athletes. Recognition of the disease and subsequent discontinuation of competitive, high- and middle-grade physical activity is likely to result in a substantial reduction of the risk of sudden death in these individuals.

In patients with HCM and syncope or cardiac arrest, curative or palliative therapy should be directed toward the removal or treatment of the precipitating cause. Among these patients, those with ventricular electrical vulnerability present the highest risk of future cardiac events during intermediate follow-up and should benefit from an implantable cardioverter-defibrillator.

## References

1. Maron BJ. Hypertrophic cardiomyopathy. Curr Probl Cardiol 1993; 18:639.
2. Braunwald E. Hypertrophic cardiomyopathy: continued progress. N Engl J Med 1989; 320:800.
3. Sherrid MV, Chu CK, Delia E, et al. An echocardiographic study of the fluid mechanics of obstruction in hypertrophic cardiomyopathy. J Am Coll Cardiol 1993; 22:816.
4. Sapp JL, Howlett SE. Density of ryanodine receptors is increased in sarcoplasmic reticulum from prehypertrophic cardiomyopathic hamster rat. J Mol Cell Cardiol 1994; 26:235.
5. Bonow RO. Left ventricular diastolic function in hypertrophic cardiomyopathy. Herz 1991; 16:13.
6. Wagner JA, Sax FL, Weisman HF, et al. Calcium-antagonist receptors in the atrial tissue of patients with hypertrophic cardiomyopathy. N Engl J Med 1989; 320:755.
7. Davies MJ, Krikler DM. Genetic investigation and counselling of families with hypertrophic cardiomyopathy. Br Heart J 1994; 72:99.
8. Watkins H. Multiple disease genes cause hypertrophic cardiomyopathy. Br Heart J 1994; 72:S4.
9. Davies MJ. Hypertrophic cardiomyopathy: one disease or several? Br Heart J 1990; 63:263.
10. Davies MJ, McKenna WJ. Hypertrophic cardiomyopathy: an introduction to pathology and pathogenesis. Br Heart J 1994; 72:S2.
11. Codd MB, Sugrue DD, Gersh BJ, Melton LJ III. Epidemiology of idiopathic dilated and hypertrophic cardiomyopathy: a population-based study in Olmsted county, Minnesota, 1975–1984. Circulation 1989; 80:564.
12. Maron BJ, Gardin JM, Flack JM, et al. Prevalence of hypertrophic cardiomyopathy in a general population of young adults: echocardiographic analysis of 4111 subjects in the CARDIA study. Circulation 1995; 92:785.
13. Corrado D, Basso C, Schiavon M, Thiene G. Screening for hypertrophic cardiomyopathy in young athletes. N Engl J Med 1998; 339:364.
14. McKenna WJ. The natural history of hypertrophic cardiomyopathy. Cardiovasc Clin 1988; 19:135.
15. Vassalli G, Seiler C, Hess OM. Risk stratification in hypertrophic cardiomyopathy. Curr Opin Cardiol 1994; 9:330.
16. Spirito P, Chiarella F, Caratino L, et al. Clinical course and prognosis of hypertrophic cardiomyopathy in an outpatient population. N Engl J Med 1989; 320:749.

17. Maron BJ, Spirito P. Impact of patient selection biases on the perception of hypertrophic cardiomyopathy and its natural history. Am J Cardiol 1993; 72:970.
18. Kofflard MJ, Waldstein DJ, Vos J, ten Cate FJ. Prognosis in hypertrophic cardiomyopathy observed in a large clinic population. Am J Cardiol 1993; 72:939.
19. Clark AL, Coats AJ. Screening for hypertrophic cardiomyopathy. Br Med J 1993; 306:409.
20. Maron BJ, Roberts WC, McAllister HA, et al. Sudden death in young athletes. Circulation 1980; 62:218.
21. Burke AP, Farb A, Virmani R, et al. Sports-related and non-sports-related sudden cardiac deaths in young adults. Am Heart J 1991; 121:568.
22. Maron BJ, Shirani J, Poliac LC, et al. Sudden death in young competitive athletes: clinical, demographic, and pathophysiological profiles. JAMA 1996; 276:199.
23. Spirito P, Bellone P. Natural history of hypertrophic cardiomyopathy. Br Heart J 1994; 72:S10.
24. Fananapazir L, Chang AC, Epstein SE, McAreavey D. Prognostic determinants in hypertrophic cardiomyopathy: prospective evaluation of a therapeutic strategy based on clinical, Holter, hemodynamic, and electrophysiological findings. Circulation 1992; 86:730.
25. Fananapazir L, Epstein SE. Hemodynamic and electrophysiologic evaluation of patients with hypertrophic cardiomyopathy surviving cardiac arrest. Am J Cardiol 1991; 67:280.
26. Almendral JM, Ormaetxe J, Martinez Alday JD, et al. Treatment of ventricular arrhythmias in hypertrophic cardiomyopathy. Eur Heart J 1993; 14:71S.
27. Clark AL, Coats AJ. Screening for hypertrophic cardiomyopathy. Br Med J 1993; 306:409.
28. DeRose JJ Jr, Banas JS Jr, Winters SL. Current perspectives on sudden cardiac death in hypertrophic cardiomyopathy. Prog Cardiovasc Dis 1994; 36:475.
29. Fananapazir L, Leon MB, Bonow RO, et al. Sudden death during empiric amiodarone therapy in hypertrophic cardiomyopathy. Am J Cardiol 1991; 67:169.
30. Gilligan DM, Missouris CG, Boyd MJ, Oakley CM. Sudden death due to ventricular tachycardia during amiodarone therapy in familial hypertrophic cardiomyopathy. Am J Cardiol 1991; 68:971.
31. Fananapazir L, Epstein SE. Value of electrophysiologic studies in hypertrophic cardiomyopathy treated with amiodarone. Am J Cardiol 1991; 61:175.
32. The Antiarrhythmic versus Implantable Defibrillators (AVID) Investigators. A comparison of antiarrhythmic drug therapy with implantable defibrillators in patients resuscitated from near-fatal ventricular arrhythmias. N Engl J Med 1997; 337:1576.

# 27

# The Implantable Cardioverter-Defibrillator As a Bridge to Transplantation: Is It Worthwhile?

*Antonio Raviele, MD*

## Introduction

Since the first human heart transplant more than 30 years ago, a great deal of progress has been made in this field, and heart transplantation is now regarded as an effective therapeutic option for patients with end-stage heart disease of various etiologies. Currently, about half of cardiac allograft recipients are still alive 10 years after transplantation and their quality of life is usually improved; exercise tolerance is good and side effects from immunosuppression are acceptable.[1-3] These results have led to a progressive broadening of the selection criteria and to an increase in the number of potential candidates for heart transplantation.[4] As consequence of this, and because of the relatively fixed supply of donor hearts, the average waiting time for heart transplantation has significantly lengthened in recent years[4-6] and has now reached 6–12 months for outpatients in some centers.[7] During this period, the risk of death is fairly high and a considerable number of subjects die while awaiting a donor heart, despite the use of pharmacological or mechanical support for circulation.[8-12]

The mortality rate of these patients has been reported by Stevenson et al. to be 22% after 6 months, 33% after 1 year, and 38% after 2 years of follow-up.[7] These figures are in agreement with other published data.[1,5,13] For example, in a meta-analysis regarding a total of 17,002 patients listed for heart transplantation, Schmidinger found a 27% overall mortality during a median follow-up of 14 months.[14] Similar results were observed by Narang et al. in a meta-analysis of 27 studies with a total of 10,137 subjects with advanced heart failure not listed for heart transplantation.[15] The 2-year mortality rate, in this meta-analysis, was 41% for patients in NYHA functional Class III or IV.[15]

From: Aliot E, Clementy J, Prystowsky EN (editors). *Fighting Sudden Cardiac Death: A Worldwide Challenge.* ©Futura Publishing Company, Armonk, NY, 2000.

Progressive pump failure is recognized as the most frequent cause of death among patients awaiting heart transplantation and accounts for more than 40% of all deaths.[14] Sudden death is also very common in these patients and is responsible for about 30% of cases.[14] The percentage of patients who die suddenly is particularly high in subjects with NYHA functional Class III: 61% compared with 21% among NYHA functional Class IV patients.[16] It is noteworthy that the etiology of underlying heart disease (ischemic versus dilated cardiomyopathy) does not influence the mode of death of heart transplant candidates.[17]

## Causes of Sudden Death in Patients Awaiting Heart Transplantation

The causes of sudden death in patients awaiting heart transplantation are manifold and include ventricular tachyarrhythmias, bradyarrhythmias, and nonarrhythmic causes, such as coronary occlusion, electromechanical dissociation, myocardial rupture, pulmonary embolism, stroke, etc.[18] In nonhospitalized pretransplant patients in stable condition, the most likely cause of sudden death is malignant ventricular arrhythmia. Indeed, in patients resuscitated following out-of-hospital cardiac arrest and in those who die outside hospital while wearing Holter devices, ventricular tachycardia or ventricular fibrillation is the rhythm usually recorded at the time of the fatal or near-fatal event (70–80% of cases).[19,20]

By contrast, in patients hospitalized for management of advanced heart failure and evaluation for heart transplantation, severe bradycardia or electromechanical dissociation is the mechanism most often (62% of cases) responsible for sudden death, with ventricular tachyarrhythmia being observed in only 38% of cases.[21]

## Rationale for Prophylactic Implantation of an Implantable Cardioverter-Defibrillator

Because malignant ventricular arrhythmia is a common cause of sudden death, and sudden death is a frequent mode of death in patients listed for heart transplantation, especially when waiting at home in stable condition, prophylactic antiarrhythmic treatment seems to be justified in the majority of these patients.[22–24] However, antiarrhythmic drugs, with the sole exception of beta blockers, are known to be ineffective or even harmful in subjects with advanced heart failure.[25–34] Moreover, catheter ablation and direct antiarrhythmic surgery are technically feasible in only a limited number of patients and are not indicated for the prevention of sudden death.

Thus, the only antiarrhythmic measure we can currently take to avoid sudden death from ventricular tachyarrhythmia in patients awaiting heart transplantation is the implantable cardioverter-defibrillator (ICD).

Many studies, including recent randomized controlled trials, have demonstrated that the ICD is highly effective in interrupting life-threatening ventricular arrhythmias and reducing both sudden death and total mortality in a variety of clinical settings.[30-35] However, up to now there is no clear-cut evidence that ICD treatment in pretransplant patients is really useful in preventing sudden death and prolonging survival until a donor heart is available and replacement of the failing heart is possible: the so-called "electronic bridge to heart transplantation."[36,37]

The possible indications of the ICD as a "bridge to transplantation" are essentially: (1) "secondary prevention" of sudden death in patients who have already survived an episode of life-threatening ventricular arrhythmias; and (2) "primary prevention" of sudden death in patients with no history of such arrhythmias but at high risk of developing them.

# ICD Therapy for "Secondary Prevention" of Sudden Death

In the literature, only a few nonrandomized, noncontrolled studies have assessed the value of ICD therapy for "secondary prevention" of sudden death in patients with sustained ventricular tachycardia or ventricular fibrillation who are awaiting heart transplantation.[36,38-40] In total, 75 patients, with a mean left ventricular ejection fraction ranging from 13% ± 7 to 20% ± 5, have been reported.[14] No case of perioperative death occurred in these patients. During a mean follow-up of 8.5 to 10.4 months, the majority of the patients (83%) received ICD discharges and only 1 (1.3%) died suddenly before transplantation; 3 subjects (4%) died of progressive heart failure, 40 (53%) underwent successful transplantation, and 31 (41%) remained on the waiting list as clinically stable patients.

In a case control study, Grimm et al.[40] analyzed the outcome of 30 patients with a history of syncopal ventricular tachyarrhythmias who were on ICD therapy at the time of registration for transplantation. These patients were compared with 30 matched patients who, for various nonmedical reasons, had not undergone ICD therapy. Both groups were comparable in terms of clinical and hemodynamic characteristics, as was the median waiting time for transplantation (5.7 and 6 months, respectively). During this period, 26 (87%) ICD patients experienced adequate ICD discharges and 12 (40%) non-ICD patients were treated successfully by means of external electrical defibrillation; moreover, 1 (3%) ICD patient died (nonsudden death), compared with 7 (23%) non-ICD patients (5 sudden deaths). Finally, in agreement with other reports,[41] ICD insertion before transplantation did not adversely affect outcome after transplantation.

The results of these studies[36,38-40] suggest that, in patients with a history of malignant ventricular tachyarrhythmias, ICD implantation as a "bridge to transplantation" is a fairly effective tool in aborting sudden death and allowing patients to live long enough to undergo successful heart transplantation. However, if the waiting time for transplantation becomes excessively long, it is likely that the initial survival benefit conferred by ICD is subsequently lost, as reported by Sweeney et al.,[42] because of the progression of heart failure and the conversion of the mode of death from sudden to nonsudden.

The high incidence of ICD shocks in heart transplant candidates is not surprising. A similar finding has been observed in patients with severely depressed ($\leq 30\%$) left ventricular ejection fraction who are not on waiting lists for heart transplantation[43,44] and confirms the high arrhythmic risk of these patients.

# ICD Therapy for "Primary Prevention" of Sudden Death

The hypothesis that prophylactic ICD implantation may be useful in heart transplantation candidates who have not yet experienced spontaneous episodes of ventricular tachyarrhythmias remains to be proved. The multicenter DEFIBRILAT trial[16] was conceived to explore this hypothesis but unfortunately was terminated before any patients were enrolled because of lack of funding.[42] It must be underlined that the favorable results reported by MADIT[33] and MUSTT[34] on the use of ICDs for "primary prevention" of sudden death in high-risk post-MI patients were obtained in a very select subgroup of subjects and, thus, cannot be extrapolated "sic et simpliciter" to any other patient population.[45]

Taking into account that the most frequent mechanism of sudden death in hospitalized patients awaiting heart transplantation is severe bradycardia and electromechanical dissociation (62% of cases),[21] and that sudden death is a relatively rare phenomenon in hospitalized patients with end-stage heart disease (21% of cases),[16] it is unlikely that ICD implantation as a "bridge to transplantation" in these patients may lead to a substantial survival benefit.

In contrast, in hemodynamically stable patients awaiting heart transplantation on an outpatient basis, ventricular tachyarrhythmia is the most common cause of sudden death (70–80% of cases),[19,20] and sudden death is a very frequent mode of death (up to 40% of cases).[39] Thus, the prophylactic use of ICD in these patients seems to be more rational. However, ICD is a costly therapy and its use should be limited to patients who are at the highest risk of dying suddenly.[46] Unfortunately, risk stratification of sudden death in patients awaiting heart transplantation is problematic. Indeed, up to now, no clinical or instrumental variables have been unequivocally shown to be helpful in identifying those pretransplant patients who are most prone to sudden death.[14,42] For example, while Lindsay et al. found that signal-averaged ECG and programmed ventricular stimulation are valuable examinations for this purpose,[47] Stevenson et al. and Middlekauff et al. have reported completely different results.[48,49]

## Conclusion

Because of the scant potential benefit in terms of survival and the current uncertainties and difficulties in identifying those candidates for heart transplantation who are at high risk of sudden death, we believe that, at present, the routine and extensive implantation of an ICD as a "bridge to transplantation" should not be performed in subjects with no history of sustained ventricular tachyarrhythmias. However, future randomized studies will have to establish whether this policy is correct.

## References

1. Pasic M, Loebe M, Hummel M, et al. Heart transplantation: a single-center experience. Ann Thorac Surg 1996; 62:1685–1690.
2. Fraund S, Pethig K, Franke U, et al. Ten-year survival after heart transplantation: palliative procedure or successful long-term treatment? Heart 1999; 82:47–51.
3. Robbins RC, Barlow CW, Oyer PE, et al. Thirty years of cardiac transplantation at Stanford University. J Thorac Cardiovasc Surg 1999; 117:939–951.
4. Mc Manus RP, O'Hair DP, Beitzinger JM, et al. Patients who die awaiting heart transplantation. J Heart Lung Transplant 1993;12:159–171.
5. Kubo SH, Ormaza SM, Francis GS, et al. Trends in patient selection for heart transplantation. J Am Coll Cardiol 1993; 21:975–981.
6. Rodeheffer RJ, Naftel DC, Stevenson LW, et al. Secular trends in cardiac transplant recipient and donor management in the United States, 1990 to 1994: a multi-institutional study. Cardiac Transplant Research Database Group. Circulation 1996; 94:2883–2889.
7. Stevenson LW, Hamilton MA, Tillisch IH, et al. Decreasing survival benefit from cardiac transplantation for outpatients as the waiting list lengthens. J Am Coll Cardiol 1991; 18:919–925.
8. Lee HR, Hershberger RE, Port JD, et al. Low-dose enoximone in subjects awaiting cardiac transplantation: clinical results and effects on beta-adrenergic receptors. J Thorac Cardiovasc Surg 1991; 102:246–258.
9. Sindone AP, Keogh AM, Macdonald PS, et al. Continuous home ambulatory intravenous inotropic drug therapy in severe heart failure: safety and cost efficacy. Am Heart J 1997; 134:889–900.

10. Pacher R, Stanek B, Hulsmann M, et al. Prostaglandin E1-bridge to cardiac transplantation: technique, dosage, results. Eur Heart J 1997; 18:318–329.
11. Murali S. Mechanical circulatory support with the Novacor LVAS: worldwide clinical results. J Thorac Cardiovasc Surg 1999; 47(Suppl 2):321–325.
12. El- Banayosy A, Korfer R., Arusoglu L, et al. Bridging to cardiac transplantation with the Thoratec Ventricular Assist Device. J Thorac Cardiovasc Surg 1999; 47(Suppl 2):307–310.
13. Lavee J, Kormos RL, Uretsky BF, et al. Prediction of mortality in patients awaiting cardiac transplantation: increased risk of sudden death in ischemic compared to idiopathic dilated cardiomyopathy. Isr J Med Sci 1996; 32:282–287.
14. Schmidinger H. The implantable cardioverter defibrillator as a "bridge to transplant": a viable clinical strategy? Am J Cardiol 1999; 83:151D-157D.
15. Narang R, Cleland JG, Erhardt L, et al. Mode of death in chronic heart failure: a request and proposition for more accurate classification. Eur Heart J 1996; 17:1390–1403.
16. DEFIBRILAT Study Group. Actuarial risk of sudden death while awaiting cardiac transplantation in patients with atherosclerotic heart disease. Am J Cardiol 1991; 68:545–546.
17. Stevenson WG, Stevenson LW, Middlekauff HR, et al. Sudden death prevention in patients with advanced ventricular dysfunction. Circulation 1993; 8:2953–2961.
18. Kjekshus J. Arrhythmias and mortality in congestive heart failure. Am J Cardiol. 1990; 65:42–48.
19. Myerburg RJ, Conde CA, Sung RJ, et al. Clinical, electrophysiologic and hemodynamic profile of patients resuscitated from prehospital cardiac arrest. Am J Med 1980; 68:568–572.
20. Bayes de Luna A, Coumel P, Leclercq JF. Ambulatory sudden cardiac death: mechanism of production of fatal arrhythmia on the basis of data from 157 cases. Am Heart J 1989; 117:151–159.
21. Luu M, Stevenson WG, Stevenson LW, et al. Diverse mechanisms of unexpected cardiac arrest in advanced heart failure. Circulation 1989; 80:1675–1680.
22. Cardiac Arrhythmia Suppression Trial (CAST) Investigators. Effect of encainide and flecainide on mortality in infarction. N Engl J Med 1989; 321:406–412.
23. Cardiac Arrhythmia Suppression Trial (CAST) Investigators. Effect of antiarrhythmic agent moricizine on survival after myocardial infarction. N Engl J Med 1992; 327:227–233.
24. Waldo AC, Camm AJ, deRuyter H, et al. Effect of d-sotalol on mortality in patients with left ventricular dysfunction after recent and remote myocardial infarction. Lancet 1996; 348:7–12.
25. Singh SN, Fletcher RD, Fisher SG, et al. Amiodarone in patients with congestive heart failure and asymptomatic ventricular arrhythmia. Survival Trial of Antiarrhythmic Therapy in Congestive Heart Failure. N Engl J Med 1995; 333:77–82.
26. Julian DG, Camm AJ, Frangin G, et al. Randomised trial of effect of amiodarone on mortality in patients with left ventricular dysfunction after recent myocardial infarction: EMIAT. Lancet 1997; 349:667–674.
27. Cairns JA, Connolly SJ, Roberts R, et al. The Canadian Amiodarone Myocardial Infarction Arrhythmia Trial Investigators. Randomised trial of outcome after myocardial infarction in patients with frequent or repetitive ventricular premature depolarizations: CAMIAT. Lancet 1997; 349:675–682.
28. Mason JW. A comparison of seven antiarrhythmic drugs in patients with ven-

tricular tachyarrhythmias: Electrophysiologic Study versus Electrocardiographic Monitoring Investigators. N Engl J Med 1993; 329:452–458.

29. Greene HL. The CASCADE Study: randomized antiarrhythmic drug therapy in survivors of cardiac arrest in Seattle. CASCADE Investigators. Am J Cardiol 1993; 72:70F-74F.

30. The Antiarrhythmics versus Implantable Defibrillators (AVID) Investigators. A comparison of antiarrhythmic drug therapy with implantable defibrillators in patients resuscitated from near-fatal ventricular arrhythmias. N Engl J Med 1997; 337:1576–1583.

31. Kuck KH. ACC NewsOnline: CASH. 1998.

32. Connolly SJ. ACC NewsOnline: CIDS. 1998.

33. Moss AJ, Hall WJ, Cannom DS, et al. Multicenter Defibrillator Implantation Trial (MADIT): design and clinical protocol. Pacing Clin Electrophysiol 1991; 14:920–927.

34. Buxton AE. ACC News Online: MUSTT, 1999.

35. Raviele A, Gasparini G. Italian multicenter clinical experience with endocardial defibrillation: acute and long-term results in 307 patients. Pacing Clin Electrophysiol 1995; 18:599–608.

36. Bolling SF, Deeb GM, Morady F, et al. Automatic internal cardioverter defibrillator: a bridge to heart transplantation. J Heart Lung Transplant 1991; 10:562–566.

37. Trappe HJ, Wenzlaff P. Cardioverter defibrillator as a bridge to heart transplantation. Pacing Clin Electrophysiol 1995; 18:622–631.

38. Jeevanandam V, Bielefeld MR, Auteri JS, et al. The implantable defibrillator: an electronic bridge to cardiac transplantation. Circulation 1992; 86:II276–279.

39. Saxon LA, Wiener I, DeLurgio DB, et al. Implantable defibrillators for high-risk patients with heart failure who are awaiting cardiac transplantation. Am Heart J 1995; 130:501–506.

40. Grimm M, Grimm G, Zuckermann A, et al. ICD therapy in survivors of sudden cardiac death awaiting heart transplantation. Ann Thorac Surg 1995; 59:916–920.

41. Novick RJ, Menkis AH, Guiraudon GM, et al. Heart transplantation after cardioverter-defibrillator implantation: a case control study. Chest 1993; 103:1710–1714.

42. Sweeney MO, Ruskin JN, Garan H, et al. Influence of the implantable cardioverter/defibrillator on sudden death and total mortality in patients evaluated for cardiac transplantation. Circulation 1995; 92:3273–3281.

43. Fogoros RN, Elson JJ, Bonnet CA, et al. Efficacy of the automatic implantable cardioverter-defibrillator in prolonging survival in patients with severe underlying cardiac disease. J Am Coll Cardiol 1990; 16:381–386.

44. Powell AC, Fuchs T, Finkelstein DM, et al. Influence of implantable cardioverter-defibrillators on the long-term prognosis of survivors of out-of-hospital cardiac arrest. Circulation 1993; 88:1083–1092.

45. Raviele A, Bongiorni MG, Brignole M, et al. Which strategy is "best" after myocardial infarction? The beta-blocker strategy plus implantable cardioverter defibrillator trial: rationale and study design. Am J Cardiol 1999; 83:104–111D.

46. Raviele A. Implantable cardioverter-defibrillator (ICD) indications in 1996: have they changed? Am J Cardiol 1996; 78:21–25.

47. Lindsay BD, Osborn JL, Schechtman KB, et al. Prospective detection of vulnerability to sustained ventricular tachycardia in patients awaiting cardiac transplantation. Am J Cardiol 1992; 69:619–624.

48. Stevenson WG, Stevenson LW, Weiss J, et al. Inducible ventricular arrhythmias

and sudden death during vasodilator therapy of severe heart failure. Am Heart J 1988; 116:1447–1454.

46. Middlekauff HL. Comparison of frequency of late potentials in idiopathic dilated cardiomyopathy and ischemic cardiomyopathy with advanced congestive heart failure and their usefulness in predicting sudden death. Am J Cardiol 1990; 66:1113–1117.

# VII

## *Pediatrics*

# 28

# Neuromuscular Disorders and Sudden Death

*Denis Duboc, MD, PhD,*
*Jean Varin, MD,*
*Henry Marc Becane, MD,*
*Gisele Bonne, PhD,*
*Zine Ounnoughenne, MD,*
*and Arnaud Lazarus, MD*

## Introduction

Many neuromuscular disorders can increase the risk of sudden cardiac death. These diseases can be acquired or genetically transmitted.[1-9] In polymyositis, heart involvement is possible with the occurrence of atrioventricular block and/or ventricular arrhythmias, increasing the risk of sudden death associated with the inflammatory process of the myocardium. On the other hand, mitochondrial disorders can also increase this risk by complete atrioventricular block. This is observed in the classic Kearns-Sayre syndrome, which is of mitochondrial origin associated with abnormal adenosine triphosphate production by the cells.

In Duchenne's muscular dystrophy, which is related to the lack of dystrophine (protein located in the inner face of the myocyte plasma membrane), severe ventricular arrhythmias can occur at the end-stage of the evolution. In this disease, it reflects the severity of left ventricular dysfunction more than a specific mechanism increasing the risk of arrhythmias. On the other hand, cardiac arrhythmias can be observed in facioscapulohumeral dystrophy (Landouzy-Déjerine), which is the second most frequent muscle disease, but sudden death has not yet been reported. This chapter focuses on two genetic neuromuscular disorders predisposing to sudden cardiac death by specific mechanisms.[18-24]

The first one is Steinert's muscular dystrophy,[1] which is the most frequent genetically transmitted muscle disorder, and Emery-Dreifuss muscular dystrophy.

From: Aliot E, Clementy J, Prystowsky EN (editors). *Fighting Sudden Cardiac Death: A Worldwide Challenge.* ©Futura Publishing Company, Armonk, NY, 2000.

## Steinert's Muscular Dystrophy

Steinert's muscular dystrophy[1-17] is the most frequent of the muscular diseases, affecting 1/7,000 persons. It is linked to a gene mutation that encodes a serine-threonine protein kinase (DMPK) that consists of an abnormal repeat of DNA in a regulatory region. One of the characteristics of this disease is the possibility of a complete dissociation between heart involvement and skeletal muscle involvement.[18,19] Some patients will present severe cardiac symptoms with moderate or absent muscular manifestations.[20-22] On the other hand, other patients will have severe disability due to muscle diseases and moderate or absent cardiac manifestation. For example, we observed a 15-year-old patient whose first manifestation of the disease was sudden death, due to ventricular fibrillation that required the implantation of a defibrillator.[15] This patient had no muscular manifestation of disease other than a moderate myotonia when the weather was cold.

Classically, heart involvement in Steinert's muscular dystrophy consists essentially of abnormal auriculoventricular conduction increasing the risk of complete atrioventricular block.[2-4] However, in this disease we also observe a myocardial involvement that predisposes to supraventricular and ventricular arrhythmias. During electrophysiological testing, atrial fibrillation or ventricular arrhythmias can frequently be initiated.

Sudden death is frequently reported in this disease. The actual incidence is not clear—5% for some authors and up to 15% for others. The mechanism of sudden death is not clear and could be attributed to ventricular arrhythmia or complete atrioventricular block in patients who did not have permanent pacemakers. In order to determine the mechanism of sudden death, we studied the long-term outcome of patients who had implantation of devices containing Holter monitoring function.[16-19]

The Holter recordings indicate a high incidence of complete atrioventricular block in patients with prolonged HV interval, but also a high incidence of ventricular and supraventricular tachycardia in such patients. Some patients died suddenly, but 2 had no evidence of arrhythmic events.

The indicators of patients who are more at risk than others for developing severe ventricular arrhythmias are still controversial. Electrophysiological testing may be helpful, but the literature is inconclusive.[23] The decrease of coronary flow reserve seems to be a reliable prognostic marker of cardiac events during follow-up. If the coronary flow reserve is severely depressed, the patient is at risk for developing ventricular and supraventricular arrhythmias. Distal ischemia is probably a marker that can initiate arrhythmias in this particular population genetically exposed to the risk of cardiac sudden death.

## Autosomal Emery-Dreifuss Muscular Dystrophy

$h1Cardiac manifestation in this dystrophy consists of atrioventricular block, atrial fibrillation, ventricular arrhythmias, and dilated cardiomyopathy.[5-8,19,20] The cardiac symptoms can be isolated and increase the risk of cardiac sudden death. Sudden death can be the first manifestation of disease. It is due to a gene mutation that encodes in the inner face of the nuclear membrane.[9] This particular disease offers new insights into the molecular mechanisms of sudden cardiac death. An abnormal protein in the nucleus is associated with ventricular arrhythmias. In families with a high incidence of sudden death, genetic testing for this mutation is recommended.

## References

1. Perloff JK, Stevenson WG, Roberts NK, Cabeen W, Weiss J. Cardiac involvement in myotonic muscular dystrophy (Steinert's disease): a prospective study of 25 patients. Am J Cardiol 1984; 54:1074–1081.
2. Cannom DS, Wyman MG, Goldreyer BN. Clinical and induced ventricular tachycardia in a patient with myotonic dystrophy. J Am Coll Cardiol 1984; 4:625–628.
3. Grigg LE, Chan W, Mond HG, Vohra JK, Downey WF. Ventricular tachycardia and sudden death in myotonic dystrophy: clinical, electrophysiologic and pathologic features. J Am Coll Cardiol 1985; 6:254–256.
4. Moorman JR, Coleman RE, Packer DL, Kisslo JA, Bell J, et al. Cardiac involvement in myotonic muscular dystrophy. Medicine 1985; 64:371–387.
5. Emery AE. Emery-Dreifuss syndrome. J Med Genet 1989; 26: 637–641.
6. Hawley RJ, Milner MR, Gottdiener JS, Cohen A. Myotonic heart disease: a clinical follow-up. Neurology 1991; 41:259–262.
7. Fragola PV, Autore C, Magni G, Antonini G, Picelli A, et al. The natural course of cardiac conduction distrurbances in myotonic dystrophy. Cardiology 1991; 79:93–98.
8. Monsegu J, Duboc D, Freychet L, Fardeau M, Becane HM, et al. L'atteinte cardiaque au cours de certaines maladies musculaires: a propos de 216 observations. Arch Mal Coeur 1993;. 86:1421–1426.
9. Annane D, Duboc D, Merlet P, Fardeau M, Guerin F, et al. Corrélation between decreased myocardial glucose phosphorylation and the DNA mutation size in myotonic dystrophy. Circulation 1994; 90:2629–2634.
10. Lazarus A, Varin J, Duboc D, Eymard B, Fardeau M, et al. Proarrhythmic effect of class 1 antiarrhythmic drugs in patients with myotonic dystrophy (abstract). Eur JCPE 1994; 4:220.
11. Melillo G, Ruggieri MP, Magni G, Fragola PV, Antonini G, et al. Malignant cardiac involvement in a family with myotonic dystrophy. G Ital Cardiol 1996; 26:853–861.
12. Annane D, Merlet P, Fardeau M, Syrota A, Duboc D. Blunted coronary reserve in myotonic dystrophy: an early and gene-related phenomenon. Circulation 1996; 94:973–977.
13. Tamura K, Tsuji H, Matsui Y, Masui A, Hikosaka M, et al. Sustained ventricular tachycardias associated with myotonic dystrophy. Clin Cardiol 1996; 19:674–677.

14. Phillips MF, Harper PS. Cardiac disease in myotonic dystrophy. Cardiovasc Res 1997; 33:13–22.
15. Goldfarb LG, Park KY, Cervenakova L, Gorokhova S, Lee HS, et al. Missense mutations associated with familial cardiac and skeletal myopathy. Nat Genet 1998; 19: 402–403.
16. Duboc D, Annane D, Becane HM, et al. Quantification of coronary flow reserve is a reliable predictor of cardiac events in myotonic dystrophy. AHA, 1998 (abstract in Circulation).
17. Lazarus A, Babuty D, Varin J, et al. Multicentric study about sudden death in myotonic dystrophy: results at two years (abstract). PACE 1998 ; 21:654.
18. Laforet P, De Toma C, Becane HM, Fardeau M, Duboc D. Cardiac involvement in genetically confirmed facioscapulohumeral muscular dystrophy. Neurology 1998; 51:1454–1456.
19. Duboc D, Bonne G, Becane HM, et al. Clinical presentation and genetic localization of a new form of autosomal dominant dilated cardiomyopathy. AHA 1998 (abstract in Circulation).
20. Nelson SD, Sparks EA, Graber HL, Boudoulas H, et al. Clinical characteristics of sudden death victims in heritable (chromosome 1p1–1q1) conduction and myocardial disease. J Am Coll Cardiol 1998; 32: 1717–1723.
21. Hiromasa S, Ikeda T, Kubota K, Hattori N, Coto H, et al. Ventricular tachycardia and sudden death in myotonic dystrophy. Am Heart J 1998; 115:914–915.
22. Duboc D, Becane HM, Bonne G, Warnous S, Lavergne T, et al. High incidence of sudden death in a new form of conduction system and myocardial disease due to lamin A/C mutation. AHA 1999 (abstract in Circulation).
23. Lazarus A, Varin J, Laforêt P, Weber S, Duboc D. Electrophysiologic testing in myotonic dystrophy: correlation with heart function and extent of DNA mutation. Circulation 1999; 99:1041–1046.
24. Hoogerwaard EM, van der Wouw PA, Wilde AA, Bakker E, Ippel PF, et al. Cardiac involvement in carriers of Duchenne and Becker muscular dystrophy. Neuromusc Disord 1999; 9:347–351.

# 29

# Sudden Cardiac Death After Surgery for Congenital Cardiac Diseases

*Elisabeth Villain, MD*

## Introduction

As postoperative survival has improved after surgery for congenital heart diseases, more attention has been paid to late postoperative problems, especially late arrhythmias, unexpected sudden death, and the relationship between them. The highest incidence of late sudden death has been found in patients with tetralogy of Fallot repair, Mustard and Senning operations for transposition of the great arteries (TGA), and in patients with aortic obstructions.[1] Most attention has been concentrated on late arrhythmias after repair of tetralogy of Fallot and TGA.

## Mustard and Senning Operations

The Mustard and Senning operations were developed to treat patients with TGA. The Mustard operation required a right atriotomy, an atrial septectomy, and the placement of a pericardium pantleg-shaped patch so as to channel blood from the pulmonary veins to the aorta and from the venae cavae to the pulmonary artery. The Senning operation had the same hemodynamic effect but used almost entirely native cardiac tissue.

These operations have an excellent immediate result, but the main concern about patients with Mustard or Senning repairs of TGA is the risk of late postoperative sudden death. By combining the results from several reports, Christopher Wren calculated a risk of sudden death of 7.9 per 1,000 patient years of follow-up after Senning or Mustard operations.[2] Loss of sinus rhythm is common after these operations, but it has not been demonstrated that bradycardia is associated with a poor long-term outcome, and pacemaker implantation does not reduce the risk of sudden death.[3–5] It seems more probable that sudden death in these patients is due to an ar-

From: Aliot E, Clementy J, Prystowsky EN (editors). *Fighting Sudden Cardiac Death: A Worldwide Challenge.* ©Futura Publishing Company, Armonk, NY, 2000.

rhythmia, and the candidate arrhythmia is atrial flutter. Although the term intraatrial reentrant tachycardia would be more appropriate, the term atrial flutter is used for uniformity. Specific factors predisposing these patients to intraatrial reentry tachycardia include sinus node dysfunction, atrial scarring caused by multiple atriotomies and suture lines, as well as high atrial wall stress and hypertrophy.[6] Atrial flutter is inducible in most Mustard and Senning patients, but routine electrophysiology cannot identify those who are at risk to develop atrial flutter and die suddenly.

The first study to demonstrate atrial flutter as a risk factor for sudden death was that of the multicenter Pediatric Electrophysiology Group.[7] It has been demonstrated that atrial flutter with 1/1 atrioventricular conduction may lead to ventricular arrhythmia.[8] However, not all patients with atrial flutter die and not all those who die have ever had an atrial arrhythmia; associated anatomic abnormalities and hemodynamic factors such as right ventricular dysfunction may be additional risk factors for late sudden death.[4,5]

Termination of atrial flutter is best obtained by overdrive pacing or cardioversion. Endocardial pacing is our preferred method because it allows atrial pacing in case of severe sinus failure, and hemodynamic and angiographic investigations can be done to look for subclinical abnormalities. We have found high doses (500–1,000 mg/m²) of oral amiodarone to be effective in restoring sinus rhythm within 24 to 48 hours. Intravenous drugs should be avoided in these patients.

Prophylactic treatment of atrial flutter is mandatory, and the main goal of therapy should be to eliminate recurrent episodes of atrial flutter since the likelihood of sudden death is increased when patients continue to have atrial flutter.[9]

Medical therapy is still considered first line but is not easy and is still empirical. It should be initiated in hospital, and implantation of a pacemaker is necessary in patients who receive antiarrhythmic drugs and have severe sinus failure. Overall, the most effective drug is amiodarone with a 70% success rate when it is given orally, with doses ranging from 200 to 250 mg/m².[9,10] However, if amiodarone is well tolerated in children, side effects increase with follow-up and age of patients so that it cannot be given lifelong to postoperative patients. IC drugs are contraindicated, and a review of the literature has shown a high incidence of cardiac arrest and sudden death in patients with atrial flutter and underlying heart diseases.[11] Beta blockers are recommended for patients who have exercise-induced atrial tachycardia, since sudden death in Mustard and Senning patients almost always occurs during exertion. Sotalol, a Class III antiarrhythmic agent with beta-blocking activity, is an effective drug to delay the recurrence of atrial flutter in adults with structural heart diseases; in young patients with postoperative atrial flutter, the success rate is approximately

50%. However, fatigue is a commonly reported adverse effect and may preclude its use in teenagers and young adults. Patients with severe sinus node function should be paced, since the risk of sotalol-induced QT interval prolongation and torsades de pointes is amplified at slow ventricular rates; high-degree block has also been reported in children.[12]

Antitachycardia atrial pacing has been proposed as a possible therapeutic option in postoperative patients. Prior to implantation of an antitachycardia device (Intertach II, Intermedics R), patients should meet the following criteria: recurrent flutter despite medical treatment including amiodarone, constant tachycardia termination with overdrive pacing, and normal atrioventricular conduction. Results are encouraging, as patients are less symptomatic, take fewer drugs and have better cardiovascular performance. However, atrial signals have low amplitude, and algorithms that constantly overdrive patients' tachycardia may be difficult to find. Finally, antitachycardia pacing should be undertaken with caution, since tachycardia acceleration by the device, followed by sudden death, has been reported.[13]

The failure of the conventional techniques of arrhythmia control has led to interest in the use of radiofrequency ablation in Mustard and Senning patients. From activation mapping, putative surgical scars may be identified (earlier site of activation, fractionated or double potentials >50 ms, confirmation by pacing to demonstrate concealed entrainment). Reentry circuits require a critical isthmus of conducting tissue between surgical scars and anatomic barriers, and it is possible to apply radiofrequency ablation lesions to interrupt this critical zone. Parts of the reentry circuit may be disrupted by single radiofrequency lesions, but recurrences are frequent, so that the most effective method is to draw ablation lines by the delivery of multiple lesions.[14] Development of new techniques, such as computerized imaging of the atrial activation, will certainly improve the results of radiofrequency ablation in postoperative flutter. However, it is sometimes difficult to interrupt reentry circuits in thick and scarred atrial tissue, and new circuits may develop with the progression of the disease.

# Tetralogy of Fallot

The occurrence of late sudden death after Fallot repair increases with follow-up duration, reaching 6% at 30 years of follow-up .[1,15] It was originally thought that late sudden death was due to development of atrioventricular block, but this is not so. However, patients with transient postoperative complete block and residual abnormalities, or with long PR interval associated with right bundle branch block and left axis deviation ("trifascicular block"), merit an electrophysiological investigation.

Sudden cardiac death after Fallot repair is attributed mainly to ventricular arrhythmias, which are related to surgery. Repair of tetralogy of Fallot involves not only closure of the ventricular septal defect, but also a right ventriculotomy and a transannular patch. Fibrosis and ventricular scars provide the substrate for ventricular tachycardia due to reentry that can be mapped to the patch or the ventriculotomy site.

Among patients who develop ventricular arrhythmias, only a small proportion will die, and risk factors for sudden death have been extensively studied. Approximately 50% of patients with long follow-up after Fallot repair have ventricular arrhythmias on 24-hour ambulatory electrocardiogram (Holter) so that their predictive value is almost nil. Although ventricular ectopy is more frequent in symptomatic patients, even complex ventricular arrhythmias detected by Holter monitoring had no prognostic significance in a long-term prospective study by Cullen, et al.[16] Inducible ventricular tachycardia at electrophysiological study is not a risk factor for sudden death. In a large multicenter study reported by the Pediatric Electrophysiology Society, ventricular tachycardia was inducible in 17% of 359 patients. There were 5 sudden deaths in nearly 2,500 patient years of follow-up, and none had inducible ventricular tachycardia.[17] Thus, it has not been proved that spontaneous or induced ventricular arrhythmia after surgical correction indicates an elevated risk of sudden death.

Recent studies from the United Kingdom have suggested a mechano-electrophysiological relation between right ventricular dilatation and ventricular arrhythmias, and sudden death. Gatzoulis et al. have found that QRS prolongation >180 ms is associated with adverse arrhythmic effects. None of their patients with QRS <180 ms had ventricular tachycardia (100% negative predictive value) and QRS >180 ms had 95% specificity for detecting clinical ventricular tachycardia.[18] After a long follow-up period, it is thought that, as the right ventricle dilates, the QRS duration is prolonged and favors reentry. Ventricular tachycardia patients also have increased QT and JT dispersion, suggesting that both depolarization and repolarization abnormalities are associated with ventricular arrhythmias.

Although there are no absolute criteria to accurately define patients at higher risk of sudden death, prophylactic treatment of postoperative ventricular arrhythmias has been recommended by Garson et al.[19] However, the use of a control group before 1978 and a treatment group after 1978 invalidates the conclusions of this study and the concept that suppression of asymptomatic ventricular arrhythmia will reduce the risk of sudden death remains to be proved. Thus, it seems appropriate to investigate and treat only symptomatic patients. As ventricular tachycardia is more likely to progress toward fibrillation in patients with a bad postoperative result, a combined hemodynamic and angiographic study as well as an invasive electrophysiological study are recommended in symptomatic patients to guide selection of the most appropriate therapeutic modality.

Patients who have significant residual abnormalities should be referred for reoperation. It is our policy to treat with amiodarone patients who have moderate symptoms such as dizziness or palpitations, with a good surgical result. In patients with more severe symptoms, such as syncope, amiodarone is also selected for in those who have no inducible arrhythmia or who refuse aggressive strategies such as implantation of an implantable cardioverter-defibrillator (ICD). Although amiodarone is the most effective agent, side effects develop increasingly with older age of patients and with long-term use, so that alternative strategies have to be found.

When programmed ventricular stimulation can reproduce the clinically documented arrhythmia, and when mapping is possible, catheter ablation has been proposed to eliminate postoperative ventricular tachycardia. At Jean Rostand Hospital in Paris, ablations have been performed in 11 patients who had drug-resistant symptomatic ventricular tachycardia, 3 to 13 years after Fallot repair.[20] In all cases, ventricular tachycardia origin was found in the right ventricle. The first patients had fulguration (DC shock), the next 6 had failure of radiofrequency ablation followed by DC shock, and the last 3 (after 1996) had only radiofrequency ablation with high-power generators and large (8-mm) electrodes. All procedures were successful and there was no immediate complication. Follow-up ranges from 1 to 8 years: 1 patient died suddenly of ventricular fibrillation 10 years after ablation and 1 needed surgery on a second tachycardia site. Thus, ablation is effective and safe for postoperative ventricular arrhythmias but usually requires high energies.

Finally, advances in the development and size of ICDs have reached the stage where pediatric implantation can now be performed. Our main indication for implantation of an ICD device is aborted cardiac death due to ventricular arrhythmia. In a series that was reported in 1993 about 125 patients less than 20 years old who underwent implantation of an ICD between 1980 and 1991, Silka et al. identified 22 patients (18%) who had repaired congenital heart diseases. There was 1 late death among postoperative patients, approximately 60% of patients experienced an "appropriate" ICD discharge within the 36 months of follow-up, and duration of follow-up was the primary variable correlated with ICD discharge.[21]

# Conclusion

Sudden death after surgery for congenital heart diseases remains unpredictable, and the optimal management of malignant postoperative arrhythmias has not yet been defined. Medical treatment is effective, but the long-term side effects of antiarrhythmic agents and the lack of compliance of patients restrict its use on a long-term basis. Radiofrequency ablation is promising when reentry circuits can be mapped, but as the disease progresses and substrates evolve, more tachycardia circuits may become active. The implantation of ICD devices is recommended in patients who were resuscitated from cardiac arrest due to postoperative ventricular arrhythmia.

## References

1. Silka MJ, Hardy BG, Menashe VD, et al. A population-based prospective evaluation of risk of sudden cardiac death after operation for common congenital heart defects. J Am Coll Cardiol 1998; 32:245–251.
2. Wren C. Late postoperative arrhythmias. In: Wren C, Campbell RWF (eds). Paediatric Cardiac Arrhythmias. Oxford University Press, 1996, pp 239–259.
3. Puley G, Siu S, Connelly M, et al. Arrhythmia and survival in patients >18 years of age after the Mustard procedure for complete transposition of the great arteries. Am J Cardiol 1999; 83:1080–1084.
4. Gewillig M, Cullen S, Mertens B, et al. Risk factors for arrhythmia and death after Mustard operation for simple transposition of the great arteries. Circulation 1991; 84(Suppl III): III-187–192.
5. Gelatt M, Hamilton RM, McCrindle BW, et al. Arrhythmia and mortality after the Mustard procedure: a 30-year single-center experience. J Am Coll Cardiol 1997; 29:194–201.
6. Vetter VL, Tanner CS, Horowitz LN. Electrophysiologic consequences of the Mustard repair of d-transposition of the great arteries. J Am Coll Cardiol 1987; 10:1265–1273.
7. Flinn CJ, Wolff GS, MacDonald D, et al. Cardiac rhythm after the Mustard operation for complete transposition of the great arteries. N Engl J Med 1984; 310:1635–1638.
8. Silka M, Kron J, McAnulty J. Supraventricular tachyarrythmias, congenital heart disease and sudden cardiac death. Pediatr Cardiol 1992; 13:116–118.
9. Garson A Jr, Bink-Boelkens M, Hesslein P, et al. Atrial flutter in the young: a collaborative study of 380 cases. J Am Coll Cardiol 1985; 6:871–878.
10. Villain E. Amiodarone as treatment for atrial tachycardias after surgery. PACE 1997; 20(PtII):2130–2132.
11. Fish FA, Gillette PC, Benson DW. Proarrhythmia, cardiac arrest and death in young patients receiving encainide and flecainide. The Pediatric Electrophysiology Group. J Am Coll Cardiol 1991; 18:356–365.
12. Pfammater JP, Paul T, Lehmann C, et al. Efficacy and proarrhythmia of oral sotalol in pediatric patients. J Am Coll Cardiol 1995; 26:1002–1007.
13. Rhodes LA, Walsh EP, Gamble WJ, et al. Benefits and potential risk of atrial antitachycardia pacing after repair of congenital heart disease. PACE 1995; 18(Pt I):1005–1116.
14. Triedman JK, Bergau DM, Saul P, Epstein MR, Walsh EP. Efficacy of radiofrequency ablation for control of intraatrial reentrant tachycardia in patients with congenital heart disease. J Am Coll Cardiol 1997; 30:1032–1038.
15. Murphy JG, Gersh BJ, Mair DD, et al. Long-term outcome in patients undergoing surgical repair of tetralogy of Fallot. N Engl J Med 1993; 329:593–599.
16. Cullen S, Celemajer DS, Franklin RCG, et al. Prognosis significance of ventric-

ular arrhythmia after repair of tetralogy of Fallot: a 12-year prospective study. J Am Coll Cardiol 1994; 23: 1151–1155.

17. Chandar JS, Wolff GS, Garson A Jr, et al. Ventricular arrhythmias in postoperative tetralogy of Fallot. Am J Cardiol 1990; 65:655–661.

18. Gatzoulis MA, Till JA, Somerville J, et al. Mechanoelectrical interaction in tetralogy of Fallot: QRS prolongation relates to right ventricular size and predicts malignant ventricular arrhythmias and sudden death. Circulation 1995; 91:231–237.

19. Garson A, Randall DC, Gillette PC, et al. Prevention of sudden death after repair of tetralogy of Fallot: treatment of ventricular arrhythmias. J Am Coll Cardiol 1985; 6:221–227.

20. Frank R, Guzman CE, Romerao L, et al. Ablation of ventricular tachycardia after Fallot repair: long-term experience on 11 cases (abstract). Eur Heart J 1999; 20:232.

21. Silka MJ, Kron J, Dunnigan A, Macdonald D II. Sudden cardiac death and the use of implantable cardioverter defibrillators in pediatric patients. Circulation 1993; 87:800–807.

# VIII

## *Etiologies*

# 30
# Sudden Death in Mitral Valve Prolapse

*Jean-Paul Fauchier, MD,*
*Dominique Babuty, MD, PhD,*
*Laurent Fauchier, MD,*
*Christian Marchal, MD,*
*Danielle Casset-Senon, PhD,*
*Pierre Cosnay, MD, and*
*Christian Neel, MD*

## Introduction

The prevalence of mitral valve prolapse (MVP) in the general population, its association with arrhythmias, and its prognosis are difficult to evaluate fully through the disparate data available from in-patients or ambulatory series, isolated "illustrative" cases, electrophysiological studies of selected patients, and/or postmortem observations. Sudden death is the most feared evolution of this condition, but its incidence is not well known and its mechanism(s) not clearly understood.

## Prevalences

More than 3 decades ago, MVP was considered to affect a large proportion of the general adult population (5–30%).[1] It is currently deemed the most common valvular abnormality in industrialized nations[1–3] but the most recent studies,[4,5] using updated echocardiographic criteria, have shown that the actual prevalence of MVP is only 3–4% in the normal adult population (about 40–60 years old). These large series and others[6,7] have underlined the fact that MVP syndrome has to be understood not as a single entity but as a spectrum of different conditions with, at one end, patients with bowing and normal-appearing leaflets (labeled "normal variant of MVP") and, at the other end, those with redundant myxomatous

From: Aliot E, Clementy J, Prystowsky EN (editors). *Fighting Sudden Cardiac Death: A Worldwide Challenge.* ©Futura Publishing Company, Armonk, NY, 2000.

and thickened leaflets with elongation of the chordal apparatus ("primary form of MVP").[8] The condition is rare in newborns and children, and is more frequent in women (2/3 of adults with MVP). One third of cases is familial (autosomal dominant inheritance pattern).[6] MVP is frequently associated with diseases of connective tissue or thoracic and skeletal abnormalities, and/or with various cardiac diseases (atrial septal defect, primitive hypertrophic cardiomyopathy, etc.).[1] About 25% of MVP patients will develop severe mitral regurgitation (MR), particularly in men (2/3 of MVP with MR), with advancing age, and in the case of posterior valve prolapse, with thicker leaflets. In addition to these risk factors, there is some evidence that high arterial blood pressure and excessive body weight may facilitate this evolution toward MR.[6]

MVP is frequently associated with arrhythmias, strokes, or syncopes, deemed classic complications of this disease, and the risk of sudden death.[9] However, these assertions are difficult to prove, because they are generally assessed from selected series of highly symptomatic patients not representative of the general population. Second, it is possible that these associations are fortuitous, resulting from the coincidental occurrence of diseases that are not rare in the general population. Third, MVP can be so mild and/or asymptomatic (occasionally revealed at autopsy) that its responsibility for certain severe complications is largely speculative. Finally, obvious or hidden cardiac diseases associated with MVP can be the actual causes of cardiac events and sudden death.

In terms of arrhythmias, we have observed that, by comparison with a control group, only repetitive atrial and complex ventricular arrhythmias are significantly more frequent in the MVP population, this difference being more evident in MVP patients with MR (Table 1), as already reported by Kligfield et al.[10]

The incidence of severe cardiac events (endocarditis, cardiac failure, cerebral ischemia, cardiac arrest, etc.) was evaluated at 0.3–1% yearly in early clinical studies,[11,12] and at 1–4% in more recent echocardiographic series.[2,7,13] According to Freed et al.,[5] the prevalence of syncope is quite similar in patients with or without MVP (3.6% versus 3%) and Gilon et al.[4] found that MVP is not more common among young patients suffering from strokes or transient ischemic attack than in a normal control group (1.9% versus 2.7%). The risk of sudden death (Table 2) was initially evaluated at 0.2–0.4% yearly,[2,13] that is, twice the incidence of sudden death from all causes (0.2% yearly) in the general adult population.[10] The risk should be 4 times greater for hospitalized patients than for nonselected ambulatory patients.[10] This risk has been recently established at about 0.1% yearly: there were 3 cases of sudden death in Zuppiroly's study (316 MVP; mean follow-up 120 ± 32 months)[7] and 1 in Kim's study (229 patients, mean follow-up 76 months).[14] In our series of 61 MVP patients, we

## Table 1

Prevalence of Arrhythmias During 24-Hour ECG Monitoring in MVP Patients Compared to a Control Group, and According to Presence or Absence of Mitral Regurgitation

| | Control n = 57 | MVP n = 58 | MVP with MR n = 27 | MVP without MR n = 31 |
|---|---|---|---|---|
| Age (mean ± SD) years | 41 ± 13.9 | 46.6 ± 17.9 | 50.8 ± 19.4 | 43 ± 15.8 |
| Sex (male/female) | 38/19 | 29/29 | 10/17 | 19/12 |
| First/second AV block (n) | 0/0 | 1/1 | 1/1 | 0/0 |
| Third degree AV block (n) | 0 | 1 | 1 | 0 |
| Sinus deficiency | 0 | 1 | 1 | 0 |
| Wolff-Parkinson-White (n) | 0 | 1 | 0 | 1 |
| Atrial tachycardia (n) | 0 | 10 | 7 | 3 |
| Supraventricular tachycardia (n) | 0 | 1 | 0 | 1 |
| PVCs (n) | | | | |
| Lown grade 0 | 25 | 13 | 2 | 11 |
| Lown grade 1 | 19 | 14 | 5 | 9 |
| Lown grade 2 | 3 | 5 | 1 | 4 |
| Lown grade 3 | 6 | 2 | 1 | 1 |
| Lown grade 4A | 4 ⎤ 17.5% | 14 ⎤ 44.8%* | 11 ⎤ 70.4%† | 3 ⎤ 22.6% |
| Lown grade 4B | 0 ⎦ | 10 ⎦ | 7 ⎦ | 3 ⎦ |
| SVT | — | 0 | 0 | 0 |

*p < 0.01 (versus control).

†< 0.05 (MR versus without MR).

MVP = mitral valve prolapse; MR = mitral regurgitation; PVC = premature ventricular contraction.

## Table 2

### The Estimated Risk of Sudden Death in Mitral Valve Prolapse

| Authors | Number of MVP | Number of Sudden Death | Mean Follow-up | Estimated per Year for Sudden Death |
|---|---|---|---|---|
| Nishimura[2] (NEJM 1985) | 237 | 3 | 6 years | 0.4 |
| Duren[13] (JACC 1988) | 300 | 3 | 6 years | 0.2 |
| Zuppiroli[7] (AJC 1995) | 316 | 3 | 102 months | 0.1 |
| Kim[14] (AHJ 1996) | 229 | 1 | 76 months | 0.1 |
| Fauchier (1999) | 61 | 1 | 71 months | 0.1 |

MVP = mitral valve prolapse.

observed only 1 case of sudden death (Table 2; Figure 1). Numerous isolated cases of sudden death or ventricular fibrillation have been published in recent years, but not in relation to the general population, and thus without defining a precise incidence of this fatal outcome in MVP.[15-24] Finally, in view of its multiple clinical and anatomical aspects,

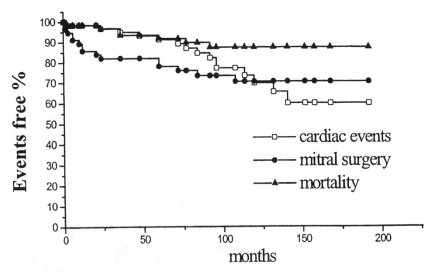

Figure 1. Follow-up of 61 MVP patients. Cumulative percentage of MVP patients with no events. Results are given using the Kaplan-Meier method. Cardiac events: sudden death (n=1), sustained VT (n=1), atrial arrhythmias (n=9), cardiac failure (n=2), cerebral event (n=1).

MVP has caused confusion concerning its true prevalence and gravity. There is probably a large prevalence of benign and asymptomatic forms in the general population, but some patients with primary MVP, particularly with MR, require increased vigilance and long-term follow-up to assess their actual prognosis.

## Clinical Profiles of MVP Patients Suffering Sudden Death

There were early attempts to define the profile of MVP patients exposed to a risk of sudden death, with an addition to these characteristics in subsequent years: according to Jeresaty[9] and others,[7,10,25] a predisposition was typically observed in women aged about 40 years, with a history of syncope or presyncope, familial occurrence of valvular disease, a late or pansystolic murmur, various ECG changes (ST-T changes in left precordial and/or inferior leads, QT prolongation), ventricular dysfunction, and/or complex arrhythmias. Sudden death frequently occurred during catecholergic stimulation, exercise, or stress.[21,22] More recent echocardiographic studies have shown that the strongest predictors of subsequent death or morbid events, associated with odds ratios of 15 to 27, were the presence of left atrial and/or ventricular enlargement, indicative of significant MR.[7,10] The importance of MR for the prognosis had already been demonstrated in initial studies: Kligfield et al.[10] reported that the risk of sudden death in MVP patients without MR was 0.01–0.02% per year, lower than the annual risk of sudden death from any cause in the general population (0.2% yearly; 0.07% for 45–54-year-old patients without coronary disease). In contrast, this risk increased to 0.9 to 2% per year in MVP patients with MR, which is 50 to 100 times greater than the risk in MVP patients without MR.[10] It was confirmed by postmortem studies that MVP with MR can be responsible for sudden death, chiefly among young patients;[24–26] however, clinical reports[19,20] and pathology studies[9,15,27] have shown that isolated MVP can also be observed, but only with significant valvular deformities (involvement of 2 leaflets, redundant mitral valve, annular dilatation, myxomatous changes, etc.) and with no or minimal MR. In such cases, the valvular malformation itself could be considered responsible for sudden death. Indeed, the direct responsibility of isolated MVP in such deaths is not clear. In 1983, Chesler et al.[15] reviewed 39 reported cases of sudden death attributed to myxomatous mitral valves. They noted that autopsy was performed in only 19 patients, and in many, the information was so sparse that other pathological abnormalities could not be excluded with certainly. They considered that undoubtedly some cases of sudden death attributed to MVP resulted from other causes or from unrecognized and unrelated disorders.[15]

## Mechanisms of Sudden Death

The causes of sudden death in MVP are not fully understood. Several mechanisms have been evoked, but few are confirmed by data obtained from the isolated cases reported or from larger series of patients.

An arrhythmic origin of sudden death is assumed, as in other cardiac diseases, in view of the high incidence of arrhythmias attributed to MVP, and the isolated cases of sudden death in MVP with demonstrative ECG before or during cardiac arrest.[15–22] Asystole can occur, due to sinus node dysfunction or to atrioventricular block (generally confined to the atrioventricular node).[28] A significant prolongation of AH interval and Wenckebach conduction at lower paced atrial rhythm can be detected during electrophysiological studies in MVP patients compared to the general population.[29] Nevertheless, in our series (Table 1) as in others,[10] higher degrees of AV block are rare and without significant excess in comparison with a control group. Thus, this mechanism of sudden death is probably fortuitous. In other respects, repetitive atrial arrhythmias and fibrillation are significantly more frequent in MVP patients than in a control group, and this difference is more marked in patients with MR (25% of atrial tachycardia in patients with MR versus 2% without MR; Table 1), increasing with age. They are generally vagally mediated and well tolerated, but syncopes due to such arrhythmias have been reported in MVP.[30] In a study of 27 MVP patients with syncope or presyncope, Brembilla-Perrot et al.[31] noted that 24 (nearly 90%) had induced atrial arrhythmias (associated with junctional tachycardia in 19) and that 90% (13/14) of spontaneous atrial arrhythmias without syncope were reinducible. This high incidence of spontaneous and induced atrial arrhythmias is not so surprising in such valvular disease frequently associated with MR, as these 2 abnormalities tend to increase spontaneously with age. Atrial arrhythmias are likely to be life-threatening, particularly in cases of rapid ventricular rate, such as in patients with abnormal rapid conduction in the atrioventricular node or associated ventricular preexcitation.[32] However, there is no excessive incidence of such abnormalities in MVP patients (no case of Wolff-Parkinson-White syndrome in 300 MVP in the Framingham study;[3] 1 case in our personal series; Table 1). Consequently, there is only a weak probability that sudden death with MVP is due to excessively rapid atrial arrhythmias.

A high incidence (50–90%) of ventricular arrhythmias is noted in all published series of MVP (Table 3), with a significant difference from nor-

Table 3

Detection of Ventricular Arrhythmias by Resting, Exercise ECG, and 24-Hour ECG Monitoring

| | Year | No. | ECG (Rest) % | ECG (Exercise) % | Holter (24-H) % |
|---|---|---|---|---|---|
| Pocok and Barlow | 1970 | — | 0 | 25 | — |
| Gooch et al. | 1972 | — | 42 | 50 | — |
| Sloman et al. | 1972 | — | 45 | 55 | — |
| Winkle et al. | 1975 | 24 | 40 | 85 | 90 |
| De Maria et al. | 1976 | 31 | 35 | 45 | 58 |
| Malcom and Ahuja | 1978 | — | — | 16 | — |
| Savage et al. | 1983 | 61 | 0 | 10 | 49 |
| Kavey et al. | 1984 | 6 | 16 | 38 | — |
| Fauchier et al. | 1999 | 58 | 28 | 50 | 90 |

mal subjects (45% versus 18%, for example, in our series, p<0.01; Table 1). However, the difference was due chiefly to MVP patients with MR; 74% of our group of 27 MVP patients with MR had Lown grades III–IV premature ventricular contractions (PVCs) versus 23% in the group of 31 patients without MR (p<0.05) (Table 1). The PVCs are frequently repetitive, but cases of sustained ventricular tachycardia (VT) are rare (Table 1).[3,9,33] Two-thirds of patients have monomorphic ventricular arrhythmias but, surprisingly for such left valvular disease, the QRS waveform just as frequently has a right as a left bundle branch block morphology.[34] A large majority (90%) of ventricular arrhythmias are predominantly diurnal with exacerbation by exercise in one-third of cases,[34] a fact perhaps correlated with exercise-induced MR in 32% of patients.[35] In our series and in various reports, the gravity of ventricular arrhythmias is not closely related to a change in the ventricular ejection fraction.[9,10,25,33,36,37] The risk of ventricular arrhythmias is significantly lower in the absence of late ventricular potentials.[38–42] In the majority of series, programmed ventricular stimulation induced sustained monomorphic VTs only in patients with spontaneous sustained VT. Nonsustained VTs are more frequently induced in patients with late ventricular potentials and/or Lown grades III–IV PVCs.[39] In a study by Rosenthal et al. of 20 MVP patients presenting with either presyncope or cardiac arrest, 14 had inducible arrhythmias.[43] However, induced polymorphic sustained VT or ventricular fibrillation are judged to be without specific prognostic value, and no relationship between the response to programmed ventricular stimulation and subsequent patient prognosis has yet been demonstrated. The available data suggest only that patients without syncope and/or who are not inducible on electrophysiological study have good short-term prognosis despite associated complex ventricular arrhythmias on ambulatory ECG.[33,43-45] Various mechanisms have been suggested for such arrhythmias:[30] afterdepolarization-induced triggered activity[22,46] or reentry provoked by stretching and excessive traction of papillary muscle,[22,45] ectopic enhanced automaticity[47] caused by alteration of ventricular systolic function, increased dispersion of ventricular refractoriness, etc. These abnormalities can occur in valvular or nonvalvular sites (papillary muscle, chordae, endocardial ventricular tissue), within or near the zones of localized friction, hemorrhagic lesions, scars, etc. It is possible that these electrophysiological changes can be modulated by sympathetic stimulation or by other autonomic disturbances,[48] combined with arrhythmias induced by prolongation of QTc interval[49] with or without electrolytic imbalance, or provoked by the deleterious effects of different drugs. Theoretically, complex ventricular arrhythmias (i.e., VT or fibrillation, torsades de pointes) could provide a valid explanation for the occurrence of sudden death in MVP. The preferential occurrence of sudden death and ventricular arrhythmias in a catecholinergic environment, the reports of illustrative ECGs with ventricular fibrillation in some MVP patients with sudden death, and the frequent detection of ventricular arrhythmias on ambulatory ECG monitoring before the occurrence of sudden death in some series of MVP (e.g., 6/7 cases in Chesler's series[15]) are all sound arguments for an arrhythmogenic origin of sudden death in MVP. Unfortunately, it proved impossible in the majority of MVP series to find a good correlation between the presence of such arrhythmias and the risk of sudden death. Likewise, the indirect markers of such arrhythmias (presence of late ventricular potentials, induction by exercise or electrical stimulation) are unable to predict such risk. One can only hope that future large series will provide confirmation (or negation) of this hypothesis.

Arrhythmias are not the only possible mechanism of sudden death; hemodynamic and/or neurohumoral dysfunction with severe hypotension, coronary spasm or embolism with myocardial or cerebral ischemia, and baroreflex abnormalities have also been suggested.[30,48,50,51] The precise role of each of these factors remains unassessed, and sudden death in MVP could perhaps have a multifactorial origin.

Whatever the mechanism(s) of sudden death, one can speculate about the primary disease directly responsible for such a fatal outcome: Is it the mitral prolapse itself?[9,15,27] Is it the mitral regurgitation, the deterioration of ventricular function, and/or the atrial or ventricular lesions?[10,26] Is occult cardiomyopathy constitutionally or fortuitously associated with MVP? The first 2 hypotheses have been discussed, each supported by above-mentioned data. The latter had been evoked as early as 1983–1984 by Chesler et al. and by Crawford et al.[52] Several arguments have been added during recent years to support this last supposition:

1. *Clinical data:* No constant and significant correlation was seen in the majority of series between the importance of MVP (or its effects on atrial regurgitation or ventricular function) and the risk of sudden death. Arrhythmias generally deemed to be the cause of sudden death are not significantly correlated with such risk and frequently (or always) have another origin. For example, in the series of La Vecchia et al., 25% of patients with idiopathic VT of left origin had MVP and most of them had increased myocardial fibrosis at endocardial biopsy.[53] Kosmas, reporting 1 case of MVP, noticed that it was possible to suppress by radiofrequency a nonsustained VT deemed to be idiopathic and originating in the right ventricular outflow tract.[45] In our series of 50 cases of idiopathic VT, we observed 5 cases of MVP; 2 had VT of left origin, but in 3 others, VT was of right ventricular origin (nonpublished data). It is also necessary to emphasize that the first illustrative cases of sudden death in MVP (60 up to 1980)[54] were reported before several arrhythmogenic deleterious diseases (arrhythmogenic right ventricular dysplasia, Brugada syndrome, torsades de pointes with brief QTc interval, etc.) were defined and/or become well known, perhaps suggesting the need for a retrospective revision of the diagnosis. Finally, relapse of severe cardiac arrhythmias[55] or occurrence of sudden death[22] after appropriate surgical correction of MVP is a good argument to suggest that valvular deformity is not directly incriminated in the fatal outcome.

2. *Electrophysiological findings:* The different QRS waveforms of ventricular arrhythmias (right or left bundle branch block morphology) are not consistent with an exclusively left valvular disease. The multiplicity of mechanisms evoked to explain life-threatening arrhythmias is rather disturbing. Above all, the abnormally high incidence of late ventricular potentials detected in all of the series of MVP (between 30% and 38%)[38-42] is not consistent with a purely valvular disease and suggests an associated myocardial disease.

3. *Isotopic study:* We have evaluated regional and overall wall motion using isotopic methods in a group of 36 patients with apparently isolated MVP. We found more marked heterogeneous right ventricular contraction in patients suffering from complex ventricular arrhythmias, suggesting right ventricular disease.[56]

4. *Pathology studies:* These studies show that isolated MVP is far from being the rule in cases of sudden death clinically attributed to this disease. In the 13 cases of sudden death with MVP studied post mortem by Davies et al., 7 had chordae rupture and 4 were suspected of having another possible cause of sudden death.[26] In a recent study of 163 cases of sudden death in young people, MVP was found in 10% of cases (17/163) but there was a high prevalence of myocardial abnor-

malities (12/17; 70%) chiefly in the right ventricle.[24] Likewise, another study concerning postmortem examination of 24 MVP patients with sudden death detected dysplasia of the atrioventricular nodal artery in 75% of cases, possibly responsible for septal ischemia, with fibrosis at the base of the ventricular septum.[51] In a postmortem study of 1,000 cases of sudden death, Loire et al.[57] observed 12.5% of PVM, of which only 1.4% were isolated, others being associated with different cardiac or vascular diseases. In 1997, Maron found isolated MVP in only 2% of 134 young competitive athletes with sudden death.[58] Even when MVP is isolated, lesions, scars, and/or atrial or left ventricle enlargement are not rare. It is thus difficult to be certain that the origin of sudden death is confined to valvular deformity.

Finally, with increased clinical and demographic experience, more appropriate invasive and noninvasive explorations, and multiplication of extended pathology studies, it seems that patients with trivial MVP dying suddenly (in fact, a rare eventuality) have another associated anatomic and/or electrophysiological disease more probably directly incriminated in this fatal event. This is hardly surprising, considering the fact that as early as 1987, Levy listed more than 50 conditions reportedly associated with MVP.[1]

## Management and Treatment

Clearly, MVP is a common and a benign condition, and the first step in its management is to reassure the majority of subjects who have moderate and/or asymptomatic valvular disease. Some patients warrant more invasive studies when they are believed to have a higher risk of fatal cardiac events (patients with MR, syncopes, or presyncopes, ventricular dysfunction, and/or life-threatening arrhythmias). Surgical correction by valve replacement or valvuloplasty of symptomatic and severe MR is indicated in a few patients (1–2%),[59] although it is obvious that such surgery does not entirely prevent complex arrhythmias or sudden death.[22,54,60–62] Surgery is thus a seldom quoted and certainly not generally accepted indication in MVP with life-threatening arrhythmias without hemodynamically significant MR because it seems unduly aggressive.[60] Rare cases of severe sinus node dysfunction or high-degree atrioventricular block need cardiac stimulation. Radiofrequency ablations are considered advisable for abnormal atrioventricular accessory pathways responsible for excessively rapid atrial arrhythmias. The prevention of ventricular arrhythmias (and sudden death, assuming that it has an arrythmogenic origin) is more problematic because no medical or surgical treatment has confirmed long-term efficacy. An approximate evaluation recently suggested that

2,000 MVP patients with repetitive or multiform PVCs (or at least 300 cases with MR) would require effective treatment for 1 year in order to prevent only 1 case of sudden death.[10] Nevertheless, when potentially lethal ventricular arrhythmias are documented (ECG, Holter monitoring), chiefly with demonstrated reproducibility and reinducibility (by exercise stress test, electrical programmed stimulation), beta blockers[22] or amiodarone[23] can be used in view of the frequent occurrence of ventricular arrhythmias and sudden death in a context of sympathetic stimulation. However, their efficacy is not established and they have to be tested with caution, with their advantages being compared to their arrhythmogenic risks. Arguing from good results obtained in other cardiac diseases (ischemic and nonischemic) with similar arrhythmogenic risk, it can be assumed that the most effective prevention of sudden death related to deleterious ventricular arrhythmias would be achieved with implantable defibrillator devices, but only a few cases have been reported.[16,20,21] In other words, the preventive treatment of sudden death in MVP seems questionable, and is more guided by the gravity of arrhythmias than by the existence of valvular disease itself. In view of the rare cases of sudden death associated with this condition, the results of this treatment have not to date been assessed, and it will be the aim of future studies to confirm the validity of such management.

## References

1. Levy D, Savage D. Prevalence and clinical features of mitral valve prolapse. Am Heart J 1987; 113:1281–1290.
2. Nishimura RA, Mc Goon MD, Shub C, et al. Echocardiographically documented mitral valve prolapse: long-term follow-up of 237 patients. N Engl J Med 1985; 13:1305–1309.
3. Savage DD, Levy D, Garrison RJ, et al. Mitral valve prolapse in the general population. 3. Dysrhythmias: the Framingham Study. Am Heart J 1983; 106:582–586.
4. Gilon D, Buonanno FS, Joffe MM, et al. Lack of evidence of an association between mitral valve prolapse and stroke in young patients. N Engl J Med 1999; 341:8–13.
5. Freed LA, Levy D, Levine RA, et al. Prevalence and clinical outcome of mitral valve prolapse. N Engl J Med 1999; 341:1–7.
6. Bella JN, Devereux RB. Mitral valve prolapse: clinically relevant aspects. Acc Curr J Rev 1998; 6:80–81.
7. Zuppiroli A, Rinaldi M, Fox RK, et al. Natural history of mitral valve prolapse. Am J Cardiol 1995; 75:1028–1032.
8. Nishimura RA, McGoon MD. Perspectives on mitral valve prolapse. N Engl J Med 1999; 341:48–50.
9. Jeresaty RM. Mitral Valve Prolapse. Raven Press, New York, 1979, pp 187–221.
10. Kligfield P, Devereux RB. Arrhythmia in mitral valve prolapse. In: Podrid PJ, Kowey PR (eds). Cardiac Arrhythmia: Mechanisms, Diagnosis and Management. Williams and Wilkins, Baltimore, 1995, pp 1253–1266.

11. Bisset GS, Schwartz DC, Meyer RA, et al. Clinical spectrum and long-term follow-up of isolated mitral valve prolapse in 119 children. Circulation 1980; 62:423–429.
12. Mills P, Rose J, Hollingsworth J, et al. Long-term prognosis of mitral valve prolapse. N Engl J Med 1977; 297:13–18.
13. Düren DR, Becker AE, Dunning AJ. Long-term follow-up of idiopathic mitral valve prolapse in 300 patients: a prospective study. J Am Coll Cardiol 1988; 11:42–47.
14. Kim S, Kuroda T, Nishinaga M, et al. Relation between severity of mitral regurgitation and prognosis of mitral valve prolapse: echocardiographic follow-up study. Am Heart J 1996; 132:348–355.
15. Chesler E, King RA, Edwards JE. The myoxomatous mitral valve and sudden death. Circulation 1983; 67:632.
16. Cristofini P, Desnos M, Funck F, et al. Défibrillateur automatique implantable pour fibrillations ventriculaires itératives sur prolapsus valvulaire mitral isolé. La Presse Médicale 1987; 16:13.
17. Jeresaty RM. Sudden death in the mitral valve prolapse click syndrome. Am J Cardiol 1976; 37:317–318.
18. Moritz HA, Parnass SM, Mitchel J. Ventricular fibrillation during anesthetic induction in a child with undiagnosed mitral valve prolapse. Anesth Anal 1997; 85:59–61.
19. Ronneberger DL, Hausmann R, Betz P. Sudden death associated with myoxomatous transformation of the mitral valve in an 8-year-old boy. Int J Legal Med 1998; 111:199–201.
20. Vlay SC. Ventricular tachycardia/fibrillation on the first day of medical school. Am J Cardiol 1986; 57:483.
21. Vlay SC. Morte d'amour with subsequent electrophysiologic studies. Am J Cardiol 1988; 61:1364.
22. Wilde AAM, Düren DR, Hauer RNW, et al. Mitral valve prolapse and ventricular arrhythmias: observations in a patient with a 20-year history. J Cardiovasc Electrophysiol 1997; 8:307–316.
23. Strasberg B, Caspi A, Kusniec J, et al. Ventricular fibrillation in a patient with "silent" mitral valve prolapse. Cardiology 1988; 75:149–153.
24. Corrado D, Basso C, Nava A, et al. Sudden death in young people with apparently isolated mitral valve prolapse. G Ital Cardiol 1997; 27:1097–1105.
25. Fukuda N, Oki T, Luchi A, et al. Predisposing factors for severe mitral regurgitation in idiopathic mitral valve prolapse. Am J Cardiol 1995; 76:503–507.
26. Davies HJ, Moore BP, Braimbridge MV. The floppy mitral valve: study of incidence, pathology and complications in surgical necropsy and forensic material. Br Heart J 1978; 40:468–481.
27. Dollar AL, Roberts WC. Morphologic comparison of patients with mitral prolapse who died suddenly with patients who died from severe valvular dysfunction or other conditions. J Am Coll Cardiol 1991; 17:921–931.
28. Leichtman D, Nelson R, Gobel F, et al. Bradycardia with mitral valve prolapse, a potential mechanism of sudden death. Ann Intern Med 1976; 85:453–455.
29. Ware JA, Magro SA, Luck JC, et al. Conduction system abnormalities in symptomatic mitral valve prolapse: an electrophysiologic analysis of 60 patients. Am J Cardiol 1984; 53:1075–1078.
30. Mc Kenna WJ, Alfonso F. Arrhythmias in the cardiomyopathies and mitral valve prolapse. In: Zipes DP, Rowlands DJ (eds). Progress in Cardiology. Lea and Febiger, Philadelphia, 1988, pp 59–75.
31. Brembilla-Perrot B, Beurrier D, Jacquemin L, et al. Syncopes associées au prolapsus mitral. Ann Cardiol Angiol 1996; 45:257–262.

32. Vesterby A, Bjerregaard P, Gregensen M, et al. Sudden death in mitral valve prolapse: associated accessory atrioventricular pathways. Forensic Sci Internat 1982; 19:125–133.
33. Babuty D, Fauchier L, Neel CH, et al. Arrhythmias and sudden death in patients with mitral valve prolapse. CEPR 1997; 1:264–267.
34. Fauchier J-P, Neel CH, Charbonnier B, et al. Les troubles du rythme du prolapsus mitral. Ann Cardiol Angiol 1980; 29:281–290.
35. Stoddard MF, Prince CR, Dillon S, et al. Exercise-induced mitral regurgitation is a predictor of morbid events in subjects with mitral valve prolapse. J Am Coll Cardiol 1995; 25:693–699.
36. Farb A, Tang AL, Atkinson JB, et al. Comparison of cardiac findings in patients with mitral valve prolapse who die suddenly to those who have congestive heart failure from mitral regurgitation and to those with fatal noncardiac conditions. Am J Cardiol 1992; 70:234–239.
37. Rosen SE, Borer JS, Hochreiter C, et al. Natural history of the asymptomatic/minimally symptomatic patient with severe mitral regurgitation secondary to mitral valve prolapse and normal right and left ventricular performance. Am J Cardiol 1994; 74:374–380.
38. Burger A, Jabi H, Orawiec B, et al. Late potentials in patients with mitral valve prolapse without ventricular tachycardia (abstract). J Am Coll Cardiol 1990; 15:38A.
39. Babuty D, Charniot J-C, Delhomme C, et al. Potentiels ventriculaires tardifs et prolapsus valvulaire mitral. Arch Mal Coeur 1994; 87:339–347.
40. Jabi H, Burger AJ, Orawiec B, et al. Late potentials in mitral valve prolapse. Am Heart J 1991; 122:1340–1345.
41. Leclercq J-F, Malergue M-C, Coumel P. Potentiels tardifs et prolapsus valvulaire mitral. Arch Mal Cœur 1993; 86:285–289.
42. Turitto G, Klonis D, Val-Mejias JE. High frequency of late potentials in mitral valve prolapse (abstract). J Am Coll Cardiol 1991; 17:387A.
43. Rosenthal ME, Hamer A, Gang ES, et al. The yield of programmed ventricular stimulation in mitral valve prolapse patients with ventricular arrhythmias. Am Heart J 1985; 110:970–976.
44. Babuty D, Cosnay P, Breuillac J-C, et al. Ventricular arrhythmias factors in mitral valve prolapse. PACE 1994; 17:1090–1099.
45. Kosmas CE, Dalessandro DA, Langieri G, et al. Monomorphic right ventricular tachycardia in a patient with mitral valve prolapse. PACE 1996; 19:509–513.
46. Shenoy MM, Hariman RJ, Balla S, et al. Triggered activity as a possible mechanism of ventricular tachycardia in mitral valve prolapse. Am Heart J 1986; 112:1339–1342.
47. Wit AL, Fenoglio JJ, Hordof AJ, et al. Ultrastructure and transmembrane potentials of cardiac muscle in the human anterior mitral valve leaflet. Circulation 1979; 59:1284–1292.
48. Slovut DP, Lurie KG. A potential mechanism for mitral valve prolapse syndrome. J Cardiovasc Electrophysiol 1998; 9:100–102.
49. Cowan MD, Fye WB. Prevalence of QTc prolongation in women with mitral valve prolapse. Am J Cardiol 1989; 63:133–134.
50. Boudoulas H. Mitral valve prolapse: etiology, clinical presentation and neuroendocrine function. J Heart Valve Dis 1992; 1:175–188.
51. Burke AP, Farb A, Tang A, Smialek J, et al. Fibromuscular dysplasia of small coronary arteries and fibrosis in the basilar ventricular septum in mitral valve prolapse. Am Heart J 1997; 134:282–291.
52. Crawford MH, O'Rourke RA. Mitral valve prolapse: a cardiomyopathic state? Prog Cardiovasc Dis 1984; 27:133–147.

53. La Vecchia S, Ometto R, Centofante P. Arrhythmic profile, ventricular function and histomorphometric findings in patients with idiopathic ventricular tachycardia and mitral valve prolapse. Clin Cardiol 1998; 21:731–735.
54. Jeresaty RM. Mitral valve prolapse: definition and implications in athletes. J Am Coll Cardiol 1986; 7:231–236.
55. Kay HJ, Krohn BG, Zubiate P, et al. Surgical correction of severe mitral prolapse without mitral insufficiency but with pronounced cardiac arrhythmias. J Thorac Cardiovasc Surg 1979; 78:259–267.
56. Delhomme C, Casset-Senon D, Babuty D, et al. Etude par tomographie cavitaire isotopique de 36 cas de prolapsus valvulaire mitral. Arch Mal C_ur 1996; 89:1127–1135.
57. Loire R, Tabib A. Mort subite cardiaque inattendue: bilan de 1,000 autopsies. Arch Mal C_ur 1996; 89:13–18.
58. Maron BJ. The young competitive athlete: causes of sudden death, detection, preparticipation screening, and standards for disqualification with cardiac abnormalities. CEPR 1997; 1:274–277.
59. Wilcken DEL, Hickey AJ. Lifetime risk for patients with mitral valve prolapse of developing severe valve regurgitation requiring surgery. Circulation 1988; 78:10–14.
60. Pocock WA, Barlow JB, Marcus RH, et al. Mitral valvuloplasty for life-threatening ventricular arrhythmias in mitral valve prolapse. Am Heart J 1991; 121:199–202.
61. Vohra J, Sathe S, Warren R, et al. Malignant ventricular arrhythmias in patients with mitral valve prolapse and mild mitral regurgitation. PACE 1993; 16(Part I):387–393.
62. Viguier E, Delahaye JP, De Gevigney G, et al. Les arythmies ventriculaires pré- et postopératoires de l'insuffisance mitrale. Arch Mal Cœur 1994; 87:439–444.

## 31

# Sudden Death in Patients with Cardiac Conduction Disorders

*Henri E. Kulbertus, MD*

## Introduction

The literature published in the 1970s and 1980s demonstrated a keen interest of the medical community in the epidemiology, etiopathogenesis, prognostic significance, and management of cardiac conduction disorders. The relationship between the latter and sudden cardiac death was repeatedly emphasized. It seems, however, that the electrocardiologists who worked on that subject rapidly had their attention drawn toward other areas, especially the newer techniques of investigation or therapy such as invasive electrophysiology, signal-averaged electrocardiography, heart rate variability, and ablation. The major medical literature databases reveal that over the last 10–15 years, very few new papers were devoted to cardiac conduction disorders, and the majority in the last few months dealt with the extremely interesting, albeit relatively not very common, Brugada.

In spite of all the knowledge accumulated about a quarter of a century ago, it is noteworthy that the fortuitous discovery of a bundle branch block or of an atrioventricular (AV) conduction disturbance at routine electrocardiography still poses even today the problem of how best to assess the significance of that finding in the clinical context of the patient in whom it is discovered.

## Atrioventricular Block

### Congenital Complete Atrioventricular Block

The initial view of the prognosis of congenital complete AV block was rather optimistic. However, this has progressively changed. Michaelsson

From: Aliot E, Clementy J, Prystowsky EN (editors). *Fighting Sudden Cardiac Death: A Worldwide Challenge.* ©Futura Publishing Company, Armonk, NY, 2000.

et al.[1] recently published an update of studies on the natural history of this disorder. They indicate that a risk for heart failure, syncope, and sudden death is present at any age, including during fetal life. Ultrasound screening (Figure 1) has shown that complete fetal AV block can be manifest and detected as early as the 16th week of pregnancy. More than 50% of the cases have associated structural disease that entails a high fetal mortality reaching up to 85%. The fetal mortality in isolated congenital complete AV block is high as well-between 11% and 25%. Admittedly, the series that have been reported to date come from large university centers whose statistics may be biased toward cases with an unfavorable prognosis. It seems, in fact, that most fetuses with an isolated complete AV block and a ventricular rate above 60/min have no problem during gestation, labor, and delivery.[1] In contrast, a low ventricular rate of (55/min, fetal hydrops, increased cardiothoracic index, AV valve regurgitation, and low aortic flow velocity indicate a poor prognosis and require anticongestive prena-

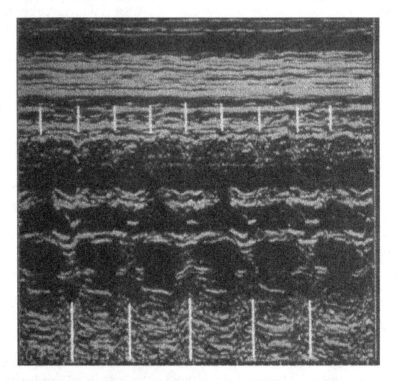

Figure 1. M-mode fetal echocardiogram showing AV dissociation (small vertical bars identify atrial contractions; longer bars = ventricular contractions) by complete AV block in a 32-week-old fetus. (Courtesy of Professor D. Soyeur, University of Liège, Belgium.)

tal therapy with, possibly, early delivery and immediate postnatal pacing. Thus, the prognosis is not good in the fetus with associated structural heart disease and it becomes very poor if the fetus is hydropic, even if the heart rate remains above 60/min.

Indications for pacing in infancy, according to Michaelsson et al.,[1] are congestive heart failure, ventricular rate below 55/min in isolated block, and below 65/min with associated disease, prolonged QTc interval, syncopal attacks, frequent ventricular ectopic beats, and alternating ventricular pacemakers. During childhood and adult life, symptoms associated with congenital AV block may appear at any age. It is interesting to note that the ventricular rate decreases with age in isolated congenital heart block. In a series published by Michaelsson,[2] the median ventricular rate was 60 in the neonate, 50 between ages 6 to 10 years, 45 between 16 and 20 years, and 38 over 40 years of age. It is therefore important to regularly assess the median ventricular rate and compare it with normal values for age. Indications for prompt pacing in childhood and adult life according to Michaelsson et al.[1] are syncope, prolonged QT interval, and mitral regurgitation. They recommend that all patients older than 15 years be prophylactically paced.[1]

## Chronic Acquired Complete Atrioventricular Block

Although complete AV block may be associated with valvular (especially aortic) heart disease or a variety of other cardiac or systemic diseases, chronic complete AV block most often results from idiopathic bilateral bundle branch fibrosis. It is a process in which conduction fibers progressively vanish from the bifurcating AV bundle and proximal bundle branches. In the form described by Lev,[3] the initial loss of conduction fibers takes place in the proximal left bundle branch and then extends into the bifurcating bundle, producing AV block. According to Lev, this disease process results from the combined effects of aging and of microtraumatic lesions to the specialized tissue provoked by the contractions of the interventricular septum. The lesions described by Lenegre[4] showed progressive loss of conduction fibers with replacement fibrosis in diffuse or focal segments of both right and left bundle branches. Extension of the loss of conduction fibers into the distal portion of the bundle branches was also seen. The hypothesis that this may result from a myopathic process selective for conduction fibers has been postulated.[5] An important feature is that in both cases, the myocardium adjacent to the conduction system is normal and the small septal arteries are almost always open. The disease is by nature progressive and its manifestations appear almost exclusively in elderly patients. They may appear at an earlier age in subjects in whom the conduction system was partially damaged, for example, by an episode of diphtheric myocarditis, and in whom idiopathic fibrosis of bundle branches associated with aging adds itself to the sequelae of the previous disease.

A proportion of patients with complete heart block survive for years without showing any symptoms. At some stage they may develop heart failure or syncopal attacks of the Adams-Stokes variety. When this happens, if left untreated, the life expectancy is usually very short, i.e., no more than a few months. It has been clearly established that symptomatic complete AV block has a mortality greater than 50% in 5 years and that it can even reach 50% in 1 year.[6] These patients often die suddenly, the cause of death being either cardiac asystole or a ventricular rhythm disorder, possibly starting with an episode of torsades de pointes, an arrhythmia that is favored by bradycardic rhythms. Ventricular pacing is known to modify the mortality of patients with symptomatic complete AV block in such a way that the life survival curve of groups of such patients after implantation closely approaches the curve obtained in the normal population of similar age.

Less information is available regarding Mobitz type II AV block. It seems, however, that it often progresses to complete AV block; then, when symptoms have developed, the outlook is poor as in unpaced patients with complete AV block. Once again, pacing restores a life expectancy similar to that of the general population.[7,8] The view is generally held that Mobitz type I AV block is rather benign. This has been questioned in a study[9] in which the incidence of symptoms, prognosis, and influence of pacing were the same in Mobitz type I AV block as those for patients with Mobitz type II block. This, of course, did not apply to young individuals with transient, nocturnal Wenckebach block due to high vagal tone, which is benign.[7]

## Atrioventricular Block Associated with Acute Myocardial Infarction

Acute myocardial infarction represents the most frequent cause of acute transient complete AV block. Its incidence may reach 30% in series of patients submitted to electrocardiographic monitoring.

### Anterior Infarction

AV blocks associated with anterior infarction are due to extensive lesions of the conduction system. The right bundle branch is almost completely destroyed in its median part by a massive necrosis of the septum. The fascicles of the left bundle branch running along the septal surface may be simultaneously involved. The conduction disorder seems to result partially from necrosis of the specific tissue, and partially from hypoxic dysfunction. The AV block is of sudden onset, but is generally preceded by the development of signs of bilateral conduction disorders. The escape rhythm is generally extremely slow and unstable. Invariably, the mortality among those patients is extremely high even if temporary pacing is used and relates to pump dysfunction due to extensive myocardial infarction.[10-12] In those who survive, AV conduction may resume, usually with persistence of a long PR interval and/or a complete right bundle branch block (RBBB) or bifascicular block. The sudden death rate among those patients is high, death occurring frequently within the first weeks or months after the acute event.

## Inferior Infarction

The incidence of AV block complicating inferior infarction varies between 14% and 20%.[13] It is generally an early complication of the infarct and occurs in 70% of patients during the first 24 hours of admission. The lesions responsible for this rhythm disorder are generally located within the Tawara node or the initial portion of the common His bundle. They are generally reversible. If AV block is complete, the escape rhythm is junctional and frequently of a satisfactory rate, and stable. Return to normal conduction often occurs within a few days. The general opinion is that the prognosis is extremely favorable. Our own experience[13] reported in 1989 indicated that, among 477 consecutive patients admitted for inferior acute myocardial infarction, second or third degree AV block developed in 20% (88 cases). Compared with the 359 without AV block, these 88 patients presented a higher incidence of Killip Class 1, pericarditis, atrial fibrillation, complete bundle branch block, and in-hospital mortality (24% versus 4%; p<0.001). Among the patients with AV block, those who died in hospital were older, and had a higher incidence of heart failure and bundle branch block. Interestingly, the 3-year mortality among hospital survivors who had had AV block in the acute phase and those who did not have this complication was superposable. Therefore, one can conclude that there is no increase of sudden cardiac death among patients who developed AV block in inferior acute myocardial infarction and survived the hospital stay.

# Bundle Branch Block

## Bundle Branch Block Not Associated with Acute Myocardial Infarction

As early as 1933, Graybiel and Sprague[14] reported on a group of 395 patients with bundle branch block generally associated with hypertension or coronary artery disease. Adequate follow-up obtained in 77% yielded

223 fatal cases with an average survival of 14 months. Perera et al.[15] studied 104 cases of right bundle branch block (RBBB) and 60 cases of left bundle branch block (LBBB). Sixty percent of the latter were dead at 1 year and over one-third of the former had died over a mean period of 4 years. Several other publications derived from observation of hospital-based series indicated that a bundle branch block was a sign of very poor prognosis. In the late 1970s, 2 major studies drew attention toward the prognostic significance of bundle branch block in terms of sudden cardiac death.

In 1978, McAnulty et al.[16] reviewed 42,000 electrocardiograms recorded at their University Hospital from 1969 to 1971. Three hundred twenty-five patients had LBBB or RBBB with axis deviation. Survival at 4 years of 164 LBBB patients (40.7 ± 4.1%) was approximately equal to that of 161 patients with RBBB and axis deviation (49.5 ± 4.2%). Patients with coronary artery disease had a particularly poor prognosis (survival at 5 years: 33.7%), especially if they had a history of previous myocardial infarction (survival at 5 years: 23.5%). Primary conduction disease was present in 20% with a survival of 50.6% at 5 years; it was therefore not without risk of its own. The same group[17] prospectively followed up 257 patients with LBBB or RBBB with axis deviation who had been submitted to His bundle studies. Over a follow-up period of 25 months, 50 patients died; 27 of them died suddenly. Actuarial analysis revealed an annual mortality rate of 29% ± 2.6% and a sudden death rate of 10.2% ± 2.6%. Length of the HV interval did not influence the outcome. This is in contrast with other publications,[18,19] indicating that a greatly prolonged HV interval identifies a subgroup of patients at high risk of sudden death, especially when heart failure is associated. In the same year (1978), Dinghra et al.[20] reported that among 102 patients with chronic LBBB followed up for 32 to 2,271 days, the cumulative mortality at 4 years was close to 70% and the mortality by sudden death was approximately 60%. The same authors[21] observed among 452 patients with RBBB and axis deviation that the cumulative mortality by sudden death was 20% ± 2.3% at 4 years. As stated earlier, these publications were all derived from observation of hospital-based series.

It was soon realized that the prognosis was much better when bundle branch block was detected in individuals without clinical evidence of cardiovascular disease. Thus, an investigation studied the prevalence and prognosis of electrocardiographic findings in 18,403 London male civil servants aged 40 to 60.[22] These subjects were followed-up for 5 years. In LBBB, the excess coronary artery disease mortality reached the 5% level of statistical significance, but the dominant impression was the low level of risk in the group with nonsymptomatic history. Among 321 patients with ventricular conduction defects, only 2 died of coronary artery disease. The contrast between the results obtained in hospital-based patients and those obtained in subjects without a symptomatic history was further confirmed by 2 other studies. The Manitoba Study[23–25] was designed to evaluate the predictive value of the electrocardiogram for sudden death in the absence of preexisting manifestations of heart disease. Three thousand nine hundred and eighty-three individuals, all former Canadian Air Force pilots, pilots in training, or licensed pilots, were followed-up for 30 years (1948–1978). Cases were selected if they fulfilled 2 criteria: (1) an electrocardiographic abnormality that was detected during a routine examination; (2) no clinical evidence of ischemic or valvular disease existed in either that examination or the previous one since entry.

Among this group, 70 died suddenly; 50 (71.4%) had electrocardiographic abnormalities. These included 22 cases (31.4%) with ST-T changes, 11 (15%) with ventricular premature beats, 9 (12.9%) with left ventricular hypertrophy, 5 (7.1%) with LBBB, and 4 (5.7%) with abnormal left axis deviation. None had RBBB. In the Manitoba cohort, LBBB without evidence of heart disease was noted in 33 cases. Among those, cardiovascular mortality, all by sudden death, was 15.2% (5/33). The age-adjusted sudden death incidence rate was 12.2 per 1,000 person years, i.e., almost 14 times the incidence in men without LBBB. Prognosis in LBBB was dependent on the age of the patient at its detection. For men aged 35 to 44, there was no increased risk of sudden death. In contrast, among men in the age range of 45 to 64, the 5-year incidence of sudden death as the first manifestation of coronary artery disease was more than 10 times higher than among men without LBBB. This difference might reflect a difference in etiology. In young people, LBBB might be due to a congenital malformation with no adverse prognosis. Thus, the results of that study indicated that LBBB is a serious finding when it develops in men after the age of 40. Several other population studies have indicated that cardiovascular mortality in newly acquired LBBB was significantly increased even after considering multivariate analysis, age, blood pressure, diabetes, coronary heart disease, and congestive heart failure.[26,27] Conversely, different population studies with control or comparison groups have demonstrated that complete RBBB with or without axis deviation is not a predictor of sudden cardiac death.

Our group also published the data obtained during an experimental community hypertension screening program carried out in Liege in the early 1970s.[28] Briefly, screening was performed in selected urban, suburban, and rural parts of the province. All individuals aged 35 or over were invited to submit themselves to a screening examination. Subjects under current treatment for cardiovascular disease were advised not to come. Each subject was asked to fill out a questionnaire dealing with smoking habits and family or personal history of cardiovascular disease and to indicate all medications taken at the time of examination. The Rose and Blackburn questionnaire for the diagnosis of effort angina was answered with the help of a nurse. The patients were also submitted to a measurement of height and weight, a standard electrocardiogram, a chest x-ray, and finally, a blood pressure measurement taken after a 10-minute period of rest in the supine position. Between October 1, 1973, and June 13, 1977, 33,001 individuals were examined (15,300–46.3% male; 17,701–53.6% female). The overall prevalence and age distribution of the various types of conduction disorders are shown in Figure 2. Generally, conduction defects increased in frequency with increasing age. The age slope for left anterior hemiblock was shallower than for RBBB and LBBB. Conduction disorders were more frequent in men than in women as far as left anterior hemiblock, RBBB, and left anterior hemiblock-RBBB were concerned. In contrast, LBBB showed a slight but statistically significant predominance in the female group (male to female ratio: 0.68; p<0.01). Three hundred and nineteen cases with isolated RBBB (197 male; 122 female), 248 cases with LBBB (85 male; 163 female), and 129 instances of left anterior hemiblock-RBBB (93 male; 36 female) were diagnosed at entry. These patients were followed up for an average of 4 years. Their outcome was compared with that of paired controls. Among patients with RBBB, no instances of sudden cardiac death were observed; total mortality was not increased at 48 months, unless in the presence of associated left anterior hemiblock. Among patients with LBBB, total mortality and cardiac mortality were significantly increased at 36 and 48 months, compared to controls. The sudden death rate (20.5% at 36 and 48 months) was higher than in controls (5% at 36 months; 10% at 48 months, respectively), but not significantly so.

It is interesting to illustrate the survival curves (Figure 3) obtained in patients with bundle branch block and without apparent heart disease.[29] There were 161 subjects with RBBB and no heart disease-110 men and 51 women. Their mean age was 61.78 ± 11.71 years and they were followed-up for an average of 39.21 ± 16.03 months. In this group, 7 deaths were observed. None was sudden, 2 were cardiac, and 5 were noncardiac. The actuarial survival curve was superposable to that of matched controls. There were 57 instances of LBBB without apparent heart disease (27 men, 30 women). They had a mean age of 60.79 ± 11.81 years and their average follow-up period was 41.22 ± 50.72 months. In that group, 4 deaths were registered-2 were sudden and 2 were noncardiac. The actuarial analysis failed to disclose any significant difference between the 2 groups regarding mortality rate. It should be noted, however, that the survival curve of LBBB patients was consistently below that of matched controls. Finally, 45 instances of RBBB with left anterior hemiblock and no apparent heart disease were discovered (35 men, 10 women). Their mean age was 67.04 ± 9.00 years and the average follow-up period was 45.88 ± 15.86 months. Three of them died, 1 from myocardial infarction and 2 from bronchial carcinoma. There was no instance of sudden death and the survival curve compared to that of the matched controls was almost superposable.

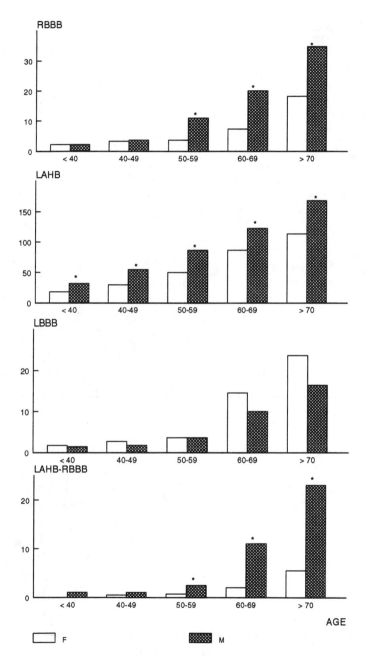

Figure 2. Age and sex distribution of conduction disorders among 33,001 individuals examined in the Province of Liège. (Used with permission from Kulbertus HE, et al.[28]) *p<0.01.

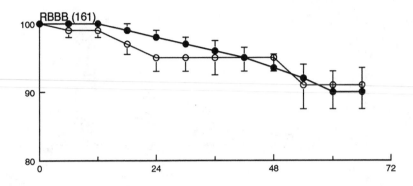

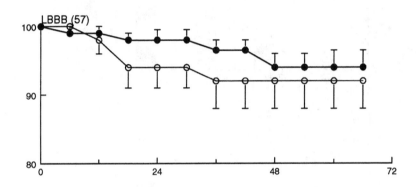

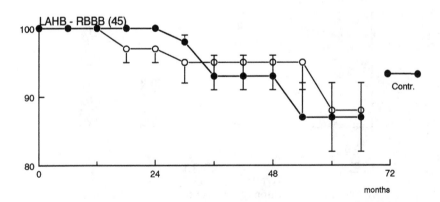

Figure 3. Survival curves of subjects with various conduction disorders compared to matched controls. (Used with permission from Kulbertus HE, et al.[29])

The projected 5-year mortality rate of all subjects with bundle branch block without apparent heart disease was 10%. Exactly the same figure was obtained for the whole group of controls. This may be compared with the annual mortality rate observed for the whole population of the French- and German-speaking part of Belgium in the late 1970s, which at the age of 65 was 1.75% for women and 4% for men.

In conclusion, these various studies have provided important but incomplete information. It is clear that in patients with overt cardiac disease, bundle branch block is an ominous sign and indicates a threat of sudden death. This is particularly evident for populations of patients culled from large cardiology departments of university hospitals. It seems to apply to all etiologies of cardiac disease (ischemic, hypertensive, valvular, or idiopathic). The prognostic significance of a bundle branch block in the individual without evidence and symptoms of cardiovascular disease still contains areas of uncertainty. It seems clear that isolated RBBB does not carry any particular risk. Conversely, LBBB, especially newly acquired in men after the age of 40, represents a serious finding that should prompt careful cardiac assessment. The literature, however, contains no guidelines indicating which type of investigation should be selected to try and identify the individual at high risk of sudden cardiac death.

## Bundle Branch Block Associated with Acute Myocardial Infarction

We have to mention from the start that the statistics on which the following paragraphs are based were obtained before the thrombolytic era. Therefore, we do not know whether they apply to patients treated with modern methods of reperfusion. The data are still of value, however, because of the fact that a sizable proportion of patients with myocardial infarction, for various reasons, are still treated without reperfusion therapy.

It has long been known that the presence of a bundle branch block in the course of an acute myocardial infarction significantly worsens the prognosis. Several series have demonstrated this phenomenon, which is illustrated by our own results[30] and by pooled results from 12 different studies,[31] One had expected that the risk would be particularly increased in patients with new versus preexisting bundle branch block; indeed, myocardial infarction patients who develop a new bundle branch block generally have larger infarcts, carrying the risk of cardiogenic shock or heart failure. This hypothesis has been confirmed by some studies[32,33] but not by others.[34] The site of the block also seems to have an influence. Norris and Woo had suggested that RBBB (both old or preexisting) had a worse hospital mortality rate than LBBB.[35] Several studies on freshly acquired RBBB[32,35] have confirmed this finding, although this was not the case in all series.[36,37] What is the relationship between bundle branch block seen during an acute phase of myocardial infarction and postmyocardial infarction sudden cardiac death? In a study published in 1980, Lie et al.[38] reported that of 1,008 hospital survivors of myocardial infarction 26 died suddenly within 1 year of the infarct. The subset of patients with bundle branch block and anteroseptal infarction seemed to behave in a particular manner since 4 of the 5 sudden deaths with this type of infarct occurred within 6 weeks after the infarction. In this series, 4 of 7 patients with early (<6 weeks after onset on infarction) sudden death had the initial characteristics of bundle branch block complicating an anteroseptal infarction.

Our group also reported on the short- and long-term prognostic significance of complete bundle branch block complicating acute myocardial infarction.[30] Among 1,013 consecutive patients with acute myocardial infarction, 104 (10%) developed complete bundle branch block. The clinical characteristics and the short- and long-term prognosis were similar in the 53 patients with right and the 51 patients with LBBB. Compared to the 909 patients without this conduction disturbance, these 104 patients were older (64 ± 9 versus 58 ± 10 years, p<0.001), more frequently women (26% versus 17%, p<0.05), had a larger infarct (peak CK 1,672 ± 1,124 versus 1,356 ± 1,089 IU/l, p<0.001), and were more frequently anterior (60% versus 37%, p<0.001). They had a higher incidence of Killip Class 1 (63% versus 38%, p<0.001), pericarditis (40% versus 23%, p<0.001), atrial fibrillation or flutter (22% versus 12%, p<0.01), ventricular fibrillation (15% versus 9%, p<0.05), and AV block (23% versus 11%, p<0.001). Both hospital mortality (32% versus 10%, p<0.001) and 3-year post-hospital mortality (37% versus 18%, p<0.001) were much higher among patients with complete bundle branch block. Transient bundle branch block had the same deleterious prognosis as bundle branch block persistent at discharge (mortality 33% versus 39%, ns). The prognostic importance of bundle branch block was more prominent during the first 6 months after infarction (mortality between 6 and 36 months: 18% with bundle branch block versus 11% without bundle branch block, ns).

# Conduction Disorders in Rarer Clinical Conditions

## Conduction Disorders and Sudden Cardiac Death in Athletes

It has sometimes been suggested that some occult abnormalities of the cardiac conduction system in the absence of other structural cardiac abnormalities may be responsible for sudden death in young athletes and young people with otherwise structurally normal hearts.[39] This must be extremely exceptional and, in the reported cases, the described morphologic abnormalities that were incriminated as the determinants of sudden death were not absolutely demonstrated to be the cause of the demise.[40]

## Brugada Syndrome[41,42]

In 1992, Brugada and Brugada[43] described a distinct group of patients with episodes of idiopathic polymorphic ventricular tachycardia or ventricular fibrillation, and the unique ECG pattern characterized by RBBB and ST elevation from $V_1$ to $V_3$ (Figure 4). They introduced the term "RBBB, persisting ST segment elevation, and sudden cardiac death syndrome." The familial occurrence of the syndrome has been underlined in several series. The syndrome almost exclusively affects male patients and manifests primarily in adult life (30–40 years). It might be responsible for 4–12% of unexpected sudden deaths and for 50% of all sudden deaths in patients with an apparently normal heart.[42]

It is noteworthy that the electrocardiographic abnormalities associated with the syndrome can vary and even completely disappear at times. These changes are probably due to modulation of the autonomic nervous system. Class Ia and Ic antiarrhythmic drugs and beta blockers increase the ST elevation, and administration of ajmaline, procainamide, or flecainide can unmask the distinctive electrocardiographic abnormalities in affected patients with intermittent changes or in familial members with apparently normal electrocardiograms. The recent discovery of a missense mutation in the cardiac sodium channel gene *SCN5A* in patients with Brugada syndrome provided important new insight to the understanding of the genetic and molecular bases of the syndrome. Genetically induced sodium channel dysfunction with current inhibition may result in loss of the epicardial action potential dome in the right ventricular epicardium with transmural dispersion of repolarization, which in turn may lead to ventricular fibrillation. Corrado et al.[41] have insisted on the fact that the diagnosis of Brugada syndrome can be made only after careful investigation to rule out the possibility of any organic heart disease. The pattern of RBBB with precordial ST elevation can indeed be encountered in patients with structural heart disease affecting the right ventricle, such as arrhythmogenic right ventricular cardiomyopathy, familial cardiac conduction and myocardial disease, and infiltrative cardiomyopathy. The only treatment for symptomatic patients with Brugada syndrome is implantation of a defibrillator.

## Late Sudden Death in Postoperative Tetralogy of Fallot[44]

Children who have undergone definitive surgical repair of tetralogy of Fallot may develop late onset ventricular arrhythmias and sudden car-

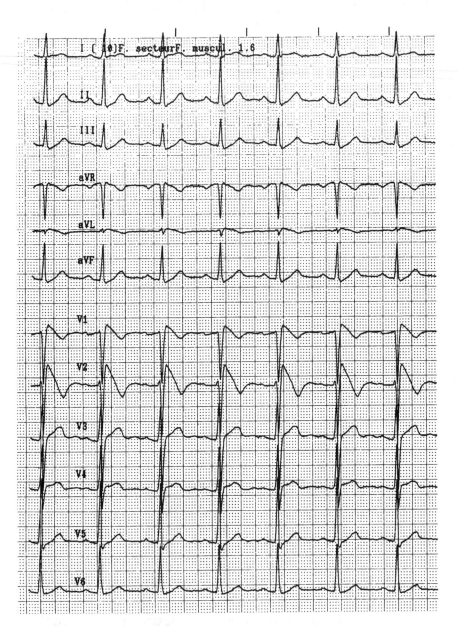

**Figure 4.** Electrocardiogram of a 32-year-old man with the Brugada syndrome.

diac death with an estimated risk ranging from 2% to 10%, possibly increasing with age or time from surgery. Following surgical repair, many patients have both depolarization and repolarization abnormalities, including RBBB possibly associated with left anterior hemiblock and QT prolongation (Figure 5). Initially, it had been expected that sudden death in these patients might result from evolution of the conduction disorders into complete AV block and asystole. Now it is generally accepted that the cause of death is a ventricular arrhythmia. Nonuniform conduction delay due to chronic ventricular hypertrophy, scars, areas of ischemia or infarction, and arterial patch materials may promote reentrant ventricular arrhythmias. The regionally inhomogeneous ventricular repolarization may also promote the arrhythmias, and there are probably multiple potential mechanisms for sudden death in these patients. Several investigations have attempted to define the best marker for the risk of sudden death in this population. QRS prolongation as a single ECG marker seems more predictive than QT duration or dispersion for identifying vulnerability to late onset ventricular arrhythmias.[45]

## Conduction Disorders in Still Rarer Conditions

Patients with cardiac primary amyloidosis[46] are prone to disease of the His-Purkinje system. Prolongation of the HV interval is common and may not be detected from the surface electrocardiogram in the presence of narrow QRS complexes. These patients have a high prevalence of sudden cardiac death, the independent predictor of which is the length of the HV interval.

Steinert's myotonia commonly affects the conduction system and congestive failure is less frequent. The site of AV conduction impairment may be difficult to identify by noninvasive electrocardiography. Patients with such abnormalities of cardiac conduction may suffer sudden cardiac death due to AV block or ventricular electrical instability. Active inflammatory processes (for example, myocarditis) and various infiltrative processes (amyloidosis, scleroderma, hematochromatosis, morbid obesity) may damage the AV node and/or the His bundle and produce AV block. Focal diseases (sarcoidosis, Whipple's disease, rheumatic arthritis) also at times involve the conduction system. These lesions of the conduction system have been implicated as possible substrates for sudden cardiac death. Focal involvement of the conduction tissue by tumors (mesothelioma of the AV node, lymphoma, carcinoma, rhabdomyoma, and fibroma) has also been reported and some cases of sudden cardiac death have been attributed to these lesions. Some authors have also described an abnormal postnatal morphogenesis of the specialized conduction tissue as a significant factor in sudden cardiac death in infants and in children.[47]

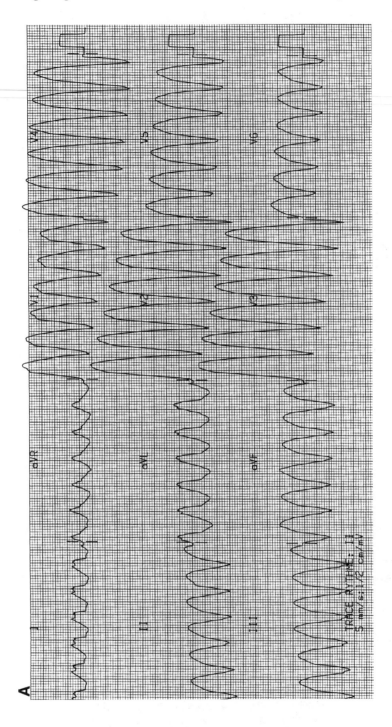

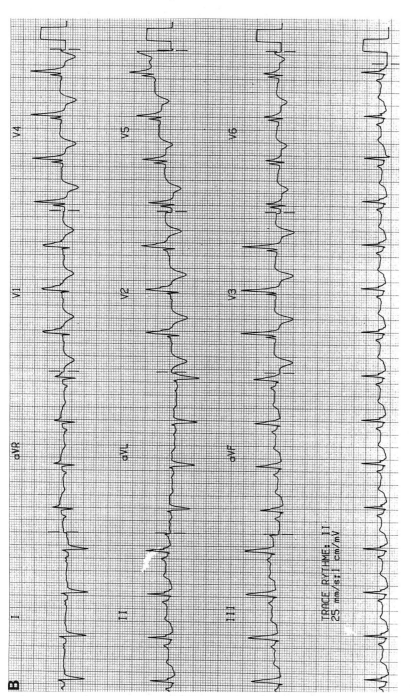

Figure 5. Electrocardiograms of 27-year-old woman who developed severe ventricular tachycardia 11 years after complete correction of a tetralogy of Fallot (A). Her postoperative tracing showed complete RBBB and inferior axis (B).

## Conclusions

Cardiac conduction disorders were intensively studied in the 1970s and 1980s. Their relationships with sudden cardiac death were strongly emphasized at the time. Progressively, however, they seem to have disappeared from the literature. Recent excellent reviews on sudden cardiac death[48] and on patients at high risk of subsequent arrhythmic death after myocardial infarction[49] hardly mention conduction disorders among their lists of risk factors.

In spite of this, the discovery of a bundle branch block still remains a sign of great prognostic significance in many different diseases; its value for identification of patients at high risk of sudden cardiac death should not be disregarded.

## *References*

1. Michaelsson M, Riesenfeld T, Jouzou A. Natural history of congenital complete atrioventricular block. PACE 1997; 20:2098.
2. Michaelsson M. Congenital complete atrioventricular block. Prog Pediatr Cardiol 1995; 4:1.
3. Lev M. The pathology of complete atrioventricular block. Prog Cardiovasc Dis 1964; 6:317.
4. Lenègre J. Etiology and pathology of bilateral branch fibrosis in relation to complete heart block. Prog Cardiovasc Dis 1964; 6:409.
5. Davies MJ, Ward DE. The pathology of arrhythmias, conduction disturbances and sudden death. In: Julian DG, Camm AJ, Fox KM, et al (eds). Diseases of the Heart. Baillière-Tindall, London, 1989, p 496.
6. Sutton R, Bourgeois I. The Foundations of Cardiac Pacing. Futura Publishing Co, Mount Kisco, NY, 1991, p 236.
7. Bennett DH. The management of bradycardias. In: Julian DG, Camm AJ, Fox KM. et al. (eds). Diseases of the Heart. Baillière-Tindall, London, 1989, p 584.
8. Shaw DB, Kekwick CA, Veale D, Gowers J, Whistance T. Survival in second degree atrioventricular block. Br Heart J 1985; 53:587.
9. Strasberg B, Amat-y-Leon F, Dhingra RC, et al. History of chronic second degree atrioventricular nodal block. Circulation 1981; 63:1043.
10. Norris RM. Heart block in posterior and anterior infarction. Br Heart J 1969; 31:352.
11. Kostuk WJ, Blanlands DI. Complete heart block associated with acute myocardial infarction. Am J Cardiol 1970; 26:1034.
12. Rosen KM, Loeb HS, Cherquimia R, et al. Site of heart block in acute myocardial infarction. Circulation 1970; 42:925.
13. Dubois C, Pierard LA, Smeets JP, Carlier J, Kulbertus HE. Long-term prognostic significance of atrioventricular block in inferior acute myocardial infarction. Eur Heart J 1989; 10:816.
14. Graybiel A, Sprague HB. Bundle branch block: an analysis of 395 cases. Am J Med Sci 1933; 185:395.
15. Perera G, Levine SA, Erlanger H. Prognosis of right bundle branch block: a study of 104 cases. Br Heart J 1942; 4:35.
16. McAnulty JH, Kauffman S, Murphy E, Kassebaum DG, Rahimtoola SH. Sur-

vival in patients with intraventricular conduction defects. Arch Intern Med 1978; 138:30.

17. McAnulty JH, Rahimtoola SH, Murphy ES, Kauffman S, Ritzmanm LW, et al. A prospective study of sudden death in "high risk" bundle branch block. N Engl J Med 1978; 299:209.

18. Narula OS, Gann D, Samet P. Prognostic value of H-V intervals in His bundle electrocardiography and clinical electrophysiology. In: Narula OS (ed). His Bundle Electrocardiography and Clinical Electrophysiology. FA Davis Co, Philadelphia, 1975, p 437.

19. Scheinman M, Peters RW, Modin G, Brennan M, Mies C, et al. Prognostic value of intranodal conduction time in patients with chronic bundle branch block. Circulation 1977; 56:240.

20. Dinghra RC, Amat-Y-Leon F, Wyndham C, Sridhar SS, Wu D, et al. Significance of left axis deviation in patients with chronic left bundle branch block. Am J Cardiol 1978; 42:551.

21. Dinghra RC, Wyndham C, Amat-Y-Leon F, Denes P, Wu D, et al. Incidence and site of atrioventricular block in patients with chronic bifascicular block. Circulation 1979; 59:238.

22. Rose G, Baxter PJ, Reid D, McCartney P. Prevalence and prognosis of electrocardiographic findings in middle-aged men. Br Heart J 1978; 40:636.

23. Rabkin SW, Mathewson FA, Tate RB. Natural history of left bundle branch block. Br Heart J 1980; 43:164.

24. Rabkin SW, Mathewson FA, Tate RB. The electrocardiogram in apparently healthy men and the risk of sudden death. Br Heart J 1982; 47:546.

25. Rabkin SW. Electrocardiographic abnormalities in apparently healthy men and risk of sudden death. Drugs 1984; 28(Suppl I):28.

26. Schneider JF, Thomas HE Jr, Kuger BE, Mc Namara FM, Kanrul WB. Newly acquired left bundle branch block: the Framingham Study. Ann Intern Med 1979; 90:303.

27. Blackburn A, Taylor HL, Key SA. The electrocardiogram in prediction of the 5-year coronary heart disease incidence among men aged forty through fifty-nine. Circulation 1970; 41 & 42(Suppl I):154.

28. Kulbertus HE, de Leval-Rutten F, Dubois M, Petit JM. Sudden death in subjects with intraventricular conduction defects. In: Kulbertus HE, Wellens HJJ (eds). Sudden Death. Martinus Nijhoff Publisher, The Hague, 1980, p 379.

29. Kulbertus HE, de Leval-Rutten F, Albert A, Dubois M, Petit JM. Electrocardiographic changes occurring with advancing age. In: Wellens HJJ, Kulbertus HE (eds). What's New in Electrocardiography? Martinus Nijhoff Publishers, The Hague, 1981, p 300.

30. Dubois C, Pierard LA, Smeets JP, Legrand V, Kulbertus HE. Short- and long-term prognostic importance of complete bundle branch block complicating acute myocardial infarction. Clin Cardiol 1988; 11:292.

31. Mullens CB, Atkins JM. Prognosis and management of ventricular conduction blocks in acute myocardial infarction. Mod Concepts Cardiovasc Dis 1976; 45:129.

32. Lie KI, Wellens HJJ, Schuilenburg RM. Bundle branch block and myocardial infarction. In: Wellens HJJ, Lie KI, Janse MJ (eds). The Conduction System of the Heart. Stenfert Kroese, Leiden, 1976.

33. Nemetz AA, Shrebooks SJ Jr, Hutter AM Jr, De Sanctis RW. The significance of bundle branch block during acute myocardial infarction. Am Heart J 1975; 90:439.

34. Gann D, Balachandran PK, El Sherif N, Samet P. Prognostic significance of

chronic versus acute bundle branch block in acute myocardial infarction. Chest 1975; 67:298.

35. Norris RM, Woo KS. Bundle branch block after myocardial infarction: short and long term effects. In: Kelley DT (ed). Advances in the Management of Arrhythmias. Telectronics, Sydney, 1978, p 364.

36. Hindman WC, Wagner GS, Ja Ro M, et al. The clinical significance of bundle branch block complicating acute myocardial infarction. Circulation 1978; 58:679.

37. Roos JC, Dunning AJ. Bundle branch block in acute myocardial infarction. Eur J Cardiol 1978; 6:403.

38. Lie KI, Manger Cats V, Durrer D. CCU findings useful for identification of sudden death candidates in the post-hospital phase of myocardial infarction. In: Kulbertus HE, Wellens HJJ (eds). Sudden Death. Martinus Nijhoff Publisher, The Hague, 1980, p 232.

39. Corrado D, Thieme G, Nava A, Rossi L, Pennelli N. Sudden death in young competitive athletes: clinicopathologic correlations in 22 cases. Am J Med 1990; 89:588.

40. Maron BJ. Heart disease and other causes of sudden death in young athletes. Curr Probl Cardiol 1998; 23:477.

41. Corrado D, Baja G, Basso C, Nava A, Thieme G. What is the Brugada syndrome? Cardiol Rev 1999; 7:191.

42. Brugada J, Brugada P, Brugada R. The syndrome of right bundle branch block, ST segment elevation in $V_1$ to $V_3$, and sudden death: the Brugada syndrome. Europace 1999; 1:156.

43. Brugada J, Brugada P. Right bundle branch block, persistent ST segment elevation and sudden cardiac death: a distinct clinical and electrocardiographic syndrome: a multicenter report. J Am Coll Cardiol 1992; 20:1391.

44. Jonsson H, Ivert T, Brodin LA, Jonassen R. Late sudden deaths after repair of tetralogy of Fallot. Scand J Cardiovasc Surg 1995; 29:131.

45. Berul CHL, Hill SHL, Geggel RL, et al. Electrocardiographic markers of late sudden death risk in postoperative tetralogy of Fallot children. J Cardiovasc Electrophysiol 1997; 8:1349.

46. Reisinger J, Dubrey SW, Lavalley M, Skinner M, Falk RH. Electrophysiologic abnormalities in AL (primary) amyloidosis with cardiac involvement. J Am Coll Cardiol 1997; 30:1046.

47. Myerburg R, Castellanos A. Cardiac arrest and sudden cardiac death. In: Braunwald E (ed). Heart Disease, 4th edition. WB Saunders, Philadelphia, 1992, p 756.

48. Zipes DP, Wellens HJJ. Sudden cardiac death. Circulation 1998; 98:2334.

49. Santoni-Rugiu FR, Gomes JA. Methods of identifying patients at high risk of subsequent arrhythmic death after myocardial infarction. Curr Probl Cardiol 1999; 24:117.

# 32

# Myocarditis:

# An Underestimated Cause of Sudden Cardiac Death

*Cristina Basso, MD, PhD,*
*Fiorella Calabrese, MD,*
*Domenico Corrado, MD,*
*and Gaetano Thiene, MD*

## Introduction

A cardiac organic substrate frequently underlies sudden cardiac death, even in the young. Despite careful clinical evaluation, subtle lesions such as focal cardiomyopathy and myocarditis may be underecognized. In other words, these diseases are frequently concealed and discovered with surprise only at postmortem examination by means of a thorough macroscopic and histological investigation. This chapter addresses the current knowledge of inflammatory heart muscle disease (myocarditis), ranging from clinical presentation to molecular pathology aspects.

## Definition, Clinical Presentation, and In Vivo Diagnosis

According to the WHO/ISFC classification of cardiomyopathies, "myocarditis is an inflammatory heart muscle disease associated with cardiac dysfunction and is diagnosed by established histological, immunological, and immunohistochemical criteria."[1] Classification may be based on *etiological* criteria (infective or noninfective myocarditis, whether isolated or in the setting of systemic inflammation), *temporal* (acute, fulminant, rapidly progressive, chronic, or persistent),[2,3] *clinical* (active, borderline, ongoing, resolving, resolved), or *histological* (lymphocitic, eosinophilic, polymor-

[1]Supported by the Veneto Region, Venice, and MURST, Rome, Italy.
From: Aliot E, Clementy J, Prystowsky EN (editors). *Fighting Sudden Cardiac Death: A Worldwide Challenge.* ©Futura Publishing Company, Armonk, NY, 2000.

phous, granulomatous, giant cell).[4] The superiority of an etiological classification as far as therapeutic implications are concerned is obvious.

Many open questions still exist regarding myocarditis. Clinical criteria of diagnosis are aspecific, since myocarditis may have disparate clinical presentations including chest pain, infarct-like necrosis, arrhythmias, congestive heart failure, cardiogenic shock, or even sudden, unexpected cardiac arrest. Titers of antiviral antibodies lack significance and are not of help; cultures are also not reliable. The diagnosis is based on histology of the myocardium, which is now feasible also in vivo, thanks to the introduction of endomyocardial biopsy in clinical practice.[5] The diagnostic criteria, based on the observation of inflammatory infiltrates in association with myocyte degeneration-necrosis in routine stains, are currently reinforced by the use immunohistochemistry, which allows precise identification and quantitation of leucocytes-macrophages, not only in acute but also in chronic phases.[6] The natural history of myocarditis is frequently characterized by the evolution in dilated cardiomyopathy[7,8]; however, it is not clear whether progression toward dilated cardiomyopathy is related to viral genome persistence within the myocytes, to the onset of antibody or cell-mediated immune mechanisms, or to the triggering of programmed cell death (apoptosis).[9] Identification of organ-specific cardiac autoantibodies (antimyosin) in some cases suggests the occurrence of autoimmune mechanisms, although whether they are a consequence of viral infection is uncertain.[10] Unfortunately, the microscopic observation of inflammatory infiltrates does not allow determination of the infectious, immune, or idiopathic nature of myocarditis. Thanks to the advent of molecular biology techniques, such as polymerase chain reaction (PCR) and in situ hybridization, it is now possible to systematically investigate the presence of viral genome in the myocardium in order to establish the precise etiology of the disease, set up targeted therapeutic strategies, and predict the course or recurrence of the inflammatory disease.[11–13] The recently published American Multicenter Treatment Trial on immunosuppressive therapy of myocarditis[14] failed because of the absence of any etiological background. Viral myocarditis, indeed, should be approached from the therapeutic standpoint with antiviral drugs, leaving immunosuppressive therapy to idiopathic or immune forms. Thus, the use of molecular diagnosis should be the gold standard not only for diagnosis but also for proper therapy.

## Epidemiology and Pathophysiology of Sudden Cardiac Death

Sudden death is a natural, unexpected fatal event occurring within 1 hour of the beginning of symptoms, in an apparently healthy subject or in one whose disease was not severe enough to predict such an abrupt outcome.[15] When sudden death occurs in adults and elderly persons, coronary atherosclerosis is the usual cause.[16,17] A larger spectrum of cardiovascular diseases, both congenital and acquired, may account for sudden death in the young.[18–23]

Unnatural causes of death such as occult trauma, drug addiction, or iatrogenic disorders should be excluded. Sudden death is a major issue in industrialized countries. In the United States, the annual incidence of sudden death in people 35–74 years of age was 191/100,000 in men and 57/100,000 in women; almost half of all sudden deaths occur in people with known coronary artery disease.[24] Despite numerous reports, there is a paucity of demographic data on sudden death in the young. Several studies have estimated the rate in people 1–20 years of 1.3 to 8.5/100,000 patient years.[25] A 30-year population-based study in 54 young adults 20–40 years of age who died suddenly in Olmsted County, Minnesota, demonstrated a sudden death rate of 4.1/100,000 in women and 8.7/100,000 in men.[26] We recently calculated in the Veneto region, in northeast Italy, an overall sudden death prevalence of 0.8/100,000/year in the young and 1.6/100,000/year in athletes, based only on autopsy reports.[27]

As far as pathophysiology is concerned, cardiac arrest may be *mechanical*, when the heart and circulatory functions are suddenly impeded by mechanical factors (i.e., aortic rupture with hemopericardium and cardiac tamponade, pulmonary thromboembolism, abrupt cardiogenic shock, etc.). Otherwise, sudden death may be *arrhythmic*, which is by far the most common mechanism; ventricular fibrillation accounts for nearly 70% of cases, followed by asystole (nearly 15%), ventricular tachycardia (nearly 10%), and electromechanical dissociation (about 5%).[28,29]

## Myocarditis and Sudden Death in the Young

Based on the Veneto region study project findings on juvenile ((35 years) sudden death, cardiovascular causes accounted for more than 80% of the collected cases and about one-third of events were due to a congenital heart defect present since birth.[23,27] Table 1 reports the main causes of cardiovascular sudden death in our series of cases collected since 1979.[27] In our experience, the most common causes include premature atherosclerosis (16.7%), arrhythmogenic right ventricular cardiomyopathy (10.8%), mitral valve prolapse (9.7%), conduction system disease (8.9%), and myocarditis (8.2%).

A recent review of major series on sudden cardiac death in the young revealed that myocarditis accounts for up to 44% of fatal events[30] (Table 2).

## Table 1

### Causes of Sudden Cardiac Death in People Aged ≤ 35 Years in the Veneto Region of Italy, 1979 to 1996*

| Cause | Total (n = 269) | Athletes (n = 49) | Non-athletes (n = 220) |
|---|---|---|---|
| Atherosclerotic coronary artery disease | 45 (16.7%) | 9 (18.4%) | 36 (16.4%) |
| Arrhythmogenic right ventricular cardiomyopathy | 29 (10.8) | 11 (22.4%) | 18 (8.2%)* |
| Mitral valve prolapse | 26 (9.7%) | 5 (10.2%) | 21 (9.5%) |
| Disease of conduction system | 24 (8.9%) | 4 (8.2%) | 20 (9.1%) |
| Myocarditis | 22 (8.2%) | 3 (6.1%) | 19 (8.6%) |
| Hypertrophic cardiomyopathy | 17 (6.3%) | 1 (2.0%) | 16 (7.3%) |
| Dissecting aortic aneurysm | 12 (4.5%) | 1 (2.0%) | 11 (5.0%) |
| Dilated cardiomyopathy | 10 (3.7%) | 1 (2.0%) | 9 (4.1%) |
| Anomalous origin of coronary artery | 7 (2.6%) | 6 (12.2%) | 1 (0.5%)° |
| Myocardial bridge | 7 (2.6%) | 2 (4.1%) | 5 (2.3%) |
| Pulmonary thromboembolism | 4 (1.5%) | 1 (2.0%) | 3 (1.4%) |
| Other | 66 (24.5%) | 5 (10.2%) | 61 (27.7%) |

*Modified from Corrado et al.[27]

Among these,[18–21,31–35] myocarditis was the most common cardiac diagnosis associated with sudden death in the article by Topaz and Edwards,[20] comprising 12 cases (24%), of which 11 were presumed to be viral and 1 sarcoid. It is noteworthy that among the cases of acute myocarditis was a 9-year-old boy with mumps who died suddenly on the third day of illness.

## Table 2

### Sudden Death from Myocarditis in Young People (≤35 Years)

| Author # and Reference No. | Age Range (years) | Total No. | % |
|---|---|---|---|
| Driscoll & Edwards (19) | 1–22 | 7 | 20% |
| Topaz & Edwards (20) | 7–35 | 50 | 24% |
| Molander et al. (31) | 1–20 | 9 | 44% |
| Neuspiel & Kuller (32) | 1–21 | 51 | 27% |
| Phillips et al. (33) | 17–28 | 20 | 42% |
| Kramer et al. (34) | 17–30 | 24 | 29% |
| Drory et al. (35) | 9–31 | 118 | 25% |
| Corrado et al. (27) | 1–35 | 269 | 8% |

A major limitation in the autopsy diagnosis of myocarditis in several series has been the lack of standardized histological criteria. The strongest evidence that subclinical myocarditis can be a cause of ventricular fibrillation comes from an autopsy series on United States Army recruits in which 42% of those who died suddenly had histological evidence of myocarditis.[33] Although myocarditis usually presents with signs of pump failure and ventricular dilatation, ventricular arrhythmias have been described in patients with myocarditis and an apparently normal heart. A recent flu-like illness is common, although the symptoms may be mild and clinical signs of heart failure subtle or absent. Cardiac involvement is unpredictable and may affect the conduction system, causing heart block, or the ordinary myocardium, causing ventricular arrhythmias. Sometimes the patient suffers previous syncopal episodes and/or palpitations. The electrocardiogram may show diffuse low voltage, ST-T changes, and often heart block or ventricular arrhythmias. A recent large-scale study that included 672 Finnish military conscripts with a mean age of 20 years showed that the usual presentation of acute myocarditis in young men mimicks myocardial infarction.[36] The results of echocardiography and endomyocardial biopsy are confirmatory.

Sudden death may occur both in the active or healed phases as a consequence of life-threatening ventricular arrhythmias that develop mostly in the setting of an unstable myocardial substrate, namely inflammatory infiltrate, interstitial edema, myocardial necrosis, and fibrosis. The gross appearance of the heart is not distinctive and its weight may be within normal values. Histology invariably discloses either a "starry-like sky" feature ($>$14 leucocytes/mm$^2$) (Figure 1 A,B) or a patchy inflammatory infiltrate (Figure 1C,D), sometimes no more than 3 foci at magnification 6x, and not necessarily associated with myocyte necrosis. This subtle substrate, together with the possible inflammatory involvement of the conduction system, seems highly arrhythmogenic and may account for unexpected arrhythmic cardiac arrest.[37] The inflammatory infiltrates are usually polymorphous and less frequently purely lymphocytic. Sudden death due to patchy giant cell myocarditis as well as eosinophilic myocarditis in the setting of an allergic condition, have also been reported. Rheumatic carditis is currently an exceptional occurrence.

Evidence of myocardial infection, whether bacterial or viral, has rarely been found. *Chlamydia pneumoniae* myocarditis was implicated in the sudden deaths of several young Swedish elite orienteers after RNA from this organism was detected in the heart of one of the victims.[38] A subsequent paper implicated this agent in one-third of sudden cardiac deaths of the 15 Swedish orienteers who died unexpectedly between 1979 and 1992.[39] Awareness of the problem and modification of "training habits and attitudes" have been effective, since no further deaths in the following years have been reported among Swedish orienteers.

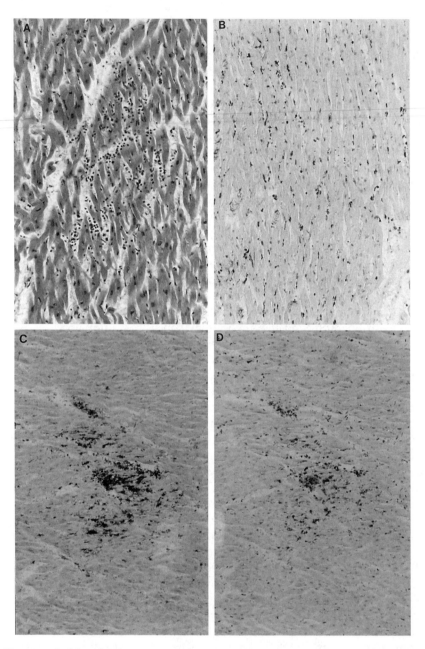

Figure 1. Sudden death at rest in a previously asymptomatic 30-year-old woman with a grossly normal heart. **A:** Inflammatory cells infiltrate with mild interstitial edema (hematoxylin-eosin ×150). **B:** Starry-like sky appearance of the myocardium due to T-lymphocyte interstitial infiltrates (CD43 ×96) **C:** Cluster of leucocytes associated with focal myocardial necrosis (CD45 ×96). **D:** Same field of (C): the inflammatory cells appear to be mostly activated T-lymphocytes (CD45RO ×96).

Nonetheless, viral infections are the most plausible cause. Application of gene amplification techniques is particularly useful in detecting viral nucleic acids in biopsies, especially when characteristic cytopathic changes cannot be observed on light microscopy, a rather frequent condition in acute fatal forms causing sudden death. Although enterovirus is the most important causative agent in the pathogenesis of myocarditis, several studies have shown that various other viruses, such as adenovirus, herpesvirus (cytomegalovirus, herpes simplex virus, Epstein-Barr virus) parvovirus, influenza virus A or B, and hepatitis C virus can be involved in myocardial infective disease, particularly in the pediatric population.[12,40] Its frequency is not so rare, especially during the influenza epidemic that occurred in 1998–99 and which has been characterized by many cases of fatal cardiogenic shock and sudden unexpected death. As far as the issue of an in vivo diagnosis of myocarditis, endomyocardial biopsy plays a key role but its interpretation is frequently challenging. First of all, it is important to keep in mind that lymphocytes can reside in the normal myocardium (normal myocardium contains less than 5 lymphocytes/high-power field ×400).[41] Moreover, endomyocardial biopsy has a low sensitivity for the detection of myocarditis because it is often focal, so that a casual and insufficient number of samples could produce a false negative (sampling error), and it is not performed in the acute phase.[42-44] Thus, to increase diagnostic sensitivity, use of immunohistochemistry is mandatory to identify and characterize the inflammatory infiltrate. Immunohistochemical analysis must always be carried out by means of CD45 (leucocyte antigen common), CD43 (T-lymphocytes), CD45RO (activated T-lymphocytes), CD68 (macrophages), CD20 (B-lymphocytes), CD4 (T-helper), and CD8 (cytotoxic T-lymphocytes) monoclonal and polyclonal antibodies (Figure 1 B-D).

Furthermore, classic morphology rarely identifies the etiological agent. The diagnosis of viral myocarditis for a long time has been based on viral culture and serology. However, these investigations are time consuming and generally fall short in specificity and sensitivity. More recently, molecular biology techniques as PCR and nested-PCR have been shown to rapidly detect the presence of infective agents, in a specific and very sensitive way, also using a very small amount of tissue such as the fragments of endomyocardial biopsies.[12,13,45] To obtain a specific molecular diagnosis of infective myocarditis, whole blood or serum is routinely analyzed to exclude "blood contamination." Different molecular strategies are now used to detect infective status of viruses: in fact, RT-PCR is usually performed instead of PCR to detect specific mRNA indicative of active viral replication and not only the presence of a latent viral form. Moreover, molecular biology techniques are successfully applied to better understand the pathogenesis of myocarditis. Until now, only a few papers have reported the evidence of hyperexpression of inflammatory cytokines in endomyocardial biopsies; their detection seems to be very important, particularly for prognostic and therapeutic implications.[12]

Studies in laboratory animals with myocarditis have shown a significant increase in mortality with strenuous physical activity.[46,47] In particular, exercise during the acute phase of the disease leads to increased viral replication, more extensive myocyte necrosis, and a worse chance of survival. Phillips et al.[33] reported that exertion may have been a precipitating factor in 7 of 8 myocarditis deaths in Air Force recruits. In the Veneto region experience, myocarditis accounted for 6% of fatalities among competitive athletes.[27] The ventricular fibrous repair following inflammatory injury may create an arrhythmogenic milieu that could be unmasked with exercise.[48] The recent Bethesda conference[49] on athletes with cardiovascular disorders recommended a convalescence period of 6 months after the onset of symptoms. Athletic participation depends on the ventricular function as assessed by echocardiography, as well as the absence of clinically significant arrhythmias. The physician who is in charge of the athlete following recovery from myocarditis should remember that persistence of ventricular arrhythmia after the resolution of myocarditis has been reported in children and young adults.[50] At present, there are no clinical variables available to stratify the risk of sudden death in these patients.

## Sudden Cardiac Death Due to Myocarditis: Peculiar Aspects

Sudden cardiac death may be ascribable to myocarditis in the setting of other pathological substrates, such as arrhythmogenic right ventricular cardiomyopathy, conduction system disease, and myocardial drug toxicity .

*Arrhythmogenic right ventricular cardiomyopathy* is one of the leading causes of sudden death in the young and in athletes in our series[21,27,51,52] and it may be a concealed abnormality in apparently healthy subjects. The disease is characterized pathologically by a peculiar myocardial atrophy with fibrofatty substitution of the right ventricular free wall in an apparently normal heart. Histology discloses the disappearance (atrophy) of the right ventricular myocardium with the fibrofatty or fatty replacement, with a wavefront extension from the epicardium toward the endocardium.[52] The intraventricular conduction delay, consequent to fibrofatty replacement, is a source of electrical instability, due to reentrant phenomena, in the shape of ventricular arrhythmias (premature ventricular beats, nonsustained or sustained ventricular tachycardia) with left bundle branch block morphology, indicating a right ventricular origin. Focal myocarditis with myocyte death was observed in all cases with fibrofatty variants; whether inflammation is primary or secondary to cell death remains to be established.[52–54] Apoptosis was detected by the TUNEL technique in a high percentage of arrhythmogenic right ventricular cardiomyopathy patients, both in autopsy and biopsy material.[9,55] Recent analysis using nested PCR for enterovirus failed to detect any viral genome in biopsies of arrhythmogenic right ventricular cardiomyopathy patients with either recent or chronic clinical onset of the disease.[56] Focal, progressive cell death may lead to either fibrous or fatty replacement, with adipocytes taking the place of dying myocytes. Patchy myocarditis, bouts of apoptosis, right ventricular aneurysms, and left ventricular involvement most probably worsen ventricular electrical vulnerability and lower the ventricular fibrillation threshold. The coexistence of myocarditis and apoptosis in arrhythmogenic right ventricular cardiomyopathy suggests that these mechanisms contribute to myocyte injury and repair in susceptible patients. Recent studies highlight complex interactions between proapoptotic proteins, proinflammatory cytokines, and other agents that modulate apoptosis and myocarditis.[57] These investigations will have important implications also for therapeutic treatment.

Sudden death in *ventricular preexcitation* is a rare event.[58] In the majority of patients it occurs as the result of atrial fibrillation with rapid response over the accessory pathway.[59] Oddly enough, 50% of young subjects who died suddenly with ECG-documented ventricular preexcitation (Wolff-Parkinson-White syndrome) had morphological evidence of focal atrial myocarditis, either polimorphous or lymphocytic.[60] Atrial myocarditis might act as a trigger of atrial fibrillation precipitating ventricular fibrillation and sudden death due to rapid response over the accessory pathway.

*Drug-related myocarditis* may be due to a direct dose-related toxic effect or may be secondary to a hypersensitivity reaction, which may occur any time during the course of therapy. Thus, in any case of unexplained myocarditis, particularly in the young and in the athlete, iatrogenic forms must be considered. For instance, in autopsy studies of patients who died from cocaine intoxication, a mononuclear infiltrate with foci of necrosis has been noted as a prominent finding.[61] Moreover, even anabolic steroid abuse and cardiac death due to myocarditis has been reported.[62]

## References

1. Richardson P, McKenna WJ, Bristow M, Maisch B, O'Connel J, et al. Report of the 1995 WHO/ISFC Task Force on the definition and classification of cardiomyopathies. Circulation 1996; 93:841–842.
2. Fenoglio JJ, Ursell PC, Kellog CF, Drusin RE, Weiss MB. Diagnosis and classification of myocarditis by endomyocardial biopsy. N Engl J Med 1983; 398:12–18.

3. Lieberman EB, Hutchins GM, Herskowitz A, Rose NR, Baughman KL. Clinicopathologic description of myocarditis. J Am Coll Cardiol 1991; 18:1617–1626.
4. Aretz HT, Billingham ME, Edwards WD, Factor SM, Fallon JT, et al. Myocarditis: the Dallas criteria. Hum Pathol 1987; 18:619–624.
5. Baroldi G, Thiene G. La biopsia endomiocardica. Piccin Editore, 1996.
6. Linder J, Cassling RS, Rogler WG, et al. Immunohistochemical characterization of lymphocytes in uninflamed ventricular myocardium: implications for myocarditis. Arch Pathol Lab Med 1985; 109:917–920.
7. Dec GW, Palacios IF, Fallon JT, Aretz HT, Mils J, et al. Active myocarditis in the spectrum of acute dilated cardiomyopathies: clinical features, histological correlates and clinical outcome. N Engl J Med 1985; 312:885–890.
8. Fallon JT. Myocarditis and dilated cardiomyopathy: different stages of the same disease? Cardiovasc Clin 1987; 18:155–162.
9. Valente M, Calabrese F, Thiene G, Angelini A, Basso C, et al. In vivo evidence of apoptosis in arrhythmogenic right ventricular cardiomyopathy. Am J Pathol 1998; 152:479–484.
10. Dec JW, Palacios I, Yasuda T, Fallon JT, Khaw BA, et al. Antimyosin antibody cardiac imaging: its role in the diagnosis of myocarditis. J Am Coll Cardiol 1990; 16:97–104.
11. Liu P. Cardiomyopathies and myocarditis: the molecular era has arrived. Curr Opin Cardiol 1995; 10:289–292.
12. Martin AB, Webber S, Fricker FJ, Jaffe R, Demmler G, et al. Acute myocarditis: rapid diagnostic by PCR in children. Circulation 1994; 90:330–339.
13. Calabrese F, Valente M, Thiene G, Angelini A, Testolin L, et al. Presence of enteroviral genome in native hearts may influence outcome of transplanted patients. Diagn Mol Pathol 1999; 8:39–46.
14. Mason JW, O'Connel JB, Herskowitz A, Rose NR, McManus BM, et al., and the Myocarditis Treatment Trial Investigators. A clinical trial of immunosuppressive therapy for myocarditis. N Engl J Med 1995; 333:269–275.
15. Goldstein S. The necessity of a uniform definition of sudden coronary death: witnessed death within 1 hour of the onset of acute symptoms. Am Heart J 1982; 103:156–159.
16. Baroldi G, Falzi G, Mariani F. Sudden coronary death: a postmortem study in 208 selected cases compared to 97 "control" subjects. Am Heart J 1979; 98:20–31.
17. Davies MJ, Thomas A. Thrombosis and acute coronary artery lesions in sudden cardiac ischemic death. N Engl J Med 1984; 310:1137–1140.
18. Lambert EC, Menon VA, Wagner HR, et al. Sudden unexpected death from cardiovascular disease in children. Am J Cardiol 1974; 34:89–96.
19. Driscoll DJ, Edwards WD. Sudden unexpected death in children and adolescents. J Am Coll Cardiol 1985; 5(Suppl B):118B-121B.
20. Topaz O, Edwards JE. Pathologic features of sudden death in children, adolescents, and young adults. Chest 1985; 87:476–482.
21. Thiene G, Nava A, Corrado D, Rossi L, Pennelli N. Right ventricular cardiomyopathy and sudden death in young people. N Engl J Med 1988; 318:129–133.
22. Corrado D, Basso C, Poletti A, Angelini A, Valente M, et al. Sudden death in the young: is coronary thrombosis the major precipitating factor? Circulation 1994; 90:2315–2323.
23. Basso C, Frescura C, Corrado D, Muriago M, Angelini A, et al. Congenital heart disease and sudden death in the young. Hum Pathol 1995; 26:1065–1072.
24. Gillum RF. Sudden coronary death in the United States: 1980–1985. Circulation 1989; 79:756–765.

25. Silka MJ, Kron J, Walance CG, et al. Assesment and follow-up of pediatric survivors of sudden cardiac death. Circulation 1990; 82:341–349.
26. Shen WK, Edwards WD, Hammil SC, Bayley KR, Ballard DJ, et al. Sudden unexpected non-traumatic death in 54 young adults: a 30 year population-based study. Am J Cardiol 1995; 76:148–152.
27. Corrado D, Basso C, Schiavon M, Thiene G. Screening for hypertrophic cardiomyopathy in young athletes. N Engl J Med 1998; 339:364–369.
28. Liberthson RR, Nagel EL, Hirshman JC, Naussenfeld SR, Blackbourne BD, et al. Pathophysiologic observations in pre-hospital ventricular fibrillation and sudden cardiac death. Circulation 1974; 49:790–798.
29. Myerburg R, Conde C, Sung R, Mayorca-Cortes A, Mallon S, et al. Clinical, electrophysiologic and hemodynamic profile of patients resuscitated from prehospital cardiac arrest. Am J Med 1980; 68:568.
30. Liberthson RR. Sudden death from cardiac causes in children and young adults. N Engl J Med 1996; 334:1039–1044.
31. Molander N. Sudden natural death in later childhood and adolescence. Arch Dis Child 1982; 57:572–576.
32. Neuspiel DR, Kuller LH. Sudden and unexpected natural death in childhood and adolescence. JAMA 1985; 254:1321–1325.
33. Phillips M, Robinowitz M, Higgins JR, et al. Sudden cardiac death in Air Force recruits: a 20-year review. JAMA 1986; 256:2696–2699.
34. Kramer MR, Drory Y, Lev B. Sudden death in young Israeli soldiers: analysis of 83 cases. Isr J Med Sci 1989; 25:620–624.
35. Drory Y, Turetz Y, Hiss Y, et al. Sudden unexpected death in persons less than 30 years of age. Am J Cardiol 1991; 68:1388–1392.
36. Karjalainen J, Heikkila J. Incidence of three presentations of acute myocarditis in young men in military service. Eur Heart J 1999; 20:1120–1125.
37. Basso C, Boffa G, Corrado D, Thiene G. Myocarditis and sudden death in the young (abstract). Circulation 1997; 96:I-698.
38. Wesslen L, Pahlson C, Friman G. Myocarditis caused by *Chlamydia pneumoniae* (TWAR) and sudden unexpected death in a Swedish elite orienteer. Lancet 1992; 240:427–428.
39. Wesslen L, Pahlson C, Lindquist O et al. An increase in sudden unexpected cardiac deaths among young Swedish orienteers during 1979–1992. Eur Heart J 1996; 17:902–910.
40. Akhtar N, Ni J, Stromberg D, et al. Tracheal aspirate as a substrate for polymerase chain reaction detection of viral genome in childhood pneumonia and myocarditis. Circulation, 1999; 99:2011–2018.
41. Tazelaar HD, Billingham ME. Myocardial lymphocytes: fact, fancy or myocarditis? Am J Cardiovasc Pathol 1987; 1:47–50.
42. Hauck AJ, Kearney DL, Edwards W. Evaluation of postmortem endomyocardial biopsy specimens from 38 patients with lymphocytic myocarditis: implications for role of sampling error. Mayo Clin Proc 1989; 64:1235–1245.
43. Chow LH, Radio SJ, Sears TD, McManus B. Insensitivity of right ventricular endomyocardial biopsy in the diagnosis of myocarditis. J Am Coll Cardiol 1989; 14:915–920.
44. Shirani J, Freant LJ, Roberts WC. Gross and semiquantitative histologic findings in mononuclear cells myocarditis causing sudden death and implications for endomyocardial biopsy. Am J Cardiol 1993; 72:952–957.
45. Ou J, Sole MJ, Butany JW, Chia WK, McLaughlin PR, et al. Detection of enterovirus RNA in biopsies from patients with myocarditis and cardiomyopathy using gene amplification by polymerase chain reaction. Circulation 1990; 82:8–16.

46. Satoh M, Tamura G. Expression of cytokine genes and presence of enteroviral genomic RNA in endomyocardial biopsy tissues of myocarditis and dilated cardiomyopathy. Virchows Arch 1996; 427:503–509.
47. Graimaitian B, Chason J, Lerner A. Augmentation of the virulence of murine coxsackie B3 myocardiopathy by exercise. J Exp Med 1970; 131:1121–1136.
48. Zeppilli P, Santini C, Palieri V, et al. Role of myocarditis in athletes with minor arrhythmias and/or echocardiographic abnormalities. Chest 1994; 106:373–380.
49. Maron BJ, Mitchell JH. 26th Bethesda Conference: recommendations for detecting eligibility for competition in athletes with cardiovascular abnormalities. J Am Coll Cardiol 1994; 24:845–899.
50. Friedman R, Kearney D, Moak J, et al. Persistence of ventricular arrhythmia after resolution of occult myocarditis in children and young adults. J Am Coll Cardiol 1994; 24:780–783.
51. Nava A, Rossi L, Thiene G (eds). Arrhythmogenic Right Ventricular Cardiomyopathy/Dysplasia. Elsevier, Amsterdam,1997.
52. Basso C, Thiene G, Corrado D, Angelini A, Nava A, et al. Arrhythmogenic right ventricular cardiomyopathy: dysplasia, dystrophy, or myocarditis? Circulation 1996; 94:983–991.
53. Thiene G, Corrado D, Nava A, Rossi L, Poletti A, et al. Right ventricular cardiomyopathy: is there evidence of an inflammatory aetiology? Eur Heart J 1991; 12 (Suppl D):22–25.
54. Valente M, Calabrese F, Angelini A, Caforio ALP, Basso C, et al. In: Nava A, Rossi L, Thiene G (eds). Pathobiology in Arrhythmogenic Right Ventricular Cardiomyopathy/Dysplasia. Elsevier Science, Amsterdam, 1997.
55. Mallat Z, Tedgui A, Fontaliran F, Frank R, Durigon M, et al. Evidence of apoptosis in arrhythmogenic right ventricular dysplasia. N Engl J Med 1996; 335:1190–1196.
56. Calabrese F, Angelini A, Thiene G, Basso C, et al. No detection of enteroviral genome in the myocardium of patients with arrhythmogenic right ventricular cardiomyopathy. J Clin Pathol (in press).
57. Tanaka M, Suda T, Takahashi T, Nagata S. Expression of the functional soluble form of human Fas ligand in activated lymphocytes. EMBO J 1995; 14:1129–1135.
58. Guize L, Soria R, Chaouat JC, Chretien JM, Houe D,et al. Prevalence and course of Wolff-Parkinson-White syndrome in a population of 138,048 subjects. Ann Med Intern Paris 1985; 136:474–478.
59. Wellens HJJ, Durrer D. Wolff-Parkinson-White syndrome and atrial fibrillation. Am J Cardiol 1974; 34:777.
60. Basso C, Corrado D, Thiene G. Ventricular preexcitation and sudden death. Eur Heart J 1996; 17:404.
61. Virmani R, Robinowitz M, Smialek J, Smyth D. Cardiovascular effect of cocaine: an autopsy study of 40 patients. Am Heart J 1988; 115:1068–1075.
62. Kennedy MC, Lawrence C. Anabolic steroid abuse and cardiac death. Med J Aust 1993; 158:346–348.

# IX

## Ischemia and Sudden Cardiac Death

# 33
# Arrhythmias in Acute Ischemia

*Michiel J. Janse, MD*

## Introduction

Approximately 150 years ago, Erichsen noted that ligation of a coronary artery in dogs caused the action of the ventricles to cease, with "a slight tremulous motion alone continuing."[1] Although McWilliam recognized the clinical importance of this experimental observation, and suggested in 1889 that ventricular fibrillation resulting from obstruction of a coronary artery could be the cause of sudden death in man, he had to recognize 34 years later that "little attention was given to this view for many years."[2,3] Most studies in the field of arrhythmias in the first half of the 20th century dealt with supraventricular arrhythmias, and a Dutch textbook in 1935 stated " . . . from that time onward (i.e., since the electrocardiograph became widely used in both the clinic and the experimental laboratory), fibrillation, and especially atrial fibrillation, became important in the clinic. Since ventricular fibrillation usually results in sudden death, it is, of course, of much less importance. Besides, ventricular fibrillation occurs much less frequently than atrial fibrillation."[4] The reasons why ventricular fibrillation was so neglected probably were that it was difficult to document its occurrence in humans by electrocardiographic recordings, and that it could not be treated. Not until the 1960s, when electrocardiograms were recorded from patients in the early phase of myocardial infarction, did the medical community begin to appreciate that ventricular fibrillation "is common in patients with acute myocardial ischemia with or without infarction."[5] After defibrillation became possible even outside the hospital,[6,7] the number of studies of arrhythmias resulting from ischemia and infarction increased enormously. A literature search over a 21/2-year period, from January 1980 to June 1982, identified 6,027 papers with the word "arrhythmia" in either the title or key words; for "ischemia" the count was 6,484, and for "infarction" 11,268.[8]

There is a great variation in the animal models used to study arrhythmogenesis in ischemia and infarction.[9,10] Roughly speaking, the hearts of

From: Aliot E, Clementy J, Prystowsky EN (editors). *Fighting Sudden Cardiac Death: A Worldwide Challenge.* ©Futura Publishing Company, Armonk, NY, 2000.

small mammals (rat, guinea pig) have been used mainly for metabolic studies and for quantifying the incidence of arrhythmias in different circumstances without recording electrophysiological parameters, whereas in the hearts of larger animals (dog, pig) recording of transmembrane potentials, mapping of spread of activation, determination of refractory periods, and conduction velocity have contributed to the understanding of arrhythmia mechanisms.

Even in a model very frequently used, the anesthetized dog with acute occlusion of a major coronary artery, there are many factors that determine whether, and if so, how often ventricular arrhythmias occur: size of the ischemic area, presence and number of preexisting collaterals, heart rate, depth and type of anesthesia, mode of coronary artery occlusion (abrupt or in 2 stages, ligation, or thrombotic occlusion), activity of the autonomic nervous system, whether or not reperfusion occurs, presence of a previous infarction, and preexisting hypertrophy.[9,10,12] In dogs there is variation in the number of preexisting collaterals, and depending on the degree of collateral flow, the incidence of ventricular fibrillation may vary from 0% to 100%.[13,14] Also, occlusion of the left anterior descending coronary artery results in a variation of the size of the ischemic area and "this can account for a substantial portion of non-drug-related variability in outcome of antiarrhythmic trials using the canine coronary occlusion or release model."[15] This statement was corroborated by a study in which data from different laboratories were collected on 658 dogs in which the left anterior descending coronary artery was suddenly ligated. When control series consisted of 10 dogs, the incidence of ventricular fibrillation varied from 0% to 70%; when the control group counted 20 animals, the incidence varied between 5% and 55%, and even in series of 100 dogs, there still was a range of 14% to 36%. These data underscore that in experimental studies on the effects of antiarrhythmic drugs, all factors determining arrhythmogenesis must be controlled.

In large mammals (pig, dog, sheep), the arrhythmias during the early, reversible phase of acute ischemia occur in 2 distinct phases, 1a (between 2 and 10 minutes following coronary occlusion) and 1b (from approximately 12 to 30 minutes). In smaller mammals, the time course is monomodal, and no distinction between 1a and 1b arrhythmias can be made.[10] It is not known whether in humans there is a bimodal time course.

From animal studies, it has become apparent that the 2 phases are associated with distinct changes in electrophysiological properties, which will be described in the next section.

## Electrophysiological Changes During the 1a Phase of Arrhythmias

This phase is characterized by a rapid change in excitability associated with metabolic acidification due to anerobic glycolysis and cellular potassium loss, resulting in extracellular accumulation of potassium ions[16,17] (Figure 1). The impacts of these changes are a reduction in resting membrane potential, and loss of amplitude, upstroke velocity, and duration of the transmembrane action potential (Figure 2). Recovery of excitability lags behind repolarization, and this so-called postrepolarization refractoriness accounts for the alternation in action potential amplitude and duration, which is frequently seen during this phase.[18,19] The ischemic myocytes are very sensitive to cycle length: alternation disappears upon slowing of heart rate, while an increase in heart rate will result in 2:1 responses or higher degrees of block. Conduction velocity decreases, but the decrease is relatively small, and conduction block, which changes its location from beat to beat, occurs early and abruptly.[20] Because of these changes (lengthening of the refractory period, conduction not slower than 50% of normal, tendency to conduction block[21]), large and unstable reentrant circuits are responsible for ventricular tachycardia, which frequently degenerates into ventricular fibrillation[22] (Figure 3).

The main factors responsible for the electrophysiological changes are severe hypoxia, acidosis, and extracellular $K^+$ accumulation. In addition, other factors may also play a role, such as accumulation of lysophosphoglycerides, and long-chain acylcarnitine. It is of interest that coronary artery obstruction by a thrombus is more arrhythmogenic than coronary artery ligation. Depolarization of resting membrane potential and conduction slowing occur more rapidly in a thrombotic occlusion, and it is possible that this is due to enhanced production of amphipathic metabolites.[23,24] A key factor for reentrant excitation is inhomogeneity in electrophysiological properties within the ischemic zone, which is largely due to inhomogeneities in extracellular $K^+$ concentration.[25] Because $K^+$ ions move from the ischemic to the normal zone, there are large gradients in extracellular $K^+$ from the lateral boundary toward the center of the ischemic zone. Since the degree of postrepolarization refractoriness is determined by the extracellular $K^+$ concentration, there are large differences in the refractory periods of ischemic myocytes (Figure 4). Close to the border with normal myocardium, refractory periods are shorter than in normal myocardium, and toward the center, they lengthen progressively. A premature depolarization, originating at the border by reexcitation by injury currents,[22] can propagate into the ischemic zone, but will encounter zones of unidirectional block where extracellular $K^+$ is high. This sets the stage for reentry (see Figure 3). In fact, extracellular $K^+$ concentrations between 8 and 13.5 mmol/L provide the conditions necessary for ventricular fibrillation.[25]

It is known that in animals with congestive heart failure, ventricular arrhythmias occur more often during acute ischemia than in healthy animals.[26] Extracellular $K^+$ concentration reaches higher values during the first 10 minutes of ischemia, action potential duration shortens more, and conduction velocity is lower in failing hearts compared to normal hearts.[27]

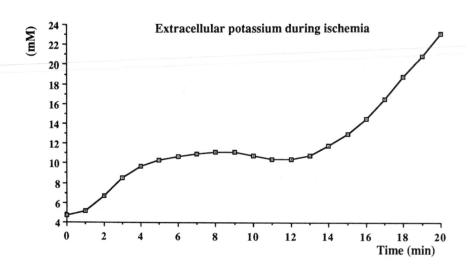

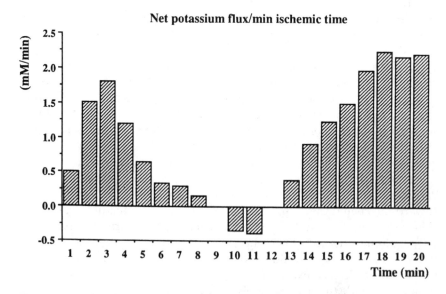

Figure 1. Panel A shows the extracellular $K^+$ concentration (ordinate) as a function of time elapsed after arrest of coronary flow (abscissa) in an isolated guinea pig heart. Panel B shows the net transfer of $K^+$ out of cells (ordinate) plotted in time windows of 1 minute (abscissa). (Reproduced with permission from Wilde AAM.[34])

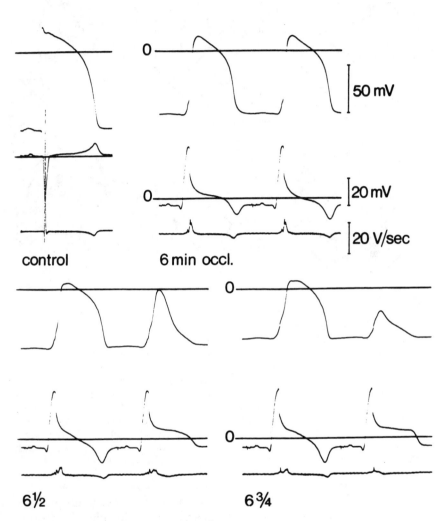

**Figure 2.** Transmembrane potentials (upper traces), local direct current electrograms (middle traces) and dV/dt ($V_{max}$) of the action potential upstroke (lowest traces) recorded in the pig heart. The top left panel shows control recordings, the top right 6 minutes after coronary artery occlusion, and the lower panels 6.5 and 6.75 minutes after onset of ischemia. Note alternation in lower panels. (Reproduced with permission from Wit AL, et al.[12])

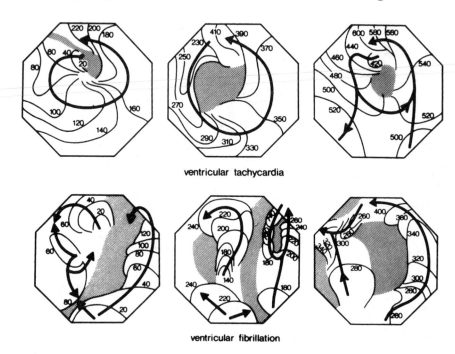

**ventricular tachycardia**

**ventricular fibrillation**

Figure 3. Top: Patterns of activation during 3 successive beats of a ventricular tachycardia that developed spontaneously 5 minutes after the onset of ischemia. An octogonal multiterminal electrode was attached to the anterior wall of the left ventricle of an isolated porcine heart, and isochrones are drawn in the area covered by the electrode (time zero is arbitrary; numbers are in ms; each limb of the octogon is 2 cm; shaded areas are zones of block). Note that basically a circus movement of fairly large dimensions is responsible for the continuation of the tachycardia, although both dimensions and the position of the reentrant circuit changes from beat to beat. Bottom: Activation pattern during ventricular fibrillation. Multiple wavelets travel along tortuous routes between islets of temporal conduction block (shaded areas). Collision and fusion of wavelets frequently occur and circus movements are rarely completed (middle). (Modified with permission from Wit AL, et al.[12])

Increased dispersion in refractoriness and a shorter wavelength may explain the higher propensity for reentrant arrhythmias in failing hearts during the 1a phase.

# Electrophysiological Changes During the 1b Phase of Arrhythmias

Whereas the 1a arrhythmias are the result of changes in excitability of ischemic myocytes, the 1b arrhythmias are related to electrical uncoupling

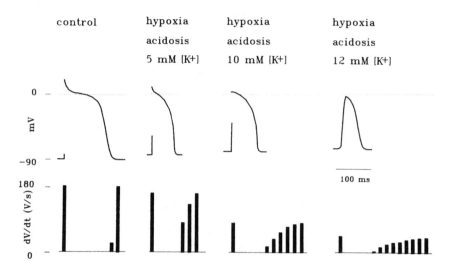

Figure 4. Schematic illustration of the changes in transmembrane potentials (top traces) and the recovery of maximal upstroke velocity, $dV/dt_{max}$ (bottom traces) following an action potential in normal ventricular myocardium (control) and in 3 different conditions of simulated ischemia in which the extracellular $K^+$ concentration is increased. Note postrepolarization refractoriness in high extracellular $K^+$. This scheme is based on results obtained by Kodama et al.[35] and Wilde.[34]

of ischemic cells.[28] At the start of the 1b phase, almost all of the epicardial cells in the ischemic zone are excitable, while less than half of midmural cells are. It appears that a critical degree of coupling between the subepicardium and the midmyocardium plays a crucial role in the genesis of these arrhythmias.[29] Although the exact mechanism of 1b arrhythmias has not yet been investigated in detail by mapping studies, it is possible that reentrant circuits are smaller than during the 1a phase, because partial electrical uncoupling allows for much smaller conduction velocities.[30]

Electrical uncoupling is associated with the start of the rise in intracellular calcium concentration and contracture and can be regarded as the beginning of irreversible injury.[31] It is known that ischemic preconditioning (brief episodes of ischemia and reperfusion preceding a prolonged ischemic period) delays electrical uncoupling, and therefore protects to a certain degree against 1b arrhythmias.[32] Interestingly, in myocardium from failing hearts, preconditioning induces an advancement of the rise in intracellular calcium and electrical uncoupling so that in the failing heart, the 1a phase and the 1b phase may occur at almost the same time.[33] In terms of ischemia-induced arrhythmias, it would appear that preconditioning may be a double-edged sword: the heart must be sick enough to need it, but healthy enough to be able to stand it.

## References

1. Erichsen JE. On the influence of the coronary circulation on the action of the heart. Lond Med Gazette 1841; 42/2:561–565.
2. McWilliam JA. Cardiac failure and sudden death. Br Med J 1889; 1:6–8.
3. McWilliam JA. Some applications of physiology to medicine. II. Ventricular fibrillation and sudden death. Br Med J 1923; August:7–43.
4. De Boer S. De pathologische physiologie en pharmacologie van den onregelmatige hartslag. Wolters, Groningen, 1935, p 346.
5. Julian DG. Treatment of cardiac arrest in acute myocardial ischaemia and infarction. Lancet 1961; 2:840–844.
6. Pantridge JF, Geddes JS. A mobile intensive-care unit in the management of myocardial infarction. Lancet 1967; 2:271–273.
7. Lown B, Amarasingham R, Neuman J. New method for terminating cardiac arrhythmias: use of synchronized capacitor discharge. JAMA 1962; 182:548–555.
8. Dialog Database, Los Angeles, 1983.
9. Janse MJ, Opthof T, Kléber AG. Animal models of cardiac arrhythmias. Cardiovasc Res 1998;39:165–177.
10. Curtis MJ. Characterization, utilization and clinical relevance of isolated perfused heart models of ischemia-induced ventricular fibrillation. Cardiovasc Res 1998;39:194–215.
11. Janse MJ, Wit AL. Electrophysiological mechanisms of ventricular arrhythmias resulting from myocardial ischemia and infarction. Physiol Rev 1989; 69:1049–1169.
12. Wit AL, Janse MJ. The Ventricular Arrhythmias of Ischemia and Infarction: Electrophysiological Mechanisms. Futura Publishing Co., Mount Kisco, NY, 1993.
13. Bolli R, Fisher DJ, Entman ML. Factors that determine the occurrence of arrhythmias during acute myocardial ischemia. Am Heart J 1986; 111:261–270.
14. Meesman W. Early arrhythmias and primary ventricular fibrillation after acute myocardial ischemia in relation to preexisting coronary collaterals. In: Parratt JR (ed). Early Arrhythmias Resulting from Myocardial Ischaemia. Macmillan Press, London, 1982, pp 93–112.
15. Austin M, Wenger TL, Harrell Jr FE, et al. Effect of myocardium at risk on outcome after coronary artery occlusion and release. Am J Physiol 1982; 243:H340–H345.
16. Hill JL, Gettes LS. Effects of acute coronary artery occlusion on local myocardial $K^+$ activity in swine. Circulation 1980; 61:768–778.
17. Wilde AAM, Aksnes G. Myocardial potassium loss and cell depolarization in ischemia and hypoxia. Cardiovasc Res 1995; 29:1–15.
18. Downar E, Janse MJ, Durrer D. The effect of acute coronary artery occlusion on subepicardial transmembrane potentials in the intact porcine heart. Circulation 1977; 56:217–224.
19. Kléber AG, Janse MJ, Van Capelle FJL, et al. Mechanism and time course of S-T and T-Q segment changes during acute regional ischemia in the pig heart determined by extracellular and intracellular recordings. Circ Res 1978; 42:603–613.
20. Kléber AG, Janse MJ, Wilms-Schopman FJG, et al. Changes in conduction velocity during acute ischemia in ventricular myocardium of the isolated porcine heart. Circulation 1986; 73:189–198.
21. Shaw RM, Rudy Y. Electrophysiological effects of acute myocardial ischemia:

a mechanistic investigation of action potential conduction and conduction failure. Circ Res 1997; 80:124–138.

22. Janse MJ, Van Capelle FJL, Morsink H, et al. Flow of "injury" current and pattern of excitation during early ventricular arrhythmias in acute regional ischemia in isolated porcine and canine hearts: evidence for two different arrhythmogenic mechanisms. Circ Res 1980; 47:151–165.

23. Goldstein JA, Butterfield MC, Olmichi Y, et al. Arrhythmogenic influence of intracoronary thrombosis during acute myocardial ischemia. Circulation 1994; 90:139–147.

24. Coronel R, Wilms-Schopman FJG, Janse MJ. Profibrillatory effects of intracoronary thrombus in acute regional ischemia of the in situ porcine heart. Circulation 1997; 96:3985–3991.

25. Coronel R, Wilms-Schopman FJG, Dekker LRC, et al. Heterogeneities in $[K^+]_o$ and TQ potential and the inducibility of ventricular fibrillation during acute regional ischemia in the isolated perfused porcine heart. Circulation 1995; 92:120–129.

26. Bril A, Forest M, Gout B. Ischemia and reperfusion-induced arrhythmias in rabbits with chronic heart failure. Am J Physiol 1991; 261:H301-H307.

27. Vermeulen JT, Tan HL, Rademaker H, et al. Electrophysiologic and extracellular ionic changes during acute ischemia in failing and normal rabbit myocardium. J Mol Cell Cardiol 1996; 28:123–131.

28. Smith WT, Fleet WF, Johnson TA, et al. The Ib phase of ventricular arrhythmias in ischemic in situ porcine heart is related to changes in cell-to-cell electrical coupling. Circulation 1995; 92:3051–3060.

29. De Groot JR, Coronel R, Wilms-Schopman FJL, et al. IB ventricular fibrillation depends on critical cellular coupling in the isolated regionally ischemic pig heart (abstract). Eur Heart J 1999; 20(Suppl):565.

30. Rudy Y, Qyan W. A model study of the effects of the discrete cellular structure on electrical propagation in cardiac tissue. Circ Res 1987; 61:815–823.

31. Dekker LRC, Fiolet JWT, Van Bavel E, et al. Intracellular $Ca^{2+}$, intercellular coupling resistance, and mechanical activity in ischemic rabbit papillary muscle: effects of preconditioning and metabolic blockade. Circ Res 1996; 79:237–246.

32. Tan HL, Mazón P, Verberne HL, et al. Ischaemic preconditioning delays ischaemia induced cellular electrical uncoupling in rabbit myocardium by activation of ATP sensitive potassium channels. Cardiovasc Res 1993; 27:644–651.

33. Dekker LRC, Rademaker H, Vermeulen JT, et al. Cellular uncoupling during ischemia in hypertrophied and failing rabbit ventricular myocardium: effects of preconditioning. Circulation 1998; 97:1724–1730.

34. Wilde AAM. Myocardial ischemia and hypoxia. Cellular ionic and electrical activity. PhD thesis, University of Amsterdam. Amsterdam, Rodopi, 1988.

35. Kodama I, Wilde AAM, Janse MJ, et al. Combined effects of hypoxia, hyperkalemia and acidosis on membrane action potential and excitability of guinea-pig ventricular muscle. J Mol Cell Cardiol 1984; 16:247–259.

# 34

# Mechanisms of Ventricular Arrhythmias in the Subacute and Late Postinfarction Period

*Nabil El-Sherif, MD,*
*Boyu Huang, PhD, and*
*Dmitry O. Kozhevnikov, MD*

## Introduction

Ventricular tachycardia and ventricular fibrillation are serious complications of myocardial infarction (MI) and ischemic heart disease. Different electrophysiological mechanisms may give rise to ventricular arrhythmias in myocardial ischemia and infarction.[1] A better understanding of these mechanisms will provide a basis for improved management. More precise information is difficult to obtain from clinical electrophysiological studies because of the limitations of the experimental protocols and techniques that can be utilized. This information could be obtained, however, from successful extrapolations from experimental studies on appropriate animal models to humans. In this chapter the electrophysiological mechanisms of ventricular arrhythmias in the subacute and late post-MI period are reviewed.

## Triggered Ventricular Rhythms in the Subacute Phase of Myocardial Infarction

Approximately 4–8 hours following coronary artery occlusion, spontaneous ventricular rhythms develop. The spontaneous multiform activity peaks 1–2 days post-MI and usually subsides by the third day.[1,2] These

[1]Supported by Veterans Affairs Medical Research Funds.
From: Aliot E, Clementy J, Prystowsky EN (editors). *Fighting Sudden Cardiac Death: A Worldwide Challenge.* ©Futura Publishing Company, Armonk, NY, 2000.

rhythms arise from surviving subendocardial Purkinje fibers overlying the infarction. In vitro studies of these surviving subendocardial Purkinje fibers have suggested that 2 mechanisms may be responsible for the activity: (1) abnormal automaticity[3] and (2) triggered activity.[2] However, the preponderance of evidence favors the second mechanism.

Delayed afterdepolarizations (DADs) giving rise to triggered activity were recorded in depolarized ischemic Purkinje fibers from a 1-day-old canine infarction.[2] The amplitude and rate of rise of the DADs were a function of both the cycle length and the number of impulses in a stimulated train. A critically timed premature impulse may be followed by a DAD that triggers activity. However, in contrast to other preparations demonstrating triggered activity, one stimulated action potential during quiescence was often able to generate a suprathreshold DAD, which in turn initiated triggered activity (Figure 1). The ease of inducing triggered activity in ischemic Purkinje fibers may explain the persistence of multiform ventricular rhythms in vivo in 1-day-old canine infarctions.

Recordings of sustained triggered activity and abnormal automaticity would have the same appearance in a transmembrane recording. The dependence of this activity on the magnitude of diastolic potential was studied directly by the application of constant depolarizing or hyperpolarizing current.[4] This was similar to Ferrier's study[5] on the digitalis-toxic Purkinje fiber. During sustained activity (maximum diastolic potential $-61 \pm 7$ mV) hyperpolarizing current decreased the DADs, rendered them subthreshold, and terminated triggered activity (Figure 2). During the quiescence

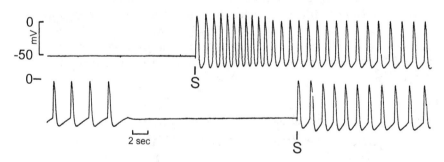

Figure 1. Initiation of triggered activity by a single stimulated action potential. Transmembrane recordings are from a Purkinje cell in the ischemic zone of an endocardial preparation from 1-day-old canine infarction. The depolarized cell (resting membrane potential, $-53$ mV) was quiescent. A single stimulated action potential initiated a run of triggered activity. In the bottom tracing, the activity slowed gradually and terminated following a subthreshold afterdepolarization. Following another quiescent period, triggered activity was again initiated by a single stimulated action potential. (Reprinted by permission of WB Saunders.[1])

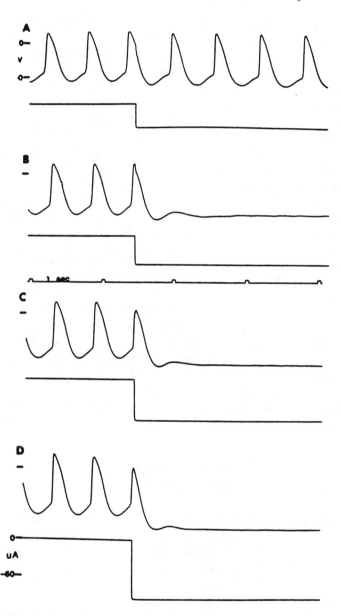

Figure 2. Effects of intermittent hyperpolarizing current during sustained activity from a canine endocardial preparation 1 day postinfarction. Hyperpolarizing current was initiated during an action potential. (A) Hyperpolarizing current prolonged the cycle length of sustained activity. (B–D) Further graded increases in hyperpolarizing current produced a graded attenuation of subthreshold delayed afterdepolarizations. Calibration for transmembrane potential is shown in A, and calibration for current is shown in D. Time calibration separates B and C. (Reprinted by permission from Gough WB, El-Sherif N. Am J Physiol 1989; 257:H770–H777.)

caused by constant hyperpolarizing current, a stimulated train of action potentials produced DADs. Decreasing the current permitted augmented DADs. In quiescent preparations (resting potential $-68 \pm 7$ mV), a train of stimulated action potentials was followed by subthreshold DADs. Depolarizing current increased the DAD amplitude. Sufficient depolarization caused triggered activity to occur (Figure 3). To exclude depolarization-induced automaticity, constant currents were applied without a previous train of stimuli. Neither DADs nor triggered activity was evoked.

The main finding of this study was that in ischemic Purkinje fibers, 1 day post-MI, there is a graded response of DADs to depolarizing currents and depolarized diastolic potentials.[4] On this basis, one can consider that the transition from nonsustained triggered activity to a sustained rhythm can be due to an enhancement of the abnormal DAD accompanying depolarization post-MI. Similarly, a sustained rhythm can become nonsustained as a consequence of repolarization accompanying recovery from ischemia. The transition from threshold to subthreshold and vice versa can be only a 1-mV change in diastolic potential. One need not invoke a separate, intrinsically oscillatory mechanism, such as abnormal automaticity, to explain the existence of sustained versus nonsustained rhythms in the same heart or isolated preparation 1 day post-MI. In addition, the DADs may become sufficiently suprathreshold that interventions such as overdrive pacing,[6] changes in temperature,[6,7] or pharmacological inhibitors[6,8] may be unable to render these DADs subthreshold and therefore will not terminate the sustained triggered activity. Caution must be applied when concluding that such interventions might differentially distinguish sustained triggered activity from abnormal automaticity.

# Ionic Mechanisms of Triggered Ventricular Rhythms

The basic hypothesis for the mechanism by which charge is carried by the transient inward current that causes the DAD is derived from studies of Purkinje and ventricular muscle cells that have been overloaded with $Ca^{2+}$ in a variety of ways. There are 2 proposed mechanisms.[9] The first mechanism, originally proposed by Kass and Tsien,[10] was a nonspecific cation channel, activated by a phasic rise in intracellular $Ca^{2+}$, which had significant permeability to $Na^+$, $K^+$, and $Ca^{2+}$. The inward current was thought to be carried predominantly by $Na^+$ with some $Ca^{2+}$ contribution. The second proposed mechanism for transient inward current is the electrogenic $Na^+$–$Ca^{2+}$ exchange pump driven by the transmembrane electrochemical gradient for $Na^+$ and $Ca^{2+}$.[11,12] The stoichiometry for charge translocation is 3 $Na^+$ to 1 $Ca^{2+}$. $Ca^{2+}$ overload produces a phasic release

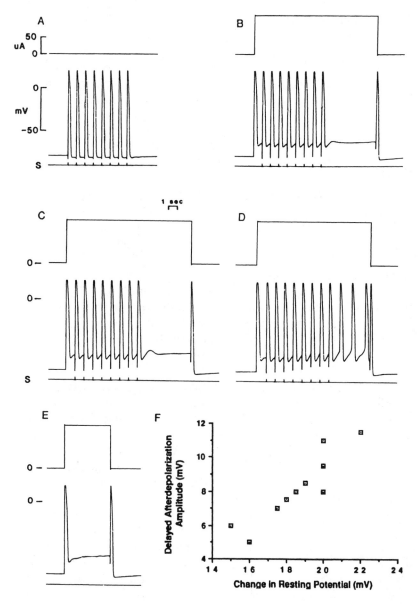

Figure 3. Effects of long depolarizing current on delayed afterdepolarization. Recordings were obtained from a canine endocardial preparation I day post-infarction. (A) Control. A train of 8 paced beats (cycle length = 1 s) produced no measurable delayed afterdepolarization. (B, C) During long graded depolarizing current pulses initiated before stimulation, delayed afterdepolarization gradually increased in amplitude. (D) Delayed afterdepolarization following the eighth beat induced triggered activity that ceased as soon as current was terminated. (E) Depolarizing current equal in amplitude to that used in D produced neither a delayed afterdepolarization nor depolarization-induced automaticity. (F) Amplitude of delayed afterdepolarization after the eighth driven beat is plotted as a function of change in resting potential. (Reprinted by permission from Gough WB, El-Sherif N. Am J Physiol 1989; 257:H770–H777.)

of $Ca^{2+}$ from the sarcoplasmic reticulum into the myoplasm. This produces a transient decrease in the transmembrane $Ca^{2+}$ gradient, which in turn facilitates $Ca^{2+}$ extrusion and $Na^+$ entry by the exchanger. The electrogenicity of the exchange produces a transient inward current.

# Reentrant Ventricular Rhythms in the Subacute Phase of Myocardial Infarction

In 1977 El-Sherif and associates made the observation that in dogs that survived the initial stage of MI arrhythmias and that were studied 3–5 days post-MI, reentrant ventricular rhythms occurred spontaneously, but were more commonly induced by programmed electrical stimulation.[13] The anatomic and electrophysiological substrates for the reentrant rhythms were later characterized in a series of reports.[14-16] These studies have shown that reentrant excitation occurred around zones (arcs) of functional conduction block. The arcs were attributed to ischemia-induced spatially nonhomogeneous lengthening of refractoriness. Sustained reentrant tachycardia was found to have a figure-8 activation pattern whereby clockwise and counterclockwise wavefronts were oriented around 2 separate arcs of functional conduction block. The 2 circulating wavefronts coalesced into a common wavefront that conducted slowly between the 2 arcs of block (Figure 4). Using reversible cooling, reentrant excitation could be successfully terminated only from localized areas along the common reentrant wavefront.[16]

Intracellular recordings from the surviving "ischemic" epicardial layer show cells with variable degrees of partial depolarization, reduced action potential amplitude, and decreased upstroke velocity. Full recovery of responsiveness frequently outlasts the action potential duration, reflecting the presence of postrepolarization refractoriness.[17] In these cells, premature stimuli could elicit graded responses over a wide range of coupling intervals (Figure 5). Isochronal mapping studies have shown that both the arcs of functional conduction block and the slow activation wavefronts of the reentrant circuit develop in the surviving electrophysiologically abnormal epicardial layer overlying the infarction.

The ionic changes induced by ischemia that explain abnormal transmembrane action potentials of myocardial cells in the subacute phase of myocardial infarction have not been fully explored. Earlier studies suggested that ischemic transmembrane action potentials may be generated by a depressed fast $Na^+$ channel. This was based on experiments that showed that ischemic cells are sensitive to the depressant effect of the fast channel blocker tetrodotoxin (TTX), but not to the slow channel blocker methoxyverapamil (D600).[17] More recent studies have shown that $I_{Na}$ is re-

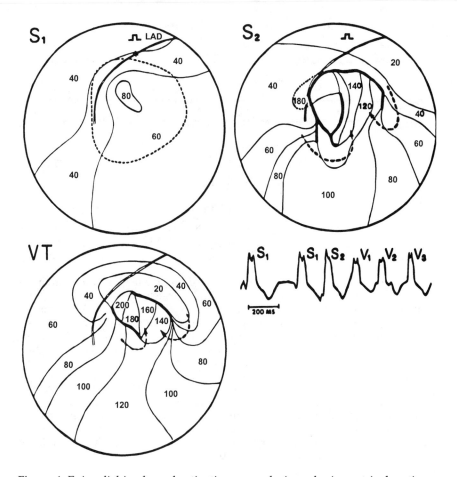

Figure 4. Epicardial isochronal activation maps during a basic ventricular stimulated beat ($S_1$), initiation of reentry by a single premature stimulus ($S_2$), and sustained monomorphic reentrant ventricular tachycardia (VT). A representative electrocardiogram is shown in the lower right panel. The recordings were obtained from a dog 4 days postligation of the left anterior descending artery (LAD). Site of ligation is represented by a double bar. Epicardial activation is displayed as if the heart is viewed from the apex located at the center of the circular map. The perimeter of the circle represents the AV junction. The outline of the epicardial ischemic zone is represented by the dotted line. Activation isochrones are drawn at 20-ms intervals. Arcs of functional conduction block are represented by heavy solid lines and are depicted to separate contiguous areas that are activated at least 40 ms apart. During $S_1$ the epicardial surface was activated within 80 ms with the latest isochrone located in the center of the ischemic zone. $S_2$ resulted in a long continuous arc of conduction block within the border of the ischemic zone. The activation wavefront circulated around both ends of the arc of block and coalesced at the 100-ms isochrone. The common wavefront advanced within the arc of block before reactivating an area on the other side of the arc at the 180-ms isochrone to initiate the first reentrant cycle. During sustained VT, the reentrant circuit had a figure-8 activation pattern in the form of clockwise and counterclockwise wavefronts around 2 arcs of functional conduction block before coalescing into a slow common wavefront that conducted between the 2 arcs of block. (Reprinted with permission of WB Saunders.[1])

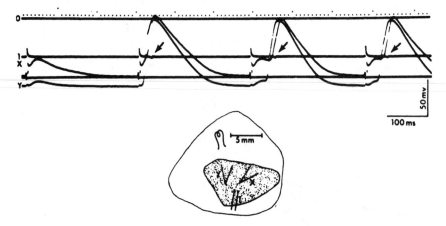

**Figure 5.** Recordings from a dog with 3-day-old infarction, illustrating action potential characteristics in ischemic epicardium. The sketch of the preparation shows 2 intracellular recordings (X and Y) and a close bipolar recording (1) from the infarction zone (hatched area). Ischemic cells had decreased upstroke velocity, reduced action potential amplitude, and a variable degree of partial depolarization. The 2 cells were recorded 5 mm apart in the infarction zone, but showed significant difference in their resting potential. The resting potential of the Y cell was only slightly reduced (−80 mV), but it still had a poor action potential upstroke. The preparation was stimulated at a cycle length of 290 ms, which resulted in a Wenckebach-like conduction pattern. Note that the pacing cycle length exceeded the action potential duration of the 2 cells, suggesting that refractoriness extended beyond the completion of the action potential (i.e., postrepolarization refractoriness). (Reprinted by permission of the American Heart Association, Inc., from El-Sherif N, Lazzara R. Circulation 1979; 6:605.)

duced and its kinetics are altered in the surviving epicardial layer from 5-day-old canine infarct.[18] The fast channel may be depressed in ischemia for various reasons. This can be only be partly explained by cellular depolarization, because the depression is usually out of proportion to the degree of depolarization of the resting potential. The $Na^+$–$K^+$ pump may be depressed in surviving ischemic myocardial cells, leading to intracellular $Na^+$ loading. This can diminish the electrochemical driving force for the inward $Na^+$ current.

Abnormal membrane properties of ischemic myocardial cells may not be the only cause for slowed conduction and block in the surviving ischemic epicardial layer. Electrical uncoupling and increase of extracellular resistance after ischemia have also been suggested.[19] Ischemia-induced increase in intracellular $Ca^{2+}$ and low pH may increase the resistance of the gap junctions of the intercalated disc. Changes in gap junctional distribution in the border zone of healing canine infarcts may define the locations of reentrant ventricular tachycardia in the surviving epicardial layer.[20]

Another factor that was considered by some authors is the anisotropic structure of the surviving epicardial layer. The normal uniform anisotropic conduction properties of the epicardial layer may be altered further following ischemia. It was suggested that the site of conduction block of premature stimuli in the ischemic epicardial layer may be determined by its anisotropic properties (i.e., premature stimuli block along the long axis of epicardial muscle fibers).[21] We have shown that functional conduction block of premature stimuli in the ischemic epicardial layer is due to abrupt and discrete change in refractoriness. The spatially nonuniform refractory distribution occurs both along and across fiber direction, the same as the arcs of conduction block.[22] We have also shown that, during sustained figure-8 monomorphic reentrant tachycardia, the 2 arcs of functional conduction block around which the reentrant wavefronts circulate are usually oriented parallel to the long axis of the epicardial muscle fibers. Other investigators have suggested that these areas represent apparent or pseudo-block, and are in fact due to very slow and possibly discontinuous conduction across the myocardial fibers.[21] Restivo et al.[22] have analyzed close bipolar electrograms obtained at high resolution (1-mm interelectrode distance) from sites of the arcs of block during sustained stable reentry. Electrograms recorded at each side of the line of block showed 2 distinct deflections; one represented local activation, and the other an electrotonus corresponding to activation recorded a 1-mm distance away. Both deflections were separated by a variable isoelectric period that correlated with the isochronal difference across the arc. In recordings obtained from the center of the arc, local activation and electrotonus were separated by 90–110 ms. This interval successively decreased toward both ends of the arc (Figure 6). These observations provide evidence that circus movement reentry is sustained around a continuous arc of functional conduction block and not very slow conduction across fibers.

## Cellular, Ionic and Molecular Basis of Arrhythmias in Postinfarction Remodeled Ventricular Myocardium

In recent years the importance of ventricular remodeling following MI on long-term survival has been better appreciated. The structural remodeling of the left ventricle post-MI involves both the region of necrosis and the noninfarcted myocardium. The noninfarcted myocardium undergoes significant hypertrophy, which is considered an adaptive universal response of the heart to increased workload from whatever cause. Clinical and experimental data strongly suggest that the risk of ventricular arrhythmias in the late post-MI period correlates with the degree and characteristics of post-MI remodeling.[23] Although post-MI remodeling is a complex time-

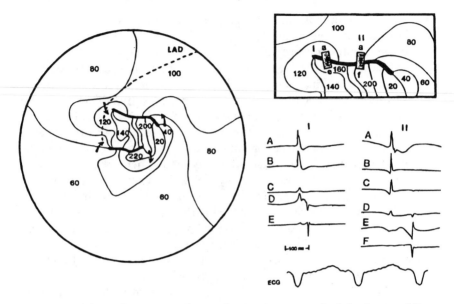

Figure 6. High-resolution recordings of activation across 1 of the 2 arcs of functional conduction block around which sustained figure-8 reentrant activation occurred. The left panel illustrates the epicardial activation pattern during a figure-8 reentrant tachycardia as obtained from a sock electrode array with 5–10 mm interelectrode distance. A high-density electrode plaque (1 mm interelectrode distance) was positioned at 2 locations across the upper arc of block. Shown on the right are an expanded map of the counterclockwise circuit around the upper arc of block and the electrograms along one row of bipolar electrodes at each location. Plaque location II was situated near the center of the arc of block. Conduction between sites A and C during the left to right wavefront on the upper side of the arc was fast. Conduction block probably occurred between sites C and D. Similarly, conduction between sites F and E during the returning wavefront on the distal side of the arc was fast, and conduction block probably occurred between sites E and D. The 2 deflections recorded at site D were separated by an isoelectric interval of 85 ms, which corresponded to isochronal activation difference across the site of 81–100 ms. Both deflections most probably represented electrotonic potentials. (Modifed from Restivo M, et al.[22])

dependent process that involves structural, biochemical, neurohumoral, and electrophysiological alterations, there is considerable evidence that electrophysiological changes associated with the hypertrophied noninfarcted myocardium play a key role in the arrhythmogenicity of the post-MI heart. For example, although beta blockers and angiotensin-converting enzyme (ACE) inhibitors have very different effects on ventricular dilatation, both agents have been shown to prevent the development of myocardial hypertrophy, and may thus decrease the susceptibility to ventricular arrhythmias.[23] On the other hand, there is a considerable amount of data from other models of hypertrophy showing that hypertrophied myocardium can generate arrhythmias more readily than can normal tissue.[24]

The most consistent electrical abnormality that has been described in association with myocardial hypertrophy is prolongation of action potential duration (APD). We have recently shown that remodeled hypertrophied left ventricular myocytes from rats 3–4 weeks post-MI have prolonged APD with marked heterogeneity of the time-course of repolarization across the left ventricular wall.[25] The prolongation of APD could be explained by the decreased density of the 2 outward $K^+$ currents, $I_{to-fast}$ and $I_{to-slow}$ (Figure 7) rather than by changes in the density or kinetics of $I_{Ca-L}$.[25]

Cardiac hypertrophy is associated with both quantitative and qualitative changes in gene expression; the latter usually represents a shift toward reexpression of fetal isogenes. Although alterations in expression of contractile and other intracellular proteins has been well characterized in a variety of experimental models of hypertrophy, little is known regarding changes in gene expression in post-MI remodeled myocardium. This is especially so regarding sarcolemmal ion channel proteins that may explain the electrophysiological alterations in these hearts. We have examined the changes in mRNA levels of the $\alpha_1$ subunit of the L-type Ca channel and the 5 K channels shown to be expressed in adult rat ventricular myocytes, in remodeled myocardium from rats 3 weeks post-MI, and compared the results with sham-operated rats. There was no statistical difference in the expression of mRNA of the $\alpha_1$ subunit of L-type Ca channel between sham and 3 weeks post-MI ventricular tissues.[26] These results are consistent with our electrophysiological studies that showed no change in the density of $I_{Ca-L}$ in ventricular myocytes obtained from sham and 3 weeks post-MI rat hearts.[25]

We have also compared the mRNA expression of Kv1.2, Kv1.4, Kv1.5, Kv2.1, Kv4.2, and Kv4.3 in ventricular tissue from sham-operated rats and from rats 3 weeks post-MI. There was a statistically insignificant increase in the expression of Kv1.2 mRNA and an insignificant decrease in the expression of Kv1.5 mRNA in post-MI hearts. On the other hand, the expression and protein levels of the Kv2.1, Kv4.2, and Kv4.3 were significantly reduced (Figure 8).[27] These data illustrate the occurrence of transcriptional regulation of voltage-gated K channels that is distinct for each channel. Recent studies suggest that the Kv4.2/Kv4.3 is the likely candidate for the native $I_{to-fast}$, while Kv2.1 may be the candidate for the $I_{to-slow}$ (also called IK).[28] However, more recently, this molecular correlate of $I_{to-slow}$ has been questioned.[29] Our data showing significant decrease in the expression and protein levels of the Kv4.2/Kv4.3 and Kv2.1 in 3 weeks post-MI remodeled ventricular myocardium correlate remarkably well with our electrophysiological observations showing significant reduction of both $I_{to-fast}$ and $I_{to-slow}$ in myocytes obtained from rats 3 weeks post-MI.

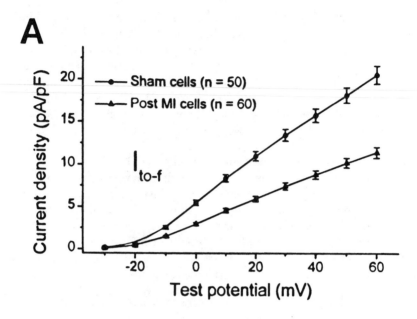

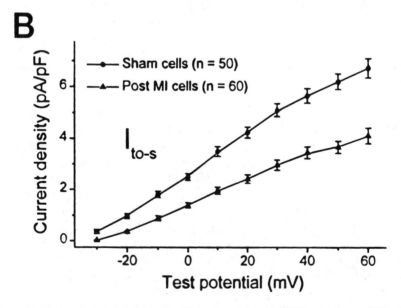

Figure 7. Comparison of the density of $I_{to\text{-}2Df}$ and $I_{to\text{-}2Ds}$ of sham and post-MI cells. When the current amplitude was normalized to membrane capacity, the density of both $I_{to\text{-}2Df}$ and $I_{to\text{-}2Ds}$ was significantly reduced in post-MI cells. (Reprinted with permission of the American Heart Association from Gin et al. Circ Res 1996; 79:461–473.)

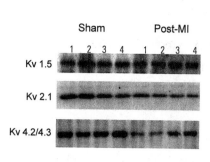 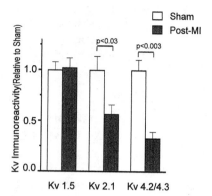

**Figure 8. left.** Western blot analysis of Kv channel subunit immunoreactive proteins (Kv1.5, Kv2.1, and Kv4.2/4.3) in LV myocardium from 3-week post-MI (n=4) and sham operated (n=4) rats. Note that different proteins were investigated in different blots. Right: Bar graph showing Kv immunoreactivities by measuring the signal for the protein (Kv1.5, Kv2.1, and Kv4.2/4.3) by densitometry. Columns represent the mean values, with error bars indicating SEM (n=4). There was no significant change in the protein level of Kv1.5, while the protein levels of Kv2.1 and Kv4.2/4.3 were significantly reduced by 43% (P<0.03) and 67% (P<0.003), respectively. (Reprinted with permission of the American Heart Association from Gidh-Jain et al. Circ Res 1996; 79:669–675.)

# Spatial Alterations in the Expression of Connexin43 in Post-MI Rat Ventricle

We have recently shown that there is a significant decrease in connexin43 (Cx43) protein level in left ventricular (LV) endocardium, septum, and right ventricle (RV) but, interestingly enough, not in LV epicardium 3 weeks post-MI.[30] The decrease in Cx43 protein level occurs as early as 3 days post-MI. The pattern of alterations in Cx43 protein level is well correlated with the patterns of collagen remodeling and ACE binding post-MI.[31] The decrease in the Cx43 protein level could be induced by myocardial damage due to myocyte necrosis, myocytes side-to-side slippage,[32] fibrosis, and/or renin-angiotensin stimulation. A widespread downregulation of Cx43 gap junction was reported to occur in myocardium distant from the infarct in the human heart as well as in other hypertrophied nonischemic myocardium.[20] However, spatial differences in Cx43 changes in post-MI remodeled LV have not been reported before and could be a significant determinant of the increased anisotropic properties of the post-MI heart. Gap junctional coupling of myocytes is an important determinant of intracellular conductance.[33] Longitudinal impedance in the heart is usually quantitatively analyzed in terms of parallel intracellular and extracellular pathways; the former has 2 series components, one attributable to the sarcoplasm and the other to the low-resistance junctions between adjacent cells. It has recently been shown that in the hypertrophied heart, there is an increased intracellular resistivity that could be attributed solely to an increase of the junctional resistance between adjacent cells.[33]

## Electrophysiological Mechanisms of Arrhythmia Generation in the Post-MI Remodeled Ventricular Myocardium

Three potential electrophysiological mechanisms for arrhythmia generation have been described in the post-MI remodeled hypertrophied ventricular myocardium as well as in other models of cardiac hypertrophy in general.[34] These are: (1) EAD-triggered activity, (2) DAD-triggered activity, and (3) reentrant excitation.

### EAD-Triggered Activity

Prolongation of APD, the universal and consistent electrophysiological abnormality described in hypertrophied myocytes, is considered the priming step for development of EAD.[35] Several changes in ionic currents that have been described in different models of hypertrophy favor both the prolongation of APD and the generation of EADs. These include a decrease of $I_{to}$ and $I_K$, shift of inactivation of L-type calcium current ($I_{Ca-L}$) to more positive potentials, and prolongation of the current inactivation. Although spontaneous generation of EADs in hypertrophied myocardium has not been reported, Aronson[36] showed that EADs were more easily induced in the hypertrophied rat myocyte when outward $K^+$ currents were suppressed by tetraethylammonium (TEA). Our group has demonstrated the development of single and repetitive EADs in isolated post-MI remodeled myocytes[25] (Figure 9). The in vivo representation of EAD-induced triggered activity is a prolonged QT interval associated with polymorphic ventricular tachycardia, known as torsades de pointes.[35]

### DAD-Triggered Activity

DADs have been shown to be more easily induced in hypertrophied myocytes under the influence of increased intracellular $[Ca^{2+}]_i$,[36] or in the presence of β-adrenergic agonists.[25,37] Higher $[Ca^{2+}]_i$ through the $Na^+–Ca^{2+}$ exchange mechanism associated with the prolonged APD and impaired $Ca^{2+}$ uptake by the SR in hypertrophied cells can favor the occurrence of DADs.[38] There is also evidence that the hyperpolarization-acti-

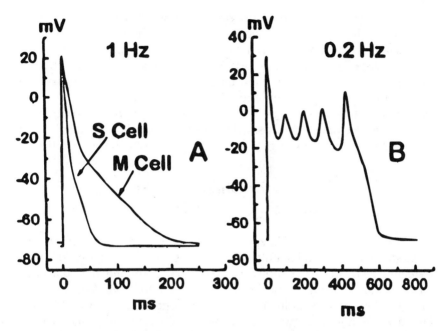

Figure 9. Action potential of an isolated postinfarction hypertrophied myocyte superimposed on action potential of an isolated sham myocyte (S) to illustrate the changes in action potential duration in MI cells. Note that APD25, APD50, APD75, and APD90 of the Ml cell were all prolonged compared to the S cell. Section B shows the development of multiple early afterdepolarizations in an isolated Ml myocyte. The early afterdepolarizations were more easily induced at 0.2 Hz stimulation than at 1 Hz. (Modified with permission.[25])

vated current ($I_f$) is increased in hypertrophied myocytes and may favor the occurrence of spontaneous action potentials.[39] Further, T-type calcium current ($I_{Ca-T}$) was shown to be reexpressed in some models of hypertrophy,[40] including the post-MI model.[41] The steady-state voltage relations for activation and inactivation of $I_{Ca-T}$ are shifted by 35 mV toward negative potentials compared to $I_{Ca-L}$, making $I_{Ca-T}$ well suited for participating in pacemaker activity. A current flowing through $I_{Ca-T}$ channels might be involved in several types of arrhythmias, including both DADs and EADs.[42]

## Reentrant Excitation

Reentrant excitation is an important potential electrophysiological mechanism of tachyarrhythmia in the post-MI remodeled myocardium. Changes in both active membrane properties[22] and passive resistivity[43] could create heterogeneity of repolarization, slowed conduction, and functional conduction block, thus providing the necessary prerequisites for reentrant excitation. There is evidence that prolongation of APD in hypertrophied remodeled ventricle is not homogeneous,[25] which provides a substrate for dispersion of refractoriness. Besides the evidence for hypertrophy-induced increase in interstitial tissue with possible impairment of intracellular coupling, evidence for quantitative changes in gap junctional proteins are of interest.[44] Regional differences in the expression of connexin in the remodeled post-MI myocardium can increase the anisotropic properties of the remodeled ventricle and predispose to reentrant excitation.

## Triggers for Changes in Gene Expression of Post-MI Heart

Previous studies on LV hypertrophy focused primarily on the effect of pressure overload[45] and spontaneous hypertension.[46] In models of hemodynamic overload, hypertrophy was accompanied by the immediate activation of early response genes (proto-oncogene c-fos, c-jun, c-myc, Hsp70, Erg-1), followed by the induction of embryonic genes (ANF, β-MHC, skeletal α-actin) and an upregulation of constitutively expressed genes (cardiac α actin and myosin light chain-2). Chronic pressure and volume overload have been shown to result in morphologically and functionally distinct forms of hypertrophy.[47] However, the cellular and molecular mechanisms that contribute to cardiac hypertrophy after MI, which has features more consistent with those of volume overload, remain unknown.

A recent study from our laboratory has emphasized the differences in cardiac gene expression in the post-MI heart compared to other overload hypertrophy models.[48] One striking difference is the continued expression of c-fos, which remains elevated up to 3 weeks post-MI while c-fos expression is generally rapid and quite short-lived in response to other cardiac stimuli causing hypertrophy.[49] The delayed activation of BNF and the return of β-MHC and $\alpha_2$ Na-K ATPase to basal levels during the compensatory phase of hypertrophy are other noteworthy differences.[48] Differences in fetal gene expression between post-MI hypertrophy and other models of overload hypertrophy have also been reported from our laboratory. For example, in post-MI remodeled myocardium, there is a significant increase in the mRNA level of the fetal isoform of the L-type $Ca^{2+}$ current, with reversion of the fetal:adult isoform ratio to the fetal phenotype.[26] Similar changes were not reported in other overload hypertrophy models. The physiological significance of these findings remains to be determined since, to our knowledge, the currents corresponding to the 2 isoforms have not, thus far, been characterized. However, a novel DHP-resistant $Ca^{2+}$ current similar to $I_{Ca-L}$ has been described in the rat fetal myocyte that disappears during development.[50] The T-type Ca current that is expressed only in fetal rat ventricular myocytes is also reexpressed in the hypertrophied myocardium after MI,[41] but not in other rat overload hypertrophy models.[42] Although the exact role of $I_{Ca-T}$ is not clear, its appearance in post-MI remodeled hypertrophy may increase total $Ca^{2+}$ influx, change the cell electrophysiological properties, and predispose for arrhythmias in the hypertrophied heart. Last but not least, Huang et al. have shown that there is differential expression of $Na^+$ channel subtypes in post-MI hypertrophied myocardium.[51] Once again, the physiological significance of these changes is unknown. However, in cardiac myocytes, the slow $Na^+$ current contributes to the plateau phase of APD. An increased $I_{Na-slow}$, due to altered gating kinetics of the $I_{Na}$ in hypertrophied myocytes, if present, can significantly contribute to prolongation of APD and arrhythmogenesis.

The differences between gene expression post-MI and other overload hypertrophy models suggest that alterations in gene expression that accompany hypertrophy post-MI may encompass other alternate pathways of gene activation. At present little is known about molecular mechanisms by which ischemic stimuli are converted into intracellular signals to regulate gene expression. Some recent preliminary data suggest that ischemia may preferentially activate specific protein kinase cascades.[52] Because of the significant consequences of altered gene expression on post-MI electrophysiological and mechanical functions of the heart, further investigations of post-MI signal transduction pathways are urgently needed.

## References

1. El-Sherif N, Gough WB, Restivo M. Boutjdir M. Electrophysiology of ventricular arrhythmias in myocardial ischemia and infarction. In: El-Sherif N, Samet P (eds). Cardiac Pacing and Electrophysiology. WB Saunders, Philadelphia,1991; pp 18–56.
2. El-Sherif N, Gough WB, Zeiler RH, Mehra R. Triggered ventricular rhythms in one-day-old myocardial infarction in the dog. Circ Res 1983; 52:566–579.
3. Friedman PL, Stewart JR, Wit AL. Spontaneous and induced cardiac arrhythmias in subendocardial Purkinje fibers surviving extensive myocardial infarction in dogs. Circ Res 1973; 33:612–626.
4. Gough WB, El-Sherif N. Dependence of delayed afterdepolarizations on diastolic potentials in ischemic Purkinje fibers. Am J Physiol 1989; 257:H770–H777.
5. Ferrier GR. Effects of transmembrane potential on oscillatory afterpotentials induced by acetylstrophanthidin in canine ventricular tissues. J Pharmacol Exp Ther 1980; 215:332.
6. LeMarec H, Dangman KH, Danilo P, Rosen MR. An evaluation of automaticity and triggered activity in canine heart one to four days after myocardial infarction. Circulation 1985; 71:1124.
7. Mugelli A, Cerbai E, Amerini S, Visentin S. The role of temperature on the development of oscillatory afterpotentials and triggered activity. J Mol Cell Cardiol 1986; 18:1313.

8. Le Marec H, Spinelli W, Rosen MR. The effects of doxorubicin I on ventricular tachycardia. Circ Res 1986; 74:881.
9. January CP, Fozzard HA. Delayed afterdepolarizations in heart muscles: mechanisms and relevance. Pharmacol Rev 1988; 30:219.
10. Kass R, Tsien RW, Weingart R. Ionic basis of transient inward current induced by strophanthidin in cardiac Purkinje fibers. J Physiol 1978; 281:208.
11. Nobel D. The surprising heart: a review of recent progress in cardiac electrophysiology. J Physiol 1984; 353:1.
12. Arlock P, Katzung BG. Effects of sodium substitute on transient inward current and tension in guinea pig and ferret papillary muscle. J Physiol 1985; 360:105.
13. El-Sherif N, Scherlag BJ, Lazzara R, Hope RR. Reentrant ventricular arrhythmias in the late myocardial infarction period: conduction characteristics in the infarction zone. Circulation 1977; 55:686–702.
14. El-Sherif N, Smith RA, Evans K. Canine ventricular arrhythmias in the late myocardial infarction period: epicardial mapping of reentrant circuits. Circ Res 1981; 49:255–265.
15. El-Sherif N. The figure-8 model of reentrant excitation in the canine postinfarction heart. In: Zipes DP, Jalife J (eds). Cardiac Electrophysiology and Arrhythmias. Grune & Stratton, Orlando, FL, 1985, pp 365–378.
16. El-Sherif N, Mehra R, Gough WB, Zeiler RH. Reentrant ventricular arrhythmias in the late myocardial infarction period: interruption of reentrant circuits by cryothermal techniques. Circulation 1983; 8:644–656.
17. El-Sherif N, Lazzara R. Reentrant ventricular arrhythmias in the late myocardial infarction period: effects of verapamil and D-600 and role of the "slow channel." Circulation 1979; 60:605–615.
18. Pu J, Boyden PA. Alterations of $Na^+$ currents in myocytes from epicardial border zone of the infarcted heart: a possible ionic mechanism for reduced excitability and postrepolarization refractoriness. Circ Res 1997;81:110–119.
19. Spear JF, Michelson EL, Moore EN. Reduced space constant in slowly conducting regions of chronically infarcted canine myocardium. Circ Res 1983; 53:176–185.
20. Peters NS, Coromilas J, Severs NJ, Wilt AL. Disturbed connexin-43 gap junction distribution correlates with the location of reentrant circuits in the epicardial border zone of healing canine infarcts that cause ventricular tachycardia. Circulation 1997; 95:988–996.
21. Dillon S. Allessie MA, Ursell PC, Wit AL. Influences of anisotropic tissue structure on reentrant circuits in the epicardial border zone of subacute canine infarcts. Circ Res 1988; 63:182–206.
22. Restivo M, Gough WB, El-Sherif N. Ventricular arrhythmias in the subacute myocardial infarction period: high resolution activation and refractory patterns of reentrant rhythms. Circ Res 1990; 66:1310–1327.
23. Belichard P, Savard P. Cardinal R, et al. Markedly different effects on ventricular remodeling result in a decrease in inducibility of ventricular arrhythmias. J Am Coll Cardiol 1994; 23:505–513.
24. Aronson RS, Ming Z. Cellular mechanisms of arrhythmias in hypertrophied and failing myocardium. Circulation 1993;87(Suppl VII) VII-76–83.
25. Qin D, Zhang Z-H, Caref EB, Boutjdir M, Jain P, et al. Cellular and ionic basis of arrhythmias in postinfarction remodeled ventricular myocardium. Circ Res 1996; 79:461–473.
26. Gidh-Jain M, Huang B, Jain P, Battula V, El-Sherif N. Reemergence of the fetal pattern of L-type calcium channel gene expression in noninfarcted myocar-

dium during left ventricular remodeling. Biochem Biophys Res Commun, 1995; 216:892–897.

27. Gidh-Jain M, Huang B, Jain P, El-Sherif N. Differential expression of voltage-gated $K^+$ channel genes in left ventricular remodeled myocardium after experimental myocardial infarction. Circ Res 1996; 79:669–675.

28. Barry DM, Trimmer JS, Merlie JP, Nerbonne JM. Differential expression of voltage-gated K channel subunits in adult rat heart, relation to function K channels. Circ Res 1995; 77:361–369.

29. Xu H, Barry DM, Nerbonne JM. Molecular correlates of functional $I_{to}$ and $I_K$ channels in rat ventricular myocytes probed with $K^+$ channel toxins and antisense oligonucleotides (abstract). Circulation 1997; 96:I-421.

30. Huang B, Qin D, Gidh-Jain M, Boutjdir M, El-Sherif N. Spatial alterations Kv channel and connexin 43 expression and K current density of post-infarction remodeled left ventricle (abstract). Circulation 1998; 98:I-697.

31. Sun Y, Weber KT. Angiotensin II receptor binding following myocardial infarction in the rat. Cardiovasc Res 1994; 28:1623–1628.

32. Olivetti G, Quaini F, Lagrasta C, Cigola E, Ricci R, et al. Cellular basis of ventricular remodeling after myocardial infarction in rats. Cardioscience 1995; 6:101–106.

33. Cooklin M, Wallis WR, Sheridan DJ, Fry CH. Changes in cell-to-cell electrical coupling associated with left ventricular hypertrophy. Circ Res 1997; 80:765–771.

34. Hart G. Cellular electrophysiology in cardiac hypertrophy and failure. Cardiovasc Res 1994; 28:933–946.

35. El-Sherif N, Craelius W, Boutjdir M, Gough WB. Early afterdepolarizations and arrhythmogenesis. J Cardiovasc Electrophysiol 1990; 1:145–160.

36. Aronson RS. Afterpotentials and triggered activity in hypertrophied myocardium from rats with renal hypertension. Circ Res 1981; 48:720–727.

37. Barbieri M, Varani K, Cerbai E, Guerra L, Li Q, et al. Electrophysiological basis for the enhanced cardiac arrhythmogenic effect of isoprenaline in aged spontaneously hypertensive rats. J Mol Cell Cardiol 1994; 26:849–860.

38. Bing OHL, Brooks WW, Conrad CH, Sen S, Perreault CL, et al. Intracellular calcium transients in myocardium from spontaneously hypertensive rats during the transition to heart failure. Circ Res 1991; 68:1390–1400.

39. Cerbai E, Barbieri M, Mugelli A. Characterization of the hyperpolarization-activated current, $I_f$ in ventricular myocytes isolated from hypertensive rats. J Physiol 1994; 481.3:585–591.

40. Nuss HB, Houser SR. T-type $Ca^{2+}$ current is expressed in hypertrophied adult feline left ventricular myocytes. Circ Res 1993; 73:777–782.

41. Qin D, Jain P, Boutjdir M, El-Sherif N. Expression of T-type calcium current in remodeled hypertrophied left ventricle from adult rat following myocardial infarction. Circulation 1995; 92(Suppl I):I-587.

42. Vassort G, Alvarez J. Cardiac T-type calcium current: pharmacology and role in cardiac tissues. J Cardiovasc Electrophysiol 1994; 5:376–393.

43. Wit AL, Dillon SM, Coromilas J. Anisotropic reentry as a cause of ventricular tachyarrhythmias in myocardial infarction. In: Zipes DP, Jalife J (eds). Cardiac Electrophysiology: From Cell to Bedside. WB Saunders, Philadelphia, 1995, pp 511–526.

44. Peters NS, Green CR, Poole Wilson PA, Severs NJ. Reduced content of connexin43 gap junctions in ventricular myocardium from hypertrophied and ischaemic human hearts. Circulation 1993; 88:864–875.

45. Izumo S, Nadal-Ginard B, Mahdavi V. Protooncogene induction and reprogramming of cardiac gene expression produced by pressure overload. Proc Natl Acad Sci USA 1988; 85:339–343.

46. Kessler-Icekson G, Barhum Y, Schlesinger H, Shohat J, Sharma H, et al. Molecular manifestations of cardiac hypertrophy in the spontaneously hypertensive rat: effects of antihypertensive treatments. In: Sideman S, Beyar R (eds). Molecular and Subcellular Cardiology: Effects of Structure and Function. Plenum Press, NY, 1995, pp 195–203.

47. Oparil S. Pathogenesis of ventricular hypertrophy. J Am Coll Cardiol 1985; 5:57B-65B.

48. Gidh-Jain M, Huang B, Jain P, El-Sherif N. Alterations in cardiac gene expression during transition to compensated hypertrophy following myocardial infarction. J Mol Cell Cardiol 1998; 30:627–637.

49. Brand T, Sharma HS, Schaper W. Expression of nuclear proto-oncogenes in isoproterenol-induced cardiac hypertrophy. J Mol Cell Cardiol 1993; 25:1325–1337.

50. Tohse N, Masuda H, Sperelakis N. Novel isoform of $Ca^{2+}$ channel in rat fetal cardiomyocytes. J Physiol (London) 1992; 451:295–306.

51. Huang B, Gidh-Jain M, Jain P, El-Sherif N. Changes in the expression of the sarcolemmal sodium channel subtypes in rat ventricle after myocardial infarction. Biophys J 1997; 72(2):A33.

52. Shimizu N, Omura T, Hanatani A, Kim S, Iwao H, et al. The time course of MAP kinase and transcription factor DNA binding activities in myocardial infarcted rats (abstract) Circulation 1997; 96(8):I-197.

# X

# *Markers of Sudden Cardiac Death in the Era of Revascularization*

# 35

# Usefulness of Premature Ventricular Contractions and Late Potentials for Risk Stratification after Myocardial Infarction in the Era of Revascularization

*Salem Kacet, MD, and Claude Kouakam, MD*

## Introduction

Sudden cardiac death (SCD) remains a major unresolved clinical and public health problem, responsible for more than 300,000 of the deaths in the United States annually, and accounting for 50% of all cardiovascular deaths.[1] In Europe, the incidence is estimated around 50 per 100,000 subjects. It is now believed that the majority of episodes of SCD occurs in patients with ventricular dysfunction secondary to previous myocardial infarction (MI), that they begin as ventricular tachycardia (VT), which may degenerate into ventricular fibrillation (VF), and that they are not associated with either acute MI or significant ischemia.[1] Epidemiological and clinical associations between premature ventricular contractions (PVCs) and potential fatal sustained arrhythmias (VT/VF) have been emphasized for many years.[2] On the other hand, many previous studies have demonstrated that patients with late potentials after MI are at high risk for SCD or sustained VT.[3]

During the past 2 decades, advanced management strategies including thrombolysis and/or acute coronary angioplasty have been shown to reduce mortality after acute MI.[4–8] A report by Stack et al.[8] showed a low sudden death mortality rate after early intravenous thrombolysis followed by emergency coronary angioplasty. In that study, 94% of 342 patients underwent successful reperfusion. Importantly, among 304 patients who survived to hospital discharge, there were only 8 cardiac deaths after discharge, for a 1-year survival rate of 98%.

From: Aliot E, Clementy J, Prystowsky EN (editors). *Fighting Sudden Cardiac Death: A Worldwide Challenge.* ©Futura Publishing Company, Armonk, NY, 2000.

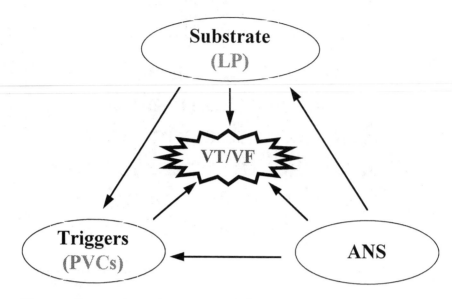

**Figure 1.** Determinants of post-myocardial infarction ventricular arrhythmias. ANS = autonomic nervous system; LP = late potentials; PVCs = premature ventricular contractions; VT/VF = ventricular tachycardia/ventricular fibrillation.

Although this effect appears to be related primarily to a decrease in infarct size after early successful reperfusion,[9] the lower mortality rate also reflects improved ventricular electrical stability.[10] Indeed, studies of thrombolytic therapy in patients with acute MI have found both decreased mortality in the absence of demonstrable myocardial salvage and a decrease in the incidence and inducibility of ventricular arrhythmia.[11] PVCs and late potentials are thought to be 2 independent markers of electrical stability (Figure 1), and previous studies have shown that each provides important prognostic information in identifying patients at risk of arrhythmic events after an MI. Thus, interest in recent years has been focused on the potentially beneficial effects of coronary reperfusion on the susceptibility to ventricular tachyarrhythmias, and risk evaluations in post-MI survivors after the widespread application of thrombolysis or coronary angioplasty have been submitted to extensive reassessment.

## Premature Ventricular Contractions in the Era of Revascularization

Thrombolysis has led to important changes in the natural history of patients after acute MI. However, despite advanced management strategies, including thrombolysis and/or coronary angioplasty, the use of PVCs for risk stratification of arrhythmogenic events after acute MI remains valid.[12]

In the prethrombolytic era, the independent predictive role of PVCs in the stratification of SCD post-MI was established by extensive multi-center trials. The prevalence of PVCs was reported as 86% of patients in the Multicenter Post-Infarction Research Group (MPIP) study,[2] and as 84% in the placebo group of the BHAT study.[13] The occurrence of complex PVCs (i.e., more than 10 per hour) was 21.2% for the MPIP, 12.9% for BHAT, and 14.6% for the MILIS Study Group[14] and nonsustained VT was reported as 11.3% in the MPIP study.

In the thrombolytic era, Maggioni et al. in the GISSI-2 study[15] reported a reduced prevalence of ventricular arrhythmias (64%), of complex PVCs (19.7%), and of nonsustained ventricular tachycardia (6.8%). The GISSI-2 study confirmed frequent PVCs as independent risk factors of sudden death in the first 6 months following the acute event; however, the significance of nonsustained VT was more controversial. Théroux et al. showed that the number of PVCs was reduced by 50% in patients who received thrombolytic therapy compared to those with conventional therapy (21 ± 61 versus 40 ± 123 per hour, p<0.05), demonstrating the long-term benefit of reperfusion.[16] More recently, Statters et al. also found that mean PVC frequency was significantly higher in patients who did not undergo thrombolysis.[12] These authors additionally found mean PVC frequency to be more highly predictive of prognosis after acute MI in patients who have undergone thrombolysis than in those who have not. At a sensitivity level of 40%, the positive predictive accuracy for cardiac mortality and arrhythmic events for the thrombolysis group was 19.4% and 25.8%, respectively, compared with 16% and 16% for those without thrombolysis. In contrast, Zimmermann et al.[17] and Pedretti et al.[18] found no difference in the rate of PVCs, and presence of couplets, runs, or nonsustained VT in patients with or without thrombolysis. Moreover, both authors found no correlation between patency of the infarct-related artery and frequency, complexity, or both, of PVCs. Differences in the size of the populations, in the timing of the Holter recordings (6–10 days in the study by Statters et al. versus 23 ± 9 days in the study by Pedretti et al.), and follow-up duration may account for some of these discrepancies.

Regarding the influence of myocardial function in patients treated by thrombolytic therapy, the number of PVCs per hour was found to depend in a linear, inverse fashion on the residual left ventricular ejection fraction, and was independent of the occurrence of reperfusion in the acute phase of infarction in the study by Marino et al.[19] They concluded that patency of the infarct-related coronary artery could contribute to reduce post-MI ventricular arrhythmias by reducing infarct size, which could minimize pump damage. Thus, early successful reperfusion could reduce areas in which mechanical stress develops and could reduce the risk of arrhythmias in patients with increased left ventricular volumes and decreased pump performance.

## Late Potentials in the Era of Revascularization

In clinical cardiology, late potentials are found in 10–50% of all cardiac disease, mainly in coronary artery disease. Late potentials correspond to delayed and fragmented ventricular activation arising typically in the border zones of MI where strands of surviving fibers are surrounded by fibrous tissue. Reentry as the major cause of malignant ventricular arrhythmias has, as a prerequisite, a zone of slow conduction, and a large number of studies in the 1990s have shown that late potentials provide important prognostic information for identifying patients who subsequently develop arrhythmic events and sudden death after acute MI.[20] Their value as a predictor of arrhythmic events is relatively low (10–30%), but very high in predicting a good outcome, showing 95% of event-free survival if late potentials are negative. Since the basis of late potentials is the changes induced by ischemia, the question in recent years has been to determine to what extent the dynamics of ischemia can be monitored or predicted by late potential analysis, especially in the setting of acute MI with or without thrombolysis and/or coronary angioplasty.

Gang et al.[21] were the first to look for a possible relationship between thrombolytic therapy and the incidence of late potentials early after MI. Within 48 hours after MI, late potentials were found in 5% of rt-PA treated patients versus 23% of patients managed conventionally. More interestingly, late potentials in the thrombolytic group were detected only if the infarct-related artery was occluded. In the conventional group, late potentials were recorded in 32% of patients with occluded infarct arteries and in 14% where the artery was patent. These findings have been confirmed by many other authors (Table 1),[22] giving insight into what occurs in acute MI with respect to the development of necrosis and arrythmogenic substrate in the field of interventional therapy. The findings also support data by de Chillou et al.,[23] who found that coronary artery patency was the most important factor decreasing the rate of late potentials after a first MI (Table 2), independent of left ventricular function. Similar data have been previously reported by Breithardt et al.[24] and were also found by Zimmermann et al.[17] and Pedretti et al.[18] Only Turitto et al. found no difference between the 2 treatment groups or in relation to coronary artery patency.[25]

Regarding the influence of the time of onset of reperfusion, Aguirre et al. reported no influence of thrombolytic therapy on the occurrence of late

## Table 1

### Prevalence of Late Potentials After Acute Myocardial Infarction and Dependence on Reperfusion

| Author/Reference No. | Patients (n) | Thrombolytic Therapy | Conventional Therapy | p |
|---|---|---|---|---|
| Gang et al. [21] | 106 | 5% | 23% | < 0.01 |
| Zimmermann et al. [17] | 223 | 10% | 24% | < 0.05 |
| Pedretti et al. [18] | 174 | 17% | 34% | < 0.05 |
| Moreno et al. [22] | 101 | 22% | 43% | < 0.05 |

potentials if they began less than 2 hours or between 2 and 6 hours after acute MI.[26] Concerning "primary" angioplasty, Maki et al.[27] showed that the prevalence of late potentials was directly correlated with the delay between the onset of symptoms and the angioplasty (Table 3), and concluded that in acute MI, reperfusion needs to be achieved within 6 hours to reduce the prevalence of late potentials. Concerning "late" coronary angioplasty, published data remain controversial. Ragosta et al.[28] reported no change in the incidence of late potentials after successful reperfusion if performed by angioplasty $12 \pm 8$ days after acute MI, contrasting with studies by Théroux et al.,[16] Vatterott et al.,[29] and Lomama et al.,[30] who showed that successful reperfusion by late angioplasty of the infarct artery contributes to a decrease in the prevalence of late potentials. Nevertheless, from all these data, it may be deduced that late reperfusion has a beneficial effect on late potentials.

## Table 2

### Influence of Infarct-Related Artery on the Prevalence of Late Potentials After Acute myocardial Infarction

| | Patent Infarct-Artery (n = 99) | Occluded Infarct-Artery (n = 68) | p |
|---|---|---|---|
| LP prevalence (thrombolysis therapy) | 16% | 37% | ns |
| LP prevalence (conventional therapy) | 0% | 35% | < 0.001 |
| | p< 0.02 | ns | |

Adapted from Moreno FL, et al.[23]
LP = late potential

### Table 3

### Relationship Between Prevalence of Late Potentials and Delay Between Onset of Symptoms and Coronary Angioplasty in 94 Patients Who Survived a First Acute Myocardial Infarction and Who Showed Total Occlusion of the Infarct-Related Artery

| Delay Angioplasty (hours) | Prevalence Late Potential (%) |
|---|---|
| < 4 | 8 |
| 4–6 | 12 |
| 6–8 | 24 |
| 8–10 | 33 |
| > 10 | 43 |

Adapted from Maki H, et al.[27]

Regarding the influence of the method used to achieve early coronary reperfusion, data from Karam et al.[31] showed that the prevalence of late potentials after acute MI was lower when reperfusion was achieved by angioplasty (either primary or as a rescue procedure after failed thrombolysis) than by thrombolysis.

## Conclusions

Patients with acute MI treated with advanced management strategies, including thrombolysis and/or coronary angioplasty, show a reduced prevalence of PVCs and late potentials when compared to those treated with conventional therapy. Reperfusion of an infarct-related artery has a beneficial effect on the markers of arrhythmias, and this effect is more pronounced in early rather than in late reperfusion, but is unrelated to left ventricular ejection fraction. Also in the thrombolytic era, PVCs and late potentials maintain their characteristic of remaining markers of electrical stability. These findings may, at least in part, explain the significantly increased rate of survival after acute MI in patients with patent infarct-related arteries. Prevention of SCD seems to be one of the major long-term benefits of reperfusion and can be predicted by prevention of PVCs and late potentials in the acute phase.

## References

1. Myerburg RJ, Kessler KM, Castellanos A. Sudden cardiac death: structure, function, and time-dependence of risk. Circulation 1992; 85(Suppl I):I-2-I-10.
2. Bigger JT, Fleiss JL, Kleiger R, Miller JP, Rolnitzky LM, the Multicenter Post-Infarction Research Group. The relationship among ventricular arrhythmias, left

ventricular dysfunction and mortality in the 2 years after myocardial infarction. Circulation 1984; 69:250–258.

3. Simson MB. Noninvasive identification of patients at high risk for sudden cardiac death: signal-averaged electrocardiography. Circulation 1992; 85(Suppl I):I-145-I-151.

4. Gruppo Italiano per lo Studio della Streptochinasi nell'Infarto Miocardico (GISSI). Effectiveness of intravenous thrombolytic therapy treatment in acute myocardial infarction. Lancet 1986; 1:397–402.

5. ISSIS-2 (Second International Study of Infarct Survival) Collaborative Group. Randomized trial of intravenous streptokinase, oral aspirin, both, or neither among 17,187 cases of suspected acute myocardial infarction: ISSIS-2. Lancet 1988; 2:349–360.

6. AIMS Trial Study Group. Long-term effects of intravenous anistreplase in acute myocardial infarction: final report of the AIMS study. Lancet 1990; 335:427–431.

7. Anglo-Scandinavian Study of Early Thrombolysis (ASSET). Trial of tissue plasminogen activator for mortality reduction in acute myocardial infarction. Lancet 1988; 2:525–530.

8. Stack RS, Califf RM, Hinohara T, et al. Survival and cardiac events rates in the first year after emergency coronary angioplasty for acute myocardial infarction. J Am Coll Cardiol 1988; 11:1141–1149.

9. White HD. Relation of thrombolysis during acute myocardial infarction to left ventricular function and mortality. Am J Cardiol 1990; 66:92–95.

10. Volpi A, Cavalli A, Santoro E, Tognoni G, and GISSI Investigators: Incidence and prognosis of secondary VF in acute myocardial infarction: evidence for a protective effect of thrombolytic therapy. Circulation 1990; 82:1279–1288.

11. Farrell T, Bashir Y, Poloniecki J, Ward D, Camm AJ. The effects of thrombolysis on risk stratification for arrhythmic events in post-infarction patients. J Am Coll Cardiol 1991; 17:17A.

12. Statters DJ, Malik M, Redwood S, Hnatkova K, Staunton A, et al. Use of ventricular premature complexes for risk stratification after acute myocardial infarction in the thrombolytic era. Am J Cardiol 1996; 77:133–138.

13. Kostis JB, Byington R, Friedman LM, Goldstein S, Furberg C, for the BHAT Study Group. Prognostic significance of ventricular ectopic activity in survivors of acute myocardial infarction. J Am Coll Cardiol 1987; 10:231–242.

14. Mukharji J, Rude RE, Pole WK et al., for the MILIS Study Group. Risk factors for sudden death after acute myocardial infarction: two-year follow-up. J Am Coll Cardiol 1984; 54:31–36.

15. Maggioni AP, Zuanetti G, Franzosi MG et al., on the behalf of GISSI-2 Investigators. Prevalence and prognostic significance of ventricular arrhythmias after myocardial infarction in the fibrinolytic era. Circulation 1993; 87:312–322.

16. Théroux P, Morisette D, Juneau M, deGuise P, Pelletier G, et al. Influence of fibrinolytic or percutaneous transluminal coronary angioplasty on the frequency of ventricular premature complexes. Am J Cardiol 1989; 63:797–801.

17. Zimmermann M, Adamec R, Ciaroni S. Reduction in the frequency of ventricular late potentials after myocardial infarction by early thrombolytic therapy. Am J Cardiol 1991; 67:697–703.

18. Pedretti R, Laporta A, Etro ME, et al. Influence of thrombolysis on signal-averaged electrocardiogram and late arrhythmic events after myocardial infarction. Am J Cardiol 1992; 69:866–872.

19. Marino P, Nidasio G, Golia G et al., on the behalf of GISSI-2 Investigators. Frequency of predischarge ventricular arrhythmias in post-myocardial infarction

patients depends on residual left ventricular pump performance and is independent of the occurrence of acute reperfusion. J Am Coll Cardiol 1994; 23:290–295.

20. Vester EG, Strauer BE. Ventricular late potentials: state of the heart and future perspectives. Eur Heart J 1994; 15 (Suppl C):34–48.

21. Gang ES, Lew AS, Hong M, et al. Decreased incidence of ventricular late potentials after successful thrombolytic therapy for acute myocardial infarction. N Engl J Med 1989; 321:712–716.

22. Moreno FL, Karagounis L, Marschall H, et al. Thrombolysis-related early patency reduces ECG late potentials after acute myocardial infarction. Am Heart J 1992; 124:558–564.

23. de Chillou C, Sadoul N, Briançon S, Aliot E. Factors determining the occurrence of late potentials on the signal-averaged electrocardiogram after a first myocardial infarction: a multivariate analysis. J Am Coll Cardiol 1991; 18:1638–1642.

24. Breithardt G, Borggrefe M, Karbenn U, Abendroth RR, Yeh HL, et al. Prevalence of late potentials in patients with and without ventricular tachycardia: correlation with angiographic findings. Am J Cardiol 1982; 4:1932–1937.

25. Turitto G, Risa AL, Zanchi E, Prati P. The signal-averaged electrogram and ventricular arrhythmias after thrombolysis for acute myocardial infarction. J Am Coll Cardiol 1990; 15:1270–1276.

26. Aguirre FV, Kern MJ, Hsia J, et al. Importance of myocardial infarct patency on the prevalence of ventricular arrhythmia and late potentials after thrombolysis in acute myocardial infarction. Am J Cardiol 1991; 68:1410–1416.

27. Maki H, Ozawa Y, Tanigawa N, et al. Effect of reperfusion by direct percutaneous transluminal coronary angioplasty on ventricular late potentials in case of total coronary occlusion at initial coronary arteriography. Jpn Circ J 1993; 57:183–188.

28. Ragosta M, Sabia PJ, Kaul S, et al. Effects of late (1 to 30 days) reperfusion after acute myocardial infarction on the signal-averaged electrogram. Am J Cardiol 1993; 71:19–23.

29. Vatterott PJ, Hammil SC, Bailey KR, Wiltgen CN, Gerah BJ. Late potentials on signal-averaged electrograms and patency of the infarct-related artery in survivors of acute myocardial infarction. J Am Coll Cardiol 1991; 17:330–337.

30. Lomama E, Helft G, Persoz A, Vacheron A. Late coronary angioplasty and ventricular late potentials. Am J Cardiol 1998; 82:985–987.

31. Karam C, Golmard J, Steg PG. Decreased prevalence of late potentials with mechanical versus thrombolysis-induced reperfusion in acute myocardial infarction. J Am Coll Cardiol 1996; 27:1343–1348.

# 36

# Baroreflex Sensitivity and Heart Rate Variability:

## State of the Art and Perspectives

*Marek Malik, MD, PhD, and Irina Savelieva, MD*

## Introduction

Experimental as well as clinical studies conducted during approximately the past 2 decades have firmly established the importance of the autonomic nervous system (ANS) in arrhythmogenesis and have provided a physiological and pathophysiological basis for consideration of different autonomic tests for stratification of arrhythmia and sudden cardiac death risk.[1-7] Sympathetic and vagal activity and their role in the genesis of ventricular tachyarrhythmias have been investigated mainly by stimulating or blocking the neural pathways to the heart or by administering various agents that are known to interfere with autonomic balance. The past years have witnessed remarkable progress in noninvasive methods aimed at the quantification of the cardiac autonomic status. Among other possibilities, heart rate variability (HRV) and baroreflex sensitivity (BRS) have received the most clinical attention and have been researched the most. Both methods provide different facets of comprehensive insight into sympathovagal cardiovascular interaction, the former representing the "tonic" and the latter assessing the "phasic" activity of ANS. HRV and BRS evaluate the integrity of cardiovascular autonomic innervation, the physiological status of autonomic activity and, consequently, the vulnerability to cardiac arrhythmias.

Promising success in identifying patients at high risk of malignant arrhythmic events has been reported when using these methods in multicenter studies involving large cohorts of myocardial infarction (MI) survivors.[8,9] However, uncertainty exists regarding methodology, predictive accuracy, relation to other known risk-stratifying factors, and the usefulness in clinical settings beyond MI. In this chapter, we discuss the current state of the art and the future potential of HRV and BRS methods. We also

From: Aliot E, Clementy J, Prystowsky EN (editors). *Fighting Sudden Cardiac Death: A Worldwide Challenge.* ©Futura Publishing Company, Armonk, NY, 2000.

attempt to put these technologies into perspective with other risk-stratification technologies, namely those based on newly emerging concepts and possibilities.

## Heart Rate Variability

The origins of the knowledge about the existence of respiratory sinus arrhythmia are difficult to trace. It was almost 70 years ago when Samaan showed that a section of vagal nerves abolishes this arrhythmia and that the ANS determined not only the rate but also the rhythm of the heart.[10] Approximately half a century later, Akselrod et al.[11] demonstrated that muscarinic and/or beta-adrenergic blockade suppressed different components of spectral heart rate fluctuations and provided a physiological basis for investigations of HRV.

The first report on the association of low HRV with poor prognosis in MI patients[12] was unfortunately almost unnoticed and was practically rediscovered only after the association of reduced HRV with poor post-MI survival was observed in the MPIP study.[8] Since then, HRV has been extensively studied in different clinical settings and recognized as a surprisingly powerful tool for arrhythmia risk stratification.[13–16] Recognizing the need to standardize the diverse variety of technologies and to systematically review the frequently conflicting reports on physiological meaning and clinical applicability, the European Society of Cardiology and North American Society of Pacing and Electrophysiology established an international Task Force in 1994 and charged with it the responsibility of providing standards in all important facets of HRV studies, that is, in measurement, physiological interpretation, and clinical use. The report of the ESC/NASPE Task Force[13] was published in 1996, and although substantial development has occurred since its publication, the report still provides a reasonable standard to follow.

## Methodology and Problems of HRV Assessment

In addition to the rather primitive formulae for HRV assessment that were used mainly in the very initial studies (e.g., the absolute or relative difference between the maximum and minimum RR intervals recorded during a variety of provocations), the most common and clinically appropriate methods of HRV measurement can be divided into time domain (which include the so-called statistical and the so-called geometrical methods), and frequency domain spectral methods. The statistical methods are based on statistical measures to quantify RR interval data variations around the mean heart rate. The simplest variable to calculate is the standard deviation of all normal RR intervals (SDNN), which represents all the cyclic components responsible for variability during the recording and corresponds to total power of spectral analysis.

Other commonly used statistical variables include the standard deviation of the average normal RR intervals calculated over 5-minute periods (SDANN), which "filters out" the fastest components of heart period modulations and, in spectral terms, expresses long-term variations with frequency below 0.0033 Hz. While SDNN and SDANN measure HRV in the sequence of RR intervals irrespective of their order, other statistical methods investigate the beat-to-beat differences between adjacent RR intervals. The RMSSD measure is the square root of the mean squared differences between adjacent RR intervals, while the pNN50 method expresses the proportion of pairs of adjacent RR intervals that differ by more than 50 ms. Both RMSSD and pNN50 estimate high-frequency variations in heart rate.

Although statistical methods have been extensively investigated and are currently being used for risk stratification and assessment of treatment modalities, the well-known difficulty with obtaining a high-quality RR interval sequence required for statistical methods limits their clinical relevance and makes, to some extent, the assessment of HRV not very practical in daily routine practice. Despite comprehensive automatic algorithms used in modern Holter equipment, misrecognition of artifacts and nondetection of QRS complexes are unavoidable and may result in a significant error of HRV measurement[14] (Figure 1). Although editing the short-term recording bears less work burden, it is unlikely that clinical and, particularly, risk-related information derived from these recording is of value similar to that obtained from complete 24-hour electrocardiograms.[15,16]

In order to overcome these limitations, geometrical methods have been proposed that are less affected by noise and artifacts in computerized processing of long-term electrocardiograms.[17] In this approach, HRV is assessed from basic measurement of a geometrical pattern, specifically from the RR interval distribution. The simplest geometrical method is the HRV triangular index, which is determined by dividing the number of all RR intervals by the number of RR intervals in a modal frequency.

Visual analysis of the patterns of RR interval dynamics can also be based on classification of images created by plotting the length of each RR interval against the length of the preceding RR interval. These images are known as the so-called Lorenz or Poincaré plots. The incorrectly measured RR intervals, the coupling intervals, and the compensatory pauses of atrial and ventricular premature beats are easily detectable in the map. Similarly, various rhythm disturbances such as atrial fibrillation can be identified. Preserved physiological HRV produces a relatively wide-spreading plot, sometimes called the "fan-shaped" plot, whereas decreased HRV results in a compact, or "narrow-shaped" plot. Terms such as "torpedo-

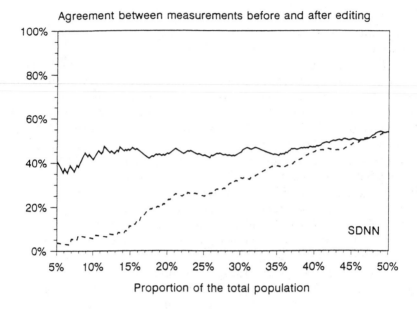

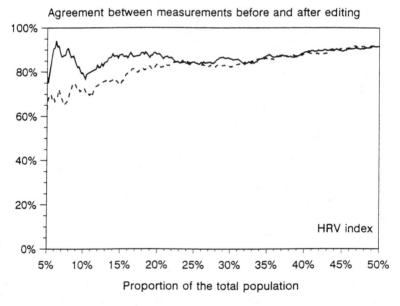

**Figure 1.** Agreement between HRV measurements based on edited and nonedited data from Holter recording. Note that the HRV index performs better than SDNN, especially in patients with reduced HRV. Solid line represents the agreement between measurements in patients with the lowest values of HRV; dashed line represents the agreement in patients with the highest values of HRV. (Used with permission from Malik M, Camm AJ, eds.[14])

shaped" and "complex-shaped" plots have also been reported by some to represent underlying rhythm abnormalities (Figure 2).[18–20] Although the classification method can provide a reasonable assessment of HRV in low-quality recordings when statistical and spectral methods cannot be applied, the approximate nature and highly subjective estimate restrict its practical use.

Spectral analysis of HRV aims at distinguishing different frequency components of sinus rhythm modulations and at quantifying each of these components in numerical terms.[21] The nonparametric approach to the computation of spectral components is most frequently based on the fast Fourier transform while the parametric approach uses autoregressive modeling. Despite mathematical differences, both methods assume relative stationarity of RR interval modulations that contain inherent periodicity during the entire analyzed period.[22] Experimental and clinical evidence has clearly established that the high-frequency spectral components reflect vagal modulations of the cardiac rhythm. The low-frequency components are associated with vasomotor modulations and sympathetic activity,[23,24] although disputes exist in relation to the interpretation of low-frequency components and to the concept of the so-called sympathovagal balance of the cardiac autonomic status.[25] The mathematical assumption of the intrinsic periodicity is highly speculative when applied to the spectral analysis of 24-hour recording, since biological signals are subject to nonperiodic modulations by environmental demands. Thus, spectral analysis is the method of choice when dealing with short-term recordings, particularly those obtained under controlled conditions when the stationarity of autonomic modulations is likely to be maintained. While spectral analysis of 24-hour recordings is also technically possible, no study has ever shown that the assessment of specific spectral components in 24-hour recordings has any advantage compared to more easily applied time domain methods. A linear slope of a 24-hour spectrogram plotted on log-log scale can be obtained as an additional measure of long-term HRV. In a seminal clinical study by Bigger et al.,[26] it has been shown to differ among normal healthy volunteers, patients with congestive heart failure, and cardiac transplant recipients.

Recently, several mathematical approaches based on nonlinear mathematics and the chaos theory have been suggested for analysis of long-term fluctuations of heart rhythm, though nonperiodic, but yet governing by deterministic laws.[27] These include geometrical methods applied to Poincaré plots,[18] scaling index method,[28] nonlinear mathematics quantification of the fractal properties,[29–31] and entropy measures.[31,32] More recently, several studies have been published suggesting that nonlinear indices of HRV have some practical and, mainly, clinical advantages compared to the more usual evaluation by time and frequency domain

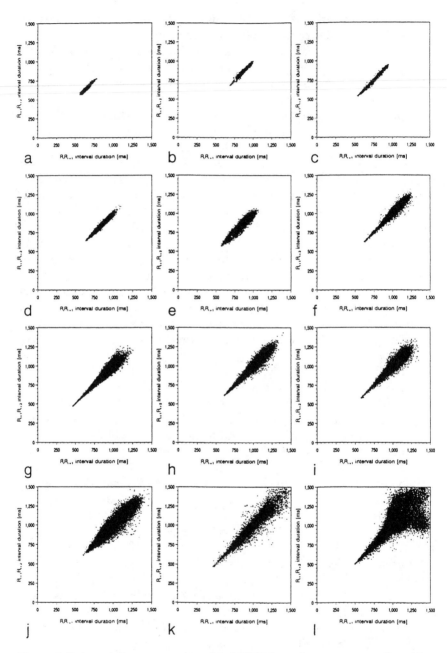

**Figure 2.** Poincaré plots presenting global HRV from the minimum values (a) to the maximum values (i). Note an obvious difference only between the extreme values, whereas no substantial differences can be seen in individual steps. (Used with permission from Malik M, ed.[57])

methods. However, none of the observations has been independently confirmed by different investigators utilizing different data. Hence, only further investigations will show whether the methodology of nonlinear dynamic analysis of HRV offers a true practical advantage or whether the present reports are subject to the bias of selective publications.

## Clinical Considerations

The early study by Wolf et al.,[12] who reported a 3-fold mortality risk associated with a decreased HRV measured as the variance of 30 successive RR intervals in 176 patients with acute MI, was, although not directly, followed by many further investigations of the prognostic significance of HRV in various clinical conditions.[33-42] In population-based Framingham and Rotterdam studies,[43-45] reduced HRV has been found to be associated with as much as a 4-fold increase in all-cause mortality as well as with a significant increase in morbidity from MI, coronary artery disease, and congestive heart failure. Although encouraging results have been obtained regarding the prognostic value of HRV in coronary artery disease,[33] congestive heart failure,[34,36] dilated and hypertrophic cardiomyopathies,[36,37] and heart transplant recipients,[42] the HRV-based risk stratification has been mainly centered around the possibility of using it as a prognostic tool in patients who survived an acute MI. The predictive power of HRV was initially recognized in 1987 when Kleiger et al.[8] evaluated 808 post-MI patients and reported a 5.3-fold mortality risk associated with SDNN <50 ms compared to those with preserved HRV (SDNN >100 ms). Data from the St. George's Post-Infarction Research Survey Programme confirmed these findings in a large cohort of post-MI patients, using an HRV index <15 as a definition of the depressed HRV.[46] Other publications of our research group by Farrell et al.[47] and Odemuyiwa et al.[48] further suggested that low HRV was not only capable of predicting total cardiac mortality but also identified patients at risk of arrhythmic events including cardiac arrest and sustained ventricular tachycardia with a sensitivity and specificity higher than that for left ventricular ejection fraction (LVEF) (Figures 3, 4).

Although data from large post-MI survival studies have repeatedly confirmed that the predictive value of HRV is independent of other known risk factors, such as frequent ventricular ectopy on 24-hour Holter, reduced LVEF, and abnormal signal-averaged ECG,[8,47-50] the predictive value of HRV taken alone is rather modest. In most studies, the positive predictive accuracy of HRV alone, although higher than many other single variables, did not exceed 20% within the range of practically relevant levels of sensitivity. A combination of HRV with other risk factors yields better positive predictive accuracy (Figure 4). Bigger et al.,[50] combining HRV with ventricular premature beats on Holter, or reduced LVEF, re-

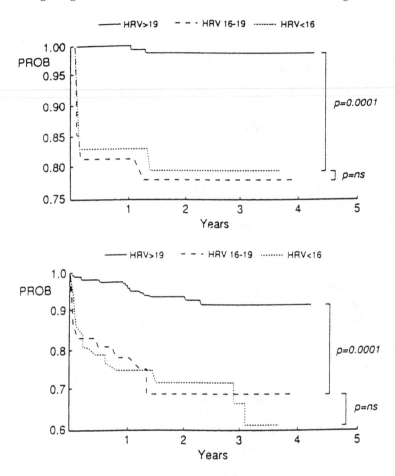

**Figure 3.** The sensitivity and specificity of left ventricular ejection fraction (LVEF; dashed line), heart rate variability index (HRV; solid line), and their combination (bold line) for the prediction of all-cause mortality, arrhythmic events, and sudden death. (Used with permission from Odemuyiwa O, et al.[48])

ported as high as 2-fold improvement of a positive predictive accuracy (50% versus 24–26%). However, this was not the case in other studies,[46,47] in which combining HRV and LVEF did not result in a remarkable change in predictive accuracy, but combining HRV with ventricular premature beats >10/h increased a positive predictive value from 17% and 16%, respectively, to 34%. A possible explanation might be that different risk factors predict specific risks. For instance, ventricular ectopy is more likely to be related to serious arrhythmic events and arrhythmic death, whereas reduced LVEF is more likely to be associated with death due to circulatory failure and electromechanical dissociation although the final lethal

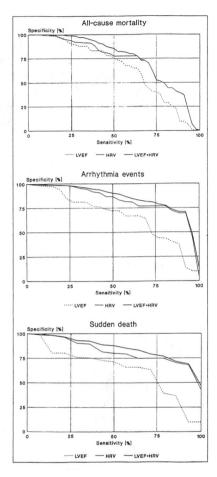

**Figure 4.** Kaplan-Meier survival curves for arrhythmic events (top) and cardiac mortality (bottom). Heart rate variability (HRV) is stratified at >19, 16–19, and <16 ms. The p values refer to differences in event rates between subgroups. PROB = probability. (Used with permission from Farrell TG, et al.[47])

episode might still be of arrhythmic character. Although reduced HRV is predictive of all-cause mortality, the autonomic background makes it more related to arrhythmic rather than circulatory death. A combination of impaired HRV (HRV triangular index <20 units), repetitive ventricular ectopic forms, and late potentials achieved a positive predictive value of 58%.[47] In a study by Hartikainen et al.,[51] depressed HRV and nonsustained ventricular tachycardia predicted both arrhythmic and nonarrhythmic post-MI death, whereas low LVEF was associated only with nonarrhythmic mortality. An important finding of this study is that information on combined risk factors can be used to identify patients with a high total mortality and a high proportion of either arrhythmic or nonarrhythmic death. By selecting patients with a high risk of arrhythmic mortality (depressed HRV) and excluding those with a high risk of nonarrhythmic mortality (low LVEF), investigators identified a patient group in which 75% of deaths were of arrhythmic nature. Similarly, a patient group having 75% of deaths due to nonarrhythmic mechanisms was defined by selecting patients with the lowest LVEF and omitting those with the lowest HRV.

# Baroreflex Sensitivity

Although HRV has become an established marker of autonomic imbalance and vulnerability to arrhythmia, it was not until 1998 when the ATRAMI study (Autonomic Tone and Reflexes in Acute Myocardial Infarction) was completed that the prognostic value of ANS cardiac measures have been shown in a prospective multicenter trial.[9]

## Methodology of BRS

While the HRV method usually provides information on the continuous basal sympathovagal balance, the BRS method is aimed mainly at quantitative assessment of ability of the ANS to react to acute stimulation that involves primarily vagal reflexes, although baroreflexes also operate in a physiological steady-state condition. Methods used for BRS assessment include the Valsalva maneuver, neck cuff, negative pressure applied to lower part of the body, carotid massage, and intravenous administration of phenylephrine. BRS measurement obtained with different methods varies widely, which is probably the result of assessment of different aspects of baroreflex function.[52] Intravenous phenylephrine ($\alpha$-adrenoreceptor agonist) administration (25–100 $\mu$g in healthy subjects, 150–350 $\mu$g in patients) is the most standardized method for the assessment. Under physiological conditions, the administration of phenylephrine causes an increase in blood pressure by 20–30 mm Hg accompanied by an increase of RR interval durations.[53] The rate-pressure response is characterized by a linear relationship, the slope of which, measured by a linear regression, is used to express the baroreflex function numerically. It was generally assumed that the slope reflects mainly vagal activity with little change in sympathetic tone. However, a flat slope, which is common in cardiac patients, may also indicate sympathetic hyperactivity (Figure 5A, B).

The normal values of BRS have been reported to be 14.8–16 ms/mm Hg,[53,54] whereas in hypertensive and post-MI patients, a significantly decreased BRS was observed (mean values of 3 and 7.5 ms/mm Hg, respec-

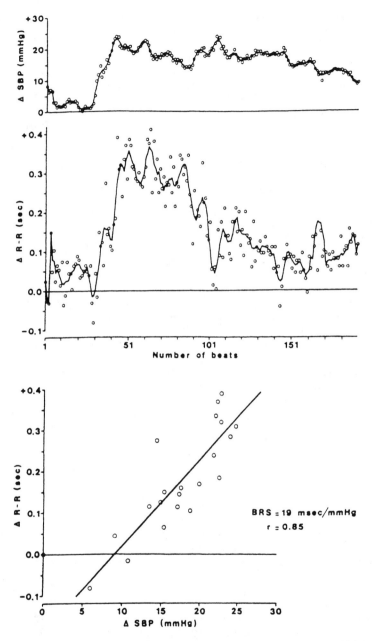

Figure 5A. Beat-to-beat changes in systolic arterial blood pressure (ΔSBP; top panel) and RR intervals (ΔRR; middle panel) after phenylephrine injection compared with baseline level. The regression line (bottom panel) is constructed using points from the first major increase in blood pressure and corresponding changes in heart rate. Note a 25-mm Hg increase in blood pressure and a marked acceleration of heart rate after phenylephrine, showing a well-preserved BRS (19 ms/mm Hg) expressed as a slope of the regression line. *Continued.*

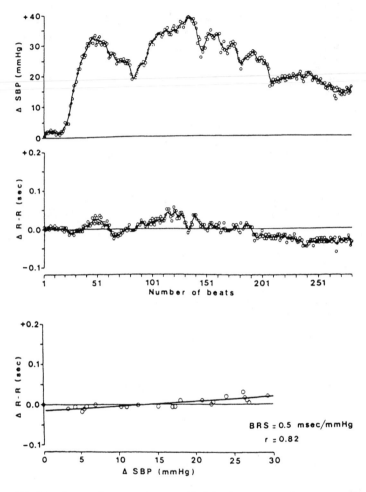

**Figure 5B.** Despite an increase in systolic blood pressure, heart rate does not change, resulting in a "flat" regression line demonstrating a remarkably reduced BRS (−0.5 ms/mm Hg). (Used with permission from La Rovere MT, et al.[55])

tively).[53–55] It is necessary to note that the dose of phenylephrine depends on the underlying heart disease and may vary from 150 to 350 µg (2–4 µg/kg) or even to 750 µg (10 µg/kg) in patients with congestive heart failure.[56] Consideration should also be given to limiting phenylephrine use for BRS evaluation such as the vasoconstrictor effect.[57]

The assessment of spontaneous changes in baroreflex function represents another attractive tool for quantification of cardiac autonomic status and dynamics. Similar to HRV, it applies statistical and spectral approaches.[58–60] However, controversies exist regarding the agreement between the spectral analysis of spontaneous BRS and the results of the phenylephrine method.[60,61]

## Prognostic Significance of BRS

Ten years prior to results of the ATRAMI study, in a small series of post-MI patients, a significant difference in BRS between survivors and the deceased was reported. With a cutoff point of 3 ms/mm Hg, a mortality increase by 47% was found.[55] At the same time Bigger et al.[62] noted a correlation between BRS and HRV. In post-MI patients, BRS <3 ms/mm Hg was found to have a 36-fold relative risk for the inducibility of ventricular tachycardia during programmed stimulation; however, 95% confidence intervals were very large (5–266).[63]

In a larger post-MI population, the same research group found decreased BRS to carry a relative risk for arrhythmic events of 23.1 and to be superior to other variables including ventricular ectopy, abnormal signal-averaged ECG, low LVEF, and HRV.[64] Data from other studies conducted in post-MI patients confirmed these observations by revealing a striking difference in BRS between aborted sudden death survivors and those with uncomplicated post-MI course (1.75 versus 9.17 ms/mm Hg[65] and 4.2 versus 8 ms/m Hg[66]). It has been suggested that low BRS in patients with ventricular tachycardia may be responsible for poor tolerability and hemodynamic collapse due to a significantly enhanced sympathetic drive during tachycardia paroxysms.[67] On the contrary, less reduced BRS may indicate more flexible cardiovascular reflexes to compensate adverse hemodynamic effects of tachycardia[68] (Figure 6).

In the ATRAMI study,[9] involving 1,284 post-MI patients, low values of HRV (SDNN <70 ms) and BRS (<3 ms/mm Hg) carried a significant risk of cardiac mortality (3.2 and 2.8, respectively). The combination of low SDNN and BRS further increased mortality risk. A 2-year death rate was 17% with both variables below cutoff points, and only 2% with both well preserved (SDNN >105 ms and BRS >6.1 ms/mm Hg). When LVEF <35% was added to low HRV or BRS, mortality risk increased to 6.7 and 8.7, respectively. In this study, HRV and BRS correlated moderately with each other, confirming that the 2 methods evaluate different aspects of ANS activity.

In a recent study by Hohnloser et al.[69] conducted in implantable cardioverter-defibrillator (ICD) recipients, although neither HRV nor BRS were found to be associated with recurrent ventricular tachycardia or ventricular fibrillation documented on electrograms, the combination of T wave alternans and BRS distinguished between patients with and without arrhythmic events with 100% sensitivity and 57% positive predictive accuracy. None of the 10 patients with BRS >3 ms/mm Hg and without T wave alternans developed ventricular tachycardia or ventricular fibrillation dur-

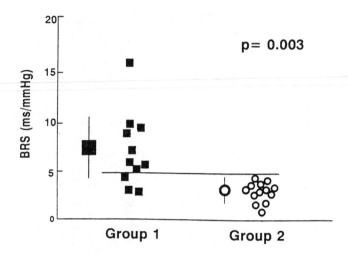

**Figure 6.** Individual and mean values of BRS in patients with ventricular tachycardia who tolerated it well (Group 1) and patients with poorly tolerated ventricular tachycardia (Group 2). Horizontal line represents a cutoff point at 5 ms/mm Hg. Note that only 3 patients with well-tolerated ventricular tachycardia had BRS below this value. (Used with permission from Landolina M, et al.[68])

ing a 2.5-year follow-up, whereas 23 of 33 patients with abnormal BRS and positive T wave alternans experienced 1 or more arrhythmic events.

## Future Perspectives

Experimental and clinical evidence that is presently available supports the value of the assessment of cardiac autonomic status and shows that methods used to quantify cardiac ANS activity represent powerful tools for arrhythmia risk stratification. In the past, this stratification has been effective mainly in post-MI patients but seminal reports of studies investigating different patient populations suggest a similar value of the cardiac autonomic assessment. In clinical studies conducted in large patient cohorts and with different underlying cardiac pathology, neither HRV nor BRS alone have been able to select high-risk groups with sufficient sensitivity and positive predictive accuracy. A combination with other known risk factors is clearly needed. Unfortunately, the methodology for such combinations[70] is far from simple, and improved understanding of multivariate risk stratification strategies, including the stepwise strategies, is badly required.

Further refinement of the technologies used to investigate the cardiac autonomic system should also be studied. Recently, the concept of so-called heart rate turbulence has been introduced.[71] It shows that low-risk post-MI patients modulate their heart rate in a rather systematic fashion following each singular spontaneous ventricular premature beat. It seems plausible to speculate that heart rate turbulence is an expression of "intrinsic" baroreflex, which is rather different from the externally induced reflexes used in BRS estimation. Combinations of heart rate turbulence with HRV and BRS measures seem to lead to particularly potent risk stratification.[72] In addition to a significant practical value, the concept of heart rate turbulence also shows very clearly that our present technology for treating ventricular premature beats in RR interval datastreams used to evaluate HRV is not appropriate.

Different methods offering insight into different facets of cardiac autonomic status must not be seen as mutual competitors. Rather, the relationship between these different facets should be intensively studied. Only in such a way will a truly comprehensive assessment of cardiac ANS reflexes and modulations be made possible. Present knowledge indicates clearly that in this way, a substantially improved risk stratification will be achieved together with substantially improved understanding of cardiac autonomic control.

## References

1. Lown B, Verrier RL. Neural activity and ventricular fibrillation. N Engl J Med 1976; 294:1165–1170.
2. Kolman BS, Verrier RL, Lown B. The effect of vagus nerve stimulation upon vulnerability of the canine ventricle: role of the sympathetic-parasympathetic interactions. Circulation 1975; 52:578–585.
3. De Ferrari GM, Vanoli E, Stramba-Badiale M, Hull SS Jr, Foreman RD, et al. Vagal reflexes and survival during acute myocardial ischemia in conscious dogs with healed myocardial infarction. Am J Physiol 1991; 261:H63-H69.
4. Malliani A, Schwartz PJ, Zanchetti A. A sympathetic reflex elicited by experimental coronary occlusion. Am J Physiol 1969; 217:703–709.
5. Rosen M, Hordof AJ, Ilvento JP, et al. Effects of adrenergic amines on electrophysiological properties and automaticity of neonatal and adult canine Purkinje fibers: evidence of alpha- and beta-adrenergic actions. Circ Res 1977; 40:390–400.
6. Verrier RL, Thomson P, Lown B. Ventricular vulnerability during sympathetic stimulation: role of heart rate and blood pressure. Cardiovascular Res 1974; 8:602–610.
7. Verrier RL. Neurogenic aspects of cardiac arrhythmias. In: El-Sherif N, Samet P (eds). Cardiac Pacing and Electrophysiology. WB Saunders Co, Philadelphia, 1991, pp 77–91.
8. Kleiger RE, Miller JP, Bigger JT Jr, Moss AJ, and the Multicenter Postinfarction Research Group. Decreased heart rate variability and its association with increased mortality after acute myocardial infarction. Am J Cardiol 1987; 59:256–262.
9. La Rovere MT, Bigger JT Jr, Marcus FI, Mortara A, Schwartz PJ, for the

ATRAMI (Autonomic Tone and Reflexes After Myocardial Infarction) Investigators. Baroreflex sensitivity and heart rate variability in prediction of total cardiac mortality after myocardial infarction. Lancet 1998; 351:478–484.

10. Samaan A. The antagonistic cardiac nerves and heart rate. J Physiol 1935; 83:332–340.

11. Akselrod S, Gordon D, Ubel FA, Shannon DC, Barger AC, et al. Power spectrum analysis of heart rate fluctuations: a quantitative probe of beat-to-beat cardiovascular control. Science 1981; 213:220–222.

12. Wolf MM, Varigos GA, Hunt D, Sloman JG. Sinus arrhythmia in acute myocardial infarction. Med J Aust 1978; 2:52–53.

13. Malik M, Bigger JT Jr, Camm AJ, Kleiger RE, Malliani A, et al. Task Force of the European Society of Cardiology and the North American Society of Pacing and Electrophysiology. Heart rate variability: standards of measurement, physiological interpretation, and clinical use. Circulation 1996; 93:1043–1065.

14. Malik M. Effect of electrocardiogram recognition artifact on time-domain measurement of heart rate variability. In: Malik M, Camm AJ (eds). Heart Rate Variability. Futura Publishing Co, Armonk, NY, 1995, pp 99–118.

15. Malik M, Camm AJ. Significance of long-term components of heart rate variability for the further prognosis after acute myocardial infarction. Cardiovasc Res 1990; 24:793–803.

16. Malik M, Farrell TG, Camm AJ. Circadian rhythm of heart rate variability after acute myocardial infarction and its influence on the prognostic value of heart rate variability. Am J Cardiol 1990; 66:1049–1054.

17. Malik M. Geometrical methods for heart rate variability assessment. In: Malik M, Camm AJ (eds). Heart Rate Variability. Futura Publishing Co, Armonk, NY, 1995; pp 47–61.

18. Huikuri HV, Seppänen T, Koistenen MJ, Airaksinen KEJ, Ikäheimo MJ, et al. Abnormalities in beat-to-beat dynamics of heart rate before the spontaneous onset of life-threatening ventricular tachyarrhythmias in patients with prior myocardial infarction. Circulation 1996; 93:1836–1844.

19. Brouwer J, van Veldhuisen DJ, Man in't Veld AJ, Haaksma J, Dijk WA, et al., for the Deutch Ibapamide Multicenter Trial Study Group. Prognostic value of heart rate variability during long-term follow-up in patients with mild to moderate heart failure. J Am Coll Cardiol 1996; 28:1183–1189.

20. Woo MA, Stevenson WG, Moser DK, Middlekauff HR. Complex heart rate variability and serum norepinephrine levels in patients with advanced heart failure. J Am Coll Cardiol 1994; 23:565–569.

21. Cerutti S, Bianchi AM, Mainardi LT. Spectral analysis of heart rate variability signal. In: Malik M, Camm AJ (eds). Heart Rate Variability. Futura Publishing Co, Armonk, NY, 1995, pp 63–74.

22. Kamath MV, Fallen EL. Power spectral analysis of heart rate variability: a noninvasive signature of cardiac autonomic function. Crit Rev Biomed Eng 1993; 21:245–311.

23. Malliani A, Pagani M, Lombardi F, Cerutti S. Cardiovascular neural regulation explored in the frequency domain. Circulation 1991; 84:482–492.

24. Pagani M, Lombardi F, Guzzetti S, Rimoldi O, Furlan R, et al. Power spectral analysis of heart rate and arterial pressure variabilities as a marker of sympathovagal interaction in man and conscious dog. Circ Res 1986; 59:178–193.

25. Eckberg DL. Sympathovagal balance: a critical appraisal. Circulation 1997; 96:3224–3232.

26. Bigger JT, Steinman RC, Rolnitzky LM, Fleiss JL, Albrecht P, et al. Power law behavior of RR-interval variability in healthy middle-aged persons, patients

with recent myocardial infarction, and patients with heart transplants. Circulation 1996; 93:2142–2151.

27. Kaplan DT, Golgberger AL. Chaos in cardiology. J Cardiovasc Electrophysiol 1991; 2:342–354.

28. Schmidt G, Morfill GE. Nonlinear methods for heart rate variability assessment. In: Malik M, Camm AJ (eds). Heart Rate Variability. Futura Publishing Co, Armonk, NY, 1995, pp 87–98.

29. Lombardi F, Sandrone G, Mortara A, Torzillo D, La Rovere MT, et al. Linear and non-linear dynamics of heart rate variability after acute myocardial infarction and reduced left ventricular ejection fraction. Am J Cardiol 1996; 77:1283–1288.

30. Butler GC, Ando S, Floras SJ. Fractal component of heart rate variability and systolic pressure in congestive heart failure. Clin Sci 1997; 92:543–550.

31. Signorini MG, Cerutti S, Guzzetti S, Parola R. Non-linear dynamics of cardiovascular variability signals. Meth Inform Med 1994; 33:81–84.

32. Pincus SM, Goldberger AL. Physiologic time-series analysis: what does regularity quantify? Am J Physiol 1994; 226:H1643-H1656.

33. Rich MW, Saini JS, Kleiger RE, Carney RM, De Velde A, et al. Correlation of heart rate variability with clinical and angiographic variables and late mortality after coronary angiography. Am J Cardiol 1988; 62:714–717.

34. Kienzle M, Ferguson DW, Birkett CL, Myers GA, Berg WJ, et al. Clinical, hemodynamic and sympathetic neural correlates of heart rate variability in congestive heart failure. Am J Cardiol 1992; 69:761–767.

35. Szabo BM, van Veldhuisen DJ, van der Veer N, Brouwer J, De Graeff PA, et al. Prognostic value of heart rate variability in chronic congestive heart failure secondary to idiopathic or ischemic dilated cardiomyopathy. Am J Cardiol 1997; 79:978–980.

36. Yi G, Goldman JH, Keeling PJ, Reardon M, McKenna WJ, et al. Heart rate variability in idiopathic dilated cardiomyopathy: relation to disease severity and prognosis. Heart 1997; 77:108–114.

37. Counihan PJ, Lü Fei, Bashir Y, Farrell TG, Haywood GA, et al. Assessment of heart rate variability in hypertrophic cardiomyopathy: association with clinical and prognostic features. Circulation 1993; 88:1682–1690.

38. Furlan R, Guzzetti S, Crivellaro W, et al. Continuous 24-hour assessment of the neural regulation of systemic arterial pressure and RR variabilities in ambulant subjects. Circulation 1990; 81:537–547.

39. Eggeling T, Osterhues H, Hoher M, Kochs M. Influence of beta-blocker therapy on heart rate variability in patients with long QT syndrome (abstract). Circulation 1993; 88:1116.

40. Lü Fei, Statters DJ, Hnatkova K, Poloniecki J, Malik M, et al. Change of autonomic influence on the heart immediately before the onset of spontaneous idiopathic ventricular tachycardia. J Am Coll Cardiol 1994; 24:1515–1522.

41. Kokovic DZ, Harada T, Shea JB, Soroff D, Friedman PL. Alterations of heart rate variability after radiofrequency catheter ablation of supraventricular tachycardia: delineation of parasympathetic pathways in the human heart. Circulation 1993; 88:1671–1681.

42. Ramaekers D, Ector H, Vanhaecke J, van Cleemput J, van de Werf F. Heart rate variability after cardiac transplantation in humans. PACE 1996; 19:2112–2119.

43. Tsui H, Larson MG, Venditti FJ Jr, Manders ES, Evans JC, et al. Impact of reduced heart rate variability on risk for cardiac events: the Framingham Heart Study. Circulation 1996; 97:2850–2855.

44. Tsui H, Venditti FJ Jr, Manders ES, Evans JC, Larson MG, et al. Reduced heart

rate variability and mortality risk in an elderly cohort: the Framingham Heart Study. Circulation 1994; 90:878–883.
45. Algra A, Tijssen JGP, Roelandt JRTC, Pool J, Lubsen J. Heart rate variability from 24-hour electrocardiography and 2-year risk for sudden death. Circulation 1993; 88:180–185.
46. Cripps TR, Malik M, Farrell TG, Camm AJ. Prognostic value of reduced heart rate variability after myocardial infarction: clinical evaluation of a new analysis method. Br Heart J 1991; 65:14–19.
47. Farrell TG, Bahir Y, Cripps T, Malik M, Poloniecki J, et al. Risk stratification for arrhythmic events in postinfarction patients based on heart rate variability, ambulatory electrocardiographic variables and the signal-averaged electrocardiogram J Am Coll Cardiol 1991; 18:687–697.
48. Odemuyiwa O, Malik M, Farrell TG, Bashir Y, Poloniecki J, et al. Comparison of the predictive characteristics of heart rate variability index and left ventricular ejection fraction for all-cause mortality, arrhythmic events and sudden death after acute myocardial infarction. Am J Cardiol 1991; 68:434–439.
49. Pedretti R, Etro MD, Laporta A, Braga SS, Carù B. Prediction of late arrhythmic events after acute myocardial infarction from combined use of noninvasive prognostic variables and inducibility of sustained monomorphic ventricular tachycardia. Am J Cardiol 1993; 71:1131–1141.
50. Bigger JT Jr, Fleiss JT, Steinman RC, et al. Frequency domain measures of heart rate variability and mortality after myocardial infarction. Circulation 1992; 85:164–171.
51. Hartikainen JEK, Malik M, Staunton A, Poloniecki J, Camm AJ. Distinction between arrhythmic and nonarrhythmic death after acute myocardial infarction based on heart rate variability, signal-averaged electrocardiogram, ventricular arrhythmias and left ventricular ejection fraction. J Am Coll Cardiol 1996; 28:296–304.
52. Goldstein DS, Horwitz D, Keiser HR. Comparison of techniques for measuring baroreflex sensitivity in man. Circulation 1982; 66:432–439.
53. Bristow JD, Honour AJ, Pickering JW, Sleight P, Smyth HS. Diminished baroreflex sensitivity in high blood pressure. Circulation 1969; 39:48–54.
54. Eckberg DL, Drabinsky M, Braunwald E. Defective cardiac parasympathetic control in patients with heart disease. N Engl J Med 1971; 285:877–883.
55. La Rovere MT, Specchia G, Mortara A, Schwartz PJ. Baroreflex sensitivity, clinical correlates and cardiovascular mortality among patients with a first myocardial infarction: a prospective study. Circulation 1988; 78:816–824.
56. Mortara A, La Rovere MT, Pinna GD, Perpa A, Maestri R, et al. Arterial baroreflex modulation of heart rate in chronic heart failure: clinical and hemodynamic correlates and prognostic implications. Circulation 1997; 96:3450–3458.
57. La Rovere MT, Pinna GD, Mortara A. Assessment of baroreflex sensitivity. In: Malik M (ed). Clinical Guide to Cardiac Autonomic Tests. Kluwer Academic Publishers, Dordrecht, 1998, pp 257–281.
58. Parati G, Di Rienzo M, Bertinieri G, Pomidossi G, Casadei R, et al. Evaluation of the baroreceptor-heart rate reflex by 24-hour intra-arterial blood pressure monitoring in humans. Hypertension 1988; 12:214–222.
59. Robbe HWJ, Mulder LJM, Ruddel H, Langewitz WA, Veldman JB, et al. Assessment of baroreceptor reflex sensitivity by means of spectral analysis. Hypertension 1987; 10:538–543.
60. Watkins LL, Grossman P, Sherwood A. Noninvasive assessment of baroreflex control in borderline hypertension: comparison with the phenylephrine method. Hypertension 1996; 28:238–243.

61. Maestri R, Pinna GD, Mortara A, La Rovere MT, Tavazzi L. Assessing barore-flex sensitivity in post-myocardial infarction patients: comparison of spectral techniques and phenylephrine. J Am Coll Cardiol 1998; 31:344–351.

62. Bigger JT Jr, La Rovere MT, Steinman RC, Fleiss JL, Rottman JN, et al. Comparison of baroreflex sensitivity and heart period variability after myocardial infarction. J Am Coll Cardiol 1989; 14:1511–1518.

63. Farrell TG, Paul V, Cripps TR, Malik M, Bennett ED, et al. Baroreflex sensitivity and electrophysiological correlates in patients after acute myocardial infarction. Br Heart J 1992; 67:129–137.

64. Farrell TG, Odemuyiwa O, Bashir Y, et al. Prognostic value of baroreflex sensitivity testing after acute myocardial infarction. Br Heart J 1992; 67:129–137.

65. Hohnloser SH, Klingenheben T, van de Loo A, et al. Reflexes versus tonic vagal activity as a prognostic parameter in patients with sustained ventricular tachycardia and ventricular fibrillation. Circulation 1994; 89:1068–1073.

66. De Ferrari GM, Landolina M, Mantica M, et al. Baroreflex sensitivity, but not heart rate variability, is reduced in patients with life-threatening ventricular arrhythmias long after myocardial infarction. Am Heart J 1995; 130:473–480.

67. Smith ML, Ellenbogen KA, Beightol LA, Eckberg DL. Human sympathetic neural responses to induced ventricular tachycardia. J Am Coll Cardiol 1995; 92:3206–3211.

68. Landolina M, Mantica M, Pessano P, et al. Impaired baroreflex sensitivity is correlated with hemodynamic deterioration of sustained ventricular tachycardia. J Am Coll Cardiol 1997; 29:568–575.

69. Hohnloser SH, Klingenheben T, Yi-Gang Li, Zabel M, Peetermans J, et al. T wave alternans as a predictor of recurrent ventricular tachyarrhythmias in ICD recipients: prospective comparison with conventional risk markers. J Cardiovasc Electrophysiol 1998; 9:1258–1268.

70. Redwood SR, Odemuyiwa O, Hnatkova K, Staunton A, Poloniecki J, et al. Selection of dichotomy limits for multifactorial prediction of arrhythmic events and mortality in survivors of acute myocardial infarction. Eur Heart J 1997; 18:1278–1287.

71. Schmidt G, Malik M, Barthel P, Schneider R, La Rovere MT, et al. Heart rate turbulence after ventricular premature beats as a predictor of mortality after acute myocardial infarction. Lancet 1999; 353:1390–1396.

72. Malik M, Schmidt G, Barthel P, Schneider R, Ulm K, et al. Heart rate turbulence is a post-infarction mortality predictor which is independent of and additive to other recognized risk factors (abstract). PACE 1999; 22:747.

# 37

# Markers of Sudden Cardiac Death and Clinical Usefulness of the QT Study:

## QT Duration, QT Dispersion, QT Dynamicity, and T Wave Alternans

*Antoine Leenhardt, MD, Pierre Maison Blanche, MD, Fabrice Extramiana, MD, Paul Milliez, MD, and Philippe Coumel, MD*

## Introduction

Identification of patients at high risk of sudden cardiac death represents one of the most challenging issues in patient care. Poor sensitivity and low predictive value are common limitations of noninvasive indexes.[1] From experimental data, the role of ventricular repolarization abnormalities in the genesis of ventricular arrhythmias is well established. Thus, surface ECG noninvasive markers of ventricular repolarization have been evaluated. However, when considered alone, these markers provide controversial added value for arrhythmic risk stratification. In this chapter, we will evaluate the value of various parameters of the ventricular repolarization (QT interval) in the identification of patients at high risk of arrhythmic events: QT duration, QT dispersion, QT dynamicity, and T wave alternans.

The QT interval corresponds to the time elapsed between the first depolarization and the last repolarization occurring in ventricular cells. Despite the lack of electrophysiological correlates, it is considered as a surrogate of cellular action potential duration. However, it yields a limited view of the complex electrogenesis of the ventricular myocardium.

From: Aliot E, Clementy J, Prystowsky EN (editors). *Fighting Sudden Cardiac Death: A Worldwide Challenge.* ©Futura Publishing Company, Armonk, NY, 2000.

# QT Duration

Some authors reported a predictive value of a prolonged QTc interval after myocardial infarction.[2,3] However, Algra et al. found that QTc duration is a predictive index only when left ventricular ejection fraction is normal.[4] These results were confirmed in a recent prospective study of 554 patients with chronic heart failure in which none of the QT parameters were shown to be independent predictors of outcome (all-cause mortality and mode of death).[5] In a recent study from our group,[6] we found no significant difference in QTc interval between patients with and patients without ventricular arrhythmias following myocardial infarction. In both groups, left ventricular ejection fraction was around 40%, and our results are in accordance with the findings of Algra.

# QT Dispersion

Evidence of T wave end inequality between leads among surface ECG traces was reported by Wilson[7] and it was revived by the concept of QT dispersion. Because of its apparent simplicity, QT dispersion became rapidly fashionable and a growing literature is now devoted to its potential prognostic value.[8,9] A good reason for the success of the concept in the cardiology community is the name coined to designate it. For clinicians, "dispersion" immediately suggests "inhomogeneity" in both the distribution of action potential duration and conduction wavefronts. All of these electrophysiological parameters are known to be highly arrhythmogenic, but we may be somewhat misled by our semantics.

The information about ventricular electrical activity is contained in a single image, the spatial QRS and T loops that can be characterized by their morphology, planarity, speed, etc. When projected on the orthogonal XYZ axes, or on the frontal, sagittal, and horizontal planes, they form the QRS-T complexes. A single structure such as a 3-dimensional loop cannot generate any "dispersion." However, any projection on a 2-dimensional plane implies the loss of a part of the information, and identifying "dispersion" from various projections may be just a way to characterize the lost information. In particular, every time the tip of the electrical vector progresses perpendicular to the plane or the axis of projection, the resulting activity becomes transiently nil, as if the original source had disappeared.

Whether or not QT dispersion is a reality or an illusion, the practical problem remains that even an illusion should be evaluated as precisely as possible in order to assess its clinical implications.

## Measurement

The definition itself of QT dispersion is not clearly established. Most studies used the range of QT intervals for all available leads, but the standard deviation of QT interval could be preferable, being less dependent of extreme values. Other studies proposed the use of the variation coefficient (QT standard deviation/mean QT). In the attempt to take into account the inability of measuring all leads, some authors corrected the QT duration range by the square root of the number of measured leads.[9] A second unsolved issue remains the exact definition of the T wave offset. If most studies consider the return to isoelectric line or the nadir between the T wave and the U wave, others claim that the method of Surawicz (intersection between the isoelectric line and the tangent to the descending limb of the T wave) is more reliable.[10] Another critical point raised by Statters is the possible use of a subset of leads, as it could be inappropriate to merge the limb lead information with that of precordial chest leads. Our group and that of Brohet in Brussels reported on the discriminant power of XYZ QT dispersion.[11,12] We compared the ECG recordings between 92 normal subjects and 71 patients following myocardial infarction, and we found that, although reduced when compared to 12 leads, dispersion in XYZ leads could discriminate.

Another matter of dispute is whether or not QT dispersion should be corrected for heart rate, although this specific issue was related mainly to the nonsimultaneous acquisition of leads typical of some poor commercial system.

## Clinical Implications

After a long series of many encouraging publications showing strong discriminant and prognostic power of QT dispersion, [13–21] the more recent literature is less enthusiastic. There is accumulated evidence that manual measures of QT dispersion on paper printouts are irrelevant. The first implication is that all previously published material based on manual measurement should be considered with extreme caution.

In contrast to these positive studies based mainly on a retrospective analysis of an ECG database, Zabel et al. prospectively collected 12-lead resting ECGs in 280 consecutive patients referred for acute MI.[22] In this study, the 12-lead ECGs were optically scanned and digitized before automatic analysis of QT dispersion and other repolarization variables. After a mean follow-up of 32 months, QT dispersion was neither predictive for global mortality nor for arrhythmic death. This contrasts with the confirmation that ejection fraction, heart rate variability, and heart rate were indeed good predictors of events.

The morphology of spatial T wave loop structure may also be of importance because findings from our group showed that the presence of an electrophysiological substrate for repolarization inhomogeneity is associated with alterations in the morphology of spatial T wave loop structure.[23]

## Potential Mechanisms

The QT dispersion addresses macroscopic rather than microscopic inhomogeneity. The potential interest in detecting susceptibility to malignant arrhythmias was highlighted some time ago[24,25] using the concept initially formulated by Han and Moe.[26] These authors, however, were referring to inhomogeneity of recovery at the cellular level, and extrapolation to ECG repolarization may not be adequate. In any case, the concept of inhomogeneity and its implication in the clinical term of dispersion can apply differently in heart diseases such as myocardial infarction, cardiomyopathy, and long QT syndrome. It remains to be seen whether the existence of layers of M cells, in particular, macroscopic areas of the ventricular myocardium,[27] may help to fill the gap between diffuse and localized electrophysiological disturbances.

## The Future of QT Dispersion

The evaluation of ventricular repolarization must be improved. Technically, only digitized recordings should be considered, a necessity that occasionally would favor prospective studies. Using automated processing does not obviate the problem of intersystem differences, and it would be utopic to look for any consensus in the recognition algorithms. A decisive advantage of computer techniques, however, is a reproducible deviation from the humanly defined reference,[28,29] a condition sufficient to make the studies more comparable. An adequate quantification of QT dispersion would probably help to better understand its significance through its pathophysiological variations. There is no doubt that resurgence of QRS-T integral mapping would be suitable, although this technique obviously suffers from practical limitations in its clinical applications.

## QT Dynamicity

QT dynamicity contains 2 important bits of information. The behavior of the cellular action potential is reflected by QT rate dependence, and the autonomic nervous system modulates both QT duration and rate dependence. QT rate dependence is one of the major properties of ventricular repolarization with demonstrated circadian modulation[30,31] and gender influences.[31,32] Studying QT dynamicity presupposes selective manipulation of thousands of QRS-T complexes over 24 hours to extract relevant information. This can be achieved, and in contrast to the study of QT dispersion, the processing offers the definite advantage of measuring changes of duration rather than absolute values. Any algorithm can reliably detect changes on the order of the millisecond simply because potential deviations from reference are fixed. The relation between QT rate dependence and ventricular arrhythmia has been evaluated by others in the long QT syndrome[33] and in idiopathic ventricular fibrillation.[34] Our experience with the long QT syndrome[34] and in patients with prior myocardial infarction[6] shows that QT dynamicity is a reliable marker of the probability of arrhythmic events.

## Measurement

Our methodology of QT analysis from Holter recordings has been previously reported.[31,35,36] Briefly, the major characteristics of this analysis were (1) selective beat averaging, using QRS-T complexes preceded by a 1-minute period of stable heart rate, (2) automatic measurement of QT interval with manual over-reading, and (3) separate analysis of 3 different circadian periods defined according to subject diaries and average hourly heart rate. The first period consisted of the 8 consecutive daily hours with fastest heart rate (awake period), the second consisted of the 4 consecutive sleeping hours with lowest heart rate (sleep period), and the third consisted of the 2 hours around the awakening heart rate acceleration (awakening period). For each individual, and for each circadian period, linear regression analysis between QT intervals obtained in stable heart rate conditions and corresponding RR intervals was performed. In addition, all data from each individual were pooled according to the group and to the circadian period, and a global linear regression analysis was performed on the pooled data. The slope of the global linear regression was used to assess QT rate dependence ($\Delta QT/\Delta RR$). QT rate dependence was also expressed in terms of QT interval duration at different RR values (600, 800, and 1,000 ms).

## Clinical Implications

The study population consisted of 68 patients with a prior history of Q wave myocardial infarction.[6] The ventricular arrhythmia group (VT) consisted of 34 patients who had a recent history of ventricular tachyarrhythmia and in whom the programmed electrical stimulation was positive, without any antiarrhythmic treatment. It was compared to a matched control group of 34 patients with a prior Q wave myocardial infarction but without a history of ventricular arrhythmia events, an arrhythmia-free survival for more than years during the follow-up, and a negative electrophysiological study.

Within the 3 circadian periods, the QT rate dependence was enhanced in patients with ventricular arrhythmias compared to the control group. This difference was more pronounced after awakening (slope differences = 0.072 [0.032; 0.112]). The lowest QT rate dependence was observed during sleep (0.138 and 0.180, respectively, in the control and VT groups).

At a fast heart rate (i.e., 90/min), the QT interval was shorter in the VT group, whereas at a lower heart rate (60/min), the QT interval was significantly longer in the VT group. The magnitude of QT shortening might have physiopathological implications. QT interval prolongation may have a potential proarrhythmic effect at a low rate, and an increase of QT shortening could induce a lack of protection against ventricular arrhythmia at a high rate.

## The Future of QT Dynamicity

This retrospective study and others recently published suggest that QT rate dependence can identify patients with or without vulnerability to ventricular tachyarrhythmias occurring after myocardial infarction. The same results have been found by our group in the Emiat patients.[37] A common characteristic of diseased myocardium is the existence of a steeper QT/RR slope. However, the predictive value of this new index should be evaluated and compared to other noninvasive risk markers in a large prospective trial.

# T Wave Alternans

T wave alternans (TWA) is characterized by beat-to-beat changes in T wave amplitude. It has been found to be an important prognostic factor for malignant ventricular arrhythmias in patients with the long QT syndrome,[38] with ischemic heart disease,[39,40] and electrolyte disturbance.[41] However, the easily recognizable pattern of visually obvious TWA is very rare, explaining the interest for techniques able to detect a low level of TWAs.

## Measurement

A spectral method and sophisticated signal-processing techniques are able to measure the TWA down to one-millionth of a volt. This technique involves measuring the amplitude of the T wave, at a fixed offset from the QRS complex, in 128 sequential beats in order to create a time series. This time series is analyzed using a fast Fourier transform to generate a power spectrum. Applying this technique to a series of points in the T wave, each with a different offset from the QRS, creates a set of power spectra. All of these power spectra are then averaged to generate a composite power spectrum for the entire T wave. As the spectrum reflects measurements taken once per beat, its frequencies are expressed in the units of cycles/beat. Alternans level is defined by a peak centered at exactly 0.5 cycles/beat, which represents oscillations occuring on an every-other-beat basis. The magnitude of TWA is expressed either as the alternans power (i.e., the height of the peak above the background noise level in microvolts) or as the alternans ratio (i.e., the ratio of the alternans power to the standard deviation of the noise). Thus, the alternans ratio is a measure of the statistical significance of the alternans peak representing the number of standard deviations by which it exceeds the background noise level.

TWA is a threshold phenomenon, tending to appear abruptly when the heart rate exceeds a patient-specific onset heart rate threshold. The onset heart rate for sustained TWA is different in patients susceptible to ventricular tachyarrhythmias (below 110 beats/min) compared to subjects not thought to be at increased risk for ventricular arrhythmias (onset of TWA between 140 and 160 beats/min). The TWA test is considered to be positive if alternans is sustained with an onset heart rate below 110 beats/min, and with an alternans voltage >1.9 microvolts and an alternans ratio exceeding 3.

Another technique has been described to analyze the TWA using a type of harmonic analysis called complex demodulation.[42] However, the applicability of this technique in clinical practice is still in the initial phase of its development.

## Mechanism of T Wave Alternans

The hypotheses proposed are related to an increased dispersion of the refractory times and spatial inhomogeneity of ventricular repolarization that lead to the development of reentry.[43]

Recent studies from both cellular and whole animal experiments suggest that T wave alternans occurs at a cellular level and is related to beat-to-beat alternation of repolarization between myocardial layers or between epicardial cells. The large electrical gradients induced allow for unidirectional block and initiation of rapid polymorphic ventricular arrhythmias.

## Clinical Implications

### Clinical Studies

In 1994, Rosenbaum et al. showed, in a group of 83 patients undergoing electrophysiological testing, that, consistent with previous experimental studies, TWA was an independent marker of vulnerability to inducible ventricular arrhythmias (sensitivity, 81%; specificity 84%; relative risk, 5.2) and clinical arrhythmic events.[44] The TWA was fully equivalent to invasive electrophysiological testing as a predictor of arrhythmia-free survival in this study.

In this study, atrial pacing was used to increase the heart rate and reduce the interbeat interval variability. In order to make measurement of microvolt-level TWA a totally noninvasive procedure, it was necessary to measure the TWA by applying other methods to increase the heart rate, such as bicycle exercise. Exercise complicates the measurement of TWA because it introduces movement artifact and because the heart rate is not fixed. Electrode systems and signal processing were developed to minimize the movement artifact, and pedaling was controlled to keep the frequency of the motion artifact far from the frequency alternans (pedaling rate at one-third to two-thirds the heart rate).

Hohnloser et al. demonstrated[43] in a series of 30 consecutive patients with ventricular tachyarrhythmias that microvolt TWA can be assessed reliably and noninvasively during exercise stress. This was confirmed by Estes et al.[45] in a series of 27 patients with syncope and/or ventricular arrhythmias: TWA predicted inducibility of ventricular arrhythmias with a sensitivity of 86%, a specificity of 75%, and overall clinical accuracy of 78% (p<0.01). Preliminary results of a multicenter study in the first 111 patients referred for electrophysiological study show that TWA is a statistically significant predictor of ventricular tachyarrhythmias or death (p=0.01). The relative risk associated with a positive versus a negative TWA test was 10.6 at 1 year of follow-up. Invasive electrophysiological study was also a significant predictor (p=0.03), but with a lower relative risk of 3.7.[46]

There are at this time only limited data in different patient populations. A recent study found, in 64 patients with hypertrophic cardiomyopathy, that TWA was significantly correlated with ventricular tachycardia or ventricular fibrillation.[47] TWA appears to identify nonischemic dilated cardiomyopathy patients at high risk for ventricular tachyarrhythmic events in a preliminary series of 56 patients.[48]

### Comparison of T Wave Alternans with Other Noninvasive Means of Risk Stratification

In a study of 27 patients with syncope and/or ventricular arrhythmias,[45] TWA was found to be an accurate predictor of risk of arrhythmia compared to the signal-averaged electrocardiogram, which was not a statistically significant predictor of arrhythmia vulnerability in the selected patient population studied. Armoundas et al.[49] found the same results in a retrospective study of the patients previously published by Rosenbaum et al.[44] They pointed out the fact that TWA was successfully measured in a larger proportion of patients than those undergoing signal-averaged electrocardiograms because an intraventricular conduction delay does not interfere with determination of the former while it makes the latter uninterpretable.

In a high-risk population of 95 patients, all of whom had an implantable cardioverter defibrillator (ICD), Hohnloser et al. prospectively compared TWA with invasive electrophysiological testing and other risk markers (electrophysiological testing, left ventricular ejection fraction, baroreflex sensitivity, signal-averaged electrocardiogram, 24-hour heart rate variability, QT dispersion) with respect to their ability to predict recurrence of ventricular tachyarrhythmias as documented by ICD electrograms.[50] Determinate TWA results were not obtained in 26 patients (27%) due to failure to achieve a heart rate of 105 beats/min or technical factors. Multivariate Cox regression analysis revealed that TWA was the only statistically independent risk factor. The sensitivity, specificity, and predictive positive accuracy of TWA were, respectively, 78%, 61%, and 67% (p< 0.003).

## The Future of T Wave Alternans

As studies confirming the strong predictive power of TWA for cardiac arrhythmias or sudden cardiac death among specific high-risk populations are being completed, prospective screening of large groups of patients at lower relative risk of sudden cardiac death will be the next step. If this technique is able to define small subgroups among large populations whose first or next cardiac event is highly likely to be an arrhythmic death, its future will be very exciting.

Some particular points need further studies. Optimal heart rate threshold cutoffs need to be defined for TWA-based risk stratification in the postmyocardial infarction population. The effect of autonomic modulation on TWA in humans is unknown. In a preliminary study, esmolol infusion decreased TWA amplitude and its sensitivity for predicting inducibility of ventricular tachycardia.[51] In all completed studies, there is a high percentage (25–28%) of patients in whom the analysis of TWA is indeterminate, and thus an improvement of the technique is needed.

## Conclusion

A new field of investigation has been opened with the study of ventricular repolarization. Several studies have been done or are ongoing on

QT duration, QT morphology (including TWA and post-pause changes), and QT dynamicity. Collecting, processing, and using this information properly would probably provide new markers of arrhythmic events.

## References

1. Farrell TG, Bashir Y, Cripps T, et al. Risk stratification for arrhythmic events in postinfarction patients based on heart rate variability, ambulatory electrocardiographic variables and the signal-averaged electrocardiogram. J Am Coll Cardiol 1991; 18:687–697.
2. Puddu PE, Bourassa MG. Prediction of sudden death from QTc interval prolongation in patients with chronic ischemic heart disease. J Electrocardiol 1986; 19:203–212.
3. Peters RW, Byington RP, Barker A, Yusuf S. Prognostic value of prolonged ventricular repolarization following myocardial infarction: the BHAT experience. J Clin Epidemiol 1990; 43:167–172.
4. Algra A, Tijssen JG, Roelandt JR, et al. QTc prolongation measured by standard 12-lead electrocardiography is an independent risk factor for sudden death due to cardiac arrest. Circulation 1991; 83:1888–1894.
5. Brooksby P, Batin PD, Nolan J, et al. The relationship between QT intervals and mortality in ambulant patients with chronic heart failure: The United Kingdom Heart Failure Evaluation and Assessment of Risk Trial (UK-Heart). Eur Heart J 1999; 20:1335–1341.
6. Extramiana F, Neyroud N, Huikuri HV, et al. QT interval and arrhythmic risk assessment after myocardial infarction. Am J Cardiol 1999; 83:266–269.
7. Wilson, Macleod AG, Barker PS, et al. The interpretation of the initial deflections of the ventricular complex of the electrocardiogram. Am Heart J 1931; 6:637–664.
8. Statters DJ, Malik M, Ward DE, et al. QT dispersion: problems of methodology and clinical significance. J Cardiovasc Electrophysiol 1994; 5:672–685.
9. Day CP, McComb JM, Matthews J, et al. Reduction in QT dispersion by sotalol following myocardial infarction. Eur Heart J 1991; 12:423–427.
10. Lepeschkin E, Surawicz B. The measurement of the Q-T interval of the electrocardiogram. Circulation 1952; 51:378–388.
11. Sainte Beuve C, Badilini F, Maison-Blanche P, et al. QT dispersion: comparison of orthogonal, quasi-orthogonal and 12-lead configurations. ANE 1999; 4(2):167–175.
12. Zaidi M, Robert A, Fesler R, et al. Computer-assisted study of the ECG indices of the dispersion of ventricular repolarization. J Electrocardiol 1996; 29:199–211.
13. Moreno FL, Villanueva T, Karagounis LA, et al. Reduction in QT interval dispersion by successful thrombolytic therapy in acute myocardial infarction. Circulation 1994; 90:94–100.
14. Manttari M, Oikarinen L, Manninen V, et al. QT dispersion as a risk factor for sudden cardiac death and fatal myocardial infarction in a coronary risk population. Heart 1997; 78:268–272.
15. Zaidi M, Robert A, Fesler R, et al. Dispersion of ventricular repolarization in hypertrophic cardiomyopathy. J Electrocardiol 1996; 26(Suppl): 89–94.
16. Hii JT, Wyse DG, Gillis AM, et al. Precordial QT interval dispersion as a marker of torsades de pointes. Circulation 1992; 6:1376–1382.
17. Buja G, Miorelli M, Turrini P, et al. Comparison of QT dispersion in hypertrophic cardiomyopathy between patients with and without ventricular arrhythmias and sudden death. Am J Cardiol 1993; 72:973–976.

18. Glancy JM, Weston PJ, Bhullar HK, et al. Reproducibility and automatic measurement of QT dispersion. Eur Heart J 1996; 17:1035–1039.
19. Zareba W, Moss AJ, le Cessie S. Dispersion of ventricular repolarization and arrhythmic cardiac death in coronary artery disease. Am J Cardiol 1994; 74:550–553.
20. Priori SG, Napolitano C, Diehl L, et al. Dispersion of the QT interval: a marker of therapeutic efficacy in the idiopathic long QT syndrome. Circulation 1994; 89:1681–1689.
21. Karagounis L, Anderson J, Moreno F, et al. Multivariate associates of QT dispersion in patients with acute myocardial infarction: primacy of patency status of the infarct-related artery. Am Heart J 1998; 135:1027–1035.
22. Zabel M, Kligenheben T, Franz M, et al. Assessment of QT dispersion for prediction of mortality or arrhythmic events after myocardial infarction: results of a prospective, long-term follow-up study. Circulation 1998; 97:2543–2550.
23. Badilini F, Fayn J, Maison-Blanche P, et al. Quantitative aspects of ventricular repolarization: relationship between three-dimensional T-wave loop morphology and QT dispersion. ANE 1997; 2(2):146–157.
24. Mirvis DM. Spatial variation of QT intervals in normal persons and patients with acute myocardial infarction. J Am Coll Cardiol 1985; 5:625–631.
25. Burgess MJ, Green LS, Millar K, et al. The sequence of normal ventricular recovery. Am Heart J 1972; 84:660–669.
26. Han J, Moe GK. Nonuniform recovery of excitability. Circulation 1964; 14:44–60.
27. Sicouri S, Antzelevitch C. A subpopulation of cells with unique electrophysiological properties in the deep subepicardium of the canine ventricle. Circ Res 1991; 68:1729–1741.
28. The CSE Working Party. A reference database for multilead electrocardiographic computer measurement programs. J Am Coll Cardiol 1987; 10:1313–1321.
29. Willems JL, Abreu-Lima C, Arnaud P, et al. The diagnostic performance of computer programs for the interpretation of electrocardiograms. N Engl J Med 1991; 325:1767–1773.
30. Viitasalo M, Karjalainen J. QT intervals at heart rates from 50 to 120 beats per minute during 24-hour electrocardiographic recordings in 100 healthy men. Circulation 1992; 86:1439–1442.
31. Extramiana F, Maison-Blanche P, Badilini F, et al. Circadian modulation of QT rate-dependence in healthy volunteers: gender and age differences. J Electrocardiol 1999; 32:33–43.
32. Stramba-Badiale M, Locati EH, Martinelli A, et al. Gender and the relationship between ventricular repolarization and cardiac cycle length during 24-h Holter recordings. Eur Heart J 1997; 18:1000–1006.
33. Merri M, Moss AJ, Benhorin J, et al. Relation between ventricular repolarization duration and cardiac cycle length during 24-hour Holter recordings. Circulation 1992; 85:1816–1821.
34. Tavernier R, Jordaens L, Haerynck F, et al. Changes in the QT interval and its adaptation to rate, assessed with continuous electrocardiographic recordings in patients with ventricular fibrillation, as compared to normal individuals without arrhythmias. Eur Heart J 1997; 18:994–999.
35. Neyroud N, Maison-Blanche P, Denjoy I, et al. Diagnostic performance of QT interval variables from 24-h electrocardiography in the long QT syndrome. Eur Heart J 1998; 19:158–165.
36. Badilini F, Maison-Blanche P, Childers R, et al. QT interval analysis on ambu-

latory ECG recordings: a selective beat averaging approach. Med Biol Eng Comput 1998; 36:1–10.
37. Milliez P, Leenhardt A, Maison-Blanche P, et al. Arrhythmic death in the EMIAT trial: role of ventricular repolarization dynamicity as a new discriminant risk marker (abstract). Circulation (in press).
38. Schwartz P, Malliani A. Electrical alternans of the T-wave: clinical and experimental evidence of its relationship with the sympathetic nervous system and with the long Q-T syndrome. Am Heart J 1975; 89:45–50.
39. Kleinfeld MJ, Rozanski JJ. Alternans of the ST segment in Prinzmetal's angina. Circulation 1977; 55:574–577.
40. Nakashima M, Hashimoto H, Kanamaru M, et al. Experimental studies and clinical report on the electrical alternans of ST segment during myocardial ischemia. Jap Heart J 1978; 19:396–408.
41. Reddy CVR, Kiok JP, Khan RG, et al. Repolarization alternans associated with alcoholism and hypomagnesemia. Am J Cardiol 1984; 53:390–391.
42. Nearing BD, Huang AH, Verrier RL. Dynamic tracking of cardiac vulnerability by complex demodulation of the T wave. Science 1991; 252:437–440.
43. Hohnloser SH, Klingenheben T, Zabel M, et al. TWA during exercise and atrial pacing in humans. J Cardiovasc Electrophysiol 1997; 8:987–993.
44. Rosenbaum DS, Jackson LE, Smith JM, et al. Electrical alternans and vulnerability to ventricular arrhythmias. N Engl J Med 1994; 330:235–241.
45. Estes III NAM, Michaud G, Zipes D, et al. Electrical alternans during rest and exercise as predictors of vulnerability to ventricular arrhythmias. Am J Cardiol 1997; 80:1314–1318.
46. Gold MR, Bloomfield DM, Anderson KP, et al. T-wave alternans predicts arrhythmia vulnerability in patients undergoing electrophysiology study. Circulation 1998; 98(Suppl):I-647–648.
47. Murda'h A, Nagayoshi H, Kautzner J, et al. TWA as an imprtant predictor of VT/VF in patients with hypertrophic cardiomyopathy (abstract). PACE 1997; 20:1084.
48. Klingenheben T, Credner SC, Grönfeld G, et al. Microvolt T-wave alternans in prediction of ventricular tachyarrhythmic events in patients with non-ischaemic dilated cardiomyopathy (abstract). Eur Heart J 1999; 20(Suppl):332.
49. Armoundas AA, Rosenbaum DS, Ruskin JN, et al. Prognostic significance of electrical alternans versus signal averaged electrocardiography in predicting the outcome of electrophysiological testing and arrhythmia-free survival. Heart 1998; 80:251–256.
50. Hohnloser SH, Klingenheben T, Yi-Gang L, et al. TWA as a predictor of recurrent ventricular tachyarrhythmias in ICD recipients: prospective comparison with conventional risk markers. J Cardiovasc Electrophysiol 1998; 9:1258–1268.
51. Kirk MM, Cooklin M, Shorofsky SR, et al. Beta adrenergic blockade decreases TWA (abstract). JACC (in press).

# 38

# Value of Programmed Ventricular Stimulation to Select Candidates at Risk for Sudden Cardiac Death

*Eric N. Prystowsky, MD*

## Introduction

Several decades of research have identified noninvasive markers for increased risk for sudden death in patients with heart disease, especially after myocardial infarction. Two important risk factors are complex ventricular ectopy such as nonsustained ventricular tachycardia (VT) and the presence of diminished left ventricular function.[1-4] This continues to be true even in the current era of revascularization during an acute myocardial infarction.[5] Drug therapy given prophylactically to patients after myocardial infarction to improve survival has had at best a checkered past. Beta blockers improve survival; amiodarone, sotalol, and dofetilide are neutral, and several drugs have worsened survival, most notably encainide and flecainide.[4,6-11] The effort to identify patients at risk for sudden death has great merit since the overwhelming majority of patients who suffer out-of-hospital cardiac arrest in the United States are unsuccessfully resuscitated.[12,13] Success rates are likely no better in most other countries in the world. Thus, the quest continues to develop methods that will enable us to identify patients at high risk for sudden death and thereby enable primary prevention for this all-too-frequent cause of death in adults. Programmed ventricular stimulation to identify patients with inducible sustained VT is another method that has been used to stratify risk in patients after myocardial infarction.[14-17] As with any screening test, one desires high sensitivity and specificity. In patients with coronary artery disease and known sustained monomorphic VT, electrophysiological testing pacing at ≥2 right ventricular sites, using ≥2 paced cycle lengths and 1 to 3 extrastimuli, yields greater than 90% inducibility of sustained VT.[18] Specificity has been assumed to be

From: Aliot E, Clementy J, Prystowsky EN (editors). *Fighting Sudden Cardiac Death: A Worldwide Challenge.* ©Futura Publishing Company, Armonk, NY, 2000.

high, although this has not been well tested. In other words, most investigators consider induction of sustained monomorphic VT to occur in patients at high risk for this arrhythmia. The Multicenter Unsustained Tachycardia Trial (MUSTT), as noted below, is the first major prospective trial to evaluate the specificity of inducible sustained VT in patients without any previous history of such an arrhythmia.[19] Two major randomized prospective control trials, the Multicenter Automatic Defibrillator Implantation Trial (MADIT)[20] and MUSTT have evaluated the use of programmed ventricular stimulation to identify patients presumably at high risk for sudden death, and have further evaluated pharmacological and implantable cardioverter-defibrillator (ICD) therapies for these individuals. The rest of this chapter reviews data from MADIT and MUSTT.

# Multicenter Automatic Defibrillator Implantation Trial

The MADIT trial enrolled patients from 32 centers: 2 in Europe, and 30 in the United States.[20] Patients were eligible for enrollment if they had a myocardial infarction 3 weeks or more before entry, nonsustained VT of 3–30 beats with a rate greater than 120/min, and a left ventricular ejection fraction 0.35 or less. Major exclusions were coronary artery bypass graft surgery within 2 months, percutaneous transluminal coronary angioplasty within 2 months, and New York Heart Association Class IV for congestive heart failure. Patients underwent a baseline electrophysiological study using up to 3 extrastimuli in an attempt to initiate sustained VT. Patients in whom sustained VT was not suppressed with intravenous procainamide, or in some patients an equivalent drug if procainamide was contraindicated, were eligible for randomization. Patients received either an ICD or "conventional" medical therapy. Unfortunately, the choice of conventional therapy was left to the discretion of the patient's attending physician, although the majority of patients received empiric amiodarone. There was no control group for this study. Of 253 qualified patients, 196 (76%) were enrolled. No data are available regarding the number of patients who met entry criteria but who were not enrolled because of patient refusal, lack of sustained VT initiated at electrophysiological study, or VT that was suppressed with drug therapy.

The primary end-point of MADIT was overall mortality, and there was an impressive survival benefit of the ICD versus conventional medical therapy. The Kaplan-Meier survival curves demonstrate an early and substantial separation that remains significant throughout the trial duration. Thus, MADIT demonstrated a remarkable superiority of the ICD for survival in high-risk patients.

Several criticisms have been leveled at MADIT. First, 2 (6%) of the centers enrolled 63 (32%) of the patients, raising the possibility of entry bias for patient enrollment. Selection of patients with failure to suppress inducible sustained VT with antiarrhythmic drugs might have preselected individuals who were at higher risk for subsequent arrhythmic events, since previous data have shown that failure to suppress with one drug often predicts subsequent failure for other antiarrhythmic drugs.[18] Although the clinical characteristics between patient groups appeared balanced, there was an apparent significant imbalance in the use of beta blockers. Only 8% of patients received beta blockers in the conventional medical group compared with 26% of patients who received an ICD. However, this disparity may actually be less since sotalol has substantial beta-blocking effects, and the use of sotalol or beta blocker occurred in 15% of patients in the conventional group. Amiodarone was prescribed for 74% of patients in the conventional therapy group, but only 45% of patients were receiving amiodarone at the last patient contact.

In summary, as is true for all randomized prospective control trials, MADIT had its blemishes but also demonstrated a major survival benefit of the ICD in high-risk patients selected by programmed ventricular stimulation. The patients did appear to be an unusual group, for example, having a mean of 9–10 beats of spontaneous nonsustained VT compared with the typical 4–5 beats noted in most postmyocardial infarction trials. As noted below, the results of MADIT combined with the data from MUSTT make a strong case for the use of programmed ventricular stimulation to stratify risk in high-risk patients, and for implanting an ICD in such patients.

## The Multicenter Unsustained Tachycardia Trial

The design of the MUSTT trial has been previously reported.[14] Recently, the results of MUSTT have been reported and submitted for publication.[19] Only those data reported will be reviewed here. In 1989, MUSTT was conceived to test the hypothesis that antiarrhythmic therapy guided by electrophysiological testing in patients with coronary artery disease, left ventricular ejection fraction of 0.40 or less, and spontaneous nonsustained VT can decrease the risk of cardiac arrest and sudden death. In essence, MUSTT tested 2 major issues concerning programmed ventricular stimulation—whether such a method was useful to identify patients at risk for sudden death who met entry criteria and, second, whether therapy directed by electrophysiological testing could reduce mortality. Patients were enrolled from 85 centers in the United States and Canada. Nonsustained VT was defined as 3 or more consecutive ventricular complexes with at least 2 consecutive intervals with a cycle length ≤550 ms, and a mean cycle length <600 ms, with the entire episode spontaneously terminating within 30 seconds. Nonsustained VT had to occur at least 4 days after the most recent myocardial infarction or revascularization procedure, and within 6 months of enrollment into the study. Patients were eligible at least 4 days after their most recent myocardial infarction. The baseline electrophysiological study included right ventricular stimulation at 2 sites using 2 paced cycle lengths and ≤3 extrastimuli. Patients considered for randomization had inducible sustained monomorphic VT or sustained polymorphic VT induced by ≤2 extrastimuli. Patients eligible for randomization underwent electrophysiologically guided therapy or were given no specific antiarrhythmic treatment. Patients who did not meet criteria for enrollment in the randomized portion of the trial were followed in a registry. All investigators were encouraged to treat patients with both beta-adrenergic blocking agents and angiotensin-converting enzyme inhibitors whenever feasible.

Serial electrophysiological-electropharmacological testing was performed in the randomized treated patients. Antiarrhythmic drugs were randomly assigned for each patient, but amiodarone therapy could be used only after 2 failed drug trials. Initial therapy was either a Class Ia agent, propafenone, or sotalol. If the initial antiarrhythmic drug was considered ineffective, a second antiarrhythmic drug could be tried, either another Class I agent, a Class Ia plus mexiletine, or an ICD could be used. Amiodarone could be prescribed only in the third round of treatment. Success with an antiarrhythmic drug was considered permissible when <15 complexes of VT were induced, no VT was initiated, or sustained VT initiated during a 5-minute observation period was hemodynamically stable with a systolic blood pressure >80 mm Hg. Patients underwent follow-up every 3 months after enrollment in the study. The primary end-point for MUSTT was arrhythmic death or cardiac arrest from which the patient was resuscitated. Secondary end-points were total mortality, cardiac death, and spontaneous sustained VT.

## Results

Of 2,202 patients enrolled, 767 (35%) had inducible sustained VT, and 704 agreed to randomization. The 63 patients who refused randomization were followed in a registry along with 1,435 patients without inducible randomizable VT. The baseline characteristics of patients randomized to specific antiarrhythmic therapy or control were similar, and the median left ventricular ejection fraction was 0.29. Approximately 25% of patients were New York Heart Association Class III for congestive heart failure. At hospital discharge, 40% of all patients were taking beta-adrenergic blocking agents, but more patients in the control group (51%) than in the electrophysiologically guided therapy group (29%) were receiving beta blockers. This discrepancy is lessened somewhat by the 9% use of sotalol in the treated group. Over 70% of patients received angiotensin-converting enzyme inhibitors and approximately 64% of patients received aspirin, without differences between groups.

Antiarrhythmic therapy in the electrophysiologically guided group was a Class Ia agent (19%), propafenone (4%), Class Ia plus mexiletine (3%), amiodarone (10%), sotalol (9%), or an ICD (46%). No antiarrhythmic therapy was given to 7% of patients, and 2% of patients died before hospital discharge. In comparison, 96% of patients in the control group were given no specific antiarrhythmic therapy.

The median follow-up was 39 months. For the primary end-point of arrhythmic death or cardiac arrest, the 2- and 5-year rates were 12% and 25%, respectively, among patients randomized to electrophysiologically guided therapy, compared with 18% and 32% (p=0.04) for patients in the control group. This yielded a hazard ratio of 0.73, which corresponds to a 27% reduction in the risk of arrhythmic death or cardiac arrest in patients undergoing antiarrhythmic therapy. Total mortality rates for 2 and 5 years were 22% and 42%, respectively, for patients randomized to electrophysiologically guided therapy compared with 28% and 48%, respectively, for patients in the control group (p=0.06; hazard ratio 0.80). Thus, reduction in total mortality approached but did not quite reach statistical significance. Further analysis demonstrated that the reduction in the primary end-point of arrhythmic death or cardiac arrest as well as in total mortality in patients randomized to electrophysiologically guided treatment was primarily attributable to therapy with the ICD. For example, patients randomized to electrophysiologically guided therapy who received an ICD had a 60-month rate of arrhythmic death or cardiac arrest of 9% compared with 37% for patients who did not receive an ICD (p<0.001). Total mortality at 60 months for patients randomized to electrophysiologically guided therapy in the ICD versus the non-ICD group was 24% versus 55%, respectively. Preliminary data from the nonrandomizable registry patients compared with inducible patients not undergoing antiarrhythmic therapy show a slight arrhythmic death or cardiac arrest advantage for patients who had nonrandomizable VT, but there was no difference in long-term total mortality.

In summary, the results of MUSTT have demonstrated a major survival advantage of an ICD given to patients with inducible sustained VT who have coronary artery disease, spontaneous nonsustained VT, and a left ventricular ejection fraction of 0.40 or less. Surprisingly, a similar survival advantage was not found for patients with antiarrhythmic drug therapy guided by electrophysiological testing. Thus, it appears reasonable and indeed advisable for patients who meet criteria of MUSTT and MADIT to undergo electrophysiological testing, and if sustained VT is initiated, an ICD should be prescribed. Unfortunately, preliminary data from MUSTT have also shown the inadequacies of electrophysiological testing to identify those individuals at low risk for cardiac mortality and sudden cardiac death. This observation raises the question of whether patients who have high-risk clinical markers, regardless of initiation of VT at electrophysiological testing, should receive an ICD. However, such an approach, while potentially desirable, requires further testing. The use of electrophysiological testing to identify patients at high risk for sudden death who have cardiac pathology other than coronary artery disease is incompletely studied.

## References

1. Chiang BN, Perlman LV, Ostrander LD, Epstein RH. Relationship of premature systoles to coronary heart disease and sudden death in the Tecumseh epidemiologic study. Ann Intern Med 1969; 70:1159.
2. Ruberman W, Weinblatt E, Goldberg JD, Frank CW, Shapiro S. Ventricular premature beats and mortality after myocardial infarction. N Engl J Med 1977; 297:750.
3. Moss AJ, David HT, DeCamilla J, Bayer LW. Ventricular ectopic beats and their relation to sudden and nonsudden death after myocardial infarction. Circulation. 1979; 60:988.
4. Cannon DS, Prystowsky EN. Modern management of ventricular arrhythmias: detection, drugs and devices. JAMA 1999; 281:172–179.
5. Maggioni AP, Zuanetti G, Franzosi MG, Rovelli F, Santoro E, et al. Prevalence and prognostic significance of ventricular arrhythmias after acute myocardial infarction in the fibrinolytic era: GISSI-2 results. Circulation 1993; 87(2):312–322.
6. Beta-Blocker Heart Attack Trial Research Group. A randomized trial of propranolol in patients with acute myocardial infarction. JAMA 1982; 247:17107–1714.
7. Julian DG, Jackson FS, Prescott RJ, Szekely P. Controlled trial of sotalol for one year after myocardial infarction. Lancet 1982; 1:1142–1147.
8. Julian DG, Camm AJ, Frangin G, et al. Randomized trial of effect of amiodarone on mortality in patients with left ventricular dysfunction after recent myocardial infarction. Lancet 1997; 349:667–674.
9. Cairns JA, Connolly SJ, Roberts R, et al. Randomized trial of outcome after myocardial infarction in patients with frequent or repetitive ventricular premature depolarizations. Lancet 1997; 349:675–682.
10. The Cardiac Arrhythmia Suppression Trial (CAST) Investigators. Preliminary report: effect of encainide and flecainide on mortality in a randomized trial of arrhythmia suppression after myocardial infarction. N Engl J Med 1989; 321:406–412.
11. The Cardiac Arrhythmia Suppression Trial II Investigators. Effect of the antiarrhythmic agent moricizine on survival after myocardial infarction. N Engl J Med 1992; 327:227–233.
12. Lombardi G, Gallagher J, Gennis P. Outcome of out-of-hospital cardiac arrest in New York City. JAMA 1994; 271:678–683.

13. Eisenberg MS, Horwood BT, Cummins RO, Reynolds-Haertle R, Hearne TR. Cardiac arrest and resuscitation: a tale of 29 cities. Ann Emerg Med 1990; 19:179–186.
14. Buxton AE, Fisher JD, Josephson ME, et al. Prevention of sudden death in patients with coronary artery disease: the Multicenter Unsustained Tachycardia Trial (MUSTT). Prog Cardiovasc Dis 1993; 36:215–226.
15. Gomes JAC, Hariman RI, Kang PS, El-Sherif N, Chowdhry I, et al. Programmed electrical stimulation in patients with high-grade ectopy: electrophysiologic findings and prognosis for survival. Circulation 1984; 70:43–51.
16. Klein RC, Machell C. Use of electrophysiologic testing in patients with nonsustained VT: prognostic and therapeutic implications. J Am Coll Cardiol 1989; 14:155–61.
17. Wilber DJ, Olshansky B, Moran JF, Scanlol PJ. Electrophysiological testing and nonsustained VT: use and limitations in patients with coronary artery disease and impaired ventricular function. Circulation 1990; 82:350–358.
18. Prystowsky EN. Electrophysiologic-electropharmacologic testing in patients with ventricular arrhythmias. PACE 1988; 11:225–251.
19. Buxton AE, Lee KL, Fisher JD, Josephson ME, Prystowsky EN, et al., for the Multicenter Unsustained Tachycardia Trial Investigators. Randomized, controlled study of the primary prevention of sudden death in patients with coronary artery disease. (submitted for publication).
20. Moss AJ, Hall WJ, Cannom DS, et al., for the Multicenter Automatic Defibrillator Implanatation Trial Investigators. Improved survival with an implanted defibrillator in patients with coronary disease at high risk for ventricular arrhythmia. N Engl J Med 1996; 335:1933–1940.

# 39

# Value of Left Ventricular Function Stratification

*Karl Isaaz, MD*

## Introduction

The extent of left ventricular dysfunction is one of the most important predictors of subsequent cardiac events after acute myocardial infarction. Although ejection fraction is the most popular index, many other parameters may be of importance for left ventricular function stratification. Table 1 summarizes the different parameters that can be measured using noninvasive methods in many cases.

## Left Ventricular Volumes

The GISSI-3 trial[1] showed, in a cohort of 8,606 patients, that a left ventricular end-diastolic volume greater than 112 mL is associated with a 2-fold increase in mortality at 6 months after acute myocardial infarction. End-systolic volume has been shown to represent also a strong independent predictor of survival after myocardial infarction.[1-4] In their study, White et al.[2] found that, compared with end-diastolic volume and ejection fraction, end-systolic volume was the best predictor of prognosis in patients after myocardial infarction. In the GISSI-3 trial, patients with an end-systolic volume greater than 57.6 mL have a 6-month mortality rate 2 to 3 times higher than those with lower end-systolic volumes.[1]

## Left Ventricular Mass

Due to remodeling, left ventricular mass often increases after myocardial infarction. Augmentation of left ventricular mass has been shown to be an independent predictor of cardiac death, in particular, sudden cardiac death, in patients with hypertensive heart disease.[4,5] Cardiac mortality in hypertensive patients might be due to ventricular arrhythmias triggered by transient myo-

From: Aliot E, Clementy J, Prystowsky EN (editors). *Fighting Sudden Cardiac Death: A Worldwide Challenge.* ©Futura Publishing Company, Armonk, NY, 2000.

**Table 1**

**Left Ventricular Function Predictors**

Left ventricular volumes
   end-diastolic volume
   end-systolic volume
Left ventricular mass
   total mass
   infarct mass
Left ventricular geometry
   cavity sphericity
   walls curvature
Baseline systolic function indices
   ejection fraction
   regional wall motion abnormalities
Baseline diastolic function indices
Left ventricular response to stress
   global ventricular response
   regional wall motion response

cardial ischemia.[5,6] Transient myocardial ischemia may result from imbalance between the oxygen demand of the hypertrophied myocardium and the reduced blood supply secondary to microcirculation abnormalities.[5,6]

Although there are few data published in the literature, left ventricular mass should probably be considered an important prognostic marker in patients after myocardial infarction. Bolognese et al.[7] measured left ventricular mass using M-mode echocardiography in 76 patients with a first myocardial infarction and 1-vessel disease at coronary angiogram who were followed-up for 32 ± 6 months. Among 12 evaluated risk factors, including left ventricular mass, age, sex, history of hypertension, smoking, dyslipidemia, infarction location, exercise stress testing, dypiridamole stress echocardiography, angiographic ejection fraction, TIMI flow grade of the infarct-related artery, and severity and location of residual stenosis, the authors found that left ventricular mass was the only independent marker of event-free survival.[7] There was no death in patients with normal left ventricular mass index ($<135$ g/m$^2$ in males and $<112$ g/m$^2$ in females) whereas death rate was 7% in those with increased left ventricular mass index. Analysis of the data presented in Table 2[7] shows that the relationship between left ventricular mass index and the incidence of cardiac events is exponential rather than linear (Figure 1), which supports the crucial prognostic value of this index.

Although coming up with important results, the study by Bolognese et al.[7] suffers from the limitations of left ventricular mass M-mode echocardiographic quantitation in patients with ischemic heart disease. The re-

### Table 2
### Left Ventricular Mass Components

Global left ventricular mass
Dysfunctional myocardium mass
  necrotic mass
  viable mass
Remote myocardium mass
  hypertrophy
  dilation
Cells mass and fibrous mass

gional wall motion abnormalities observed in these patients make difficult the evaluation of left ventricular mass through simple M-mode echocardiographic measurements. Moreover, as shown in Table 2, different components of the myocardial mass can contribute to the global left ventricular mass increase after myocardial infarction. It would be interesting to separate these different mass components and to evaluate their relative contribution to the increase of global left ventricular mass after myocardial infarction as well as their individual prognostic weight. M-mode echocar-

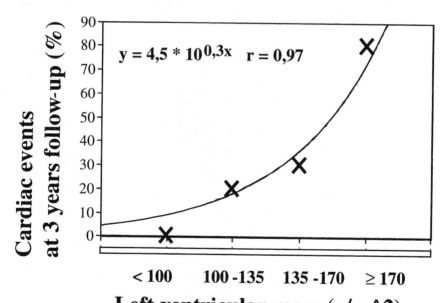

Figure 1. Relationship between left ventricular mass and cardiac events (extrapolated from curve-fitting analysis of the data presented in Table 2.)[7]

diography does not distinguish the relative contribution of each of the components to the increase of global left ventricular mass.

Attempts to estimate the infarct mass based on the quantitation of dysfunctional regional left ventricular mass have been made recently in canine experimental studies using 2- and 3-dimensional echocardiography.[8,9] However, estimates of the infarct mass from baseline echocardiographic quantitation of dysfunctional mass do not allow separating the noncontractile but viable myocardial mass from the irreversible necrotic myocardial mass. Mass estimation based on echocardiographic measurements performed during baseline as well as under a low dose of dobutamine would permit circumventing this limitation. However, poor echogenicity, often observed in humans, especially in patients with ischemic heart disease, still remains a technical limitation for a systemic stratification in a clinical setting. In the future, one can expect that improved noninvasive imaging technologies, with improvement in volume quantitation and tissue characterization by ultrasound and magnetic resonance imaging, will provide a more precise assessment of left ventricular mass in patients after myocardial infarction.

## Left Ventricular Geometry

Remodeling of the infarct and noninfarct regions after myocardial infarction leads to dilation of the left ventricular cavity, which becomes more spherical with regional endocardial curvature abnormalities.[8,10–14] The prognostic role of a left ventricular spherical shape has been demonstrated in patients with dilated cardiomyopathy, the mortality being higher in patients with a greater left ventricular diastolic short axis to long axis ratio.[15,16] Lamas et al.[14] reported data from the SAVE trial concerning the prognostic role of left ventricular geometry after myocardial infarction. From the initial SAVE trial cohort, 727 patients underwent left ventriculography 16 days after myocardial infarction. Left ventriculograms were analyzed for volumes, extent of regional wall motion abnormality, global left ventricular sphericity, and endocardial curvature. Among the 727 patients, mitral regurgitation was present in 141 patients but was severe in only 2 patients. Regurgitation was grade I in 106 patients and grade II in 33 patients. The presence of mitral regurgitation, which was mild in the vast majority of patients, was found by the authors to be an independent predictor of cardiovascular mortality during a follow-up of 3.5 years.[14] Patients with mitral regurgitation did not differ from those without regurgitation regarding ejection fraction and the total degree of wall motion abnormalities but they had more spherical chambers and greater regional endocardial curvature abnormalities.[14] Therefore, the authors[14] suggested that the poorer prognosis of patients with mitral regurgitation was not due to a larger infarct size but that subtle geometric abnormalities must be considered.

# Baseline Systolic Left Ventricular Function

## Ejection Fraction

Among the indices of left ventricular systolic function, ejection fraction is widely used since it is relatively easy to measure. Many studies have demonstrated the central role of ejection fraction as a prognosis predictor after myocardial infarction. The relationship between ejection fraction and mortality is curvilinear, the cardiac mortality increasing exponentially when ejection fraction decreases below 40%.[17,18]

However, although ejection fraction appears to be a good predictor of mortality after myocardial infarction, this global index suffers from significant limitations that may alter its prognostic significance in some cases. Indeed, load condition changes induced by blood pressure or volemia modifications, or hyperkinesia of the remote normal walls, may lead to transient modifications of ejection fraction and make difficult the interpretation of this prognostic index. Other parameters of systolic function should probably be considered for stratification.

## Regional Wall Motion Abnormalities

Investigators of the GISSI-3 trial showed, using univariate analysis, that patients with wall motion asynergy <27% at predischarge had a lower 6-month mortality (2.2%, 173/7,810) than patients with wall motion asynergy ≥27% (6.6%, 222/3,358, p<0.001).[1] In a smaller population of 95 patients with a follow-up of 32 ± 17 months, Nijland et al. also reported, using univariate analysis, an increased mortality rate in patients with a wall motion score index >1.76 when compared to patients with a score index ≤1.76 (p<0.0001).[3]

## Do Measures of Regional Wall Motion Abnormalities Add Independent Prognostic Information to Ejection Fraction?

Despite identical ejection fraction, patients may have different scores of regional wall motion abnormalities. Weissler et al.[17] showed that measures of regional wall motion abnormalities augmented the mortality risk discriminating power of left ventricular ejection fraction early after myocardial infarction. More recently, Miller et al.[18] confirmed that quantitative measurements of regional asynergy add independent prognostic information to global left ventricular ejection fraction. These authors[18] showed that the strength of the association between overall mortality and one index of nonuniform segmental contractility based on the calculation of regional ejection fraction dispersion was stronger than for the association between mortality and global ejection fraction ($\times 2 = 26.4$, p<0.001 versus $\times 2 = 21.5$, p<0.001). For patients with global ejection fraction <40%, 4-year survival was 87% for those with a low asynergy index versus 65% for those with a high asynergy index (p = 0.016).[18]

## Baseline Diastolic Left Ventricular Function

Recent studies have stressed the prognostic role of left ventricular diastolic dysfunction evaluated by Doppler echocardiography after myocardial infarction.[3,19,20] Sakata et al.,[20] in a study of 206 patients after myocardial infarction, showed that the 5-year mortality rate was significantly higher in patients with a low Doppler transmitral atrial wave, (< mean–2SD of age-adjusted normal subjects) compared to those with an atrial wave of normal magnitude (p<0.001). Nijland et al.,[3] in their series of 95 patients after myocardial infarction, on a follow-up of 32 ± 17 months, found that a restrictive left ventricular filling pattern (defined as peak velocity of early diastolic filling wave/peak velocity of late filling wave ≥2 or between 1 and 2 with a deceleration time ≤140 ms) was associated with a lower survival rate. Among all indices including enzymatic infarct size, heart failure during hospital stay, left ventricular volumes, ejection fraction, and wall motion score index, restrictive filling pattern was found to be the only independent predictor of all-cause cardiac mortality using multivariate Cox analysis.[3]

## Left Ventricular Response to Stress

Corbett et al.[21] showed, 18 years ago, that left ventricular abnormal response to exercise characterized by an increase in end-systolic volume, a decrease in wall motion score, and a failure of ejection fraction to increase with exercise was predictive of major cardiac events at 6 months with high sensitivity and specificity. Sensitivity in predicting death was 100% for absence of ejection fraction increase, for increase of end-systolic volume, and for decrease in wall motion score.[21] Specificity was 96% for absence of ejection fraction increase and for increase of end-systolic volume and was 89% for decrease in wall motion score.[21] More recently, Coletta et al.[22] reported that an abnormal end-diastolic volume response during dobutamine stress echocardiography (<10% decrease in volume) was an independent predictor of all cardiac events including cardiac death, nonfatal myocardial infarction, congestive heart failure, and unstable angina.

Quintana et al.[23] studied the prognostic value of regional wall motion abnormalities during exercise in 75 patients who had had a myocardial infarction; exercise stress testing was performed at 7 ± 4 days after myocardial infarction and a 2-dimensional echocardiography study was obtained at baseline and during exercise. ST depression and heart rate variability during ambulatory electrocardiography at 4 ± 2 days were also evaluated; the follow-up was 36 ± 15 months. Twenty-three variables derived from clinical history and examination, ambulatory electrocardiography, baseline echocardiography, exercise stress testing, and stress echocardiography appeared to be predictors of mortality by univariate analysis.[23] Among these 23 covariables, the only remaining independent predictors of mortality found by multivariate analysis were the presence of a new-onset wall motion abnormality during stress echocardiography (p<0.0001, relative risk 13.5, 95% confidence interval 3.6–51.3), ST depression during ambulatory electrocardiography (p=0.003, relative risk 5.0, 95% confidence interval 1.7–15.7), and a decreased heart rate variability (p=0.007).[23]

## Conclusion

Evaluation of left ventricular function is essential in postmyocardial infarction risk stratification. Ejection fraction, an important parameter that is widely used, suffers from limitations that may alter the actual prognostic significance of this index in some cases. The percent of infarct mass evaluated by low-dose dobutamine echocardiography might conceptually represent a prognosis-relevant parameter, but this deserves further study. Evaluation of diastolic function appears to be promising. The role of new imaging techniques in current practice, such as 3-dimensional echocardiography and magnetic resonance imaging, has to be defined in the future. Although there are many studies published in the literature, the heterogeneity of the methods does not allow definitive ranking of the various left ventricular indices that have been reported so far. There is a need for further studies, based on a follow-up of large cohorts of patients in whom all the previously reported prognostic parameters would be systematically evaluated. Finally, when analyzing the prognostic role of left ventricular function indices from current published data, it still remains difficult to differentiate sudden cardiac death from death due to a progressive and irreversible deterioration of pump function.

## References

1. The GISSI-3 Trial Investigators. The prognostic value of predischarge quantitative two-dimensional echocardiographic measurements and the effects of early lisinopril treatment on left ventricular structure and function after acute myocardial infarction in the GISSI-3 trial. Eur Heart J 1996; 17:1646–1656.
2. White HD, Norris RM, Brown MA, et al. Left ventricular end-systolic volume as the major determinant of survival after recovery from myocardial infarction. Circulation 1987; 76:44.

3. Nijland F, Kamp O, Karreman AJP, et al. Prognostic implications of restrictive left ventricular filling in acute myocardial infarction: a serial Doppler echocardiographic study. J Am Coll Cardiol 1997; 30:1618–1624.
4. Levy D, Garrison RJ, Savage DD, Kannel WB, Castelli WP. Prognostic implications of echocardiographically determined left ventricular mass in the Framingham Heart Study. N Engl J Med 1990; 322:1561–1566.
5. Zehender M, Faber T, Koscheck U, Meinertz T, Just H. Ventricular tachyarrhythmias, myocardial ischemia, and sudden cardiac death in patients with hypertensive heart disease. Clin Cardiol 1995; 18:377–383.
6. Scheler S, Motz, W, Strauer BE. Transiente myokardischamie bei hypertonikern. Z Kardiol 1989; 78:197–203.
7. Bolognese L, Dellavesa P, Rossi L, et al. Prognostic value of left ventricular mass in uncomplicated acute myocardial infarction and one-vessel coronary artery disease. Am J Cardiol 1994; 73:1–5.
8. Jugdutt BI, Khan MI, Jugdutt SJ, et al. Combined captopril and isosorbide dinitrate during healing after myocardial infarction: effect on ventricular remodeling, function, mass and collagen. J Am Coll Cardiol 1995; 25:1089–1096.
9. Yao J, Cao QL, Masani N, et al. Three-dimensional echocardiographic estimation of infarct mass based on quantification of dysfunctional left ventricular mass. Circulation 1997; 96:1660–1666.
10. Jugdutt BI, Warnica JW. Intravenous nitroglycerin therapy to limit myocardial infarct size, expansion, and infarct location. Circulation 1988; 78:906–919.
11. Pfeffer MA, Braunwald E. Ventricular remodeling after myocardial infarction. Circulation 1990; 81:1161–1172.
12. Jugdutt BI. Prevention of ventricular remodeling post-myocardial infarction: timing and duration of therapy. Can J Cardiol 1993; 9:103–114.
13. Jugdutt BI, Khan MI. Effect of prolonged nitrate therapy on left ventricular remodeling after canine acute myocardial infarction. Circulation 1994; 89:2297–2307.
14. Lamas GA, Mitchell GF, Flaker GC, et al. Clinical significance of mitral regurgitation after acute myocardial infarction. Circulation 1997; 96:827–833.
15. Douglas PS, Morrow R, Ioli A, et al. Left ventricular shape, afterload and survival in idiopathic dilated cardiomyopathy. J Am Coll Cardiol 1989; 13:311–315.
16. Matitiau A, Perez-Atayde A, Sanders SP, et al. Infantile dilated cardiomyopathy: relation of outcome to left ventricular mechanics, hemodynamics, and histology at the time of presentation. Circulation 1994; 90:1310–1318.
17. Weissler AM, Miller BI, Granger CB, et al. Augmentation of mortality risk discriminating power of left ventricular ejection fraction by measures of nonuniformity in systolic emptying on radionuclide angiography. J Am Coll Cardiol 1990; 16:387–395.
18. Miller TD, Weissler AM, Christian TF, et al. Quantitative measures of regional asynergy add independent prognostic information to left ventricular ejection fraction in patients with prior myocardial infarction. Am Heart J 1997; 133:640–647.
19. Pozzoli M, Capomolla S, Sanarico M, et al. Doppler evaluations of left ventricular diastolic filling and pulmonary wedge pressure provide similar prognostic information in patients with systolic dysfunction after myocardial infarction. Am Heart J 1995; 129:716–725.
20. Sakata K, Kashiro S, Hirato S, et al. Prognostic value of Doppler transmitral flow velocity patterns in acute myocardial infarction. Am J Cardiol 1997; 79:1165–1169.
21. Corbett JR, Dehmer GJ, Lewis SE, et al. The prognostic value of submaximal ex-

ercise testing with radionuclide ventriculography before hospital discharge in patients with recent myocardial infarction. Circulation 1981; 64:535–544.

22. Coletta C, Galati A, Sestili A, et al. Prognostic value of left ventricular volume response during dobutamine stress echocardiography. Eur Heart J 1997; 18:1599–1605.

23. Quintana M, Lindvall K, Brolund F, et al. Markers of risk after myocardial infarction: a comparison of clinical variables, ambulatory and exercise electrocardiography, echocardiography, and stress echocardiography. Coronary Artery Dis 1997; 8:327–334.

## 40

# Nonsustained Ventricular Tachycardia: Prognostic and Therapeutic Considerations

*Nadir Saoudi, MD, Frederic Anselme, MD, Maxime Chalumeau, MD, Arnaud Savoure, MD, and Alain Cribier, MD*

## Introduction

In cardiology textbooks, the electrocardiograhic diagnosis of ventricular tachycardia (VT) is suggested by the occurrence of a series of 3 or more consecutive, bizarrely shaped premature ventricular complexes whose duration exceeds 120 ms, with the ST-T vector pointing opposite to the major QRS deflection.[1] When VT is not prolonged beyond 30 seconds or does not require an intervention for termination, it is called nonsustained ventricular tachycardia (NSVT). The clinical interest in this pathological condition increased considerably when it was suggested that it was frequently associated with increased mortality. In this chapter, we review the potential importance of NSVT in various clinical conditions and address the still controversial issue of its treatment.

## Prognostic Value of Spontaneous NSVT in Various Clinical Conditions

### Chronic Coronary Artery Disease

Studies assessing the potential impact on prognosis of NSVT in coronary artery disease were published mainly in the early 1980s. During this period (which was before the thrombolytic era), it was shown that the presence of frequent and/or complex ventricular arrhythmias was an independent risk factor for subsequent mortality in patients recovering from

From: Aliot E, Clementy J, Prystowsky EN (editors). *Fighting Sudden Cardiac Death: A Worldwide Challenge.* ©Futura Publishing Company, Armonk, NY, 2000.

acute myocardial infarction (MI),[2-5] yet fibrinolysis is known to affect the natural history of infarction. As a consequence, it has been suggested that it could also alter the clinical relevance of this risk factor.[6]

In a subanalysis of the GISSI-2 patients cohort, Maggioni et al. studied the outcome of 8,676 patients with a first MI.[6] Twenty-four-hour Holter recordings obtained before hospital discharge were analyzed for the presence of ventricular arrhythmias and patients were followed for 6 months. Overall ventricular arrhythmias were present in 64.1% of the cases and NSVT was present in 6.8% of the patients. There were 256 deaths, 84 of which were sudden cardiac deaths. Mortality rates were 2% in patients without ventricular arrhythmias, 2.7% in patients with 1–10 premature ventricular beats (PVBs)/hour, 5.5% in those with more than 10 PVBs/hour, and 4.8% in those with complex PVBs. The presence of >10 PVBs/hour was significantly associated with a higher mortality rate independently of the ejection fraction. But, importantly, after adjusting for other risk factors, the presence of more than 10 PVBs/hour remained a significant and independent predictor of total and sudden cardiac death whereas NSVT was not. It was concluded from this particularly wide-scale and well-conducted study that if frequent PVBs are confirmed as independent risk factors of total and sudden death in the first 6 months following acute infarction, the significance of the presence of NSVT appears more controversial.

The impact on nonsustained ventricular arrhythmia on sexual activity of patients with chronic coronary artery disease has also been addressed in one study.[7] It was found that in 88 male patients aged 36–66, rhythm disturbances were not exacerbated during intercourse with the regular partner in most patients. If ventricular ectopic activity occurred during intercourse, it was most often simple and essentially similar to disturbances in daily activity.

Other prognosis factors related to the characteristics of NSVT have been studied. Beat-to-beat changes in the cycle lengths of NSVT or ventricular rate variability have been suggested as prognosis factors in patients with malignant ventricular arrhythmias or sudden cardiac death in the late post-MI period. In a cohort of 165 men and 26 women who had NSVT runs on 24-hour Holter monitoring obtained at least 30 days after myocardial infarction, descriptors such as gender, age ≥60 years, left ventricular ejection fraction (LVEF) of less than 40%, ventricular rate variability <30 ms, frequent PVBs (≥30/hour), NSVT rate ≥150 beats/min, and duration of NSVT ≥10 beats were evaluated. In this study, it was shown that in patients who died suddenly, ventricular heart variability was significantly reduced compared to those patients without sudden death. When all-cause mortality was considered, ventricular heart variability was again markedly lower in patients who died than in survivors.[8]

## Acute Myocardial Infarction

The incidence of sustained monomorphic VT within the first 48 hours of acute MI ranges from 0.3% to 1.9%, whereas in its nonsustained form, the incidence in acute MI has generally been reported to be in the range of 1% to 7%.[9,10] Since Eldar did not observe any adverse effect on either in-hospital or 1-year survival of primary NSVT in 49 patients, it has been suggested that its prognostic significance in acute MI was more similar to that of PVC than to that of sustained VT.[11] In a prospective study, 112 patients with NSVT within 72 hours of acute MI were compared to a control group of matched patients. Thrombolytic therapy was administered in about one-third of patients in each group. In-hospital ventricular fibrillation occurred more frequently in the NSVT group (9% versus 0%), but total in-hospital (10% versus 4%) and 34-month mortality (10% versus 17%) did not differ between the 2 groups. Multivariate analysis identified time from presentation to occurrence of NSVT as the strongest predictor of mortality. The increased relative risk of NSVT was first significant when it occurred 13 hours from presentation and continued to increase as the time from presentation to occurrence of NSVT increased, plateauing at a relative risk of 7.5 at 24 hours. From this study, it was concluded that although NSVT that occurs within the first several hours of presentation does not have an associated adverse prognosis, NSVT that occurs later is associated with a significant increase in risk. The reason for this is unclear, but since most of the mortality in this study was early mortality, NSVT that occurred beyond 13 hours may be a marker of persistent ischemia, left ventricular dysfunction, or electrophysiological instability. Another explanation could be a protective effect of early nonsustained ventricular arrhythmias on reperfusion-induced arrhythmia as suggested in animal models.[12]

## Congestive Heart Failure

Heart failure patients with ventricular arrhythmia and NSVT have a significantly increased risk of premature cardiac death.[13,14] Similar to coronary artery disease, it has been discussed whether these arrhythmias are expressions of a severely compromised ventricle or are independent risk factors. In the GESICA study, the predictive value of NSVT as a marker for sudden death or death due to progressive heart failure was studied in 516 patients among whom 33.4% had NSVT.[14] After a follow-up of 2 years, approximately 50% of the patients with and 30% of those without NSVT had died. Sudden death significantly increased from 8.7% to 23.7%, whereas heart failure death rose nonsignificantly from 17.5% to 20.8%. From this study it was concluded that NSVT in the setting of heart failure is an independent marker for increased overall mortality rate and sudden death. In contrast, in an analysis of the CHF-STAT data, Singh et al. showed that NSVT was present in 80% of patients with PVCs and heart failure while on vasodilator therapy.[15] Patients without NSVT had significantly fewer beta-adrenergic blocking agents and a higher ejection fraction. Survival analysis showed a greater risk of death among patients with NSVT. However, after multiple variables adjustment, only ejection fraction and NYHA Class were shown to be independent predictors of survival. The fact that NSVT was not an independent predictor suggests that suppression of this arrhythmia may indeed not improve survival. The reason for the discrepancies between both studies have been attributed to patient population differences, but mostly to methodological differences since ejection fraction does not seem to have been included in the multivariate analysis in GESICA.[16] In addition, the reproducibility of NSVT on serial Holter recordings makes in difficult to use these parameters for risk stratification. In a recent article dealing with a particularly large cohort of 1,080 patients with Class III/IV NYHA symptoms and ejection fraction <35%, the presence of NSVT did not again add significant information beyond the clinical variables.[17] In fact, many authors now think that NSVT is not a specific marker for death in congestive heart failure (CHF).

## Hypertrophic Cardiomyopathy

Similar to what has been discussed for CHF, the prognostic significance of ventricular arrhythmias identified on 24-hour ambulatory electrocardiographic monitoring is still controversial in patients with hypertrophic cardiomyopathy (HCM). In the early 1980s, in a population of 99 patients with HCM, high-grade ventricular arrhythmias (grade 3 and above) were seen at baseline in 66% of the patients, and 19% had episodes of asymptomatic VT.[18] After 3 years of follow-up under various forms of therapy including surgery, sudden cardiac death was significantly more common in patients with asymptomatic NSVT (24%) than in patients without VT (3%). It was concluded from this observational study that the finding of VT on Holter identifies a subgroup of patients at high risk for sudden death.[18] Similar observations were made in the European literature at the same time.[19] These observations frequently led to the initiation of antiarrhythmic drug therapy, but more recently this concept has been revisited. In a population of 151 mildly or asymptomatic patients with HCM, 42 had episodes of NSVT, with 35 patients (83%) having between 10 and 19 NSVT beats.[20] Almost 90% of the patients with VT had infrequent episodes of NSVT (≤5 episodes/24 hours). Follow-up averaged 4.8 years. During this period 6 patients died suddenly: 3 in the group with VT and 3 in the group without VT. Thus the sudden death rate was 1.4% per year in patients with and 0.6% in those without VT. The total cardiac mortality rate was 1.4% per year in the patients with VT and 0.9% in those without VT. This study showed that cardiac mortality is low in patients with HCM who are asymptomatic or only mildly symptomatic and have brief NSVT on Holter monitoring. This suggests that NSVT may not be considered, per se, as an indication for antiarrhythmic treatment in such patients.

Another very recent retrospective multicenter study dealing with the outcome of patients with HCM suggests that in high-risk patients implanted defibrillators may be useful for prevention of sudden death.[21] Out of 128 patients, defibrillators have been implanted in 83 cases for primary prevention of sudden death and followed for a mean of 3.1 years. Reasons for implantation included NSVT in 32 cases, sometimes associated with other risk factors. Only 2 patients in this subgroup had appropriate discharges during follow-up. Due to the retrospective design and the lack of control group in this study, and as acknowledged by the authors, it is difficult to draw any firm conclusions regarding primary prevention of sudden death in this subgroup, but it seems that occasionally NSVT precedes sustained ventricular arrhythmias for which defibrillators may be lifesaving.

## Indications for Ambulatory ECG Arrhythmia Detection to Assess Risk for Future Cardiac Events in Patients without Symptoms from Arrhythmia

In 1999 the American College of Cardiology and the American Heart association jointly published guidelines for ambulatory electrocardiographic monitoring that are pertinent to this review.[22] As expected because of the low positive predictive value of NSVT for prediction of future arrhythmic event or death in the various types of heart disease in which it has been assessed, there is no Class I indicator for Holter monitoring in asymptomatic patients. Patients with marked LV dysfunction after MI and patients with CHF or idiopathic HCM may benefit from ambulatory ECG recording for risk assessment, but this is considered a Class IIb indication. Class II means that there is conflicting evidence and/or divergence of opinion about the usefulness of the procedure. Within the Class II indications, Class IIa means that the weight of opinion is in favor of usefulness whereas for Class IIb it is less well established by evidence/opinion.[23] Interestingly, in these practice guidelines, there is no indication of ambulatory recording for risk stratification in patients with systemic hypertension and LV hypertrophy in patients with valvular heart disease or in postinfarction patients with normal LV function.

# Role of Electrophysiological Study in Risk Stratification in Patients with Spontaneous NSVT

## Electrophysiological Study and NSVT in Chronic Coronary Artery Disease

As discussed above, information about pump function is of prime importance to construct a risk profile after MI. The combination of frequent and complex ventricular ectopies as independent markers of increased risk of sudden death and the disappointing results of the CAST study prompted the search for an additional specific test for risk stratification in patients with NSVT.[24] In 1990, a baseline electrophysiological study (EPS) was performed in 100 patients with spontaneous asymptomatic NSVT, chronic coronary artery disease (CAD), and ejection fraction below 40%.[25] Sustained monomorphic VT was induced in 37 patients, and polymorphic VT or ventricular fibrillation in 6 patients. Fifty-seven patients without inducible sustained ventricular arrhythmias were discharged on no antiarrhythmic therapy. Twenty inducible patients were discharged on drug therapy that resulted in suppression of inducible sustained ventricular arrhythmias. The remaining patients with persistently inducible sustained arrhythmias were discharged on drug therapy, resulting in maximal rate slowing of the induced tachycardia. During a follow-up of 16.7 months, the 2-year actuarial incidence of recurrent cardiac arrests or sudden death was 6% in patients without inducible sustained ventricular arrhythmias, 11% in patients in whom inducible arrhythmias were suppressed, and 50% in patients with persistently inducible sustained ventricular arrhythmias. Multivariate analysis identified only the persistence of inducible sustained ventricular arrhythmias as a significant independent predictor of sudden death or recurrent sustained arrhythmias. Like others, these authors suggested in the early 1990s that in this patient population, programmed stimulation could be used to identify a low-risk population or the best possible antiarrhythmic treatment.[26,27]

## Dilated Cardiomyopathy

Contrary to coronary artery disease, the role of EPS in assessing the prognosis of dilated cardiomyopathy remains controversial. Early studies encompassed relatively small numbers of patients (the largest one being 92)[28] with varying protocols, and discordant results.[29–31] More recently, this issue has been readdressed in the light of the powerful analysis tool that is the implantable defibrillator.[33] Thirty-four patients with dilated cardiomyopathy, a LVEF ≤35%, and spontaneous NSVT underwent EPS and were prospectively followed for 24±13 months. Sustained ventricular arrhythmias were induced in 13 patients (38%). Prophylactic implantation of an ICD with electrogram storage capability was performed in all inducible patients and in 9 others who were not inducible. Serious arrhythmic events during follow-up occurred in 31% of inducible patients and in 24% who were not, the difference being nonsignificant. It seems, therefore, that EPS does not appear to be helpful for arrhythmia risk stratification in patients with dilated cardiomyopathy, a low LVEF, and spontaneous NSVT.

## Indications for EPS in NSVT

In 1995, guidelines for clinical intracardiac electrophysiological and catheter ablation procedures were developed and published by the American College of Cardiology/American Heart Association Task Force on Practice Guidelines in collaboration with the North American Society of Pacing and Electrophysiology.[33] As suggested by the low positive predictive value of NSVT alone, there was no Class I indication.

Two sets of patients were considered as Class II indication for EPS. In patients with other risk factors for future arrhythmic events (such as low LVEF, positive signal-averaged ECG, NSVT on Holter), EPS may be used for further risk assessment, and for guiding therapy in patients with inducible VT. EPS may be proposed in these patients with highly symptomatic uniform morphology PVC, couplets, and NSVT who are considered potential candidates for catheter ablation.

## Therapeutic Interventions in NSVT

### Drug Therapy

#### Beta-Blocker Therapy in NSVT

There is compelling evidence that occurrence of ventricular arrhythmia and survival are influenced by stimulation or blockade of the autonomic nervous system in various clinical conditions, mostly, but not exclusively, in the context of impaired ventricular function.[34–36] They have been shown to reduce mortality in children with polymorphic VT.[37] Although there is no study directly addressing the prognosis as a function of the use of these drugs in the context of purely NSVT, it has been shown that they are cost effective in the context of coronary artery disease.[38] In the CAST study, beta-blocker therapy was independently associated with longer time to occurrence of new or worsened CHF, supporting the secondary preventive benefit of beta-blocker therapy in high-risk post-MI patients, and calling attention to its possible preventive benefit against proarrhythmic events.[39] It appears wise to advise adrenergic blockade as first-line therapy whenever possible in heart disease with impaired ventricular function associated with NSVT.

## Amiodarone and NSVT

In the early 1990s, amiodarone was considered useful in symptomatic complex arrhythmias with a possible beneficial influence on mortality.[40,41] In the GESICA study, the effect of low-dose amiodarone on the mortality in 516 patients with severe chronic heart failure but without symptomatic ventricular arrhythmias was evaluated. Patients were randomized to 300 mg/day amiodarone or to standard treatment. There were 87 deaths in the amiodarone group and 106 in the control group. Both sudden and heart failure death were significantly reduced, with fewer patients in the amiodarone group being admitted to hospital due to worsening heart failure. The decrease in mortality and hospital admission was, however, independent of the presence of NSVT.[14] The authors pointed out that the decrease in mortality that was obtained was greater than would be expected from a drug that reduces death only through an antiarrhythmic effect.

Another large mortality trial using amiodarone was published approximately at the same period.[42] Six hundred seventy-four patients with CHF, 10 or more PVBs/hour, and a LVEF $\leq 40\%$ were randomly assigned to receive amiodarone or placebo. After a median follow-up of 45 months, contrary to the GESICA trial, there was no significant difference in overall mortality between the 2 treatment groups. The 2-year actuarial survival rate was 69.4% for the patients in the amiodarone group and 70.8% in the placebo group. At 2 years, the sudden death rate was not significantly different between both groups (15% in the amiodarone group and 19% in the placebo group). Yet amiodarone was significantly effective in suppressing ventricular arrhythmias. In the placebo group, 76% of the patients continued to have episodes of VT 2 weeks after randomization, whereas in the amiodarone group, only 33% of the patients had VT episodes at 2 weeks (77% at baseline). Similarly, there was no significant difference in mortality between the group of 111 patients in whom episodes of VT were eliminated by amiodarone at 2 weeks and the group of 65 patients in whom such episodes continued to occur. The lack of benefit of amiodarone on survival in patients with complex ventricular arrhythmias had already been reported in a smaller trial,[43] yet other earlier small trials had reported results similar to that of GESICA.[44,45] As explained above, the differences in outcome between GESICA and CHF-STAT has been explained mostly in terms of population differences since the proportion of patients with coronary artery disease in the GESICA trial was smaller (39%) than in the other study (70%). This difference is important, since in CHF-STAT there was a trend toward a reduction in mortality among the patients with non-ischemic cardiomyopathy.

## Nonpharmacological Therapy: The Implantable Automatic Cardioverter-Defibrillator

The use of electrophysiological testing for stratification of patients at high risk for severe arrhythmia in patients with NSVT logically prompted the start of studies on the effect of the defibrillator in these populations.[24,27]

### The Multicenter Automatic Defibrillator Implantation Trial

Prophylactic therapy with an ICD was compared to conventional medical therapy in 196 patients with prior MI, an LVEF ≤0.35, documented episodes of asymptomatic NSVT, and inducible, nonsuppressible ventricular tachyarrhythmia on EPS. Ninety-five patients were randomly assigned to receive an ICD and 101 were assigned to conventional medical therapy. During a follow-up of 27 months, there were 15 deaths in the defibrillator group (11 from cardiac causes) and 39 deaths in the conventional therapy group (27 from cardiac causes). There was no evidence that amiodarone, beta blockers, or any other antiarrhythmic therapy had a significant influence on the observed outcome. This study was the first one to clearly and nonambiguously show an improved survival in patients with a high risk for ventricular tachyarrhythmia when prophylactic therapy with an ICD was compared with conventional medical therapy. A follow-up to MADIT, MADIT-2, is currently enrolling patients with prior MI, LVEF ≤0.30, and arrhythmias no more advanced than premature ventricular contractions or couplets.

Another study, the Coronary Artery Bypass Graft (CABG) Patch Trial, evaluated the prophylactic use of ICDs in patients undergoing coronary revascularization surgery.[47] In this study, the high risk of death due to arrhythmia was considered to be indicated by a noninvasive marker—an abnormal signal-averaged electrocardiogram—and by an ejection fraction below 36%. No benefit was conferred by ICD in this trial. In this study, no attention was paid to the presence of NSVT. It would be helpful to the clinician to be able to generalize indications for defibrillator therapy based on noninvasive markers. However, as emphasized by Myerburg, on the basis of the few trials reported so far, the opposing outcomes of the MADIT and the CABG Patch Trial warn us to be careful in implantation decision.[48]

## The Multicenter Unsustained Tachycardia Trial

The hypothesis that antiarrhythmic therapy guided by electrophysiological testing can reduce the risks of sudden death and cardiac arrest among patients with coronary artery disease, LVEF ≤40%, and spontaneous NSVT has been addressed in the recently published Multicenter Unsustained Tachycardia Trial (MUSTT).[49] This study was a controlled trial in which patients were randomly assigned to receive either antiarrhythmic therapy (including drugs and ICDs) as indicated by the results of electrophysiological testing, or no antiarrhythmic therapy. After a median time between MI and enrollment of 39 months, 2,002 patients were enrolled, among which 764 were inducible. Finally, the study incorporated 704 patients in whom sustained ventricular tachyarrhythmias were induced by programmed stimulation. The median follow-up duration was 39 months. Interestingly, patients assigned to the "no antiarrhythmic therapy" group more often received agents with beta-blocking properties than those in the "electrophysiologically guided" group (51% versus 29%). In this latter group, 202 patients (58%) received defibrillators whereas among the patients assigned to no antiarrhythmic therapy only 3% had received a defibrillator by the last follow-up. Total mortality rates after 2 and 5 years were 28% and 48%, respectively, for the patients in the "no antiarrhythmic therapy" group, and 22% and 42% for those assigned to electrophysiologically guided therapy. This difference in survival did not reach statistical significance. However, the 5-year rate of cardiac arrest or death from arrhythmia was 9% among the patients assigned to electrophysiologically guided therapy who received a defibrillator, compared to 37% among those in this group who did not receive a defibrillator (p<0.001). The overall mortality rates at 5 years were 24% among the patients who received defibrillators and 55% among those who did not. The survival benefit associated with defibrillator treatment remained significant after adjustments for all available prognostic clinical factors. Similar to what had previously been reported, it was shown in this study that the inducibility rate of sustained tachyarrhythmia in patients presenting with NSVT and chronic coronary disease was 20–45%.[25,26,50,51] The MUSTT study demonstrated that the risk of cardiac arrest or death from arrhythmia is 18% among patients with inducible sustained tachyarrhythmia when no antiarrhythmic therapy was administered over the follow-up period. In this patient population, it appears that electrophysiologically guided antiarrhythmic therapy with ICDs only, but not electrophysiologically guided antiarrhythmic therapy with antiarrhythmic drugs or empiric therapy, reduces the risk of sudden death.

### *Indications for ICD therapy in NSVT*

A recent report of the ACC/AHA task force on device implantation addressed the issue of NSVT.[52] After the MADIT study, NSVT occurring in the setting of coronary disease, prior MI, LV dysfunction, and inducible VF or sustained VT at electrophysiological study that is not suppressible by a Class I antiarrhythmic drug was ranked as Class I with a level of evidence B. Evidence level B means that data, on which the expert opinion is based, were derived from a limited number of trials involving comparatively small numbers of patients or from well-designed data analysis of nonrandomized studies or observational data registries. The same situation but without the notion of suppression by a Class I antiarrhythmic drug was ranked Class IIb with a B level of evidence.

# Conclusion

If NSVT is associated in various clinical conditions with a poor prognosis, it is inconstantly an independent risk marker. However, it may be used as a marker for test selection for further risk stratification.

## References

1. Zipes DP. In: Braunwald E (ed). Heart Disease. Specific Arrhythmias: Diagnosis and Treatment. WB Saunders Co, Philadelphia, 1997.
2. Ruberman W, Weinblatt E, Goldberg JD, Frank CW, Chaudhary BS, et al. Ventricular premature complexes and sudden death after myocardial infarction. Circulation 1981; 64:297–305.
3. The Multicenter Postinfarction Research Group. Risk stratification and survival after myocardial infarction. N Engl J Med 1983; 309:331–336.
4. Kostis JB, Byington R, Friedman LM, Goldstein S, Furberg C, for the BHAT Study Group. Prognostic significance of ventricular ectopic activity in survivors of acute myocardial infarction. J Am Coll Cardiol 1987; 10:231–242.
5. Bigger JT, Weld FM, Rolnitzky LM. Prevalence, characteristics and significance of VT (three or more complexes) detected with ambulatory electrocardiographic recording in the late hospital phase of acute myocardial infarction. Am J Cardiol 1981; 48:815–823.
6. Maggioni AP, Zuanetti G, Franzosi MG, Rovelli F, Santoro E, et al. Prevalence and prognostic significance of ventricular arrhythmias after acute myocardial infarction in the fibrinolytic era: GISSI-2 results. Circulation 1993; 87:312–322.
7. Drory Y, Fisman EZ, Shapira Y, Pines A. Ventricular arrhythmias during sexual activity in patients with coronary artery disease. Chest 1996; 109(4):922–924.
8. Dabrowski A, Kramarz E, Piotrowicz R. Low variability of cycle lengths in

nonsustained ventricular tachycardia as an independent predictor of mortality after myocardial infarction. Am J Cardiol 1997; 80(10):1347–1350.

9. Eldar M, Sievner Z, Goldbourt U, Reicher-Reiss H, Kaplinsky E, et al. Primary ventricular tachycardia in acute myocardial infarction: clinical characteristics and mortality. Ann Intern Med 1992; 117:31–36.

10. Campbell R, Murray A, Julian D. Ventricular arrhythmias in the first 12 hours of acute myocardial infarction. Br Heart J 1981; 46:351–357.

11. Cheema AN, Sheu K, Parker M, Kadish AH, Goldberger JJ. Nonsustained ventricular tachycardia in the setting of acute myocardial infarction: tachycardia characteristics and their prognostic implications. Circulation 1988; 98(19):2030–2036.

12. Sik Na H, Kim YI, Yoon YW, Chul Han H, Nahm SH, et al. Ventricular premature beat driven intermittent restoration of coronary blood flow reduces the incidence of reperfusion induced ventricular fibrillation in a cat model of regional ischemia. Am Heart J 1996; 132:78–83.

13. Packer M. Lack of relation between ventricular arrhythmias and sudden death in patients with chronic heart failure. Circulation 1992; 85(Suppl I):I-50–I-56.

14. Doval H, Nul D, Grancelli H, Varini S, Soifer S, et al., for the GESICA-GEMA Investigators. Nonsustained ventricular tachycardia in severe heart failure: independent marker of increased mortality due to sudden death. Circulation 1996; 94:3198–3202.

15. Singh SN, Fisher SG, Carson PE, Fletcher RD. Prevalence and significance of nonsustained ventricular tachycardia in patients with premature ventricular contractions and heart failure treated with vasodilator therapy. Department of Veterans Affairs CHF STAT Investigators. J Am Coll Cardiol 1988; 32(4):942–947.

16. Singh SN, Carson PE, Fisher SG. Nonsustained ventricular tachycardia in severe heart failure. Circulation 1997; 96(10):3794–3795.

17. Teerlink JR, Jaladuddin M, Anderson S, Kukin ML, Eichorn EJ, et al., on behalf of the PROMISE investigators. Circulation 2000; 101:40–46.

18. Maron BJ, Savage DD, Wolfson JK, Epstein SE. Prognostic significance of 24-hour ambulatory electrocardiographic monitoring in patients with hypertrophic cardiomyopathy: a prospective study. Am J Cardiol 1981; 48(2):252–257.

19. McKenna WJ, England D, Doi YL, Deanfield JE, Oakley C, et al. Arrhythmia in hypertrophic cardiomyopathy. I: Influence on prognosis. Br Heart J 1981; 46(2): 168–172.

20. Spirito P, Rapezzi C, Autore C, Bruzzi P, Bellone P, et al. Prognosis of asymptomatic patients with hypertrophic cardiomyopathy and nonsustained ventricular tachycardia. Circulation 1994; 90(6):2743–2747.

21. Maron BJ, Shen WK, Link MS, Epstein AE, Almquist AK, et al. Efficacy of implantable cardioverter-defibrillators for the prevention of sudden death in patients with hypertrophic cardiomyopathy. N Engl J Med 2000; 342:365–373.

22. Crawford MH, Bernstein SJ, Deedwania PC, DiMarco JP, Ferrick KJ, et al. ACC/AHA guidelines for ambulatory electrocardiography: executive summary and recommendations: a report of the American College of Cardiology/American Heart Association Task Force on Practice Guidelines (Committee to Revise the Guidelines for Ambulatory Electrocardiography). Circulation 1999; 100:886–893.

23. Gregoratos G, Cheitlin MD, Epstein CA, Fellows C, Ferguson BT, et al. ACC/AHA guidelines for implantation of cardiac pacemakers and antiarrhythmia devices: a report of the American College of Cardiology/American Heart Association Task Force on Practice guidelines (Committee on Pacemaker Implantation). J Am Coll Cardiol 1998; 31:1175–1209.

24. The Cardiac Arrhythmia Suppression Trial (CAST) Investigators. Preliminary

report: effect of encaïnide and flecaïnide on mortality in a randomized trial of arrhythmia suppression after myocardial infarction. N Engl J Med 1989; 321: 406–412.

25. Wilber DJ, Olshansky B, Moran JF, Scanlon PJ. Electrophysiological testing and nonsustained ventricular tachycardia: use and limitations in patients with coronary artery disease and impaired ventricular function. Circulation 1990; 82(2):350–358.

26. Buxton AE, Marchlinski FE, Flores BT, Miller JM, Doherty JU, et al. Nonsustained ventricular tachycardia in patients with coronary artery disease: role of electrophysiologic study. Circulation 1987; 75:1178–1185.

27. Spielman SR, Greenspan AN, Kay HR. Electrophysiologic testing in patients at high risk of sudden cardiac death: nonsustained ventricular tachycardia and abnormal ventricular function. J Am Coll Cardiol 1985; 6:31–39.

28. Brembilla-Perrot B, Donetti J, de la Chaise AT, Sadoui N, Aliot E, et al. Diagnostic value of ventricular stimulation in patients with idiopathic dilated cardiomyopathy. Am Heart J 1991; 121:1124–1131.

29. Meinertz T, Treese N, Kasper W, Geibel A, Hofmann T, et al. Determinants of prognosis in idiopathic dilated cardiomyopathy as determined by programmed electrical stimulation. Am J Cardiol 1985; 56(4):337–341.

30. Wellens HJ, Brugada P, Stevenson WG. Programmed electrical stimulation of the heart in patients with life-threatening ventricular arrhythmias: what is the significance of induced arrhythmias and what is the correct stimulation protocol? Circulation 1985: 72(1):1–7.

31. Turrito G, Ahuja RK, Caref EB, El Sherif N. Risk stratification for arrhythmic events in patients with nonischemic dilated cardiomyopathy and nonsustained ventricular tachycardia: role of programmed stimulation and the signal-averaged electrocardiogram. J Am Coll Cardiol 1994; 24:1523–1528.

32. Grimm W, Hoffmann J, Menz V, Luck K, Maisch B. Programmed ventricular stimulation for arrhythmia risk prediction in patients with idiopathic dilated cardiomyopathy and nonsustained ventricular tachycardia. J Am Coll Cardiol 1998; 32(3):739–743.

33. Zipes DP, DiMarco JP, Gillette PC, Jackman WM, Myerburg RJ, et al. Guidelines for clinical intracardiac electrophysiological and catheter ablation procedures. A report of the American College of Cardiology/American Heart Association Task Force on Practice Guidelines (Committee on Clinical Intracardiac Electrophysiologic and Catheter Ablation Procedures), developed in collaboration with the North American Society of Pacing and Electrophysiology. J Am Coll Cardiol 1995; 26(2):555–573.

34. Haim M, Shotan A, Boyko V, Reicher-Reiss H, Benderly M, et al. Effect of betablocker therapy in patients with coronary artery disease in New York Heart Association classes II and III. The Bezafibrate Infarction Prevention (BIP) Study Group. Am J Cardiol 1998; 81(2):1455–1460.

35. Waagstein F, Bristow MR, Swedberg K, Camerini F, Fowler MB, et al., for the Metoprolol in Dilated Cardiomyopathy (MDC) Trial Study Group. Beneficial effects of metoprolol in idiopathic dilated cardiomyopathy. Lancet 1993; 342:1441–1456.

36. Lampert R, Jain D, Burg M, Batsford WP, MacPherson CA. Destabilizing effect of mental stress on ventricular arrhythmias in patients with implantable cardioverter-defibrillators. Circulation 2000; 101:158–164.

37. Leenhardt A, Lucet V, Denjoy I, Grau F, Ngoc DD, et al. Catecholaminergic polymorphic ventricular tachycardia in children: a 7-year follow-up of 21 patients. Circulation 1995; 91(5):1512–1519.

38. Goldman L, Sia ST, Cook EF, Rutherford JD, Weinstein MC. Costs and effectiveness of routine therapy with long-term beta-adrenergic antagonists after acute myocardial infarction. N Engl J Med 1988; 319:152–157.
39. Kennedy HL, Brooks MM, Baker MM, Bergstrandt R, Huther ML, et al., for the CAST Investigators. Beta-blocker therapy in the cardiac arrhythmia suppression trial. Am J Cardiol 1994; 74:674–680.
40. Ceremuzynski L, Kleczar E, Krzeminska-Pakula M, et al. Effect of amiodarone on mortality after myocardial infarction: a double-blind, placebo-controlled, pilot study. J Am Coll Cardiol 1992; 20:1056–1062.
41. Burkart F, Pfisterer M, Kiowski W, et al. Effect of antiarrhythmic therapy on mortality in survivors of myocardial infarction with asymptomatic complex ventricular arrhythmias: Basel Antiarrhythmic Study of Infarct Survival (BASIS). J Am Coll Cardiol 1990; 16:1171–1178.
42. Singh SN, Fletcher RD, Fisher SG, Singh BN, Lewis HD, et al. Amiodarone in patients with congestive heart failure and asymptomatic ventricular arrhythmia. Survival Trial of Antiarrhythmic Therapy in Congestive Heart Failure. N Engl J Med 1995; 333(2):77–82.
43. Nicklas JM, McKenna WJ, Stewart RA, et al. Prospective, double-blind, placebo-controlled trial of low-dose amiodarone in patients with severe heart failure and asymptomatic frequent ventricular ectopy. Am Heart J 1991; 122:1016–1021.
44. Cleland JGF, Dargie HJ, Findlay IN, et al. Clinical, haemodynamic and antiarrhythmic effects of long-term treatment with amiodarone of patients in heart failure. Br Heart J 1987; 57:436–445.
45. Chatterjee K. Amiodarone in chronic heart failure. J Am Coll Cardiol 1989; 14:1775–1776.
46. Moss AJ, Hall WJ, Cannom DS, Daubert JP, Higgins SL, et al. Improved survival with an implanted defibrillator in patients with coronary disease at high risk for ventricular arrhythmia: Multicenter Automatic Defibrillator Implantation Trial Investigators. N Engl J Med 1996; 335(26):1933–1940.
47. Bigger JT Jr. Prophylactic use of implanted cardiac defibrillators in patients at high risk for ventricular arrhythmias after coronary-artery bypass graft surgery. N Engl J Med 1997; 337:1569–1575.
48. Myerburg RJ, Castellanos A. Clinical trials of implantable defibrillators. N Engl J Med 1997; 337(22):1621–1623.
49. Buxton, AE, Lee KL, Fisher JD, Josephson ME, Prystowsky EN, et al., for the Multicenter Unsustained Tachycardia Trial Investigators. A randomized study of the prevention of sudden death in patients with coronary artery disease. N Engl J Med 1999; 341:1882–1890.
50. Gomes JAC, Hariman RI, Kang PS, El-Sherif N, Chowdhry I, et al. Programmed electrical stimulation in patients with high-grade ventricular ectopy: electrophysiologic findings and prognosis for survival. Circulation 1984; 70:43–51.
51. Klein RC, Machell C. Use of electrophysiologic testing in patients with nonsustained ventricular tachycardia: prognostic and therapeutic implications. J Am Coll Cardiol 1989; 14:155–161.
52. Gregoratos G, Cheitlin MD, Conill A, Epstein AE, Fellows C, et al. ACC/AHA Guidelines for implantation of cardiac pacemakers and antiarrhythmia devices. Executive summary: a report of the American College of Cardiology/American Heart Association Task Force on Practice Guidelines (Committee on Pacemaker Implantation). Circulation 1998; 97(13):1325–1335.

# XI

## *Prevention*

## 41

# The Role of Stress in Sudden Death:

## Can It Be Prevented?

*Philippe Coumel, MD*

## Introduction

After having been ignored for a long time as a major factor in determining of sudden death (SD), the role of the autonomic nervous system (ANS) is now recognized in many arguments of various natures. Initially, direct evidence came from the attentive analysis of Holter recordings[1,2] displaying consistent heart rate behavior before the terminal event. At the other extreme, the preventive effect of beta blockers on SD[3,4] replaced the belief in the potential of antiarrhythmic drugs. Realizing that any tachyarrhythmia, whatever its electrophysiological mechanism, includes the intervention of an autonomic factor[5] contributed to the inclusion of this parameter in the conception of experimental models and their interpretation in terms of mechanism and treatment.[6,7] The term *stress* in the title of this chapter refers to a particular modality of adrenergic stimulation, implying a notion of suddenness, and neurogenic rather than only humoral adrenergic stimulation that may become particularly crucial in certain situations. Obviously, the question of whether stress *can* be prevented should be understood in terms of consequences rather than occurrence. We will pay particular attention to the way the role of adrenergic stimulation can be detected and how its consequences can be prevented by adequate treatment.

## Sudden Death and the Role of the ANS

### Recorded Sudden Death

The experience reported from large series of recorded SD is very consistent.[1,2] The causal heart disease most often was coronary artery disease

From: Aliot E, Clementy J, Prystowsky EN (editors). *Fighting Sudden Cardiac Death: A Worldwide Challenge.* ©Futura Publishing Company, Armonk, NY, 2000.

and, to a lesser extent, various forms of cardiomyopathy. In our experience as well as that of Olshausen, heart rate changes preceding arrhythmias form the best indicator of the role of adrenergic stimulation. We studied 12 cases of primary ventricular fibrillation and 37 cases of ventricular tachycardia degenerating into fibrillation. We compared the heart rates in the hour and the 3 minutes immediately preceding the arrhythmia onset. The trend of acceleration was marked and highly significant (from 85 ± 22.8 beats/min to 99.1 ± 31.1, p<0.001) in the 27 cases in which the arrhythmia started without being preceded by any occasional pause. In 22 cases, a pause was present and triggered the arrhythmic event. In those cases, the trend of heart rate acceleration was present but did not reach a level of significance; a balance existed between the contribution of the ANS and the specific role of the pause. Finally, the deterioration of ventricular tachycardia into fibrillation was usually preceded by an acceleration that may be related to a feedback effect of hemodynamics on the ANS. The apparent contrast of an opposite trend of heart rate deceleration before death was observed in cases where the terminal event was an acquired torsades de pointes. In such a situation, a progressively slowing heart rate consistently ended with the well-known short-long phenomenon, and one is tempted to conclude the absence of any adrenergic stimulation. In fact, a more refined study of torsades de pointes demonstrated that in the last minute preceding the event, the evidence of an adrenergic stimulation is indeed present.[8]

## Specific Considerations

Arrhythmias in mitral valve prolapse frequently have an "adrenergic profile," that is, they look more frequent and severe in the context of sympathetic predominance. This pattern has long been suspected to be associated with a hyperadrenergic state, a hypothesis that was never definitely verified; the increased plasma level of catecholamines[9] or an increased heart rate variability[10] that were claimed in early studies have not been further confirmed. Determining whether the substrate sensitivity or the ANS behavior really is the cause applies in fact to numerous situations once one pays attention to the relationships between these 2 determinants[11] in the absence of heart failure. Ventricular tachyarrhythmias of right ventricular dysplasia frequently appear for the first time during strenuous exercise. According to the adrenergic paradox (see below), this would suggest a low sensitivity of the substrate to catecholamines rather than a typical example of an adrenergic dependence of the arrhythmia, which is more apparent than real. During the course of the disease, this character progressively vanishes as the arrhythmogenic properties of the substrate develop.

## The Long QT Syndrome and Its Variants

The arrhythmia substrate in the congenital long QT syndrome is of a purely electrophysiological nature. If it is clearly heralded by abnormal ventricular repolarization, it is not demonstrated that this pattern forms a necessary condition for the occurrence of tachyarrhythmias. Variants of the congenital form may include intermittent aspects of prolonged QT interval,[12] or intermittent and intermediate aspects of long QT in severe catecholinergic idiopathic ventricular tachycardias,[13] or authentic torsades de pointes but without any evidence of QT abnormality. Finally, the acquired long QT syndrome itself more and more frequently appears as a latent form of the congenital long QT, revealed by occasional factors (bradycardia, potassium depletion, or drug sensitivity) if one refers to dynamic rather than basic behavior of repolarization.12 At variance from numerous hypotheses formulated in the past, there is no evidence of any abnormality of the ANS in the long QT syndrome. Rather, it appears that the various "channelopathies" responsible for the various genetic forms are more (for the K+ channels of LQT1 and LQT2) or less (for the Na+ channel of LQT3) dependent on the adrenergic stimulation that in any case should be neurogenic (stress) rather than humoral (exercise, isoprenaline infusion) to exert their most deleterious effects. Figure 1 demonstrates how it takes no more than a few seconds for the neurogenic stimulation to trigger the arrhythmogenic substrate of the long QT syndrome, whereas it would take much longer for a humoral stimulation.

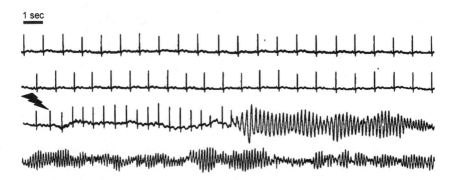

Figure 1. Stress-induced ventricular fibrillation in a long QT syndrome. The stress was induced by a telephone call at night in a patient with a long QT syndrome. This form of neurally mediated sympathetic stimulation provokes the tachyarrhythmia whereas exercise and isoprenaline infusion were ineffective. The lag time between the stress and the tachyarrhythmia was very short, as shown by the sudden heart rate acceleration of about 10 seconds.

## The Presence or the Absence of Heart Failure

In all of the preceding causes of SD, the presence or the absence of heart failure must be considered as an important parameter in order to interpret the role of the ANS. Not only are myocardial hypertrophy and heart failure arrhythmogenic on their own,[14,15] but they are associated with modifications of the autonomic nervous system itself.

In the absence of any structural heart disease, the ANS is supposed to function normally, and except for cases in which it is pathologically disturbed (e.g., diabetes mellitus), the indications obtained from the heart rate are supposed to reliably reflect its reactions to the environment. The situation is different when a heart disease alters the hemodynamic conditions. The failing heart causes activation of the sympathetic system through intramyocardial receptors and baroreceptor perception of hemodynamic alterations reflecting decreased ventricular performance. Many compensatory mechanisms involve the ANS that modify cardiac physiology. Plasma catecholamines are increased, while myocardial stores of catecholamines are decreased. Subsensitivity to beta-adrenergic stimulation develops with advancing heart failure, and the downregulation of the beta-adrenergic receptors coexists with increased neural traffic.[16] There is a decreased sensitivity to catecholamines as well as to atropine,[17] which contrasts with an enhanced sensitivity to beta blockade.

# The Autonomic Paradox

Two determining factors are essential to clinical arrhythmia: the electrophysiological substrate, and the ANS that can make it active by conditioning the adequate environment. The respective weight of these 2 factors is essential to consider in any clinical arrhythmia, and we tried to model the problem in Figure 2. There must be a balance between the substrate's sensitivity to the ANS and the impact of the latter. The stronger the autonomic stimulation, but also the greater the substrate sensitivity, the more likely the clinical arrhythmia. This is indicated by the size of the arrows that represent the respective importance of the factors. The arrhythmia manifests every time the substrate has been activated by a sufficient autonomic imbalance or an adequately sensitive substrate. This schema applies to either vagal or adrenergic stimulation at the atrial level. In the ventricle, it looks as if only the adrenergic limb of the ANS would be involved. The interaction between the substrate sensitivity and the ANS balance is in fact a reverse relationship, and is the reason we proposed the term *adrenergic paradox* to designate some consequences of this situation.[5]

Heart rate changes are indicative of a modification of the vagosympathetic balance, and, for instance, one tends to ascribe to adrenergic in-

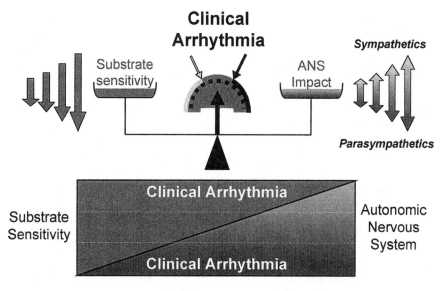

Figure 2. The 2 factors of arrhythmogenicity. The upper part of the figure represents the balance of the respective importance of the arrhythmogenic factors: the electrophysiological substrate and the autonomic nervous system. The substrate sensitivity is supposed to be more or less important as indicated by arrows of different size. The impact of the ANS can be exerted in either direction, depending on whether the vagal or the sympathetic limb of the system is involved. The autonomic stimulation disequilibrates the system so that at a certain threshold in either direction, the substrate is activated and the clinical arrhythmia is induced. The lower part of the figure is another representation of the inverse relationship between the substrate sensitivity and the ANS influence. The arrhythmia becomes clinically manifest when the thresholds are reached due to either combination.

fluences tachyarrhythmias appearing at the peak of exercise, which is most probably correct. However, considering only those arrhythmias that appear in the context of a marked heart rate acceleration is probably wrong if one refers to the notion of substrate sensitivity. The concept of adrenergic paradox logically implies that the higher the substrate sensitivity to adrenergic influences, the lower the necessary amount of adrenergic stimulation to activate the substrate, and therefore the less evident the sympathetic activation as detected from heart rate trends (Figure 3). Another aspect of the adrenergic paradox is that, to trust the heart rate trend as a marker of the ANS balance supposes that its reliability is adequate, and we just saw that myocardial dysfunction alters it. In the context of heart failure, limited heart rate variations may reflect relatively important modifications of the ANS balance that should not be overlooked. The adrenergic paradox concept calls attention to the risk of under- or overestimating the substrate sensitivity and the ANS relationships. It is our experience that

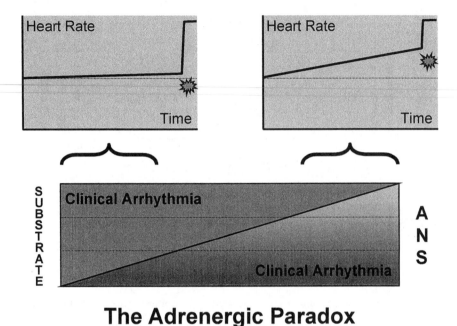

## The Adrenergic Paradox

Figure 3. The adrenergic paradox. The lower part of the figure represents the inverse relationship between the substrate sensitivity and the ANS influence, and the upper part displays the clinical arrhythmia that results from the different proportions of these factors. In the upper right panel, a limited substrate sensitivity is combined with a strong adrenergic stimulation heralded by a marked heart rate acceleration before the arrhythmia onset. In the upper left panel, the situation is the opposite, with a marked substrate sensitivity, so that the arrhythmia is triggered by a limited adrenergic stimulation demonstrated by a quite moderate heart rate increase.

even limited heart rate and heart rate variability changes must be taken into account when they are observed in the context of heart failure. Ignoring this phenomenon historically explains why it took so long to recognize the importance of using beta blockers in cardiac arrhythmias in general, and more precisely in heart failure.

### Sensitivity to Beta Blockers and Their Correct Use

The clinical effects of beta blockers on sinus rhythm and their indications for preventive treatment of tachyarrhythmias are directly linked to the concept of the adrenergic paradox. A trivial observation that is, however, rarely referred to is that the faster the heart rate, that is, the stronger the adrenergic stimulation, the more marked the slowing effect of beta blockers. The experience we had with nadolol compared with propranolol is shown in Figure 4.[18] The message is that if one expresses in percentage the beta blocker-induced heart rate slowing, this effect is more marked on higher than on lower rates. Another finding refers to the relative effect of nadolol and propranolol in the same patients: nadolol is significantly more effective than propranolol, a difference that is all but ignored in the literature. One reason is that propranolol is supposed to be the reference point of beta-blocking drugs, and with the exception of beta blockers with an intrinsic sympathetic activity, a difference in the heart rates obtained by various beta blockers is never looked for in pharmacological studies.[19] Another reason is that the difference between nadolol and propranolol is not obvious for the clinician. Its absolute value is approximately 3 bpm, which can be easily missed, although it is indeed significant if one considers 24-hour paired values.

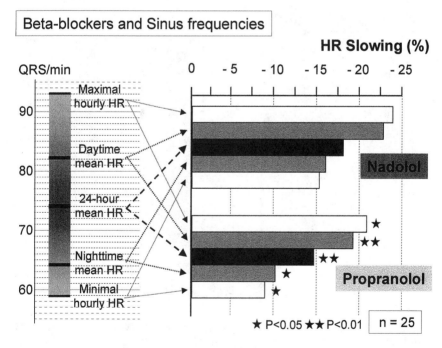

Figure 4. Different effects of 2 beta blockers on the sinus rate over a 24-hour period. In a group of 25 patients, 5 different rates are considered in the 24-hour recordings: 24-hour mean heart rate, daytime and nighttime rates, maximal and minimal hourly rates. The slowing effect of nadolol and propranolol is expressed in percentage, and it is clearly more marked for higher than lower rates. In addition, the effect of propranolol is significantly less marked than that of nadolol.

Figure 5 displays another aspect of the corollaries of the concept of adrenergic paradox. The effect of a beta blocker not only depends on its own pharmacological characteristics but on the patient's status. Two series of patients were considered according to the characteristics of the ventricular arrhythmias they were suffering from.[20] None of them had heart failure, but in one group with clearly adrenergic-dependent arrhythmias, the 24-hour heart rate was slightly (although not significantly) higher than in the other group suffering from nonadrenergic-sensitive ventricular arrhythmias. Patients in both groups received nadolol and propranolol, and the percentage of heart rate slowing was studied. Not only was it more marked with nadolol than with propranolol as previously mentioned, but it was significantly greater in the "adrenergic" than in the "nonadrenergic" group. Such behavior clearly demonstrates that

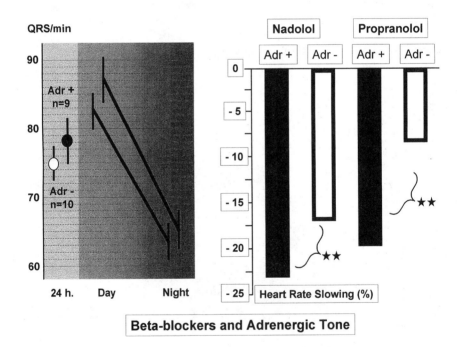

**Beta-blockers and Adrenergic Tone**

Figure 5. Different patients' sensitivity to beta blockers. Two groups of patients have been considered according to the greater ("Adr+," n= 9) or smaller ("Adr−," n=10) sensitivity of their ventricular arrhythmias to adrenergic stimulation. Their basic heart rates during the 24-hour, the day, and the night periods tended to be higher in the Adr+ than in the Adr− group, but not significantly so. Both groups received nadolol and propranolol. Not only was the effect of nadolol more marked than that of propranolol, but the heart rate slowing was significantly greater ($p<0.01$) in the Adr+ than in the Adr− group.

the response to beta blockade depends on the patient's characteristics in terms of adrenergic tone.

The dependence of the beta-blocking effect on the target can be easily verified according to the presence or the absence of myocardial hypertrophy or heart failure.[21] It is firmly established that heart disease and more precisely heart failure alters heart rate variability,[22] but little attention, however, has been paid to the behavior of sinus rate in myocardial hypertrophy and heart failure when beta blockade is applied. We studied[21] heart rate in 3 groups: 15 normal adults, 13 patients with left ventricular hypertrophy, and 13 patients with heart failure. In control conditions the mean heart rate was $77.1 \pm 1.9$ beats/min (mean ± SEM) in normals, $76.8 \pm 3.3$ bpm in patients with hypertrophy, and $79.3 \pm 3.5$ bpm in heart failure (p=NS). Acebutolol always significantly (p<0.001) slowed the heart rate, but the important finding was that the percentage of slowing was different in the 3 groups: 9.5% in normals, 18.1% in patients with myocardial hypertrophy, 19.1% in patients with heart failure.

The fact that the heart rate slowing was twice as marked in diseased patients compared to normals is not reported in the literature, with the exception of the interesting observation of Kjekshus.[23] Analyzing beta-blocker trials in heart failure, this author observed that the more marked the heart rate slowing, the more important the benefit in terms of survival. The differences could be partly explained by the presence of an intrinsic sympathetic activity for drugs such as acebutolol or oxprenolol. This does not apply, however, to other compounds. Kjekshus' explanation was that the benefit was directly linked to the degree of sinus rate slowing, which may be partially true. An alternative explanation, however, is that a greater benefit in severely diseased patients simply is heralded by the sensitivity of the sinus rate to beta blockade, due to a more marked adrenergic stimulation.

## Practical Consequences

With the noticeable exception of 2 syndromes responsible for sudden death in the absence of structural heart disease, the short coupled variant of torsades de pointes[24] and the syndrome described by Brugada,[25] one can state that all tachyarrhythmias responsible for sudden death have something to do with stress, and more generally with adrenergic stiumulation. However, they do not all depend on the stress factor to the same extent, and the adrenergic paradox may be responsible for some misleading patterns. The counterpart of the adrenergic paradox is the notion that the effect of treatment depends on both the drug used and the patient to whom it is given. As a consequence, once beta blockade is indicated, it must be as effective as possible, and the best marker of its efficacy is the amount of heart rate slowing it provokes.

## References

1. Leclercq JF, Maison-Blanche P, Cauchemez B, Coumel P. Respective roles of sympathetic tone and of cardiac pauses in the genesis of 62 cases of ventricular fibrillation recorded during Holter monitoring. Eur Heart J 1988; 9:1276–1283.
2. Olshausen KV, Witt T, Pop T, et al. Sudden cardiac death while wearing a Holter monitor. Am J Cardiol 1991; 67:381–386.
3. Yussuf S, Peto R, Lewis J, et al. Beta-blockade during and after myocardial infarction: an overview of the randomized trials. Prog Cardiovasc Dis 1985; 77:335–350.
4. The Beta-Blocker Pooling Project Research Group. The beta-blocker pooling project (BBPP): subgroup findings from randomized trials in post-infarction patients. Eur Heart J 1988; 9:8–16.
5. Coumel P. The management of clinical arrhythmias : an overview on invasive versus non-invasive electrophysiology. Eur Heart J 1987; 8:92–99.
6. Schwartz PJ, Vanoli E, Stramba-Badiale M, et al. Autonomic mechanism of sudden death: new insights from analysis of baroreflexes in conscious dogs with and without myocardial infarction. Circulation 1988; 78:969–979.
7. Patterson E, Sherlag BJ, Lazzara R. Mechanism of prevention of sudden death by nadolol: differential actions on arrhythmia triggers and substrate after myocardial infarction in the dog. J Am Coll Cardiol 1986; 8:1365–1372.
8. Locati EH, Maison-Blanche P, Dejode P, et al. Spontaneous sequences of onset of torsades de pointes in patients with acquired prolonged repolarization: quantitative analysis of Holter recordings. J Am Coll Cardiol 1995; 25:1564–1575.
9. Boudoulas H, Reynolds JC, Mazzaferri E, Wooley CF. Metabolic studies in mitral valve prolapse syndrome. Circulation 1980; 61:1200–1205.
10. Leclercq JF, Malergue MC, Milosevic D, et al. Troubles du rythme ventriculaires et prolapsus mitral: a propos de 35 observations. Arch Mal Coeur 1980; 73:276–287.
11. Coumel P, Rosengarten MD, Leclercq JF, Attuel P. Role of sympathetic nervous system in non-ischaemic ventricular arrhythmias. Br Heart J 1982; 47:137–147.
12. Neyroud N, Maison Blanche P, Denjoy I, et al. Diagnostic performance of QT interval variables from 24-hour electrocardiography in the long QT syndrome. Eur Heart J 1998; 19:158–165.
13. Leenhardt A, Lucet V, Denjoy I, et al. Catecholaminergic polymorphic ventricular tachycardia in children: a 7-year follow-up of 21 patients. Circulation 1995; 91:1512–1519.
14. Aronson RS. Mechanisms of arrhythmias in ventricular hypertrophy. J Cardiovasc Electrophysiol 1991; 2:249–261.
15. Coumel P. Pathophysiology of ventricular arrhythmias during myocardial hypertrophy and cardiac insufficiency. In: Swynghedauw B (ed). Cardiac Hypertrophy and Failure. Inserm/John Libbey Publ., 1990, pp 647–664.
16. Leimbach WN, Wallin BG, Victor RG, et al. Direct evidence from intraneural recordings for increased central sympathetic outflow in patients with heart failure. Circulation 1986; 73:913–919.
17. Eckberg DL, Drabinski M, Braunwald E. Defective cardiac sympathetic control in patients with heart disease. N Engl J Med 1971; 285:877–883.

18. Coumel P, Escoubet B, Attuel P. Beta-blocking therapy in atrial and ventricular tachyarrhythmias: experience with nadolol. Am Heart J 1984; 108:1098–1108.
19. Escoubet B, Leclercq JF, Maison-Blanche P, et al. Dose-related effect of four beta-blockers on heart rate assessed by 24-hour recordings. Clin Pharmacol Ther 1986; 39:361–368.
20. Coumel P, Rosengarten MD, Leclercq JF, Attuel P. Role of sympathetic nervous system in non-ischaemic ventricular arrhythmias. Br Heart J 1982; 47:137–147.
21. Coumel P, Hermida JS, Wennerblöm B, et al. Heart rate variability in myocardial hypertrophy and heart failure, and the effects of beta-blocking therapy : a non-spectral analysis of heart rate oscillations. Eur Heart J 1991; 12:412–422.
22. Casolo G, Bali E, Taddei T, et al. Decreased spontaneous heart rate variability in congestive heart failure. Am J Cardiol 1989; 64:1162–1167.
23. Kjekshus J. Heart rate reduction : a mechanism of benefit? Eur Heart J 1987;8L: 115–122.
24. Leenhardt A, Glaser E, Burguera M, et al. Short-coupled variant of torsades de pointes : a new electrocardiographic entity in the spectrum of idiopathic ventricular tachyarrhythmias. Circulation 1994; 89:206–215.
25. Brugada P, Brugada J. Right bundle branch block, persistent ST segment elevation and sudden cardiac death: a distinct clinical and electrocardiographic syndrome. A multicenter report. J Am Coll Cardiol 1992; 20:1391–1396.

# 42

# Can Diet Prevent Sudden Cardiac Death?

*Michel de Lorgeril, MD*

## Introduction

Sudden cardiac death (SCD) is defined as a death from a cardiac cause occurring about 1 hour from the onset of symptoms.[1] SCD is currently attributed to cardiac arrhythmia although it is now well recognized that a classification based on clinical circumstances is often misleading.

The magnitude of the problem is considerable because SCD is the most common and often the first manifestation of coronary heart disease (CHD) and is responsible for about 50% of cardiovascular mortality in the developed countries.[1] In most cases, SCD occurs without prodromal symptoms and out of hospital. Since up to 80% of patients with SCD have CHD, the epidemiology, as well as the potential preventive approaches of SCD, parallel those of CHD. Theoretically, any treatment to reduce CHD should reduce the incidence of SCD. In fact, only a few studies have addressed the hypothesis that nonantiarrhythmic intervention may reduce the risk of SCD. Also, few trials have been adequately powered to address the mechanistic question of the preventive effect of any therapy on this mode of death. In fact, if we exclude the implantable cardioverter-defibrillator (ICD) among the antiarrhythmic treatments, only amiodarone (by meta-analysis) was shown to reduce mortality from SCD[2] and the effect seems to be restricted to patients with nonischemic cardiomyopathy.

Among the nonantiarrhythmic drugs used in secondary prevention of CHD, only beta blockers were potentially protective,[3] but these drugs have many side effects and the rate of discontinuation is quite high in clinical practice. The use of aspirin may be questioned in patients at high risk of SCD because it was shown to increase the incidence of SCD in certain trials[4] (Table 1), and a proarrhythmic effect was also suggested by some animal studies.[5] On the other hand, a recent meta-analysis of randomized clinical trials of ACE inhibitors suggested that reduction in SCD might be a component of the survival benefit observed in CHD patients receiving this

From: Aliot E, Clementy J, Prystowsky EN (editors). *Fighting Sudden Cardiac Death: A Worldwide Challenge.* ©Futura Publishing Company, Armonk, NY, 2000.

### Table 1

### Causes of Death and Corresponding Relative Risks (RRs) in the Final Report of the Aspirin Component of the Physicians' Health Study*

| Causes of death | Aspirin | Placebo | Relative Risk | P Value |
|---|---|---|---|---|
| Cardiovascular mortality | 81 | 83 | 0.96 | NS |
| Acute myocardial infarction | 10 | 28 | 0.31 | 0.005 |
| Other ischemic heart diseases | 24 | 25 | 0.97 | NS |
| Sudden cardiac death | 22 | 12 | 1.96 | 0.09 |

*Despite a significant reduction in fatal myocardial infarction, cardiovascular mortality was similar in the 2 groups because of a higher rate of sudden cardiac death rate in patients taking aspirin.
NS = not significant.

type of drug.[6] Finally, in addition to a limited use of antiarrhythmic drugs (because of their proarrhythmogenic effects),[7] there is today growing recognition of a limited effect of ICD therapy on total mortality in patients implanted in accordance with the classic SCD risk stratifiers.[8,9] Thus, new, well-tolerated, and effective means for the primary prevention of SCD have to be discovered. In the present chapter, we examine whether diet (more precisely, certain dietary factors) may prevent (or help to prevent) SCD. In fact, a large body of literature exists, including experimental and clinical studies, that provide valuable information to answer this question.

## Fish, Omega-3 Polyunsaturated Fatty Acids, and SCD

The hypothesis that fish consumption may be protective in relation to SCD is derived from the results of a secondary prevention trial published in 1989, the Diet And Reinfarction Trial (DART), which showed a significant reduction in total and cardiovascular mortality (both by about 30%) in patients who consumed at least 2 servings of fatty fish per week.[10] Although SCD was not among the end-points prospectively described for the trial, the authors suggested that the protective effect of fish may be due to preventing ventricular fibrillation (VF) since no benefit was observed in the incidence of nonfatal acute myocardial infarction.

The hypothesis was consistent with experimental evidence suggesting that the n-3 fatty acids, the main fatty acids of fish oil and fatty fishes, have an important effect on the occurrence of VF in the setting of myocardial ischemia and reperfusion in various animal models both in vivo and in vitro (11–15). Recently, Billman and colleagues, using an elegant in vivo model of SCD in dogs surviving a previous acute myocardial infarction, demonstrated a striking reduction of VF after intravenous administration of pure n-3 fatty acids, including the long chain fatty acids present in fish oil and their parent n-3 fatty acid in some vegetable oils, alpha-linolenic acid.[16] These authors have found the mechanism of this protection to result from the electrophysiological effects of the free, nonesterified, n-3 fatty acids when they are simply partitioned into the phospholipids of the sarcolemma without covalently bonding to any constituents in that cell membrane[15] When they are ingested in the diet, these fatty acids are preferentially incorporated into membrane phospholipids and stored triglycerides, and in this form they are not antiarrhythmic. But with ischemia or major sympathetic adrenergic discharge, phospholipases and lipases quickly liberate the stored fatty acids which can, in their free form, exert their antiarrhythmic effect. The presence of the free form of the n-3 fatty acids into the membrane phospholipids of every cardiomyocyte make them resistant to arrhythmias. They accomplish this by modulating the conduction of several membrane ion channels.[17] Thus far, it seems that the very potent inhibitory effects of n-3 fatty acids on the fast sodium current, $I_{Na}$,[18,19] and the L-type calcium current, $I_{CaL}$,[20] are the major contributors to their antiarrhythmic actions in ischemia. Briefly, the effects of the n-3 fatty acids are to shift the steady-state inactivation potential to more negative values, and this was also observed in other excitable tissues such as neurons.[21]

Of additional interest are clinical data showing suppression (by more than 70%) of ventricular premature complexes in middle-aged patients with frequent ventricular extrasystoles who were randomly assigned to take either fish oil (suppression was obtained in 44% of the patients) or sunflower oil (in only 15% of the patients, p=0.01).[22]

Support for the DART hypothesis of a clinically significant antiarrhythmic effect of n-3 fatty acids in secondary prevention of CHD came from 2 randomized trials testing the effect of ethnic dietary patterns (instead of that of a single nutrient)—a Mediterranean type of diet and an Asian vegetarian diet—in secondary prevention of CHD.[23,24] In contrast with DART, SCD was prospectively included as a secondary end-point in both trials. The 2 experimental diets included high intake of the essential alpha-linolenic acid, the main vegetable n-3 fatty acid. Whereas in both trials the incidence of SCD was markedly reduced, the number of cases was quite small and the antiarrhythmic effect cannot be entirely attributed to alpha-linolenic acid since these experimental diets also included a high intake of other nutrients, in particular various antioxidants, with potential antiarrhythmic properties (see below). These findings were extended by the population-based case control study conducted by Siscovick and colleagues examining the intake of n-3 fatty acids among patients with primary cardiac arrest compared with that of age- and sex-matched controls.[25] Their data indicated that the intake of approximately 5 to 6 grams of n-3 fatty acids per month (equivalent to 1 fatty fish meal per week) was associated with a 50% reduction of the risk of cardiac arrest after adjustment for potential confounding factors. In their study, the use of a biomarker, the red blood cell membrane level of n-3 fatty acids, considerably enhanced the validity of the findings that were also consistent with results of many (not all) cohort studies, suggesting that consumption of 1 to 2 servings of fish per week is associated with a marked reduction in CHD mortality when compared with no fish intake.[26,27]

In a recent large prospective study (more than 20,000 participants with a follow-up of 11 years), the specific point that fish has antiarrhythmic properties and may prevent SCD was examined by Albert et al.[28] They found that men who consumed fish at least once per week had a 50% lower risk of SCD compared with those who consumed fish less than once per month. Interestingly, fish consumption was not related to nonsudden cardiac death, suggesting that the main protective effect of fish (or n-3 fatty acids) was through their effects on arrhythmias. These results differed from those of the Chicago Western Electric Study in which there was a significant inverse association between fish consumption and nonsudden cardiac death but not with SCD.[29] Several factors may explain the discrepancy between the 2 studies, in particular, as emphasized above, the way of classifying the deaths.[30] This again underlies the limitations of the observational studies. Only controlled trials can definitely provide a clear demonstration of causal relationships between the intake of any nutrient and beneficial health effects. It was the purpose of the GISSI-Prevenzione trial to help to solve the question of the health benefits of foods rich in n-3 fatty acids (and also in vitamin E) and their pharmacological substitutes.[31] Patients (n=11,324) surviving a recent infarction (<3 months) were randomly assigned supplements of n-3 fatty acids (1 g daily), vitamin E (300 mg daily), both, or none (control) for 3.5 years. The primary efficacy endpoint was the combination of death and nonfatal myocardial infarction and stroke. Secondary analyses included overall mortality, cardiovascular mortality and SCD. Treatment with n-3 fatty acids significantly lowered the risk of the primary end-point (the relative risk decreased by 15%). Secondary analyses provided a clearer profile of the clinical effects of n-3 fatty acids. Overall mortality was reduced by 20% and cardiovascular mortality by 30%. However, it is the effect on SCD (reduced by 45%) that accounted for most of the benefits seen in the primary combined end-point and both overall and cardiovascular mortality (Table 2). There was no difference across the treatment groups for nonfatal cardiovascular events, a result comparable to that of DART.[10] Thus, the results obtained in that randomized trial are consistent with previous controlled trials[10,23,24] and

## Table 2
### Clinical Efficacy of n-3 Fatty Acids in the GISSI-Prevenzione Trial

|  | Relative Risk (95% CI) |
| --- | --- |
| Death, nonfatal AMI and stroke | 0.85 (0.70–0.99) |
| Overall mortality | 0.80 (0.67–0.94) |
| Cardiovascular mortality | 0.70 (0.56–0.87) |
| Sudden cardiac death | 0.55 (0.40–0.76) |
| Nonfatal cardiovascular events | 0.96 (0.76–1.21) |
| Fatal and nonfatal stroke | 1.30 (0.87–1.96) |

CI = confidence interval; AMI = acute myocardial infarction.

large-scale observational studies[25–29] and with animal studies,[11–20] which together strongly support a role for n-3 fatty acids in relation with SCD.

Based on the current knowledge of the effect of n-3 fatty acids on SCD, what should clinicians do (or advise) in relation to primary prevention of SCD in the context of secondary prevention of CHD? The existing evidence suggests that consumption of n-3 fatty acids (about 1 g daily), in the form of supplements or alternatively by eating at least 2 large (about 200 g) servings of fatty fish per week, will help to prevent SCD in low-risk patients. The dosage to be recommended in high-risk patients and in secondary prevention of SCD warrants further investigation, which should be designed without delay.

## Vitamin E and SCD

The question of the effect of vitamin E on SCD is more controversial. Discrepant findings between expectations of benefit based on epidemiological observations[32,33] and results of clinical trials[34,35] have been published. However, in a recent controlled trial, a significant decrease in nonfatal myocardial infarction and a nonsignificant increase in cardiovascular mortality (in particular in the rate of SCD) were reported with a daily regimen of 400–800 mg vitamin E in patients with established CHD.[36] Because of severe weaknesses in the methods,[37,38] this trial was said to confuse rather than clarify the question of the usefulness of vitamin E supplementation in CHD.[31,38] In that context, the GISSI-Prevenzione trial brings new and major information. In contrast to n-3 fatty acids, the results of vitamin E studies do not support a significant effect on the primary end-point, a combination of death and nonfatal myocardial infarction and stroke.[31] However, the secondary analysis again provides a clearer view of the clinical effect of vitamin E in CHD patients that cannot be easily dismissed. In fact, among the 193 and 155 cardiac deaths that occurred in the control and vitamin E groups, respectively, during the trial (a difference of 38, p<0.05), there were 99 and 65 SCDs (a difference of 34, p<0.05), which clearly indicated that the significant decrease in cardiovascular mortality (by 20%) in the vitamin E group was almost entirely due to a decrease in the incidence of SCD (by 35%). In contrast, nonfatal cardiovascular events and nonsudden cardiac deaths were not influenced.[31] The vitamin E data of the GISSI trial do not stand in isolation. In an in vivo dog model of myocardial ischemia,[39] we also reported a protective effect of vitamin E on the incidence of VF (the main mechanism of SCD) with a 16% rate in the vitamin E group and a 44% rate in the placebo group (p<0.05). Also in line with the GISSI results, infarct size, the main determinant of acute heart failure and nonsudden cardiac death, was larger in the supplemented group (58.5% of the ischemic area) than in the placebo group (41.9%, p<0.05). Worthy of mention is the fact that the antiarrhythmic effect of vitamin E was not seen in experiments with short periods (less than 30 minutes) of ischemia,[40] suggesting that the effect was dependent on the severity of the myocardial injury. Such ambivalent effects of vitamin E may explain, at least partly, why in many studies the effects of vitamin E were neutral or nonsignificant, the negative effects masking the beneficial ones. It remains that in the GISSI trial, cardiovascular mortality and SCD were significantly reduced by vitamin E and the effect on overall mortality showed a favorable trend (p=0.07). Thus, further clinical and experimental studies, specifically designed to test the antiarrhythmic effect of vitamin E during myocardial ischemia, are obviously needed. Another point to be clarified is whether the potential antiarrhythmic effect of vitamin E is specific to vitamin E or could be extended to other antioxidants. For instance, it has been recently questioned whether the cardioprotective effect of amiodarone could be dependent on a nonspecific free radical scavenging action of the compound.[41]

## Alcohol in Moderation and SCD

The question of the effect of alcohol on cardiovascular diseases has been the subject of intense controversy in recent years. There is now a consensus to say that moderate alcohol drinking is associated with reduced cardiovascular mortality whereas the exact mechanism(s) by which alcohol is protective remains to be clarified. In contrast, chronic heavy drinking has been implicated in the occurrence of atrial as well as ventricular arrhythmias in humans. This effect has been called the "holiday heart."[42] Studies in animals have shown varying and apparently opposing effects of alcohol on cardiac rhythm and conduction, depending on the animal species, experimental model, and alcohol dosage. Given acutely to nonalcoholic animals, ethanol may even have antiarrhythmic properties.[42] In humans, few studies have investigated the effect of alcohol specifically on SCD. It seems that it is the hyperadrenergic state resulting from binge drinking and withdrawal that is the main mechanism by which alcohol induces arrhythmias in humans.[42] In the British Regional Heart Study, the relative risk of SCD in heavy drinkers (>6 drinks per day) was 2-fold higher than in occasional or light drinkers.[43] The effect of binge drinking on SCD was, however, more evident in men free of preexisting CHD than in those with established CHD. In the Honolulu Heart Program,[44] the risk of SCD among healthy middle-aged men was positively related to blood pressure, serum cholesterol, smoking, and left ventricular hypertrophy, but inversely related to alcohol intake (Table 3). In fact, the effect of moderate "social" drinking on arrhythmias in nonalcoholic subjects has been addressed thus far in only 1 study. Investigators of the Physicians' Health Study assessed whether light-to-moderate alcohol drinkers apparently free of CHD at baseline have a decreased risk of SCD.[45] After controlling for multiple confounders, men who consumed 2–4 drinks per week or 5–6 drinks per week at baseline had a significantly reduced risk of SCD (by 60–80%) compared to those who rarely or never consumed alcohol. The relationship for SCD was U-shaped (p=0.002), whereas the relationship with nonsudden CHD death was L-shaped (p=0.02).[45] Analyses were repeated after excluding deaths occurring in the first 4 years of follow-up (to exclude the possibility that some men who refrained from drinking at baseline did it because of early symptoms of cardiovascular diseases) and also using the updated measure of alcohol intake ascertained at year 7 to address potential misclassification at the baseline evaluation of alcohol drinking. These secondary analyses basically provided the same results and confirmed the potential antiarrhythmic effect of moderate drinking.

### Table 3
### Predictors of Sudden Cardiac Death Among Healthy Middle-Aged Men in the Honolulu Heart Program

| Predictors | Relative Risk # | 95% CI* |
|---|---|---|
| Systolic blood pressure | 2.7 | 1.7–4.3 |
| Serum cholesterol | 1.8 | 1.1–2.8 |
| Smoking | 1.7 | 1.0–2.7 |
| LVH | 4.9 | 2.7–8.6 |
| Alcohol intake | 0.5 | 0.3–0.9 |

For the 4th versus the 1st quartile.
LVH = left ventricular hypertrophy; CI = confidence interval.

Despite limitations (the selected nature of the cohort, no women, no information on beverage type and drinking pattern), this study suggests that a significant part of the cardioprotective effect of moderate drinking is related to the prevention of SCD. Further research should be directed toward understanding the mechanism(s) by which moderate alcohol drinking may prevent ventricular arrhythmias and SCD. Finally, the present knowledge suggests that in CHD patients at risk of SCD, there is no reason not to allow moderate drinking.

## Summary and Conclusion

Experimental studies have shown that saturated fatty acids (usually from animal foods) are proarrhythmic. For obvious practical and ethical reasons, clinical studies are not feasible. However, human trials testing dietary patterns low in saturated fatty acids also suggested that dietary prevention of SCD (as well as of CHD in general) should primarily include a low intake of saturated fat.

Experimental, clinical, and epidemiological studies and several trials did clearly demonstrate that n-3 fatty acids are antiarrhythmic and reduce the risk of SCD. Their clinical use is now encouraged[46,47] and prescription of n-3 fatty acids should logically be included in the treatment and prevention of ventricular arrhythmias in CHD patients. They should be tested in secondary prevention of SCD.

There is now quite good evidence that vitamin E may be antiarrhythmic in certain CHD patients in certain conditions. Further studies are needed, however, to determine the mechanisms of this effect and also how it should be used (in particular, at which dosage) in the clinical setting.

Alcohol in moderation also seems to be antiarrhythmic, whereas the mechanism(s) of this action remains to be elucidated.

## References

1. Zipes DP, Wellens HJ. Sudden cardiac death. Circulation 1998; 98:2234–2251.
2. Amiodarone Trials Meta-Analysis (ATMA) investigators. Effect of prophylactic amiodarone on mortality after acute myocardial infarction and in congestive heart failure: meta-analysis of individual data from 6500 patients in randomized trials. Lancet 1997; 350:1417–1424.
3. Kendall MJ, Lynch KP, Hjalmarson A, Kjekshus J. Beta blockers and sudden cardiac death. Ann Int Med 1995; 123:358–367.
4. Steering Committee of the Physicians' Health Study Research Group. Final report on the aspirin component of the ongoing Physicians' Health Study. N Engl J Med 1989; 321:129–135.
5. Dhein S, Gottwald M, Gottwald E, et al. Acetylsalicylic acid enhances arrhythmogenicity in a model of local ischemia of isolated rabbit hearts. Eur J Pharmacol 1997; 339:129–139.

6. Domanski MJ, Exner DV, Borkowf CB, et al. Effect of angiotensin converting enzyme inhibitors on sudden cardiac death in patients following acute myocardial infarction: a meta-analysis of randomized clinical trials. J Am Coll Cardiol 1999; 33:598–604.
7. Podrid PJ. Redefining the role of antiarrhythmic drugs. N Engl J Med 1999; 340:1910–1912.
8. Thomson PE, Huikuri H, Kober L, et al. Lessons from the Nordic ICD pilot study. Lancet 1999; 353:2130–2131.
9. Bigger JT, Whang W, Rottman J, et al. Mechanisms of death in the CABG Patch trial: a randomized trial of implantable cardiac defibrillator prophylaxis in patients at high risk of death after coronary artery bypass surgery. Circulation 1999; 99:1416–1421.
10. Burr ML, Fehily AM, Gilbert JF, et al. Effects of changes in fat, fish, and fibre intakes on death and myocardial reinfarction: Diet And Reinfarction Trial (DART). Lancet 1989; 2:757–761.
11. McLennan PL, Abeywardena MY, Charnock JS. Reversal of arrhythmogenic effects of long-term saturated fatty acid intake by dietary n-3 and n-6 polyunsaturated fatty acids. Am J Clin Nutr 1990; 51:53–58.
12. McLennan PL, Abeywardena MY, Charnock JS. Dietary fish oil prevents ventricular fibrillation following coronary occlusion and reperfusion. Am Heart J 1988; 16:709–716.
13. Isensee H, Jacob R. Differential effects of various oil diets on the risk of cardiac arrhythmias in rats. J Cardiovasc Risk 1994; 1:353–359.
14. Billman GE, Hallaq H, Leaf A. Prevention of ischemia-induced ventricular fibrillation by omega-3 fatty acids. Proc Natl Acad Sci USA 1994; 91:4427–4430.
15. Weylandt KH, Kang JX, Leaf A. Polyunsaturated fatty acids exert antiarrhythmic actions as free fatty acids rather than in phospholipids. Lipids 1996; 977–982.
16. Billman GE, Kang JX, Leaf A. Prevention of sudden cardiac death by dietary pure omega-3 polyunsaturated fatty acids in dogs. Circulation 1999; 99:2452–2457.
17. Kang JX, Xiao Y-F, Leaf A. Free, long-chain, polyunsaturated fatty acids reduce membrane electrical excitability in neonatal rat cardiomyocytes. Proc Natl Acad Sci USA 1995; 92:3997–4001.
18. Xiao Y-F, Kang JX, Morgan JP, Leaf A. Blocking effects of polyunsaturated fatty acids on Na channels of neonatal rat ventricular myocytes. Proc Natl Acad Sci USA 1995; 92:1100–1104.
19. Xiao Y-F, Wright SN, Wang GK, Morgan JP, Leaf A. N-3 fatty acids suppress voltage-gated Na currents in HEK293t cells transfected with the alpha-subunit of the human cardiac Na channel. Proc Natl Acad Sci USA 1998; 95:2680–2685.
20. Xiao Y-F, Gomez AM, Morgan JP, Lederer WJ, Leaf A. Suppression of voltage-gated L-type Ca currents by polyunsaturated fatty acids in neonatal and adult cardiac myocytes. Proc Natl Acad Sci USA 1997; 94:4182–4187.
21. Vreugdenhil M, Breuhl C, Voskuyl RA, Kang JX, Leaf A, et al. Polyunsaturated fatty acids modulate sodium and calcium currents in CA1 neurons. Proc Natl Acad Sci USA 1996; 93:12559–12563.
22. Sellmayer A, Witzgall H, Lorenz RL, Weber PC. Effects of dietary fish oil on ventricular premature complexes. Am J Cardiol 1995; 76:974–977.
23. Singh RB, Rastogi SS, Verma R, Laxmi B, Singh R, et al. Randomised controlled trial of cardioprotective diet in patients with recent acute myocardial infarction: results of one year follow-up. Br Med J 1992; 304:1015–1019.
24. de Lorgeril M, Renaud S, Mamelle N, Salen P, Martin JL, et al. Mediterranean alpha-linolenic acid-rich diet in secondary prevention of coronary heart disease. Lancet 1994; 343:1454–1459.

25. Siscovick DS, Raghunathan TE, King I, et al. Dietary intake and cell membrane levels of long-chain n-3 polyunsaturated fatty acids and the risk of primary cardiac arrest. JAMA 1995; 274:1363–1367.
26. Kromhout D, Bosschieter EB, de Lezenne Coulander C. The inverse relation between fish consumption and 20-year mortality from coronary heart disease. N Engl J Med 1985; 312:1205–1209.
27. Shekelle RB, Missel L, Paul O, Shryock AM, Stamler J. Fish consumption and mortality from coronary heart disease. N Engl J Med 1985; 313:820.
28. Albert CM, Hennekens CH, O'Donnel CJ, et al. Fish consumption and the risk of sudden cardiac death. JAMA 1998; 279:23–28.
29. Daviglus ML, Stamler J, Orencia AJ, et al. Fish consumption and the 30-year risk of fatal myocardial infarction. N Engl J Med 1997; 336:1046–1053.
30. Albert CM, Manson JE, Hennekens CH. Fish consumption and the risk of myocardial infarction. N Engl J Med 1997; 337:497.
31. GISSI-Prevenzione Investigators. Dietary supplementation with n-3 polyunsaturated fatty acids and vitamin E after myocardial infarction: results of the GISSI-Prevenzione trial. Lancet 1999; 354:447–455.
32. Rimm EB, Stampfer MJ, Ascherio A, et al. Vitamin E consumption and the risk of coronary heart disease in men. N Engl J Med 1993; 328:1450–1456.
33. Stampfer MJ, Hennekens CH, Manson JE, et al. Vitamin E consumption and the risk of coronary heart disease in women. N Engl J Med 1993; 328:1444–1449.
34. The Alpha-Tocopherol, Beta-Carotene Cancer Prevention Study Group. The effect of vitamin E and beta-carotene on the incidence of lung cancer and other cancers in male smokers. N Engl J Med 1994; 330:1029–1035.
35. Rapola JM, Virtamo J, Ripatti S, et al. Randomised trial of alpha-tocopherol and beta-carotene supplements on incidence of major coronary events in men with previous myocardial infarction. Lancet 1997; 349:1715–1720.
36. Stephens NG, Parsons A, Schofield PM, et al. Randomised controlled trial of vitamin E in patients with coronary heart disease: The Cambridge Heart Antioxidant Study (CHAOS). Lancet 1996; 347:781–786.
37. Mitchinson MJ, Stephens NG, Parsons A, et al. Mortality in the CHAOS trial. Lancet 1999; 353:381.
38. Ness A, Davey Smith G. Mortality in the CHAOS trial. Lancet 1999; 353:1017–1018.
39. Sebbag L, Forrat R, Canet E, Renaud S, Delaye J, et al. Effect of dietary supplementation with alpha-tocopherol on myocardial infarct size and ventricular arrhythmias in a dog model of ischemia and reperfusion. J Am Coll Cardiol 1994; 24:1580–1585.
40. Forrat R, de Lorgeril M, Haddour G, et al. Effect of chronic oral supplementation with alpha-tocopherol on myocardial stunning in the dog. J Cardiovasc Pharmacol 1997; 29:457–462.
41. Ide T, Tsutui H, Kinugawa S, Utsumi H, Takeshita A. Amiodarone protects cardiac myocytes against oxidative injury by its free radical scavenging action. Circulation 1999; 100:690–692.
42. Kupari M, Koskinen P. Alcohol, cardiac arrhythmias and sudden death. Novartis Found Symp 1998; 216:68–79.
43. Wannamethee G, Shaper AG. Alcohol and sudden cardiac death. Br Heart J 1992; 68:443–448.
44. Kagan A, Yano K, Reed DM, MacLean CJ. Predictors of sudden cardiac death among Hawaiian-Japanese men. Am J Epidemiol 1989; 130:268–277.
45. Albert CM, Manson JE, Cook NR, et al. Moderate alcohol consumption and the

risk of sudden cardiac death among US male physicians. Circulation 1999; 100:944–950.

46. Kromhout D. Fish consumption and sudden cardiac death. JAMA 1998; 279:65–66.
47. Stone NJ. Fish consumption, fish oil, lipids and coronary heart disease. 1996; 94:2337–2340.

# XII

## Medical Therapy

# 43

# Mechanisms of Defibrillation

*Nipon Chattipakorn, MD, PhD,*
*and Raymond E. Ideker, MD, PhD*

## Introduction

Ventricular fibrillation (VF) is responsible for most cases of sudden cardiac death in the industrialized world.[1] Currently, electrical defibrillation is the only successful clinical therapy for patients with this lethal arrhythmia. Despite the wide application of transthoracic and intracardiac defibrillators, the mechanisms by which the electrical shock terminates fibrillation are still not clear. In this chapter, we present some possible mechanisms to explain how an electric shock succeeds or fails in halting VF.

## Electrical Stimulation and Cardiac Responses

Unlike the action potential in nerve or in skeletal muscle, which is a brief and biphasic event, the cardiac action potential lasts longer, and the cardiac cell responds differently to an electrical stimulus than a nerve cell does.[2] Depending on the stimulation strength and the phase of the action potential at the time of stimulation, 3 possible responses can be observed:[2] (1) no response, (2) a new action potential, and (3) a graded response. When the stimulus is too weak or the cardiac cell is too refractory, no response is observed. When the stimulus is stronger (above threshold) and the cell is fully recovered or relatively refractory, a new action potential will be generated (Figure 1A).[3] When the stimulus is very strong and the cell is highly refractory, a graded response occurs (Figure 1B). The size of the graded response increases as the stimulus magnitude and/or coupling interval increases. This graded response prolongs the action potential duration as well as the refractory period of the cardiac cell.4 This type of response is thought to be important in the defibrillation process since it can prevent an activation front from propagating into or arising in this region.[4,5]

Supported in part by National Institutes of Health research grants HL-28429 and HL-42760.

From: Aliot E, Clementy J, Prystowsky EN (editors). *Fighting Sudden Cardiac Death: A Worldwide Challenge.* ©Futura Publishing Company, Armonk, NY, 2000.

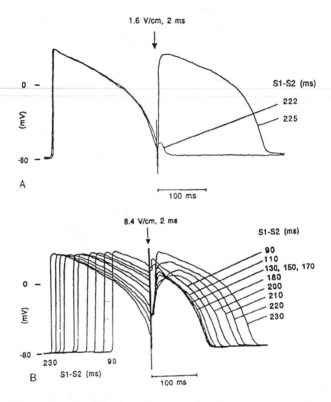

**Figure 1. (A)** Single-cell recordings illustrating the response to an S2 shock field stimulus with a potential gradient strength of 1.6 V/cm at the cell. The S1–S2 stimulus intervals for each of the responses are shown to the right of the recordings. The responses were markedly different, depending on a change in the S2 timing of only 3 ms. S2 given at an S1–S2 interval of 222 ms produced almost no response, whereas S2 given at an S1–S2 interval of 225 ms produced a new action potential. **(B)** Recordings from the same cell as in **A**, illustrating a range of action potential prolongation produced by an S2 field stimulus having a strength of 8.4 V/cm. The recordings, obtained from one cellular impalement, are aligned with the S2 time. The longest and shortest S1–S2 intervals tested, 230 and 90 ms, are indicated with their respective S1 phase-zero depolarizations. The S1–S2 intervals for each of the responses after S2 are indicated to the right of the recordings. The degree of action potential extension increased as the S1–S2 interval increased. (Reproduced with permission from Circulation Research.[3])

# The Probabilistic Nature of Defibrillation

During different VF episodes and at different times during the same VF episode, activation sequences are not constant and can differ markedly.[6,7] Cardiac responses to the same strength shocks, therefore, can be different from one shock to the next, depending on the state of the ventricles when the shock

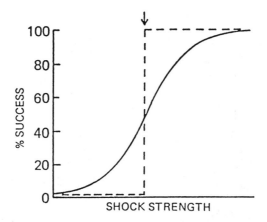

Figure 2. The probability of defibrillation success curve. There is not a discrete threshold (dashed line), above which shocks always succeed and below which shocks always fail. Instead, a sigmoid- shaped dose-response curve exists, in which shocks of higher strength are associated with greater odds of defibrillation success. (Modified by permission from American Heart Journal.[10])

is given. Since cardiac responses are crucial in determining defibrillation success, shocks of the same strength can sometimes succeed and other times fail in halting fibrillation. Other factors that may contribute to the probability of success for defibrillation include changes in autonomic tone and changes in heart volume during VF.[8] As a result, there is no definite threshold in shock strength that demarcates successful from failed defibrillation. Therefore, the relationship between the shock strength and defibrillation success is best characterized as probabilistic. The dose-response curve of this relationship (Figure 2) indicates that the greater the shock strength, the greater the percent defibrillation success for both transthoracic and intracardiac defibrillation.[9,10]

## The Importance of Potential Gradients Created by the Shock

Defibrillation success is believed to occur if a sufficient current density is achieved throughout the ventricular myocardium.[11] Although in vivo measurements of current density have been made, it is more difficult to measure experimentally than in the potential gradient.[12] Therefore, the potential (voltage) gradient, i.e., the change of potential with distance, is more commonly measured.[13] Potential gradients in the heart are calculated from the potentials created by the shock and the distances between recording electrodes. The potential gradient may be an important factor in determining the cellular responses to defibrillation shocks.[14,15]

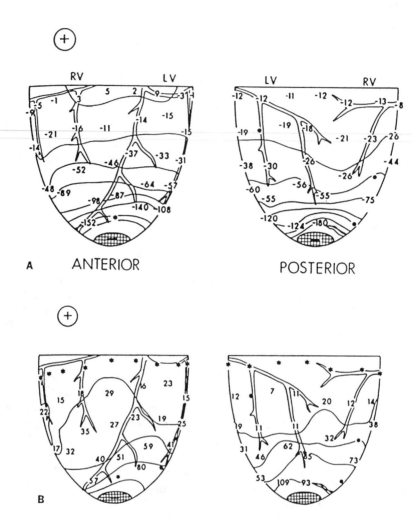

Figure 3. The epicardial potential and potential gradient distribution created by a shock delivered from electrodes (cross-hatched circles) at the apex (cathode[−]) and right atrium (anode [+]). The maps are displayed as 2 complementary projections of the ventricles with anterior left ventricular (LV) and right ventricular (RV) epicardium shown in the left diagram and the posterior LV and RV epicardium in the right diagram. Numbers represent the potential (**A**, mV) and potential gradient (**B**, mV/cm) for those electrode locations. Closed circles indicate electrode sites where adequate recordings were not obtained. Asterisks indicate electrode sites for which no gradient was calculated because there were neighboring electrodes on only one side. The isopotential lines are 25 mV per shock volt (25 mV/V) apart; the isogradient lines are 25 mV/cm/V apart. (**A**) The isopotential map during a 1-V shock given during diastole. The voltage drop across the heart was 189 mV, 18.9% of the potential difference delivered to the electrodes. The isopotential lines were closer together at the apex than at the base of the heart, indicating a higher gradient at the apex as calculated in **B**. (**B**) The isogradient map of the same shock. The higher gradient area was near the apex and the lower gradient area was at the base. There was a 102 mV/cm/V difference between the maximal and minimal gradients on the surface of the heart. (Reproduced with permission from Circulation.[16])

When the shock is delivered, the distribution of the change in shock potential over space is not uniform across the heart. Figure 3A shows an epicardial potential distribution recorded from a dog for a 1-V shock delivered from electrodes on the right atrium (anode) and left ventricular apex (cathode).[16] The voltage drop was marked at the apical portion of the ventricles close to the site where the ventricular defibrillation electrode was located. The potential gradients (Figure 3B) calculated from this potential distribution are markedly uneven. For this right atrial and left ventricular apical electrode configuration, the potential gradient is much larger and changes faster (as indicated by narrow spacing between isogradient lines) in the api-

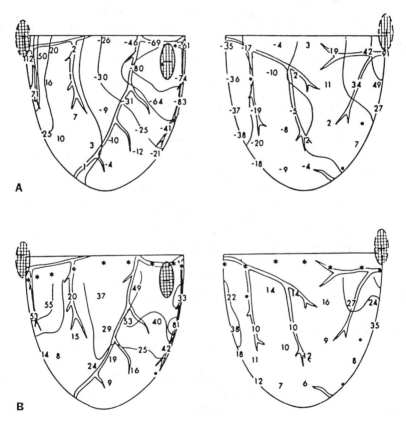

A

B

Figure 4. The epicardial potential and potential gradient distribution created by a 1.5-V shock delivered from electrodes (cross-hatched circles) at the right (anode [+]) and left (cathode[−]) ventricular bases. (A) The voltage drop between electrodes was 195 mV/V, 19.5% of the voltage given. The isopotential lines were closer together near the 2 defibrillation electrodes. (B) The isogradient map for the same shock. High gradient areas were located near the 2 defibrillation electrodes. There was a 75 mV/cm/V difference between the maximal and minimal gradients on the surface of the heart. (Reproduced with permission from Circulation.[16])

cal portion than in the basal portion of the ventricles. The pattern of the potential and potential gradient distributions depends on the location of the shocking electrodes. Figure 4 shows the potential and potential gradient distributions for a shock delivered from electrodes at the lateral base of the right (anode) and left (cathode) ventricles. For this electrode configuration, the highest gradient areas were in the basal portion of the ventricles near the electrodes and the weakest gradient areas were near the apex.[16]

Thus, the potential gradient distribution has a similar pattern for most shocking electrode configurations in that the high potential gradient region with rapidly changing gradients is always near the defibrillation electrodes and the low potential gradient region with fewer changes in gradient frequently occurs at regions distant from the shocking electrode.[16,17] Other factors that also have a direct effect on the potential gradient distribution include conductivity differences of different organs, fiber orientation,[18] myocardial connective tissue barriers,[19,20] blood vessels, scar tissue, and ischemia.[21,22]

## Sites of the Earliest Postshock Activation

The relationship between sites of early postshock activation and the potential gradient distribution are well correlated. Figure 5 demonstrates the results from the same animal as shown in Figures 3 and 4. The site of the earliest recorded postshock activation was at the base of the ventricles for the shock given from the right atrial and ventricular apical electrodes (Figure 5A) and was at the apex of the ventricles for the shock given from the right and left ventricular basal electrodes (Figure 5B). Both sites correspond to the low potential gradient region created by each shocking electrode configuration. These results indicate that the potential gradient field is important in determining the response of the myocardium to defibrillation shocks. To defibrillate, it has been proposed that it is necessary to raise the potential gradient throughout all or almost all of the ventricular myocardium to a certain minimum level that is different for different shock waveforms.[23] Since the potential gradient field created by the shock is markedly uneven, a strong shock is required to achieve this minimum level when the gradient field is weakest in the ventricles. However, this strong shock creates an excessively high field in the high gradient region near the electrodes, and it may damage the myocardium,[24,25] resulting in postshock conduction block and arrhythmias.[26]

## Activation Fronts After Unsuccessful Shocks

Two possible mechanisms have been proposed for the earliest postshock activation that occurs in the low potential gradient regions follow-

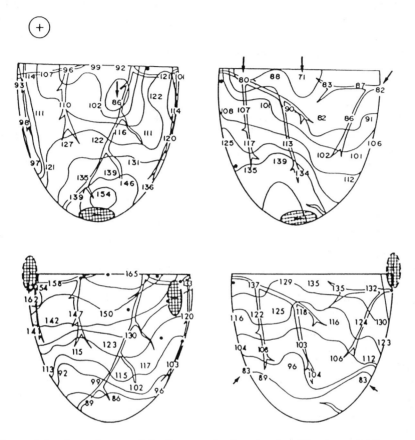

**Figure 5.** Isochronal maps of the first postshock activation. The thin solid lines are isochrones spaced 10 ms apart. Numbers represent activation times at each recording electrode in ms timed with respect to the onset of the shock. (**Top**) A 4.9-J unsuccessful defibrillation shock given during fibrillation via the electrodes placed at the right atrium and the apex. The early sites of activation were located at the base of the ventricles (arrows), the region where the shock field was weak as indicated by the gradient map shown in Figure 3 for this shocking electrode configuration. Activation then spread away from the base so that the apex was the last region to be activated. (**Bottom**) A 23.2-J unsuccessful defibrillation shock given during fibrillation via the electrodes placed at the right and left ventricular bases. The early sites of activation were located at the posterior and apical aspects of the ventricles (arrows), the region where the shock field was weak as indicated by the gradient map shown in Figure 4 for this shocking electrode configuration. The base was the last region to be activated. (Reproduced with permission from Circulation.[16])

ing shocks of a strength near the defibrillation threshold that fail to defibrillate: (1) the gradient field created by the shock is too weak to halt the fibrillatory wavefronts present in those regions at the time of the shock,[27–29] or (2) the shock halts these fibrillatory wavefronts but creates new activation fronts in these regions.[30–32] For either mechanism, activation then spreads out from the regions of low potential gradient, causing disorganized activation in the remainder of the ventricles, allowing fibrillation to resume. Since the direct effect of the shock at each cardiac site depends on both the strength of the shock (i.e., the potential gradient) and the phase of the cardiac cycle at the time the shock is delivered, the shock potential gradient must be sufficiently high to stop fibrillatory fronts on the ventricles and/or not create new activations that allow fibrillation to resume.[30–32]

## The Critical Point Hypothesis

One explanation for the relationship among the shock potential gradient, shock delivery time, and fibrillation induction was proposed theoretically by Winfree[33] and demonstrated experimentally by Frazier et al.[34] This relationship is known as the critical point hypothesis and is based on the different responses of cardiac tissue to an electrical stimulation. Some regions of the myocardium can be directly activated by the shock field to undergo a new action potential while other regions can undergo refractory period extension caused by a graded response of the action potential.[3,4,35,36] If a directly activated region is adjacent to a region with refractory period extension, no activation front can arise in the directly activated region and propagate through the region of refractory period extension because the latter region will be refractory.[37,38] However, an activation front can arise and propagate away from other portions of a directly activated region where it is not bordered by refractory tissue.[34,37] This front can later propagate to activate the region with a refractory period extension that has in the interim had time to recover and from there propagate into the region earlier directly activated by the shock, forming a reentrant circuit that may break down into VF.

Frazier and colleagues34 have investigated this phenomenon by mapping while a shock is delivered to the heart during paced rhythm (Figure 6). Figure 6A illustrates the distribution of activation times and recovery times during the last S1 pacing beat in a dog. S1 pacing was delivered from a row of epicardial stimulating wires on the right of the recording region. Solid lines represent the spread of the activation front away from the S1 electrodes while dashed lines represent the recovery times estimated from the refractory period to a local 2-mA stimulus. Approximately parallel isochronal lines and isorecovery lines indicate minimal inhomogeneity of refractoriness.

Figure 6B shows the potential gradients created by a large premature S2 shock delivered through a long narrow electrode placed near the bot-

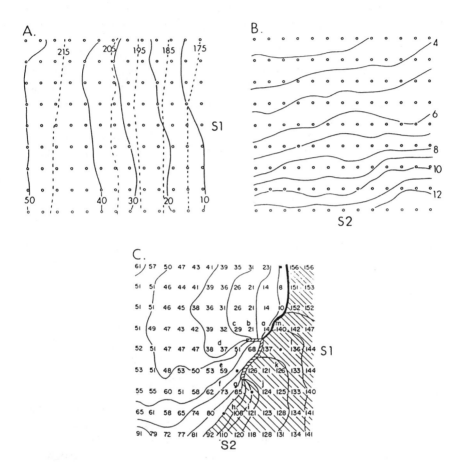

**Figure 6.** Initiation of reentry and VF following orthogonal interaction of myocardial refractoriness and the potential gradient field created by a large S2 stimulus. (**A**) The distribution of activation times during the last S1 beat (solid lines) and recovery times to a local 2-mA stimulus (dashed lines). (**B**) The potential gradient field of the S2 stimulus. (**C**) The initial activation pattern just after the S2 stimulus. The hatched area represents portions of the array thought to be directly activated by the S2 stimulus field. The heavy black line depicts the transition between successive activation maps and is known as a frame line. The frame line also represents the origin of the activation front propagating away from the directly activated region. The hatched line delineates a zone of functional conduction block, and the solid lines portray isochronal lines spaced at 10-ms intervals. (Reproduced with permission from The Journal of Clinical Investigation.[34])

tom of the mapped region perpendicular to the activation front arising from the S1 pacing stimulus. The potential gradient was high close to the S2 electrode and weakened with distance away from the S2 electrode. The isogradient lines were approximately perpendicular to the recovery lines after S1 pacing.

S2 shocks were delivered to scan the vulnerable period following the last S1. At an appropriate S1–S2 coupling interval, a reentrant circuit was formed that degenerated into VF. Figure 6C shows the initial pattern of activation when the reentrant circuit was formed. Following the strong S2 stimulation, activation did not arise close to the S2 electrode and propagate away as in the case of the weaker S1 stimulus. Instead, an activation front first appeared a few centimeters away from the S2 electrode, with one end terminating blindly at a point in the center of the mapped region, where the S2 potential gradient was approximately 6 V/cm and where the tissue was just passing out of its absolute refractory period.[34] This point is called the critical point for reentry. The value of the S2 potential gradient and the degree of recovery at the critical point may be different for different waveforms. This activation front then propagated away from the S1 electrode, pivoted around the critical point, and later spread through the lower left quadrant, and formed a reentrant circuit as it entered the right lower quadrant.

This phenomenon is thought to occur because of the simultaneous occurrence of different cardiac tissue responses to the S2 shock field in different cardiac regions. The mapped region can be divided into 4 quadrants (centered at the critical point) based on the cardiac tissue responses to the S2 shock. Myocardium at the top and bottom right quadrants (hatched region) had recovered enough at the time of the shock to be directly activated. Myocardium at the top left quadrant was still refractory at the time the S2 was delivered and was not directly activated by the S2 shock. Also, the refractoriness of the myocardium in this quadrant was not extended since the potential gradient created by the S2 shock in this region was too weak to induce this type of response. However, the refractoriness of cardiac tissue in the bottom left quadrant was prolonged since it was close to the S2 electrode and thus was exposed to a potential gradient large enough to induce a graded response. Therefore, the activation front forming in the directly excited region (hatched) could propagate only within the mapped region from the top right to the top left quadrant. Activation in the directly activated tissue in the bottom right quadrant could not propagate to the left since it was blocked by cardiac tissue in a prolonged refractory state. As this tissue recovered, the activation front from the top left quadrant entered the bottom left quadrant and propagated through it to reenter the directly activated tissue in the lower right quadrant, which had by this time recovered excitability, forming a counterclockwise reentrant circuit around the critical point.

Figure 7A is an idealized diagram representing this type of critical point formation. A region of direct activation (DA) is close to the S1 electrode and a region that has refractory period extension (RPE) is close to the S2 electrode. Thus, the activation from the DA region is blocked in the RPE region, resulting in clockwise unidirectional propagation around the critical point.

A recent study by Efimov et al.,[39] using an optical mapping technique to investigate the mechanism of failed defibrillation, demonstrated an-

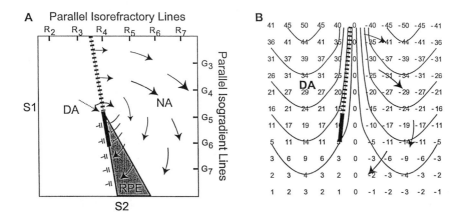

Figure 7. Two types of hypothesized critical points. **(A)** Idealized diagram corresponding to the experiment shown in Figure 6 is shown with a critical point formed at the intersection of a critical shock potential gradient of G5 and a critical tissue refractoriness of R4. S1 pacing is performed from the left to cause a dispersion of refractoriness at the time of the S2 shock with R2 representing less and R7 more refractoriness. The S2 shock is given during the vulnerable period from the bottom of the region with large gradient G7 at the bottom and small gradient G3 at the top. The region labeled DA is sufficiently recovered so that it is directly activated by the gradient field. The area in the stippled region, although more refractory, is exposed to a higher gradient and undergoes refractory period extension, RPE, so that activation in the DA tissue cannot propagate through this region. The region NA is too refractory to be affected even with a large gradient. Thus, propagation conducts unidirectionally from the DA to NA region at the top, encircling the critical point, reentering the DA region to create a reentrant circuit. **(B)** An idealized diagram is shown of a critical point caused by adjacent regions of depolarized and hyperpolarized transmembrane potential changes. Numbers represent transmembrane changes with isolines spaced every 10 mV beginning at $-45$ mV. DA occurs to the left of the frame line where depolarized transmembrane potential changes are suprathreshold. Where the gradient in transmembrane potential is high, as indicated by the closely spaced isolines at the top center of the panel, conduction can occur into the hyperpolarized region. Below, where the gradient in transmembrane potential is smaller, propagation cannot occur. A critical point is formed at the intersection of the frame and block lines where one end of the propagating activation front terminates in both panels.

other interpretation of reentrant circuit formation at a critical point. Instead of the critical potential gradient and the refractoriness, formation of this critical point depends on the magnitude and distribution of depolarization and hyperpolarization of the transmembrane potential, as graphically illustrated in Figure 7.

Figure 7B is an idealized diagram of this type of critical point formation caused by adjacent regions of depolarization and hyperpolarization.[19,40] In the DA region, the magnitude of depolarization is high and gradually decreases from top (large positive numbers) to bottom (small positive numbers). In the adjacent region of hyperpolarization caused by the shock, the magnitude of hyperpolarization is also high at the top (large negative numbers) and gradually decreases toward the bottom (small negative numbers). This distribution creates a large gradient of transmembrane potentials between the depolarized and hyperpolarized regions as indicated by the closely spaced isolines at the top center of the panel, allowing an activation front to propagate from the depolarized region into the hyperpolarized region (arrow at the top). In the bottom half of the panel where the gradient in transmembrane potentials is smaller, propagation does not occur. Hence, a critical point is formed at the intersection of the frame and block lines (indicated by hatched and solid black lines, respectively) where one end of the propagating activation front terminates.

These different interpretations of critical point formation suggest that the relationship between the shock delivered to a fibrillating heart and the cardiac responses to the shock is complex. Whatever causes the formation of a critical point, both interpretations suggest that a reentrant pattern is responsible for fibrillation after a failed shock. However, most cardiac mapping studies using a large-animal model indicate that a focal activation pattern is most commonly observed after a shock fails to defibrillate.[29,31,38,41,42] It is possible that transmural or Purkinje-myocardial reentry could exist since most studies have included only epicardial mapping.[29,31,38,42] However, a transmural mapping study has shown that only some episodes of fibrillation following a failed defibrillation shock were initiated by a reentrant pattern.[41] These findings suggest that the current interpretations of critical point formation may only partially explain defibrillation mechanisms.

## The Upper Limit of Vulnerability

In 1940, Wiggers and Wegria demonstrated that VF can be induced when a sufficiently strong electrical stimulus is given during the repolarization interval of normal rhythm, the so-called "vulnerable period."[43] This stimulus strength is known as the VF threshold (Figure 8). As the stimulation strength is increased above this threshold, VF can still be induced until the stimulus strength reaches a much higher threshold above

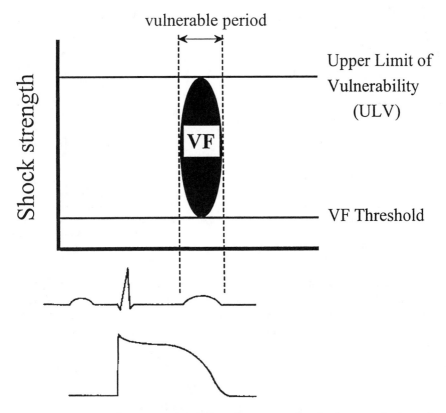

Figure 8. Diagram illustrating the relationship among the shock strength, the vulnerable period, and VF. Shocks of a strength at or above the VF threshold induce VF (filled oval) when delivered at an appropriate time during the vulnerable period (corresponding to a portion of the T wave on the ECG or the repolarization phase of the action potential). Shocks stronger than the upper limit of vulnerability, however, no longer induce VF when given at any time during the cardiac cycle.

which VF again can no longer be induced. This higher stimulus threshold above which VF is no longer induced no matter when the stimulus is delivered during the vulnerable period is known as the upper limit of vulnerability (Figure 8).[44]

During the reentry of VF, activation and repolarization are present simultaneously in different portions of the myocardium. Some portions of myocardium, therefore, should be in the vulnerable period during the delivery of any defibrillation shock. If an upper limit of vulnerability did not exist, then a defibrillation shock, which almost certainly exceeds the fibrillation threshold in this region, would be expected to reinduce VF in the region. This consideration raises the possibility that the upper limit of vulnerability and the defibrillation threshold are related and share the same

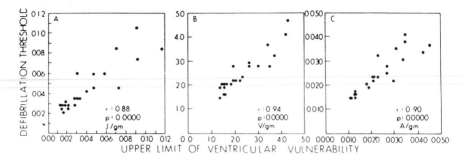

**Figure 9.** Correlation of the approximate strength of the shock required to defibrillate (the defibrillation threshold) and the upper limit of vulnerability for electrodes on the right atrium (anode) and the left ventricular apex (cathode) in 22 dogs. Results are expressed in units of energy (**A**), voltage (**B**), and current (**C**). All units are expressed per gram of heart weight. (Reproduced with permission from Circulation.[45])

mechanism. Indeed, studies on the relationship between the upper limit of vulnerability shock strength and the defibrillation threshold have shown that they are highly correlated (Figure 9),[45,46] also suggesting that the upper limit of vulnerability may be used to explain the defibrillation mechanism.[30,31,44,47]

# The Upper Limit of Vulnerability Hypothesis for Defibrillation

The upper limit of vulnerability hypothesis for defibrillation states that to successfully defibrillate, the shock must: (1) halt VF activation fronts, and (2) not create new activations that reinduce VF.[48,49] The relationship between the defibrillation threshold and the upper limit of vulnerability can be explained partially by the critical point hypothesis. Figure 10 illustrates the concept that links together the critical point, the vulnerable region, and defibrillation. When a weak shock (i.e., at the VF threshold) is delivered to the heart, it creates the critical potential gradient near the shocking electrode (line a). Thus, the formation of a critical point, i.e., the intersection between the isogradient line and the isorecovery line, is also close to the S2 electrode. When the strength of the shock is stronger, the critical gradient will be farther away from the shocking electrode (lines b–h). Therefore, the formation of critical points and reentrant circuits will move farther away from the shocking electrode. However, when the shock is strong enough that the potential gradients created by the shock are greater than the critical value throughout the entire ventricular myocardium (line i), no critical point will be created in the ventricles and no reen-

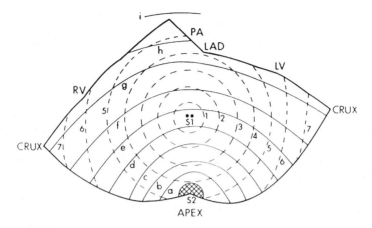

**Figure 10.** Hypothesized relationship between the critical point, the vulnerable period, and defibrillation. The epicardial surface of the canine heart is depicted as if the ventricles were folded out after an imaginary cut was made from the crux to the apex. Isorecovery lines (dashed lines 1–7), representing different degrees of refractoriness, are concentric about the pacing site labeled S1. Large premature stimuli are delivered from the apex of the heart through the electrode labeled S2 with the return electrode located elsewhere in the body away from the heart. Isogradient lines (solid lines a–i), representing different levels of extracellular potential gradient, are concentric about the S2 electrode, with the smallest values in the ventricles occurring in the small region at the top of the ventricles representing the pulmonary outflow tract. RV = right ventricle; LV = left ventricle; PA = pulmonary artery; and LAD = left anterior descending coronary artery. (Modified with permission from Cardiac Pacing and Electrophysiology.[49])

trant circuit will be formed. This shock strength therefore reaches the level of the upper limit of vulnerability and will successfully defibrillate. This concept has recently been tested and is supported experimentally by a study from Idriss and colleagues.[50]

The upper limit of vulnerability hypothesis for defibrillation also states that failed defibrillation has a mechanism similar to VF induction by shocks given during the vulnerable period.[49] The 2 critical point hypotheses discussed above are possible mechanisms by which shocks can induce VF and defibrillation failure. Other mechanisms are also possible. For example, recent VF induction studies, using shocks of a strength near the upper limit of vulnerability in a large-heart model,[51,52] indicate that a rapid repetitive focal pattern of early postshock activations arising from the low gradient region is responsible for VF induction. Other studies suggest that shock-induced automaticity or triggered activity may be responsible for this early postshock activation.[53–56] Hence, in addition to reentrant activation, focal activity caused by the shock is also a possible mechanism responsible for failed defibrillation according to the upper limit of vulnerability hypothesis.

## Postshock Isoelectric Window and Refractoriness

Early cardiac mapping studies found that, following defibrillation shocks, the time until the first activation was recorded after the shock that propagated globally across the ventricles was longer for successful than for failed defibrillation.[30,31] This interval between the shock and the first recorded postshock activation was thought to be electrically silent and was known as the "isoelectric window."[30] Later studies demonstrated that the degree of refractory period extension caused by the shock is greater and occupies a larger area for successful than for failed defibrillation.[57]

An optical mapping study extended the refractory period extension concept by demonstrating that shocks can cause refractory period extension even when given very early in the fibrillatory action potential just after completion of the upstroke. In this study, the shock caused all of the myocardium to repolarize at the same time after the shock regardless of its fibrillating electrical activity just prior to the shock.[58] This constant repolarization time after the shock creates a uniformly prolonged postshock response duration (an isoelectric window) as well as a reduction in dispersion of refractoriness, which is thought to prevent reentry in successful defibrillation. This concept is known as the synchronized repolarization hypothesis for defibrillation.[58] Against the hypothesis is the finding from a recent mapping study that activations occur during the isoelectric window that only propagate locally for a short distance and disappear before the first postshock activation that propagates globally across the heart is observed. These activations are known as "locally propagated activations" and occur following both successful and failed defibrillation shocks (Figure 11).[38] The existence of locally propagated activation indicates that the isoelectric window is not completely electrically silent and suggests that a uniform degree of refractoriness throughout the ventricles is not absolutely necessary for successful defibrillation.

Recently, a new defibrillation hypothesis known as the "progressive depolarization" hypothesis has been proposed by Dillon and Kwaku.[59] This hypothesis also attempts to unify the mechanisms of defibrillation and fibrillation induction by shocks. It emphasizes the influence of the progressive increase in depolarization with an increase in shock strength as a factor causing an increased prolongation of the refractory period, resulting in synchronized repolarization and less dispersion of refractoriness, caused by defibrillation as well as VF induction shocks. This hypothesis postulates that the immediate postshock tissue responses, i.e., the immediate postshock activation pattern, are key determinants for defibrillation or VF induction outcome.

Recent studies of both defibrillation and VF induction disagree with

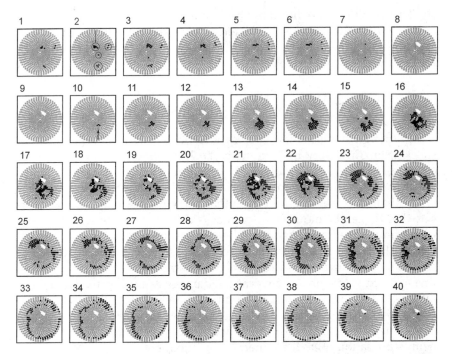

Figure 11. The presence of locally propagated activation (LPA) following a failed defibrillation shock. Each map represents a polar view of the ventricles. The interval between consecutive maps is 2 ms. Each black dot represents local activation at 1 of 504 epicardial electrodes. LPAs were detected 48 ms after the shock (circles, frame 1), propagated locally and disappeared after which a first globally propagated activation (GPA) was observed (arrow, frame 10). The GPA wavefront blocked without propagating through one LPA region (circle with arrow in frame 2). White dots from frames 8–40 indicate the LPA region in which this block occurred. (Reproduced with permission from Circulation.[38])

this hypothesis. Defibrillation studies using shocks of identical strength near the defibrillation threshold demonstrated that the immediate postshock activation pattern was not significantly different between successful and failed shocks.[29,38,42] Similarly, VF induction studies using shocks of the same strength delivered at the same time during the T wave also demonstrate that the first postshock activations are indistinguishable between episodes in which shocks did and did not induce VF.[51,52] These recent findings suggest that the progressive depolarization observed in previous studies is shock strength-dependent and may not have a direct cause and effect relationship with defibrillation outcome. These findings are consistent with the upper limit of vulnerability hypothesis since the activation patterns following defibrillation and VF induction shocks demonstrate similar behavior as predicted by this hypothesis.[49] These results also suggest that when the shock strength and timing are constant, factors in addition to the immediate response after the shock are important in determining the shock outcome.[51,52]

## Detrimental Effects of Strong Shocks

Although defibrillation success is probabilistic and dependent on shock strength, a very high-strength shock does not always assure successful defibrillation. An early study by Schuder et al.[60] has shown that if the shock strength is increased too high, defibrillation success decreases rather than increases (Figure 12). Studies using high-strength shocks indicate that VF can be induced when shocks considerably stronger than the upper limit of vulnerability are delivered at any point in the cardiac cycle.[46,61] The low probability of success for defibrillation and the high chance of VF induction at excessively high-strength shocks are probably due to electroporation and myocardial damage caused by the large magnitude (above approximately 50 V/cm) of the shock field.[57,62,63] This myocardial dysfunction, which is characterized by loss of intracellular potassium, membrane depolarization, decreased conduction velocity, and neurostimulation of both adrenergic and cholinergic fibers,[64,65] may lead to fibrillation after the shock.

Since the potential gradient distribution is markedly uneven for the shocking electrode configurations used with implantable defibrillators, a high shock strength is required to generate the minimum potential gradi-

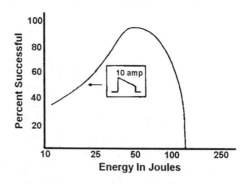

Figure 12. The relationship between success of transthoracic ventricular defibrillation and energy content of a trapezoidal shock in dogs. The energy of the 10-ampere leading edge shock is increased by increasing the duration of the shock. (Modified with permission from Circulation Research.[60])

ent needed for defibrillation at regions far from the shocking electrodes. If the shock is too strong, myocardium close to the shocking electrodes experiences an excessively high gradient and may become transiently dysfunctional or damaged, leading to refibrillation. Following failed defibrillation shocks near the defibrillation threshold delivered from the electrodes at the right ventricular apex and superior vena cava, Walker et al.66 demonstrated that the earliest postshock activation arose at the left apical and anterolateral left ventricles where the potential gradient was weak. For shocks a few hundred volts higher than the defibrillation threshold, the earliest postshock activation arose from the right ventricle and the posterior left ventricle near the right ventricular electrode, where the potential gradient was high but did not induce VF. For a few shocks that were even a few hundred volts higher, tachyarrhythmias were induced after the shock that arose from the high gradient region.

## Mechanisms of Defibrillation Are Not Completely Understood

In the past several decades, the mechanism of defibrillation has been extensively explored. Much has been discovered and defibrillation techniques have improved, yet the mechanism of defibrillation is still only incompletely understood. Recent findings suggest that the determinant for defibrillation and VF induction by shocks near the defibrillation threshold could be the number and rapidity of repetitive activations arising from the low potential gradient region, rather than the characteristics of the immediate postshock activation.[51,52] More studies need to investigate how these activations arise and why they sometimes stop and at other times continue. Application of drugs both in vitro and in vivo are a further step to study the mechanism of defibrillation and how fibrillation occurs after the shock.[67,68]

The continuing debate on whether reentry, a focus, or both are responsible for fibrillation after the shock needs to be settled. Several questions are unanswered. It is important to know where and why activation arises after the shock. Although the epicardial patterns of activation have been investigated extensively after defibrillation and VF induction, the exact intramural origin of these activations is still vague. Three-dimensional cardiac mapping should be pursued to reveal the origin.

## *References*

1. Zipes DP, Wellens HJJ. Sudden cardiac death. Circulation 1998; 98:2334–2351.
2. Katz AM. The cardiac action potential. In: Physiology of the Heart. Raven Press Ltd., New York, NY, 1992, pp 438–472.
3. Knisley SB, Smith WM, Ideker RE. Effect of field stimulation on cellular repo-

larization in rabbit myocardium: implications for reentry induction. Circ Res 1992; 70:707–715.

4. Dillon SM. Optical recordings in the rabbit heart show that defibrillation strength shocks prolong the duration of depolarization and the refractory period. Circ Res 1991; 69:842–856.

5. Tovar OH, Jones JL. Relationship between "extension of refractoriness" and probability of successful defibrillation. Am J Physiol 1997; 272:H1011–H1019.

6. Janse MJ, Wilms-Schopman FJG, Coronel R. Ventricular fibrillation is not always due to multiple wavelet reentry. J Cardiovasc Electrophysiol 1995; 6:512–521.

7. Huang J, Rogers JM, KenKnight BH, Rollins DL, Smith WM, et al. Evolution of the organization of epicardial activation patterns during ventricular fibrillation. JCE 1998; 9:1291–1304.

8. Strobel JS, Kay GN, Walcott GP, Smith WM, Ideker RE. Defibrillation efficacy with endocardial electrodes is influenced by reductions in cardiac preload. J Intervent Cardiac Electrophys 1997; 1:95–102.

9. Gold JH, Schuder JC, Stoeckle H. Contour graph for relating percent success in achieving ventricular defibrillation to duration, current, and energy content of shock. Am Heart J 1979; 98:207–212.

10. Davy JM, Fain ES, Dorian P, Winkle RA. The relationship between successful defibrillation and delivered energy in open-chest dogs: reappraisal of the "defibrillation threshold" concept. Am Heart J 1987; 113:77–84.

11. Witkowski FX, Kerber RE. Currently known mechanisms underlying direct current external and internal cardiac defibrillation. J Cardiovasc Electrophysiol 1991; 2:562–572.

12. Jarzembski WB. Current density measurement in living tissue. In: Myklebust JB, Cusick JF, Sances A, Jr, Larson SJ (eds). Neural Stimulation. CRC Press, Boca Raton, FL, 1985, pp 33–45.

13. Lepeschkin E, Jones JL, Rush S, Jones RE. Local potential gradients as a unifying measure for thresholds of stimulation, standstill, tachyarrhythmia and fibrillation appearing after strong capacitor discharges. Adv Cardiol 1978; 21:268–278.

14. Frazier DW, Krassowska W, Chen P-S, Wolf PD, Dixon EG, et al. Extracellular field required for excitation in three-dimensional anisotropic canine myocardium. Circ Res 1988; 63:147–164.

15. Krassowska W, Pilkington TC, Ideker RE. Periodic conductivity as a mechanism for cardiac stimulation and defibrillation. IEEE Trans Biomed Eng 1987; 34:555–560.

16. Chen P-S, Wolf PD, Claydon FJ, III, Dixon EG, Vidaillet HJ Jr, et al. The potential gradient field created by epicardial defibrillation electrodes in dogs. Circulation 1986; 74:626–636.

17. Tang ASL, Wolf PD, Claydon FJ, III, Smith WM, Pilkington TC, et al. Measurement of defibrillation shock potential distributions and activation sequences of the heart in three dimensions. Proc IEEE 1988; 76:1176–1186.

18. Eason J, Trayanova N. The effects of fiber curvature in a bidomain tissue with irregular boundaries. Proc of the 15th Annual Internat'l Conf of the IEEE Engineering in Medicine and Biology Society, 1993, pp 744–745.

19. Gillis AM, Fast VG, Rohr S, Kléber AG. Spatial changes in transmembrane potential during extracellular electrical shocks in cultured monolayers of neonatal rat ventricular myocytes. Circ Res 1996; 79:676–690.

20. Fast VG, Rohr S, Gillis AM, Kléber AG. Activation of cardiac tissue by extracellular electrical shocks: formation of 'secondary sources' at intercellular clefts in monolayers of cultured myocytes. Circ Res 1998; 82:375–385.

21. Mizumaki K, Fujiki A, Tani M, Misaki T. Effects of acute ischemia on anisotropic conduction in canine ventricular muscle. PACE 1993; 16:1656–1663.
22. White JB, Walcott GP, Pollard AE, Ideker RE. Myocardial discontinuities: a substrate for producing virtual electrodes to increase directly excited areas of the myocardium by shocks. Circulation 1998; 97:1738–1745.
23. Ideker RE, Chen P-S, Zhou X-H. Basic mechanisms of defibrillation. J Electrocardiol 1991; 23(Suppl):36–38.
24. Dahl CF, Ewy GA, Warner ED, Thomas ED. Myocardial necrosis from direct current countershock: effect of paddle size and time interval between discharge. Circulation 1974; 50:956–961.
25. Jones JL, Lepeschkin E, Jones RE, Rush S. Response of cultured myocardial cells to countershock-type electric field stimulation. Am J Physiol 1978; 235:H214-H222.
26. Jones JL, Jones RE. Postshock arrhythmias: a possible cause of unsuccessful defibrillation. Crit Care Med 1980; 8:167–171.
27. Zipes DP, Fischer J, King RM, Nicoll A, Jolly WW. Termination of ventricular fibrillation in dogs by depolarizing a critical amount of myocardium. Am J Cardiol 1975; 36:37–44.
28. Witkowski FX, Penkoske PA, Plonsey R. Mechanism of cardiac defibrillation in open-chest dogs with unipolar DC-coupled simultaneous activation and shock potential recordings. Circulation 1990; 82:244–260.
29. Zhou X, Daubert JP, Wolf PD, Smith WM, Ideker RE. Epicardial mapping of ventricular defibrillation with monophasic and biphasic shocks in dogs. Circ Res 1993; 72:145–160.
30. Chen P-S, Shibata N, Dixon EG, Wolf PD, Danieley ND, et al. Activation during ventricular defibrillation in open-chest dogs: evidence of complete cessation and regeneration of ventricular fibrillation after unsuccessful shocks. J Clin Invest 1986; 77:810–823.
31. Shibata N, Chen P-S, Dixon EG, Wolf PD, Danieley ND, et al. Epicardial activation following unsuccessful defibrillation shocks in dogs. Am J Physiol 1988; 255:H902-H909.
32. Chen P-S, Wolf PD, Ideker RE. Mechanism of cardiac defibrillation: a different point of view. Circulation 1991; 84:913–919.
33. Winfree AT. When Time Breaks Down: The Three-Dimensional Dynamics of Electrochemical Waves and Cardiac Arrhythmias. Princeton University Press, Princeton, NJ, 1987.
34. Frazier DW, Wolf PD, Wharton JM, Tang ASL, Smith WM, et al. Stimulus-induced critical point: mechanism for electrical initiation of reentry in normal canine myocardium. J Clin Invest 1989; 83:1039–1052.
35. Zhou X, Knisley SB, Wolf PD, Rollins DL, Smith WM, et al. Prolongation of repolarization time by electric field stimulation with monophasic and biphasic shocks in open-chest dogs. Circ Res 1991; 68:1761–1767.
36. Jones JL, Jones RE, Milne KB. Refractory period prolongation by biphasic defibrillator waveforms is associated with enhanced sodium current in a computer model of the ventricular action potential. IEEE Trans Biomed Eng 1994; 41:60–68.
37. Kwaku KF, Dillon SM. Shock-induced depolarization of refractory myocardium prevents wavefront propagation in defibrillation. Circ Res 1996; 79:957–973.
38. Chattipakorn N, KenKnight BH, Rogers JM, Walker RG, Walcott GP, et al. Locally propagated activation immediately after internal defibrillation. Circulation 1998; 97:1401–1410.

39. Efimov IR, Cheng Y, Van Wagoner DR, Mazgalev T, Tchou PJ. Virtual electrode-induced phase singularity: a basic mechanism of defibrillation failure. Circ Res 1998; 82:918–925.
40. Efimov IR, Cheng YN, Biermann M, Van Wagoner DR, Mazgalev TN, et al. Transmembrane voltage changes produced by real and virtual electrodes during monophasic defibrillation shocks delivered by an implantable electrode. J Cardiovasc Electrophysiol 1997; 8:1031–1045.
41. Chen P-S, Wolf PD, Melnick SD, Danieley ND, Smith WM, et al. Comparison of activation during ventricular fibrillation and following unsuccessful defibrillation shocks in open-chest dogs. Circ Res 1990; 66:1544–1560.
42. Usui M, Callihan RL, Walker RG, Walcott GP, Rollins DL, et al. Epicardial shock mapping following monophasic and biphasic shocks of equal voltage with an endocardial lead system. J Cardiovasc Electrophysiol 1996; 7:322–334.
43. Wiggers CJ, Wégria R. Ventricular fibrillation due to single, localized induction and condenser shocks applied during the vulnerable phase of ventricular systole. Am J Physiol 1940; 128:500–505.
44. Shibata N, Chen P-S, Dixon EG, Wolf PD, Danieley ND, et al. Influence of shock strength and timing on induction of ventricular arrhythmias in dogs. Am J Physiol 1988; 255:H891–H901.
45. Chen P-S, Shibata N, Dixon EG, Martin RO, Ideker RE. Comparison of the defibrillation threshold and the upper limit of ventricular vulnerability. Circulation 1986; 73:1022–1028.
46. Lesigne C, Levy B, Saumont R, Birkui P, Bardou A, et al. An energy-time analysis of ventricular fibrillation and defibrillation thresholds with internal electrodes. Med Biol Eng 1976; 14:617–622.
47. Chen P-S, Wolf PD, Dixon EG, Danieley ND, Frazier DW, et al. Mechanism of ventricular vulnerability to single premature stimuli in open-chest dogs. Circ Res 1988; 62:1191–1209.
48. Walcott GP, Walcott KT, Ideker RE. Mechanisms of defibrillation. J Electrocardiol 1995; 28:1–6.
49. Ideker RE, Tang ASL, Frazier DW, Shibata N, Chen P-S, et al. Ventricular defibrillation: basic concepts. In: El-Sherif N, Samet P (eds). Cardiac Pacing and Electrophysiology. W.B. Saunders Co., Philadelphia, PA, 1991, pp 713–726.
50. Idriss SF, Wolf PD, Smith WM, Ideker RE. Effect of pacing site on the upper limit of vulnerability determinations. Am J Physiol (in press).
51. Chattipakorn N, Rogers JM, Ideker RE. Influence of postshock epicardial activation patterns on the initiation of ventricular fibrillation by shocks near the upper limit of vulnerability. Circulation 2000; 101:1329–1336.
52. Chattipakorn N, Fotuhi PC, Sreenan KM, White JB, Ideker RE. Pacing-induced epicardial activation patterns after upper limit of vulnerability shocks: impact on fibrillation induction. Circulation. (In press).
53. Li HG, Jones DL, Yee R, Klein GJ. Defibrillation shocks produce different effects on Purkinje fibers and ventricular muscle: implications for successful defibrillation, refibrillation and postshock arrhythmia. J Am Coll Cardiol 1993; 22:607–614.
54. Sano T, Sawanobori T. Mechanism initiating ventricular fibrillation demonstrated in cultured ventricular muscle tissue. Circ Res 1970; 26:201–210.
55. Antoni H, Tagtmeyer H. Die Wirkung starker Ströme auf Errungsbildung und Kontraktion des Herzmuskels. Beitr Ersten Hilfe Bei Unfaellen Durch Elekt Strom 1965; 4:1.
56. Antoni H, Berg W. Wirkungen des Wechselstroms auf Erregungsbildung und

Kontraktion des Saugetiermyocards. Beitr Ersten Hilfe Bei Unfaellen Durch Elekt Strom 1967; 5:3.

57. Jones JL, Tovar OH. The mechanism of defibrillation and cardioversion. Proc IEEE 1996; 84:392–403.

58. Dillon SM. Synchronized repolarization after defibrillation shocks: a possible component of the defibrillation process demonstrated by optical recordings in rabbit heart. Circulation 1992; 85:1865–1878.

59. Dillon SM, Kwaku KF. Progressive depolarization: a unified hypothesis for defibrillation and fibrillation induction by shocks. J Cardiovasc Electrophysiol 1998; 9:529–52.

60. Schuder JC, Rahmoeller GA, Stoeckle H. Transthoracic ventricular defibrillation with triangular and trapezoidal waveforms. Circ Res 1966; 19:689–694.

61. Fabiato A, Coumel P, Gourgon R, Saumont R. Le seuil de réponse synchrone des fibres myocardiques: application à la comparaison expérimentale de l'efficacité des différentes formes de chocs électriques de défibrillation. Arch Mal C_ur 1967; 60:527–544.

62. Jones JL, Proskauer CC, Paull WK, Lepeschkin E, Jones RE. Ultrastructural injury to chick myocardial cells in vitro following "electric countershock." Circ Res 1980; 46:387–394.

63. Tung L. Detrimental effects of electrical fields on cardiac muscle. Proc IEEE 1996; 84:366–378.

64. Moore EN, Spear JF. Electrophysiologic studies on the initiation, prevention, and termination of ventricular fibrillation. In: Zipes DP, Jalife J (eds). Cardiac Electrophysiology and Arrhythmias. Grune & Stratton, Inc, Orlando, FL, 1985, pp 315–322.

65. Koning G, Veefkind AH, Schneider H. Cardiac damage caused by direct application of defibrillator shocks to isolated Langendorff-perfused rabbit heart. Am Heart J 1980; 100:473–482.

66. Walker RG, Walcott GP, Smith WM, Ideker RE. Sites of earliest activation following transvenous defibrillation. Circulation 1994; 90:I-447.

67. Ujhelyi MR, Schur M, Frede T, Bottorff MB, Gabel M, et al. Mechanisms of antiarrhythmic drug-induced changes in defibrillation threshold: role of potassium and sodium channel conductance. J Am Coll Cardiol 1996; 27:1534–1542.

68. Ujhelyi MR, Schur M, Frede T, Gabel M, Markel ML. Differential effects of lidocaine on defibrillation threshold with monophasic versus biphasic shock waveforms. Circulation 1995; 92:1644–1650.

---
# 44

# Can Nonantiarrhythmic Drugs Prevent Sudden Cardiac Death?

*E. Aliot, MD, C. de Chillou, MD,*
*I. Magnin-Poull, MD, and N. Sadoul, MD*

---

## Introduction

Sudden cardiac death (SCD) accounts for about 40% of the mortality in patients with chronic heart failure (CHF) and about 50% in patients with a previous myocardial infarction (MI). Since CAST, the use of antiarrhythmic drugs has been limited by hazardous side effects such as the potential for proarrhythmia and a negative chronotropic action. Some post-MI patients and CHF patients are at high risk for SCD, and prophylactic amiodarone has been shown to reduce the likelihood of arrhythmic SCD in such patients.[1] However, for clinical practice, it could be useful to consider the potential electrophysiological effect of "nonantiarrhythmic" drugs such as β blockers, ACE inhibitors, antialdosterone agents, etc. In this chapter, we will review the role of nonantiarrhythmic drugs on SCD in post-MI patients and in patients with CHF.

## β-Blocking Agents

### Myocardial Infarction

The beneficial cardioprotective, antiischemic, and antifibrillatory effects of β blockers have been recognized for a long time. They probably control factors predisposing to electrical instability such as myocardial ischemia, high cardiac sympathetic tone, and decreased vagal tone. In addition, a retarding effect on the progression rate of the underlying disease process has been suggested from experimental data.[2-4] The role of β blockers in increasing the threshold for ventricular fibrillation (VF) has been

From: Aliot E, Clementy J, Prystowsky EN (editors). *Fighting Sudden Cardiac Death: A Worldwide Challenge.* ©Futura Publishing Company, Armonk, NY, 2000.

clearly demonstrated by the reduced incidence of VF in the early phase of MI.[5] Actually, the mechanism by which early mortality is decreased by IV β blockers is not clear. A certain part of the mortality reduction may be explained by a reduction of myocardial rupture in the first days of MI. A meta-analysis of available data from 30 trials indicates a 15–25% reduction of reinfarction, sudden death, and lethal ventricular arrhythmias (ventricular arrhythmias) (15% reduction in the incidence of VF).[5]

Several broad trials with different β-blocking agents have demonstrated the long-term effects of β blockers that improve survival with about three-fourths of the mortality reduction explained by a reduction in SCD and presumably VF. An overview of the results of 25 trials including 24,298 patients indicates a 23% reduction in total mortality and a 32% reduction in sudden death[5,6] (Figure 1). The possibility that ancillary properties of the various agents may differentially affect their benefits has been raised. In fact, there is no statistically significant heterogeneity among benefits observed in the trials that use β blockers with intrinsic sympathomimetic activity and those without in terms of mortality and sudden death.[2,7] Finally, the benefits of β-blocking agents appear to be greater among high-risk patients such as those with a low ejection fraction than among low-risk patients.[5] Last but not least, β-blocking agents may also be useful in patients taking other antiarrhythmic drugs. Retrospective studies of the CAST and of the amiodarone trials have shown that patients tak-

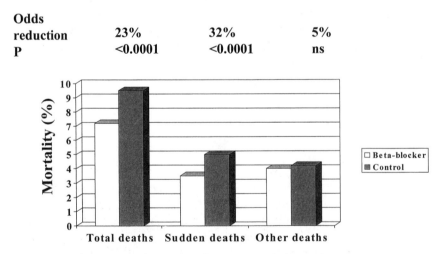

Figure 1. Long-term beta-blocking therapy after myocardial infarction. An overview of the results of 25 trials including 24,298 patients indicates a 23% reduction in total mortality and a 32% reduction in sudden death. (Used with permission from Held et al.[5])

ing β blockers were likely to have fewer incidents of sudden death and nonfatal arrest than those receiving only antiarrhythmic drugs.[8,9]

## Congestive Heart Failure

Twenty-five years ago, it was known that CHF was associated with an increase in sympathetic nervous activity. It was thought that this was a compensatory increase in order to counteract depressed myocardial function and that the β-blocking agents might cause worsening CHF. Actually, in the last 15 years, data have been accumulated to support the beneficial effect of β blockers in cases of CHF.[10]

Activity of the sympathetic nervous system is one of the cardinal pathophysiological abnormalities in patients with CHF. Norepinephrine can exert adverse effects on the circulation, both directly and indirectly, and interference with its activity can retard the progression of CHD. Previous studies with different β-blocking agents have shown that these drugs can reduce symptoms, improve left ventriclular (LV) function and increase functional capacities, but the effects of β blockers on morbidity and mortality in patients with CHF were not classified.[11]

The efforts made in examining the effects of carvedilol (a nonselective β receptor antagonist that also blocks α-1-receptors and has antioxidant effects) on CHF patients have been important in raising interest in β blockers for this condition.[12] In a double-blind placebo-controlled study, 1,094 patients with CHF and left ventricular ejection fraction (LVEF) ≤35% were enrolled in which patients were assigned to 1 of the 4 treatment protocols on the basis of their exercise capacity (mild, moderate, severe CHF). They randomly received either placebo (n=398) or carvedilol (n=696). Although this trial was not designed and powered to examine mortality as a predefined efficacy variable, there was an impressive survival benefit. It was consistent in all evaluated groups, including patients with ischemic heart disease, and was reflected in a decrease in the risk of death from progressive CHF as well as in the risk of SCD. The overall mortality rate was 7.8% in the placebo group and 3.2% in the carvedilol group, of which there were 15 (3.8%) SCDs in the placebo group and 12 (1.7%) in the carvedilol group.

CIBIS II (13) was a multicenter double-blind randomized placebo-controlled study that investigated the efficacy of bisoprolol, a β-1-selective adrenoreceptor blocker, in decreasing all-cause mortality in CHF. In this study, 2,647 symptomatic patients in NYHA Class III or IV with LVEF ≤35% receiving standard therapy with diuretics and ACE inhibitors were randomly assigned to either bisoprolol (1.25 mg to a maximum of 10 mg/day) (n=1,327) or placebo (n=1,320). Patients were followed for a mean of 1.3 years and the study was stopped early because bisoprolol showed a significant mortality benefit. All-cause mortality was significantly lower with bisoprolol than with placebo (156 [11.8%] versus 228 [17.3%] with a hazard ratio of 0.66 (0.54–0.80). Sudden death was decreased by 44% with fewer sudden deaths among patients on bisoprolol (48 [3.6%] than among those on placebo (83 [6.3%]).

The MERIT HF[14] study investigated whether metoprolol controlled release/extended release (CR/XL) once daily would lower mortality in patients with decreased LV function and symptoms of CHF. In this study, 3,991 patients with CHF, NYHA functional Class II-IV, LVEF ≤40%, stabilized with optimum standard therapy, were enrolled in a double-blind randomized control study; 1,990 patients were randomly assigned to metoprolol CR/XL 12.5 mg (NYHA III–IV) or 25 mg once daily (NYHA II) and 2,001 were assigned to placebo. The larger dose was 200 mg once a day. This study was also stopped early after a mean follow-up of 1 year. All-cause mortality was lower in the metoprolol group than in the placebo group (147 [7.2% per patient year of follow-up] versus 217 deaths 11%; RR: 0.66). Again, sudden death was decreased by 41% with fewer sudden deaths in the metoprolol group than in the placebo group (79 versus 132, RR 0.59 [0.45–0.78]).

Decreases in sudden death were similar in the 2 studies (41% in MERIT HF and 44% in CIBIS II). These results suggest an important antiarrhythmic effect. Evidence suggests that substantial proportions of sudden deaths are due to VF.[15] Although a similar difference was not seen in CIBIS,[11] a significant trend has been shown in the US carvedilol study.[12] In CIBIS, the rate of ventricular tachycardia was lower in a substudy in which vagally dependent variability in heart rate was higher in the bisoprolol group than in the placebo group, an effect linked to improved long-term prognosis after MI and CHF.[16] Moreover, the lower rate of admission to hospital for ventricular tachycardia or VF in CIBIS II bisoprolol group suggests the drug's potential antiarrhythmic effect.[13]

Metoprolol has protective effects on SCD after acute MI,[2] and has similar effects in hypertensive patients.[2,17] These data and the results of MERIT HF suggest an antifibrillatory effect of metoprolol.[14] In theory, β blockade of β-1-adrenoreceptors and β-2-adrenoreceptors should provide more complete protection against the harmful effects of catecholamines, but the results of CIBIS II and MERIT HF suggest that selective inhibition of β-1-receptors is sufficient to lower the rate of sudden death presumed to be associated with arrhythmias (Figure 2). The difference in effects according to the pharmacological profiles of β blockers is, however, important and other trials with different agents will provide essential information.[13]

The message of these 2 studies is clear. Sudden death, the most common mode of death from CHF, is reduced by more than 40% by β-1-blockers, thereby being complementary to angiotensin-converting enzyme (ACE) in-

| | CIBIS II (Bisoprolol) | | | MERIT HF (Metoprolol) | | | US Carvedilol (Carvedilol) | |
|---|---|---|---|---|---|---|---|---|
| | P (n=1320) | B (n=1327) | Risk Reduction | P (n=2001) | M (n=1990) | Risk Reduction | P (n=398) | C (n=696) |
| Total deaths | 228 (17%) | 156 (12%) | 34% | 217 (10.8%) | 145 (7.3%) | 34% | 31 (7.8%) | 22 (3.2%) |
| Pump Failure deaths | 47 (4%) | 36 (3%) | 26% | 58 (2.8%) | 30 (1.5%) | 49% | 13 (3.3%) | 5 (0.7%) |
| SCD | 83 (6%) | 48 (4%) | 44% | 132 (6.6%) | 79 (3.9%) | 41% | 15 (3.8%) | 12 (1.7%) |

Figure 2. Beta-blocking agents, chronic heart failure, and sudden cardiac death: a comparison of bisoprolol, metoprolol, and carvedilol. See text for further details.

hibitor therapy, which has no proven effect on sudden death among such patients.[10] The continued accumulation of information about β blockers in CHF is important to hasten the use of β blockade in clinical practice outside specialized departments. At the present time, addition of a β blocker to standard therapy can be recommended in appropriate stable ambulatory patients who have CHF caused by impaired LV function[13] (Figure 2).

# ACE Inhibitors

## Antiarrhythmic Properties of ACE Inhibitors

There is no doubt that ACE inhibitors profoundly affect myocardial loading conditions. However, whether or not this is the basis of ACE inhibitor electrophysiological effects remains unclear.[18] Remodeling is associated with changes in the function and distribution of cardiac myocytes and cardiac interstitium.[19,20] These changes lead to dilation, hypertrophy, and reduced contractility. They may contribute to the generation of ventricular arrhythmias as well as the alteration of LV function.

Dilation of the left ventricle and myocardial ischemia predict ventricular arrhythmias during both acute and chronic phases after acute MI. Despite the lack of placebo control, the results of the Holter subgroup of V-HeFT II deserve attention.[21] Enalapril-treated patients had fewer complex arrhythmias than did their hydralazine isosorbide dinitrate-treated counterpart. In a Holter substudy of SAVE patients, fewer premature ventricular contractions were reported in the ACE inhibitor-treated patients. In post-MI patients with LV dysfunction, this study has shown that captopril has a beneficial effect on both the number of ventricular arrhythmias as well as the number of patients who develop ventricular arrhythmias during the chronic phase.[22] This seems in all probability mediated through the effects on LV remodeling, LV function, and myocardial ischemia in patients who are exposed to an increased risk of undergoing progressive dilation of the LV. Actually, ACE inhibitors have a powerful hemodynamic effect and might reverse ventricular hypertrophy and decrease LV size, both of which are determinant factors in the genesis of arrhythmias.

A reduction in refractoriness will increase the incidence of ventricular arrhythmias, increasing the incidence of sudden death. In an electrophysiological study comparing ACE inhibitors, or captopril with a combination of hydralazine and isosorbide dinitrate, the ACE inhibitor modifications of loading prolonged ventricular refractoriness and repolarization while non-ACE inhibitor vasodilators did not, possibly reflecting a combination of mechanoelectrical effects with a restraining influence of ACE inhibitors on reflex sympathetic stimulation.[23] This is consistent with experimental data suggesting that ACE inhibitors interfere with $i_K$ currents and the L-type calcium current.[24] Further support for the clinical relevance of ACE inhibitors' calcium channel effects comes from research in isolated guinea pig hearts, but this work emphasized other factors that were likely to be contributory such as loading effects, electrolyte stabilization, and regression of LV hypertrophy.[25]

Elevated level of angiotensin II may be deleterious not only in the progression of atherosclerosis but in electrical stability of the heart, increasing the incidence of ventricular arrhythmias. Angiotensin II increases junction gap resistance, resulting in an increase in muscle resistance for electrical conduction. This will increase ventricular arrhythmias through reentry. Enalapril has been shown to decrease intracellular resistance and increase conduction velocity.[26,72] It has also been shown that in ischemia and hypertrophy, junctional conductance of myocytes increases, leading to an increase of arrhythmias as well as a higher incidence of CHF due to the uncoupling of heart cells.[27] It has been observed that an intrinsic renin angiotensin system in the heart is involved in the control of junction gap conductance in cardiac muscle. The use of ACE inhibitors and angiotensin II receptor blockers (losartan) may improve and stabilize the electrical status of the myocytes, reducing the incidence of arrhythmias and CHF.[27,72] Clinical data have also shown that ACE inhibitors may increase ventricular activity conduction in humans[28] and reduce QT dispersion, thereby reducing the cardiac electrical instability.[29,72] The electrophysiological effects of ACE inhibitors are also a consequence of their antagonism to determine effects of angiotensin II on the autonomic nervous system, of their mild β-blocking properties, and of the decrease of sympathetic tone. In fact, ACE inhibitors also have β-blocking properties, and it is possible that for some patients ACE inhibitor modification of sympathetic tone has a useful antiarrhythmic effect.[30-32] Indeed, sympathetic activity increases the risk of ventricular arrhythmias. Treatment with ACE inhibitors may reduce circulating norepinephrine as well as angiotensin II, which is a facilitator of adrenergic neurotransmission.[32] ACE inhibitors may also increase prostacycline synthesis, which reduces local epinephrine release.[33] Improvement in the hemodynamic state may also result in sympathetic withdrawal, reducing sympathetically mediated vasoconstriction. In addition, baroreflex sensitivity is increased by ACE inhibitors, and this may be an important mechanism of reducing sympathetic and enhancing vagal tone, potentially reducing SCD.[32–34] The influence of some ACE inhibitors on HRV (heart rate variability), which is a strong predictor of ventricular arrhythmias and SCD, may be beneficial in reducing the risk of SCD in post-MI patients.[35]

Last, but not least, ACE inhibitors also stabilize electrolyte concentrations, and this, too, may be relevant.[36,37] The use of ACE inhibitors may also provide some protection against potassium depletion, since it may offset the potential adverse effect of diuretics.

In summary, the reduction in propensity to ventricular arrhythmias afforded by the ACE inhibitors is likely related to attenuation of the remodeling process, reduction in potassium depletion, sympatholytic properties, decrease of LV hypertrophy, β-negative action, and other properties that are not well understood. On the other hand, SCD may also result from the electrical instability to coronary occlusion and resultant MI. Chronic ACE inhibitor therapy in patients with LV dysfunction has been shown to reduce the incidence of MI in both SAVE[38] and SOLVD[46] studies. Other mechanisms of SCD such as ventricular rupture may be prevented by the ventricular remodeling effect of ACE inhibitors.

## ACE Inhibitors in Post-MI Patients

ACE inhibitors have been tested in different clinical populations, such as post-MI patients (major trials: SAVE, AIRE, TRACE, CONSENSUS II)[38–41] and patients with CHF, with a different selection of these patients in 4 major trials (CONSENSUS, V-HeFT II, and SOLVD prevention and treatment).[44–47] Although the classification of death in CHF is complex, data are consistent which have shown that ACE inhibitors decrease the risk of sudden death after MI, with a reduction in SCD as an important component of this survival benefit. The SAVE, TRACE, and AIRE[38–40] studies (Figure 3) investigated the role of ACE inhibitors on mortality and morbidity in patients with LV dysfunction after MI. In SAVE,[38] 2,231 patients with EF ≤40% but without symptoms of overt heart failure or symptoms of ischemia were randomly assigned to receive double blind treatment either with placebo (1,116) or captopril (1,115) within 3–16 days after MI. During a follow-up of an average of 42 months, mortality from all

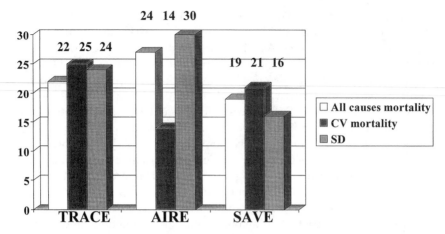

Figure 3. ACE inhibitors: mortality reduction in post-MI patients as investigated in the SAVE, TRACE, and AIRE[38–40] trials. See text for further details.

causes was significantly reduced in the captopril group (228 deaths, 20%) compared with the placebo group (275 deaths, 25%), with a reduction in risk of 19%. Sudden death, with or without preceding symptoms, showed only a trend to reduction in the captopril group without a statistically significant difference (105 deaths in the ACE inhibitors group versus 125 in the placebo group; OR: 0.83, 0.63–1.08).

TRACE[40] for the first time has shown a significant reduction of sudden death with ACE inhibitors (trandolapril) in 1,749 patients with MI and echocardiographic evidence of LV dysfunction (EF ≤35%). Three to 7 days after MI, they received either oral trandolapril (876 patients) or placebo (873 patients). During the follow-up of 24–50 months, in the trandolapril group, the relative risk (RR) of death compared with the placebo group was 0.78. One hundred five patients died suddenly in the trandolapril group versus 133 in the placebo group (OR: 0.76 [0.58–1.00]). The importance of the effects on sudden death of ACE inhibitors after MI was confirmed by the detailed results of the AIRE study.[40,42] This study randomized 2,006 patients with clinical or radiological evidence of heart failure 2–9 days after MI to receive ramipril 5 mg bid (1,014) or matching placebo (992). At an average follow-up of 15 months, mortality from all causes was significantly lower in the ramipril group (170 deaths, 17%) than in the placebo group (222 deaths, 23%) with an overall 27% reduction in the risk of death. Ramipril reduced the risk of sudden death by 30% (89 in the ramipril group versus 121 in the placebo group; OR: 0.69 [0.52–0.93]). However, overall, 45% of patients who died suddenly had severe or worsening heart failure prior to their deaths and only 30% of sudden deaths were considered to be arrhythmic. Therefore, retarding the progression of heart failure appears to be a major factor contributing to the reduction in mortality both by reducing circulatory failure and sudden death, at least in this study.

These 3 major studies are included in a recent meta-analysis on the effect of ACE inhibitors on sudden death in patients following MI.[43] In this analysis, from 15 trials including 15,104 patients, 2,356 patients died, with 900 deaths being sudden. A significant reduction or trend in SCD risk was observed in all of the larger (n>500 patients) trials (OR: 0.80 [0.70–0.92]). These results suggest that a reduction in SCD with ACE inhibitors is an important component of the survival benefice (OR: 0.83 [0.71–0.97]).

## ACE Inhibitors in Chronic Heart Failure

Defining death as sudden in patients with CHF is difficult. It is possible that an effect of ACE inhibitors on sudden presumptively arrhythmic death might be missed or overestimated. Until V-HeFT II,[44] there was nothing to suggest an ACE inhibitor's effect on sudden death in CHF. In this trial, enalapril demonstrated a favorable trend toward less arrhythmic deaths, especially in patients with relatively preserved LV function.[44] The reduction in mortality associated with enalapril compared to hydralazine/isosorbide therapy was due to a reduction in the incidence of sudden death (risk reduction, 39%). This is different from the results of the CONSENSUS trial in which mortality only from pump failure was reduced by enalapril.[45] If myocardial stretch were the mechanism of these arrhythmias, it would be expected to be more readily modified before widespread fibrosis had become established.[18] This may be due to a non-vasodilator mechanism. Again, it is difficult to interpret data as sudden death in the setting of progressive heart failure, and progressive heart failure alone may not be differentiated as in the SOLVD trials[46,47] (Figure 4).

Actually, the SOLVD trials, prevention, and treatment have studied the effects of enalapril: (1) on total mortality and mortality from cardiovascular causes, the development of heart failure, and hospitalization for heart failure in patients with EF ≤35% who were not receiving treatment for CHF (prevention);[46] and (2) on mortality and hospitalizations in patients with CHF and EF ≤35% (treatment).[47] There was a trend toward fewer deaths due to cardiovascular causes among the patients who received enalapril in the prevention study[46] and a significant reduction of mortality and hospitalization for heart failure among patients who received enalapril in the treatment study.[47] As far as sudden death is concerned, it is difficult to interpret data because it is not possible to differentiate sudden death in the setting of progressive heart failure and progressive heart failure alone. Enalapril reduced the number of arrhythmias without worsening heart failure in both studies: prevention: 98 versus 105 in the placebo group, reduction in risk 7%, NS; treatment: 105 versus 113 in the placebo group, risk

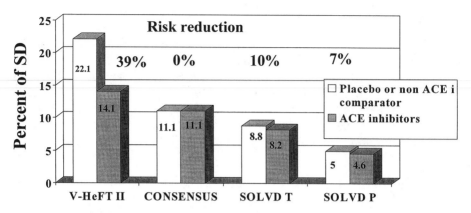

**Figure 4.** The effects of ACE inhibitors on sudden cardiac death in chronic heart failure: a comparison of results in the V-HeFT II, CONSENSUS, SOLVD T, and SOLVD P trials. See text for further details.

reduction 10%. Enalapril also reduced the number of progressive heart failures (pump failure or arrhythmias with CHF): prevention: 85 versus 106 in the placebo group, risk reduction 21%, p=0.1; treatment: 209 versus 215 in the placebo group, risk reduction 22%, p<0.004).

Even though these data are not as impressive as in post-MI patients, they are nevertheless consistent with the fact that the predominant effect of ACE inhibitors might be to prevent sudden death in this setting. On the other hand, the question remains whether a differentiation between circulation failure and SCD can be achieved with accuracy especially if the patients died out of the hospital.[73] "Retarding the progression of heart failure appears to be a major factor contributing to the reduction in mortality both by reducing circulation failure and SCD."[42] It might well be that possible reduction in sudden death reflects the same beneficial effect of ACE inhibitors on LV function. The difference in the mode of death might be due to the definitions and the assessment performed.[73]

## Angiotensin II Inhibitors

The benefits of ACE inhibitors have been attributed mainly to blockade of angiotensin II production and/or to a decrease in the breakdown of bradykinin. Nonpeptide angiotensin II type I receptor antagonists, such as losartan, can block this receptor, especially with increasing bradykinin levels, and since angiotensin II may be produced by alternate pathways, such drugs may have additional advantages over ACE inhibitors where blockade of the effects of angiotensin II is incomplete.[48]

The ELITE[48] study was a prospective double-blind randomized parallel-controlled clinical trial to determine whether specific angiotensin II receptor blockade with losartan offers safety and efficacy advantages in the treatment of CHF over ACE inhibitors with captopril. Seven hundred twenty-two ACE inhibitor-naïve patients with NYHA Class II–IV heart failure and EF ≤40% were assigned to double-blind losartan (n=352) titrated to 50 mg once a day or captopril (n=370) titrated to 50 mg 3 times a day. Even though it was only a secondary end-point, death and/or heart failure admissions occurred in 33 losartan-treated patients (9.4%) and 49 captopril-treated patients (13.2%). The risk reduction of 32% was due primarily to a decrease in all-cause mortality. Moreover, analysis by cause suggested that although the numbers of events were small, the lower total mortality in the losartan group was primarily due to a reduction in SCD (5 [1.4%]) versus 14 (3.8%), risk reduction 0.64 (0.03–0.86). These data from ELITE do not seem to be confirmed by ELITE II, designed to compare as a primary effect the effect of losartan and captopril on all-cause mortality. This study did not show any difference in total mortality between patients in the losartan group and in the captopril group, including SCD (unpublished communication, AHA, 1999, B. Pitt).

Even though losartan does not appear to be more effective than captopril, it seems to reduce the risk of SCD in patients over age 65 with CHF. Whether this property is specific to agents that may have some direct or indirect antiarrhythmic activity independent of angiotensin II receptor blockade in simulated ventricular arrhythmias and ischemia,[49] or whether it is due only to the blockade of angiotensin II, has to be confirmed. As mentioned above, the use of ACE inhibitors and angiotensin II receptor blockers may improve and stabilize the electrical status of the myocytes, reducing the incidence of arrhythmias and CHF.[27]

The effects of losartan and captopril have been studied in an elite subpopulation.[50] QT duration increased in the captopril-treated patients but did not in the losartan-treated patients. It is possible that the reduction in sudden death might be due to a more direct and effective blocking of the arrhythmogenic effect of angiotensin II by losartan. Losartan and its active metabolite E3174 have been shown experimentally to prevent ventricular dysrhythmias. This effect could be mediated through more effective suppression of sympathetic tone. No definite conclusion can be drawn from this limited retrospective study or from the ELITE I and II studies.

## Antialdosterone

The frequency of sudden death is greater in patients with CHF than in any other definable subset of patients in cardiovascular medicine. When sufficient myocardial damage is sustained to cause a decrease of myocardial output, several compensatory mechanisms become activated. Among these, the renin-angiotensin-aldosterone system plays a major role. The stimulation of the renin-angiotensin-aldosterone system with increased circulating aldosterone causes the distal renal tubules to secrete potassium. The use of diuretics, especially nonpotassium-sparing diuretics, further stimulates the release of aldosterone and can be additive, leading to hypokalemia and excretion of magnesium as well, increasing the risk of ventricular arrhythmias. Both neurohormonal systems not only aggravate ventricular loading conditions by causing systemic vasoconstriction, but also may induce ventricular arrhythmias by the direct and indirect action on myocardial conduction and excitability.[51]

A retrospective analysis of the SOLVD studies has recently been conducted to assess the relation between diuretic use at baseline and the subsequent risk of arrhythmic death in 6,797 patients with an EF ≤35%.[52] Interestingly, the use of nonpotassium-sparing diuretics was independently associated with arrhythmic death. Use of a potassium-sparing diuretic alone or in combination with a nonpotassium-sparing diuretic was not independently associated with an increased risk of arrhythmic death. These data suggest that diuretic-induced electrolyte disturbances may result in fatal arrhythmias in patients with systolic LV dysfunction and suggest that the use of a potassium-sparing diuretic may either be protective when a nonpotassium-sparing diuretic is needed or should be considered when diuretic therapy is required.

The RALES study enrolled 1,663 patients who had severe heart failure and LVEF ≤35% who were being treated with an ACE inhibitor, a loop diuretic, and in most cases, digoxin.[53] Eight hundred twenty-two patients were randomly assigned to receive 25 mg spironolactone daily and 841 to receive placebo. The trial was discontinued early after a mean follow-up of 24 months because an interim analysis determined that spironolactone reduced the number of deaths of all causes (386 [46%]) deaths in the placebo group versus 284 [35%] in the spironolactone group, RR: 0.70). This reduction was attributed to a significantly lower risk of both progressive heart failure deaths and SCDs: 110 SCDs in the placebo group versus 82 in the spironolactone group (RR: 0.71; 0.54–0.95). These results are consistent with the current understanding of the effects of aldosterone in patients with heart failure.

As mentioned previously, in addition to promoting sodium and fluid retention, aldosterone enhances urinary potassium excretion, aggravating the hypokalemia and magnesium depletion caused by treatment with loop diuretics. The consequence of these electrolyte disturbances can include myocardial electric instability and death of cardiac myocytes.[54] In hypertensive patients, potassium loss due to the chronic use of thiazide diuretics has been associated with excess mortality resulting from cardiac arrest. Such an excess mortality was reduced by using combination therapy with potassium-sparing drugs.[55] Aldosterone receptor blockade may prevent SCD by averting potassium loss and by increasing the myocardial uptake of norepinephrine. Spironolactone may also prevent myocardial fibrosis by blocking the effects of aldosterone on the formation of collagen,[56] which in turn could play a part in reducing the risk of SCD since myocardial fibrosis could predispose to variations in ventricular conduction times and hence to reentrant ventricular arrhythmias.[54–57]

Among various expressions of autonomic nervous system abnormalities in CHF, depression of baroreflex sensitivity has been associated with a poor prognosis and a high incidence of ventricular arrhythmias. Recent data suggest that aldosterone may contribute to depression of baroreflex sensibility.[55,58] Both acute administration of aldosterone in the carotid sinus and chronic infusion of aldosterone in the dog model depress baroreceptor and baroreflex without inducing hypertension. These effects are prevented by the pretreatment of animals with spironolactone.[58]

## Other Drugs

Thrombolytic therapy is beyond the scope of this chapter since it is considered as an early intervention in acute MI rather than a true postinfarction therapy. Nevertheless, early intervention, such as thrombolytic therapy, reduces ventricular arrhythmias and improves electrical stability. This is probably due to the reduction of myocardial damage and the patency of the infarct-related artery that limits ventricular dilation and prevents left ventricular aneurisms, and obviates the development of electrophysiological alterations that can predispose to arrhythmias such as the presence of late potentials.[59,60]

Aspirin has proved to be a beneficial drug for the primary and secondary prevention of coronary events. The antiplatelet effects of this agent are thought principally to mediate its efficacy in preventing acute coronary thrombosis and preventing atherosclerosis.[61,62] On the other hand, aspirin may reduce systemic vasodilation reserve, and its effect on prostaglandins may adversely affect hemodynamic function.[63] Antiplatelet agents may have other effects that are important in the setting of myocardial injury and healing, inducing reduction of fibrocellular response and remodeling in the noninfarcted myocardium (both involved in the mechanism of ventricular arrhythmias in patients with CHF),[64] and inhibition of inducible nitric oxide synthetase reduction, which is augmented in patients with heart failure.[65]

Two interesting substudies from the SOLVD trials suggest the effect of antithrombotic agents on the risk of total mortality in sudden coronary death in patients with CHF.[66,67] A first retrospective database analysis of the SOLVD trials (prevention and treatment) focused on a total of 424 deaths classified as "probable arrhythmias with no antecedent of worsening heart failure," excluding those "probable arrhythmias with some antecedent heart failure." In a multivariate analysis, antiplatelet agents and anticoagulant therapy remained independently associated with a reduction in the risk of SCD: antiplatelet with a 24% reduction (RR: 0.76; 95%; CI: 0.61–0.95), anticoagulation with 32% reduction (RR: 0.68; 95%; CI: 0.48–0.96). The combination of both therapies was not associated with a reduction in sudden coronary death.[66] A second substudy retrospectively reviewed the data on antiplatelet agents in both SOLVD trials with end-points all-cause mortality as well as the combined end-point of death or hospital admissions for heart failure. After adjusting for confounding factors, antiplatelet agents use emerged as a significant predictor of favorable outcome. As far as sudden death not preceded by worsening heart failure was concerned, antiplatelet agents reduced significantly the mortality (RR: 0.78; 0.63–0.97) with no reduction other than in the group of deaths associated with worsening of HF.[67] At this time, further investigations are warranted to explore the basis of the observed benefit associated with antithrombotic agents and for the action between antiplatelet agents and ACE inhibitors.

The overview of published randomized trials of statin drugs demonstrates a large reduction in cholesterol and a reduction of stroke and total mortality with a large and significant decrease in cardiovascular death.[68] Most of these studies did not approach SCD as a specific cause of cardiovascular death, but as they have clearly shown a reduction of coronary death, a reduction of SCD might be expected. For example, in the 4S study,[69] there was a 42% reduction in the risk of coronary death, which accounts for the improvement of total survival in the simvastatin group. There were 18% deaths in the placebo group compared to 11% in the simvastatin group. Among the coronary deaths, 68 were related to a definite or probable acute MI in the placebo group compared to 35 in the simvastatin group. Sixty-three deaths were reported to be instantaneous or within 1 hour (acute MI nonconfirmed) in the placebo group compared to 37 in the simvastatin group.

No definite data regarding reduction of total mortality and sudden death mortality were observed in post-MI patients treated with calcium antagonists.[5] On the other hand, similar results were observed in CHF patients in the PRAISE[70] or V-HeFT III[71] trials with amlodipine and felodipine, respectively (even though the possibility of amlodipine to prolong survival in patients with nonischemic cardiopathy has been suggested).

## Conclusion

Non-"classic" antiarrhythmic drugs are an important part of therapy after MI and in patients with CHF. They have been shown to reduce total mortality, and one of its principal components, SCD. The reason for this is not always clear and the mechanisms are multiple. They are related to direct and indirect effects that possibly lead to a reduction of ventricular arrhythmias. These drugs are important in the management of such patients, and are definitely preferable to antiarrhythmic agents in this setting, with the exception of amiodarone, since Class I and IV drugs are contraindicated.

## References

1. Amiodarone Trials Meta-Analysis Investigators. Effect of prophylactic amiodarone on mortality after acute myocardial infarction and in congestive heart failure: meta-analysis of individual data from 6500 patients in randomised trials. Lancet 1997; 350:1417–1424.
2. Olsson G, Wikstrand J, Warnold I, et al. Metoprolol-induced reduction in postinfarction mortality: pooled results from five double-blind randomized trials. Eur Heart J 1992; 13:28–32.
3. Östlund-Lindqvist A-M, Lindqvist P, Bräutigam J, et al. The effect of metoprolol on diet-induced atherosclerosis in rabbits. Arteriosclerosis 1988; 8:40–45.
4. Ablad B, Björkman J-A, Gustafsson D, et al. The role of sympathetic activity in atherogenesis: effects of beta-blockade. Am Heart J 1988; 116: 322–327.
5. Held PH, Yusuf S. Effects of β-blockers and calcium channel blockers in acute myocardial infarction. Eur Heart J 1993; 14(Suppl F):18–25.
6. Beta-Blocker Pooling Project Research Group. The Beta-Blocker Pooling Project (BBPP): subgroup findings from randomized trials in postinfarction patients. Eur Heart J 1998; 9:8–16.
7. Boissel J-P, Leizorovicz A, Picolet H, et al. Secondary prevention after high-risk acute myocardial infarction with low-dose acebutolol. Am J Cardiol 1990; 66:251–260.
8. Kennedy HL, et al., and the CAST Investigators. Beta-blocker therapy in the Cardiac Arrhythmia Suppression Trial. Am J Cardiol 1994; 74:674–680.
9. Boutitie F, Boissel JP, Connolly SJ, et al. Amiodarone interaction with beta-blockers: analysis of the merged EMIAT and CAMIAT databases. Circulation 1999; 99:2268–2275.
10. Fagerberg B. The merit of beta-blockade in heart failure. Eur Heart J 1999; 20:1761–1763.
11. CIBIS Investigators and Committees. Design of the Cardiac Insufficiency Bisoprolol Study (CIBIS). Circulation 1994; 90:1765–1773.
12. Packer M, Bristow MR, Cohn NN, et al. The effect of carvedilol on morbidity and mortality in patients with chronic heart failure. N Engl J Med 1996; 334:1349–1355.
13. CIBIS-II Investigators and Committees. The Cardiac Insufficiency Bisoprolol Study II (CIBIS-II): a randomised trial. Lancet 1999; 353:9–13.
14. MERIT-HF Study Group. Effect of metoprolol CR/XL in chronic heart failure: Metoprolol CR/XL Randomised Intervention Trial in Congestive Heart Failure (MERIT-HF). Lancet 1999; 353:2001–2007.
15. Rankin AC, Cobbe SM. Arrhythmias and sudden death in heart failure: can we prevent them? Clin Practice 1996; 185–205.
16. Pousset F, Copie X, Lechat P, et al. Effects of bisoprolol on heart rate variability in heart failure. Am J Cardiol 1996; 77:612–617.

17. Olsson G, Tuomilehto J, Berglund G, et al. Primary prevention of sudden cardiovascular death in hypertensive patients: mortality results from the MAPHY study. Am J Hypertens 1991; 4:151–158.
18. Campbell RWF. ACE inhibitors and arrhythmias. Heart 1996(Suppl 3);76:79–82.
19. Weisman H, Bush D, Mannisi J, et al. Cellular mechanisms of myocardial infarct expansion. Circulation 1988; 78:106–201.
20. Weber K, Brilla C, Janicki J. Myocardial fibrosis: functional significance and regulatory factors. Cardiovasc Res 1993; 27:341–348.
21. Fletcher RD, Cintron GB, Johnson G, et al., for The V-HeFT II Ventricular Arrhythmia Cooperative Studies Group. Enalapril decreases prevalence of ventricular tachycardia in patients with chronic congestive heart failure. Circulation 1993; 87:149–155.
22. Sogaard P, Gotzsche CO, Ravkilde J, et al. Ventricular arrhythmias in the acute and chronic phases after acute myocardial infarction: effect of intervention with captopril. Circulation 1994; 90:101–107.
23. Bashir Y, Sneddon JF, O'Nunain S, et al. Comparative electrophysiological effects of captopril or hydralazine combined with nitrate in patients with left ventricular dysfunction and inducible ventricular tachycardia. Br Heart J 1992; 67:355–360.
24. Racke HF, Koppers D, Lemke P, et al. Fosinoprilate prolongs the action potential: reduction of $i_K$ and enhancement of the L-type calcium current in guinea pig ventricular myocytes. Cardiovasc Res 1994; 28:201–208.
25. Stark G, Stark U, Nagl S, et al. Acute effects of the ACE inhibitor lisinopril on cardiac electrophysiological parameters of isolated guinea pig hearts. Clin Cardiol 1991; 14:579–582.
26. Demello WC, Crespo MJ, Altieri PI. Effect of enalapril on intracellular resistance and conduction velocity in rat ventricular muscle. J Cardiovasc Pharmacol 1993; 22:259–263.
27. Demello WC, Altieri PI. Enalapril, an inhibitor of angiotensin converting enzyme, increases the junctional conductance in isolated heart cell pairs. J Cardiovasc Pharmacol 1993; 22:229–263.
28. Altieri PI, Gonzalez R, Escobales N, et al. Myocardial remodeling in hypertensive patients: the role of converting enzyme inhibitors and angiotensin II receptor blockers in reducing ventricular arrhythmias. G Ital Cardiol 1998; 28:353–356.
29. Gonzales R, Altieri PI, Fernadez-Martinez J, et al. Reduction in conduction velocity delay by angiotensin converting enzyme inhibitors in hypertensive patients with left ventricular hypertrophy: detection by signal-averaged electrocardiogram. Am J Hypertens 1992; 5:896–899.
30. Townend JN, Virk SF, Qiang FX, et al. Lymphocyte beta adrenoceptor upregulation and improved cardiac response to adrenergic stimulation following converting enzyme inhibition in congestive heart failure. Eur Heart J 1993; 14:243–250.
31. Clough DP, Collis MG, Conway J, et al. Interaction of angiotensin-converting enzyme inhibitors with the function of the sympathetic nervous system. Am J Cardiol 1982; 49:1410–1414.
32. Grassi G, Cattaneo BM, Sevaralle G, et al. Effects of chronic ACE inhibition on sympathetic nerve traffic and baroreflex control of circulation in heart failure. Circulation 1997; 96:1173–1179.
33. Mc Kenna W, Haywood G. The role of ACE inhibitors in the treatment of arrhythmias. Clin Cardiol 1990; 13:49–52.
34. Ebert T. Captopril potentiates chronotropic baroreflex responses to carotid stimuli in humans. Hypertension 1985; 7:602–606.

35. Kontopoulos AG, Athyros VG, Papageorgiou AA, et al. Effect of angiotensin-converting enzyme inhibitors on the power spectrum of heart rate variability in post-myocardial infarction patients. Coronary Artery Dis 1997; 8:517–524.
36. Ikram H. Arrhythmias, electrolytes, and ACE inhibitor therapy in the elderly. Gerontology 1987; 33(Suppl 1):42–47.
37. Poquet F, Ferguson J, Rouleau JL. The anti-arrhythmic effect of the ACE inhibitor captopril in patients with congestive heart failure largely is due to its potassium sparing effects. Can J Cardiol 1992; 8:589–595.
38. Pfeffer MA, Braunwald E, Moyé LA, et al. Effect of captopril on mortality and morbidity in patients with left ventricular dysfunction after myocardial infarction. N Engl J Med 1992; 327:669–677.
39. The Acute Infarction Ramipril Efficiency (AIRE) Study Investigators. Effect of ramipril on mortality and morbidity of survivors of acute myocardial infarction with clinical evidence of heart failure. Lancet 1993; 342:821–828.
40. Kober L, Torp-Pederson C, Carlsen JE, et al. A clinical trial of the angiotensin-converting-enzyme inhibitor trandolapril in patients with left ventricular dysfunction after myocardial infarction. N Engl J Med 1995; 333:1670–1676.
41. Sewdburg K, Held P, Kjekshus J, et al. On behalf of the CONSENSUS II Study Group. Effects of early administration of enalapril on mortality in patients with acute myocardial infarction: results of the Cooperative North Scandinavian Enalapril Survival Study II (CONSENSUS II). N Engl J Med 1992; 327:678–684.
42. Cleland JGF, Erhardt L, Murray G, et al. Effect of ramipril on morbidity and mode of death among survivors of acute myocardial infarction with clinical evidence of heart failure. Eur Heart J 1997; 18:41–51.
43. Domanski MJ, Exner V, Borkowf CB, et al. Effect of angiotensin converting enzyme inhibition on sudden cardiac death in patients following acute myocardial infarction. J Am Coll Cardiol 1999; 33:598–604.
44. Cohn JN, Johnson G, Ziesche S, et al. A comparison of enalapril with hydralazine-isosorbide dinitrate in the treatment of chronic congestive heart failure. N Engl J Med 1991; 325:303–310.
45. The Consensus Trial Study Group. Effects of enalapril on mortality in severe congestive heart failure. N Engl J Med 1987; 316:1429–1435.
46. The SOLVD Investigators. Effect of enalapril on mortality and the development of heart failure in asymptomatic patients with reduced left ventricular ejection fractions. N Engl J Med 1992; 327:685–691.
47. The SOLVD Investigators. Effect of enalapril on survival in patients with reduced left ventricular ejection fractions and congestive heart failure. N Engl J Med 1991; 325:293–302.
48. Pitt B, Segal R, Martinez FA, et al. Randomised trial of losartan versus captopril in patients over 65 with heart failure (Evaluation of Losartan in the Elderly Study, ELITE). Lancet 1997; 349:747–752.
49. Thomas GP, Ferrier GR, Howlett SE. Losartan exerts antiarrhythmic activity independent of angiotensin II receptor blockade in stimulated ventricular ischemia and reperfusion. J Pharm Exp Therapeut 1996; 278:1090–1097.
50. Brooksby P, Robinson PJ, Segal R, et al. Effects of losartan and captopril on QT dispersion in elderly patients with heart failure. Lancet 1999; 354:395–396.
51. Helfant RH. Short- and long-term mechanisms of sudden cardiac death in congestive heart failure. Am J Cardiol 1990; 65:41K-43K.
52. Cooper AH, Dries DL, Davis CE, et al. Diuretics and risk of arrhythmic death in patients with left ventricular dysfunction. Circulation 1999; 100:1311–1315.
53. Pitt B, Zannad F, Remme W, et al. The effect of spironolactone on morbidity and mortality in patients with severe heart failure. N Engl J Med 1999; 341:709–717.

54. Zannad F. Aldosterone and heart failure. Eur Heart J 1995; 16:98–102.
55. Siscovick DS, Raghunathan TE, Psaty BM, et al. Diuretic therapy for hypertension and the risk of primary cardiac arrest. N Engl J Med 1994; 330:1852–1857.
56. Brilla CG, Kramer B, Hoffmeister M, et al. Low-dose enalapril in severe chronic heart failure. Cardiovasc Drugs Ther 1989; 3:211–218.
57. Klug D, Robert V, Swynghedauw B. Role of mechanical and hormonal factors in cardiac remodeling and the biologic limits of myocardial adaptation. Am J Cardiol 1993; 71(Suppl):46A–54A.
58. Wang W. Chronic administration of aldosterone depresses baroreceptor reflex function in the dog. Hypertension 1994; 24:571–575.
59. Bracchetti D, Nacarella F, Palmieri M, et al. Long-term treatment after acute MI. J Cardiovasc Pharmacol 1989; 14:S79-S83.
60. De Chillou C, Sadoul N, Briançon S, et al. Factors determining the occurrence of late potentials in the signal-averaged electrocardiogram after a first myocardial infarction: a multivariate analysis. J Am Coll Cardiol 1991; 18:1638–1642.
61. Fuster V, Badimon L, Badimon JJ, et al. The pathogenesis of coronary artery disease and the acute coronary syndrome. N Engl J Med 1992; 326: 242–250.
62. Fuster V, Badimon L, Badimon JJ, et al. The pathogenesis of coronary artery disease and the acute coronary syndrome. N Engl J Med 1992; 326:310–318.
63. Houston MC. Nonsteroidal anti-inflammatory drugs and antihypertensives. Am J Med 1991; 90:42S–47S.
64. Kalkam EAJ, van Suylen RJ, van Dijk JPM, et al. Chronic aspirin treatment affects collagen deposition in non-infarcted myocardium during remodeling after coronary artery ligation in the rat. J Mol Cell Cardiol 1995; 27:2483–2494.
65. Farivar RS, Chobanian AV, Brecher P. Salicylate or aspirin inhibit the induction of the inducible nitric oxide synthase in rat cardiac fibroblasts. Circ Res 1996; 78:759–768.
66. Dries DL, Domanski MJ, Waclawiw MA, et al. Effect of antithrombotic therapy on risk of sudden coronary death in patients with congestive heart failure. Am J Cardiol 1997; 79:909–913.
67. Al-Khadra AS, Salem DN, Rand WM, et al. Antiplatelet agents and survival: a cohort analysis from the studies of left ventricular dysfunction (SOLVD) trial. J Am Coll Cardiol 1998; 31: 419–425.
68. Hebert PR, Gaziano JM, Ki Sau Chan, et al. Cholesterol lowering with statin drugs, risk of stroke, and total mortality. JAMA 1997; 278:313–321.
69. Scandinavian Simvastatin Survival Study Group. Randomised trial of cholesterol lowering in 4444 patients with coronary disease: the Scandinavian Simvastatin Survival Study. Lancet 1994; 344:1383–1389.
70. Packer M, O'Connor C, Ghali J, et al. Effect of amlodipine on morbidity and mortality in severe chronic heart failure. N Engl J Med 1996; 335:1107–1114.
71. Cohn JN, Ziesche S, Smith R, et al. Effect of the calcium antagonist felodipine as supplementary vasodilator therapy in patients with chronic heart failure treated with enalapril (V-HeFT III). Circulation 1996; 96:856–863.
72. Altieri P, Crespo M, Escobales N, et al. Arrhythmias and "nonclassic" antiarrhythmic drugs. G Ital Cardiol 1999; 29(Suppl 5):442–444.
73. Kübler W. ACE inhibitors in heart failure: effect on mode of death. Eur Heart J 1997; 18:3–4.

# XIII

## Nonmedical Therapy

# 45

# Ventricular Tachycardia Antiarrhythmic Surgery:

## The Legacy

*Gerard M. Guiraudon, MD, George J. Klein, MD, and Colette M. Guiraudon, MD*

## Introduction

Surgical approaches to ventricular arrhythmias on an empirical basis[1] and then on documented pathophysiology[2,3] were developed in the late 1970s. Although surgical approaches contributed significantly to the body of knowledge, their indications were limited by the morbidity and mortality inherent to surgical delivery. The expected benefit from arrhythmia control was outweighed by surgical side effects.

Therefore, the question "what is left of surgery for ventricular arrhythmia to prevent sudden cardiac death?" can be understood and answered 2 ways. What is left in terms of practical use of the therapeutic interventions is negligible. But what is left in terms of scientific legacy is not negligible. Surgical rationales and techniques based on electrophysiological studies and guided by intraoperative mapping still provide the current framework for other interventions, namely catheter delivery.[4]

This chapter is organized around a series of theses. Each thesis addresses a specific legacy from experience gained by surgical approaches to ventricular arrhythmias.

## Ventricular Tachycardia

Ventricular tachycardia can be interrupted using interventions based on preoperative electrophysiological testing and intraoperative cardiac mapping.[5,6] The initial experience was based on 3 patients operated on in 1973. One patient had an idiopathic dilated cardiomyopathy, and 2 had

From: Aliot E, Clementy J, Prystowsky EN (editors). *Fighting Sudden Cardiac Death: A Worldwide Challenge.* ©Futura Publishing Company, Armonk, NY, 2000.

what would be identified as arrhythmogenic right ventricular dysplasia. In the 3 patients, an incision (ventriculotomy) performed at the earliest epicardial activation site during ventricular tachycardia interrupted the ventricular tachycardias. The surgical rationale was similar to the one used in ablation of the atrioventricular accessory pathway in the Wolff-Parkinson-White syndrome.[7] Although at that time our depth of knowledge was rather shallow, good fortune brought us success and the opportunity to advance.

## The Concept of Arrhythmogenic Substrate

The area of myocardium located around the early activation during ventricular tachycardia, as well as the area where slow conduction or delayed or fragmented (fractionation) activation were recorded, were identified as the part of myocardium where the reentrant mechanism was located. These areas were defined as arrhythmogenic.[8]

Cardiac mapping was a critical guide to identifying the arrhythmogenic substrate. Cardiac mapping could be carried out epicardially or endocardially. Unfortunately, technology and intraoperative conditions for mapping were severe limitations to the quality of information obtained. It was exceptionally possible to pinpoint the reentrant loop with its necessary slow conduction segment. Mapping essentially identified an area around the earliest activation during the tachycardia or an area where abnormal activation was recorded. Mapping, despite its limitations, was definitely established as a critical guide.[9,10]

A better definition of the arrhythmogenic substrate was achieved. It was defined as the segment of ventricular myocardium necessary but not sufficient for the tachycardia to be initiated and sustained. The necessary segment of the reentrant loop is very rarely anatomically delineated (as a bundle) but is usually functionally defined. The link may have complex morphology, with ramifications associated with either dead-end pathways or multiple vicarious pathways. These so-called "necessary links" associated with slow conduction are found mostly in pathological myocardium that exhibits a nonhomogeneous structure with excess of fibrosis or other connective tissue and a disarray of myocardial cells and/or bundles. The anatomy of the substrate can be viewed at the micro- and macrolevels. At the micro-level, the anatomic substrate appears complex and small. At the macro-level, 2 major observations can be made: (1) the slow conduction pathway appears unique and has the form of a simple channel (figure-8 model),[11] and (2) the greater the mass of pathological tissue, the greater the arrhythmogenicity.[12] This is particularly true for the infarct scar and for arrhythmogenic right ventricular dysplasia.

Arrhythmogenicity varies over time. The pathology can be progressive and/or is modified by other factors. These other factors, which are included in unnecessary and nonsufficient factors, may involve the rest of the ventricles, the autonomic nervous system, the blood supply (coronary artery disease), and various other factors. These other factors can actually be major determinants in setting the condition for arrhythmias to initiate and/or sustain. Arrhythmogenicity, in other words, is not confined to the substrate as defined above.[13]

Identification and localization of the substrate can be achieved by using either electrophysiological testing and/or anatomic landmarks.

## The Therapeutic Triad: the Target, the Bullet, the Gun

Our experience with surgery for arrhythmias helped us to understand the anatomy of every therapeutic intervention, which reconciles 3 elements: the target, the bullet, and the gun.[14–16]

The *target* is the arrhythmogenic substrate, as defined above, and is based on the documented pathophysiology of disease or symptoms to be addressed. As far as ventricular tachycardias are concerned, the target is not discrete and nonprogressive as is the atrioventricular accessory connection of the Wolff-Parkinson-White syndrome. The target is elusive and multiple, with vicarious targets at different sites. The target is difficult to localize with certainty using the current technologies.

The *bullet* is the physical agent aimed at neutralizing the target. Because of the pathophysiology and the absence of a discrete target, large "bullets" were used to neutralize as large a target as possible. Two rationales for interventions were described:

- *The concept of ablation,* aimed at neutralizing a certain mass of myocardium, and using incision, excision, or modification of targeted tissue (ablation) by various energies: cryoablation, radiofrequency current, microwave energy, laser energy, etc.[2,3]
- *The concept of exclusion,* aimed at confirming the arrhythmia mechanism within a large substrate, where the substrate is too large to be resected or ablated without severe compromise of cardiac function.[2,17]

The *gun* is the way to deliver the bullet on target. There are many methods of delivery. As far as cardiological interventions are concerned, there are, to date, the surgical route and the catheter route.

The surgical route for ventricular arrhythmias, especially those associated with coronary artery disease, requires a number of steps: general anesthesia with tracheal intubation, median sternotomy, cardiac mapping used to delineate the substrate, cardiopulmonary bypass, aortic cross-clamping with concomitant myocardial preservation, and left ventriculotomy. At that point, the management of the substrate (bullet) can be delivered according to rationale and surgical technique. Each step (including the management of the substrate) is associated with inherent risks.[18,19] The overall risk is the summation of each "elementary risk."

Surgical risk was less for patients with arrhythmogenic right ventricular dysplasia, because aortic cross-clamping was not used, and essentially the left ventricle was left intact. Side effects were effects that do not affect the target. This definition showed us that (1) most of the surgical delivery meets the definition of side effect and is associated with major mortality and morbidity, and (2) a poorly defined target is associated with the risk of undue collateral damages to myocardium, and to postoperative left ventricular dysfunction and death. Unfortunately, less invasive techniques could not be described as for the Wolff-Parkinson-White syndrome.

## Arrhythmogenic Right Ventricular Dysplasia

Although surgery for control of ventricular tachycardia associated with arrhythmogenic right ventricular dysplasia was limited to a very small number of patients, the surgical experience with arrhythmogenic right ventricular dysplasia has made dramatic contributions to the understanding of ventricular tachycardia mechanisms and the associated substrate. The rationale for surgical "ablation" and/or exclusion were initially developed for and applied to patients with arrhythmogenic right ventricular dysplasia.[2,17]

Arrhythmogenic right ventricular dysplasia is a recently identified clinical entity.[20] The lesions involve essentially the right ventricular free wall and, to a lesser extent, the left ventricle. The right ventricular free wall is dilated and presents with large dome-shaped bulges over the infundibulum, apex, and basal portion of the inferior right ventricular wall. These bulging areas are akinetic or dyskinetic. The right ventricular trabeculation is increased in size and number. The subepicardial fat is abundant, and the myocardium is infiltrated or replaced by fat. This fatty infiltration gives the myocardium its characteristic appearance. Microscopic examination shows fatty infiltration and hypertrophy or degeneration of myocardial cells. Patchy subendocardial fibrosis may be present.

Clinical characteristics are now well recognized and make identification of disease easy. Surgery for arrhythmogenic right ventricular dysplasia has evolved over time. During the 1973–1981 period, we operated on 12 patients with problematic drug-resistant tachycardias.[3] A discrete ventriculotomy/resection at the site of epicardial breakthrough (origin) of ventricular activation during ventricular tachycardia and/or at the site of late diastolic activation during sinus rhythm (arrhythmogenic area) was performed. There were no intraoperative complications. All patients were discharged free of tachycardia. During long-term follow-up (mean 36 months), 5 patients had recurrences. In 2 patients, tachycardias were not problematic and were not treated. Long-term recurrence of tachycardia was likely associated with the large amount of abnormal right ventricular wall left intact. Consequently, the entire right ventricular wall was isolated after 1981.[17] Since then, we carried out a right ventricular free wall disconnection in 10 patients.[21] Surgical indication was based on failure of nonsurgical electrophysiological interventions. One patient died perioperatively of malignant hyperthermia. One patient had early recurrence of left ventricular tachycardia. During long-term follow-up, 3 patients with a low left ventricular ejection fraction preoperatively (0.44, 0.35, 0.30) died of congestive heart failure 5 months, 3 years, and 11 years postoperatively. The 6 other patients with good left ventricular function had excellent control of arrhythmia with preserved cardiac function.

Right ventricular free wall disconnection for arrhythmogenic right ventricular dysplasia is feasible and associated with long-term good results in selected patients,[22,23] as corroborated by others' experience. Our experience suggests that patient selection is essentially based on left ventricular function. A normal left ventricular ejection fraction implies that the left ventricle is not involved in the pathological process and that good cardiac function can be anticipated postoperatively as well as arrhythmia control.

Right ventricular free wall disconnection is confined to a small number of patients with preserved left ventricular function after well-documented failure of nonsurgical electrophysiological interventions.

## Ventricular Tachycardias after Acute Myocardial Infarction: The Elusive Target

In the 1970s, attempted approaches to ventricular tachycardia after acute myocardial infarction were based on a rationale similar to the one used successfully for arrhythmogenic right ventricular dysplasia: (1) It was anticipated that cardiac mapping would be an effective guide, and (2) that interrupting ventricular tachycardia would prolong life.

These assumptions were made without a correct appreciation of the magnitude of myocardial pathology, complexity of substrate, and associated left ventricular dysfunction.

Epicardial mapping failed to provide reliable guidance, but at least pointed out that the arrhythmogenic substrate was endocardial, and that the endocardium should be mapped.[8] Unfortunately, failure to interrupt the tachycardia after epicardial mapping was blamed on mapping instead of the mapper (blame the messenger), and the pursuit of experience using endocardial mapping was stalled.

Surgical pathology documented that the lesions were mostly endocardial and that the endocardial fibrosis was a discrete landmark for subendocardial lesions.[24,25]

This series of attempted map-guided interventions was productive and allowed us to describe the first direct surgical approach to ventricular tachycardias after acute myocardial infarction based on exclusion of the entire potentially arrhythmogenic myocardium, i.e., the border zone identified by the endocardial fibrosis. The encircling endocardial ventriculotomy was based on, but did not require, mapping guidance at the time of surgery.[24] Shortly thereafter, Josephson in Philadelphia would describe a more limited endocardial approach based on intraoperative mapping.[26]

In the following decades, the acceptance of surgery as a safe and effective therapeutic system was hampered by: (1) the complexity of the substrate and inherent mismatch between target and bullet, and (2) severe side effects associated with surgical techniques on left ventricular function.

The dilemma was compounded by the fact that the patients with resistant life-threatening ventricular arrhythmias usually present with associated severe left ventricular dysfunction. The less invasive interventions used to control ventricular arrhythmias, i.e., transvenous implantable cardioverter-defibrillator (ICD) implantation, confirmed the initial hypothesis that surgical approaches failed to document: control of ventricular arrhythmias in patients with significant left ventricular dysfunction prolongs life (MADID, AVID trials).[27,28] In cardiac physiology, pacing and pumping are 2 sides of the same coin, with equal value: pacing (rhythm) cannot be restored at the expense of pumping.

## Current Status of Surgery for Ventricular Tachycardia after Acute Myocardial Infarction

Surgery for ventricular arrhythmia has declined dramatically in the recent years. Two recent surgical papers were eulogies in praise of direct surgery for ventricular tachycardias associated with coronary artery disease,[29,30] mourning the disappearance of referrals. Two comments can be made:

- Surgery for ventricular tachycardia never developed. The number of patients operated on was negligible compared to the patient population. The most active centers rarely performed more than 10 operations a year.
- The advent of new nonsurgical interventions are the accepted reasons for the decline: (1) better, less invasive, effective interventions to control arrhythmia, i.e., ICD, catheter ablation, and drugs; (2) better prevention

of arrhythmia associated with aggressive management of acute coronary artery thrombosis to avoid myocardial necrosis. The patient population characteristics changed and, therefore, their management.

Surgical indications for ventricular tachycardia are ruled by an imperative No-No rule, i.e., no mortality, no failure to control the arrhythmia.

Patient selection to avoid surgical mortality has been exemplified by van Hemel et al.[31,32] Using the left ventricular score system of the CASS study, they were able to operate on more than 100 patients without a mortality. Arrhythmia surgery can be safely carried out if 3 or more of the 9 segments identified on the LAO and RAO views are contracting normally. Other authors have successfully selected patients using similar methods—excess ejection fraction[33] or centerline chord motion analysis.[34] This patient population with preserved left ventricular function has a low surgical risk, but also good long-term survival, whatever the therapy.[35]

Amiodarone has been suggested as a risk factor. In a recent retrospective study, Mickleborough reported that amiodarone was the only cause of death.[36] Although consistent with other experience, these results remained questionable because large surgical series using amiodarone preoperatively in large doses did not report any excessive morbidity or mortality.[37]

Criteria for successful surgical ablation of arrhythmias are not well defined and vary from one series to the other. Monomorphic sustained ventricular tachycardia of 1 of 2 morphologies associated with a discrete arrhythmogenic scar (aneurysm) are ideal indicators. The site of origin of the tachycardia and/or the location of the infarct scar are associated with inconsistent results. Septal origin is reported as either difficult to ablate[38] or easy.[33] The inferior wall location is reported as either a risk for failure[33] or not.[38]

Surgical techniques deal with 2 issues: value of intraoperative mapping and best ablative techniques associated with minimal damages to contracting myocardium and left ventricular function.

Intraoperative mapping has 2 roles: a guide for surgical ablation and a research tool to retrospectively analyze surgical failures or explore pathophysiology of the scar. As a research tool, comprehensive intraoperative mapping has dramatically contributed to basic as well as to applied science. For example, the identification of epicardial breakthrough in inferior scars,[38] or the understanding of activation of deep septal origin of the tachycardias[37] or subendocardial arrhythmogenic pathways.[39]

As an intraoperative guide, cardiac mapping has significant limitations. Cardiac mapping is not feasible in all patients (between 15% and 50%), and when feasible, it is frequently incomplete. Promoters of intraoperative mapping explain surgical failure to control the arrhythmia by incomplete or misleading mapping.[40] Some authors did not observe any improvement in arrhythmia control after starting to use a better sophisticated mapping system. Rokkas reported a new way to map ventricular tachycardia using multiplexed electrodes epicardial sock, and/or endocardial balloon using potential distribution mapping, which can be available to the surgical team almost on line.[41] In simple terms, better results are associated with extensive comprehensive mapping when multiple tachycardia morphologies associated with multiple sites of origin are identified, and extensive ablation of arrhythmogenic scar is performed accordingly[42]: the more ablation, the better. All potentially arrhythmogenic tissues should be ablated as long as it can be done without damaging normal myocardium with or without supporting mapping data. This concept has been successful at our institution[43,44] and many others.[45,46] This approach is used successfully when mapping is not feasible or deemed incomplete.[32–34,38,43]

The ablative technique did not seem critical: excision, incision, cryoablation, and laser photocoagulation seem to accomplish similar goals and could be used selectively or in combination. Recently, Moosdorf documented that laser photocoagulation can be applied successfully epicardially on the closed beating heart.[47] If confirmed, these results can encourage epicardial laser ablation of ventricular tachycardias using minimally invasive techniques.

Does refinement in patient selection allow surgical ablation to fare better? All surgical series are cohort descriptive studies. However, a 5-year survival and freedom from arrhythmia does not seem dramatically better than with other interventions. Van Hemel and colleagues have recently published a randomized study comparing antiarrhythmia drug therapy and surgical therapy.[40] They could not document any advantage to the surgical technique, which was associated with a higher risk of total cardiac death. Despite inherent limitations, this remarkable study by a well-experienced center shows that surgical ablation, even in a very selected patient population with preserved left ventricular function, is not a first choice, but just an option.

Our current approach is: a patient with ventricular arrhythmia associated with coronary artery disease must have a complete assessment in terms of cardiac functional anatomy and electrophysiology. When indicated, myocardial revascularization must be performed and has been documented to decrease arrhythmia death,[48] especially in patients with ischemia-induced arrhythmia.[49] In a small group of patients, concomitant ablation of ventricular arrhythmia can be carried out if it is associated with no additional risk and it is deemed highly effective. After successful revascularization, patients are reassessed, and the appropriate electrophysiological intervention is selected. Surgical ablation of arrhythmia in patients who do not require coronary artery bypass grafting can be indicated in very few patients.

# Future Surgical Approaches

Future surgical approaches can be anticipated at 2 levels: the minimalist and the maximalist.

At the minimalist level, video-assisted thoracic surgery combined with developing sophisticated robotic technologies may allow a safe delivery of ablative energy on target with minimal side effects.[50,51]

At the maximalist level, mechanical cardiac assist, including permanently implanted left ventricular assist devices,[52-55] may describe a fundamentally different rationale. Prolonged mechanical assist can be associated with myocardial remodeling and reversal of myocardial lesions and restoration of left ventricular contractility. Concomitant remodeling of the substrate can either disable the current arrhythmogenic substrate, or the arrhythmogenic substrate can be ablated, safely under mechanical assist, using less invasive approaches, i.e., catheter ablation.

## References

1. Couch OA. Cardiac aneurysm with ventricular tachycardia and subsequent excision of aneurysm. Circulation 1959; 20:251–253.
2. Guiraudon G, Frank R, Fontaine G. Interet des cartographies dans le traitement chirurgical des tachycardies ventriculaires rebelles recidivantes. Nouv Presse Med 1974; 3:321.
3. Guiraudon G, Fontaine G, Frank R, et al. Surgical treatment of ventricular tachycardia guided by ventricular mapping in 23 patients without coronary artery disease. Ann Thorac Surg 1981; 32:439–450.
4. Morady F, Frank R, Kou WH, et al. Identification and catheter ablation of a zone of slow conduction in the reentrant circuit of ventricular tachycardia in humans. J Am Coll Cardiol 1988; 11:775–782.
5. Boineau JP, Cox JL. Slow ventricular activation in acute myocardial infarction: a source of reentrant premature ventricular contractions. Circulation 1973; 48:702.
6. Fontaine G, Guiraudon G, Frank R, Coutte R, Dragodanne C. Epicardial mapping and surgical treatment in 6 cases of resistant ventricular tachycardia not related to coronary artery disease. In: Wellens HJJ, Lie KL, Janse MJ (eds). The Conduction System of the Heart. Stenfert Kroese Pub, Leiden, 1976, p 545.
7. Guiraudon GM. Surgical treatment of Wolff-Parkinson-White syndrome: a retrospectroscopic view. Ann Thorac Surg 1994; 58:1254–1261.
8. Fontaine G, Guiraudon G, Frank R, Vedel J, Grosgogeat Y, et al. Stimulation studies and epicardial mapping in ventricular tachycardia: study of mechanisms and selection for surgery. In: Kulbertus HE (ed). Reeintrant Arrhythmias. MPT Publishing, Lancaster, 1977, pp 334–350.
9. Klein GJ, Ideker RE, Smith WM, Harrison LA, Kasell J, et al. Epicardial mapping of the onset of ventricular tachycardia initiated by programmed stimulation in the canine heart with chronic infarction. Circulation 1979; 60:1375–1384.
10. de Bakker JMT, Janse MJ, Van Capele FJL, Durrer D. Endocardial mapping by simultaneous recording of endocardial electrograms during cardiac surgery for ventricular aneurysm. J Am Coll Cardiol 1983; 2: 947–953.

11. El Sherif N, Mehra R. Gough WB, Zeiler RH. Ventricular activation pattern of spontaneous and induced ventricular rhythms in canine one-day-old myocardial infarction: evidence of focal and reentrant mechanisms. Circ Res 1982; 51:152–166.
12. Blanchard SM, Walcott GP, Wharton JM, Ideker RE. Why is catheter ablation less successful than surgery for treating ventricular tachycardia that results from coronary artery disease? PACE 1994; 17(Part I):2315–2335.
13. Coumel P. Cardiac arrhythmias and the autonomic nervous system. J Cardiovasc Electrophysiol 1993; 4(3): 338.
14. Guiraudon GM, Klein GJ, van Hemel N, et al. Atrial flutter: lessons from surgical interventions (musing on atrial flutter mechanism). PACE 1996; 19(Pt II):1933–1938.
15. Guiraudon GM. Surgery without interventions? PACE 1998; 21(Pt II): 2160–2165.
16. Guiraudon GM. Musing while cutting. J Cardiac Surg 1998; 13:156–162.
17. Guiraudon GM, Klein GJ, Gulamhusein S, Painvin GA, Del Campo C, et al. Total disconnection of right ventricular free wall: surgical treatment of right ventricular tachycardia associated with right ventricular dysplasia. Circulation 1983; 67:463–470.
18. Kirklin JW. The science of cardiac surgery. Eur J Cardiothorac Surg 1990; 4:63–71.
19. Buckberg GD. Myocardial protection: an overview. Semin Thorac Cardiovasc Surg 1993; 5:98–106.
20. Marcus FI, Fontaine GH, Guiraudon G, Frank R, Laurenceau JL, et al. Right ventricular dysplasia: a report of 24 cases. Circulation 1982; 65:384.
21. Guiraudon GM, Klein G, Guiraudon C, Yee R, Sharma A, et al. Long-term prognosis of patients with right ventricular free wall disconnection for arrhythmogenic right ventricular dysplasia: left ventricular ejection fractions as a marker of outcome. PACE 1996; 19:II:628.
22. Misaki T, Watanabe G, Iwa T, Tsubota M, Ohtake H, et al. Surgical treatment of arrhythmogenic right ventricular dysplasia: long-term outcome. Ann Thorac Surg 1994; 58:1380–1385.
23. Doig C, Nimkhedkar K, Bourke JP, et al. Acute and chronic hemodynamic impact of total right ventricular disarticulation. PACE 1991; 14(Part II):1971–1975.
24. Guiraudon G, Fontaine G, Frank R, et al. Encircling endocardial ventriculotomy: a new surgical treatment for life-threatening ventricular tachycardias resistant to medical treatment following myocardial infarction. Ann Thorac Surg 1978; 26:438–444.
25. Mallory CK, White PD, Salgedo-Salgar J. The speed of healing of myocardial infarction. Am Heart J 1931; 18:647.
26. Josephson ME, Harden AH, Horowitz LN. Endocardial excision: a new surgical technique for the treatment of recurrent ventricular tachycardia. Circulation 1979; 60:1430–1439.
27. Moss AJ, Hall WJ, Cannon DS, et al. For the multicenter automatic defibrillator implantation trial investigators: improved survival with an implanted defibrillator in patients with coronary disease at high risk for ventricular arrhythmia. N Engl J Med 1996; 335:1933–1940.
28. The Antiarrhythmics Versus Implantable Defibrillators (AVID) Investigators. A comparison of antiarrhythmic drug therapy with implantable defibrillators in patients resuscitated from near-fatal ventricular arrhythmias. N Engl J Med 1997; 337:1576–1583.
29. Page PL. Surgical treatment of ventricular tachycardia. Arch Mal Coeur 1996; 89(1):115–121.

30. Selle JG. Reflections on definitive surgical treatment of postinfarction ventricular tachycardia. Ann Thorac Surg 1994; 58:1287–1290.
31. van Hemel NM, Kingma JH, Defauw JAM, et al. Left ventricular segmental wall motion score as a criterion for selecting patients for direct surgery in the treatment of post-infarction ventricular tachycardia. Eur Heart J 1989; 10:304–315.
32. van Hemel NM, Defauw JAM, Kingma JH, van Swieten HA, Beukema WP, et al. Risk factors of map-guided surgery for postinfarction ventricular tachycardia: a 12-year experience (abstract). Eur Heart J 1992; 13:1662.
33. Lee R, Mitchell JD, Garan H, Ruskin JN, McGovern BA, et al. Operation for recurrent ventricular tachycardia. J Thorac Cardiovasc Surg 1994; 107:732–742.
34. Nath S, Haines DE, Kron IL, Barber MJ, DiMarco JP. Regional wall motion analysis predicts survival and functional outcome after subendocardial resection in patients with prior anterior myocardial infarction. Circulation 1993; 88:70–76.
35. Willems AR, Tijssen JGP, Van Capelle FJI, et al. Determinants of prognosis in symptomatic ventricular tachycardia or ventricular fibrillation late after myocardial infarction. J Am Coll Cardiol 1990; 16:521–530.
36. Mickleborough LL, Maruyama H, Mohamed S, Rappaport DC, Downar E, et al. Are patients receiving amiodarone at increased risk for cardiac operations? Ann Thorac Surg 1994; 58:622–629.
37. Kawamura Y, Page PL, Cardinal R, Savard P, Nadeau R. Mapping of septal ventricular tachycardia: clinical and experimental correlations. J Thorac Cardiovasc Surg 1996; 112:914–925.
38. Selle JG, Svenson RH, Gallagher JJ, Littman L, Sealy WC, et al. Surgical treatment of ventricular tachycardia with Nd:YAG laser photocoagulation. PACE 1992; 15:1357–1361.
39. de Bakker JMT, van Capelle FJL, Jansen MJ, et al. Macroreentry in the infarcted human heart: the mechanism of ventricular tachycardia with a "focal" activation pattern. J Am Coll Cardiol 1991; 18:1005–1014.
40. van Hemel NM, Kingma JH, Defauw JJAM, Hoogteijling-van Dusseldrop E, et al. Continuation of antiarrhythmic drugs, or arrhythmia surgery after multiple drug failures: a randomized trial in the treatment of postinfarction ventricular tachycardia. Eur Heart J 1996; 17:564–573.
41. Rokkas CK, Nitta T, Schuessler RB, Branham BH, Cain ME, et al. Human ventricular tachycardia: precise intraoperative localization with potential distribution mapping. Ann Thorac Surg 1994; 57:1628–1635.
42. Miller JM, Kienzle MG, Harken AH, Josephson ME. Morphologically distinct sustained ventricular tachycardias in coronary artery disease: significance and surgical results. J Am Coll Cardiol 1984; 4:1073–1079.
43. Guiraudon GM, Thakur RK, Klein GJ, Yee R, Guiraudon CM, et al. Encircling endocardial cryoablation for ventricular tachycardia after myocardial infarction: experience with 33 patients. Am Heart J 1994; 128:982–989.
44. Thakur RK, Guiraudon GM, Klein GJ, Yee R, Guiraudon CM. Intraoperative mapping is not necessary for VT surgery. PACE 1994; 17(Pt II): 2156–2162.
45. Ostermeyer J, Gorggrefe M, Breithardt G, Bircks W. Direct, electrophysiology-guided operations for malignant ischemic ventricular tachycardia. PACE 1994; 17(Pt II): 550–551.
46. Niebauer MJ, Kirsh M, Kadish A, Calins H, Morady F. Outcome of endocardial resection in 33 patients with coronary artery disease: correlation with ventricular tachycardia morphology. Am Heart J 1992; 124:1500–1506.
47. Moosdorf R, Pfeiffer D, Schneider C, Jung W. Intraoperative laser photocoagulation of ventricular tachycardia. Am Heart J 1994; 127:1133–1138.

48. Kelly P, Ruskin JN, Vlahakes GJ, Buckley MJ Jr, Freeman CS, et al. Surgical coronary revascularization in survivors of prehospital cardiac arrest: its effects on inducible ventricular arrhythmias and long-term survival. J Am Coll Cardiol 1990; 15:267–273.
49. Berntsen RF, Gunnes P, Liet M. Rasmussen K. Surgical revascularization in the treatment of ventricular tachycardia and fibrillation exposed by exercise-induced ischaemia. Eur Heart J 1993; 14:1297–1303.
50. Benetti FJ. Cirurgia coronaria directa con bypass de vena safena sin circulation extracorporea o parada cardaca: communicacion previs. Arg Cardiol 1980; 8:3.
51. Buffolo E, Andrade JC, Suzzi J, Leao LE, Galluci C. Direct myocardial revascularization without cardiopulmonary bypass. Thorac Cardiovasc Surg 1985; 33:26–29.
52. Bergsland J, Hasnan J, Lewin N, Bhayana J, Lajos TZ, et al. Coronary artery bypass grafting without cardiopulmonary bypass: an attractive alternative in high-risk patients. Eur J Cardiothorac Surg II 1997; 876–880.
53. Mancini Donna M, Beniaminovitz A, Levin H, Catanese K, Flannery M, et al. Low incidence of myocardial recovery after left ventricular assist device implantation in patients with chronic heart failure. Circulation 1998; 98:2382–2389.
54. Rose EA, Moskowitz AJ, Packer M, Sollano JA, et al. The REMATCH Trial: rationale, design and end-points. Ann Thorac Surg 1999; 67:723–730.
55. Mussivand TM, Masters RG, Hendry PJ, Keon WJ. Totally implantable intrathoracic ventricular assist device. Ann Thorac Surg 1996; 61:444–447.

# XIV

# *Automatic Implantable Cardioverter-Defibrillators*

# 46

# A Critical Appraisal of Implantable Cardioverter-Defibrillator/Drug Trials in the Secondary Prevention of Sudden Cardiac Death

*Gerald V. Naccarelli, MD, Deborah L. Wolbrette, MD, Hemantkumar T. Patel, MD, and Jerry C. Luck, MD*

## Introduction

Sudden cardiac death, usually due to a ventricular tachyarrhythmia, accounts for 350,000–400,000 deaths annually in the United States. Less than 20% of patients will survive a cardiac arrest and be discharged alive from a hospital.[1] Of the survivors, 50% will be dead within 3 years.[1] Since survivors of a cardiac arrest are at high risk for a recurrent arrhythmic event, aggressive management of this group of patients is mandatory. Unfortunately, patients with previous sustained ventricular tachyarrhythmias account for only <1% of patients dying suddenly. Given the high subsequent event rate and the low chance of surviving another cardiac arrest, antiarrhythmic drugs, in an attempt to prevent arrhythmia recurrence, and implantable cardioverter-defibrillators (ICDs), to successfully convert a sustained ventricular tachyarrhythmia, have been aggressively prescribed.[2]

Previous trials have suggested that amiodarone and sotalol are the most effective antiarrhythmic agents in patients with sustained ventricular tachycardia (VT)/ ventricular fibrillation (VF).[3,7] Although Class I agents appear to have a deleterious effect on survival,[8] beta blockers improved survival in the same retrospective trial. Amiodarone is effective in preventing VT recurrences in over 60% of patients with drug-refractory sustained VT/VF (5,6). In the CASCADE trial,[7] patients treated with empiric amiodarone had better "cardiac survival" (defined as cardiac mor-

From: Aliot E, Clementy J, Prystowsky EN (editors). *Fighting Sudden Cardiac Death: A Worldwide Challenge.* ©Futura Publishing Company, Armonk, NY, 2000.

tality, syncope/ICD shock, resuscitated cardiac arrest) than the conventionally treated group guided by serial electrocardiographic or electrophysiological testing (p=0.007). In addition, the amiodarone patients had a greater survival free of sustained arrhythmias (p=0.001). The ESVEM trial demonstrated that guided sotalol therapy was superior to other drugs tested in the prevention of VT recurrence, sudden death, and total mortality.[3] Findings from ESVEM are limited since there was no placebo control limb of the study. In addition, active control comparisons against a pure beta blocker or amiodarone were not made. A substudy of ESVEM[9] demonstrated that the addition of a beta blocker to the Class I treatment arms improved efficacy to that achieved by d,l-sotalol. These data suggest that the beta-blocker component of d,l-sotalol and beta blockers in general have a role in treating sustained VT/VF.

ICDs have had a significant impact in the prevention of sudden cardiac death in patients with sustained ventricular tachyarrhythmias. Uncontrolled studies suggested that ICD therapy reduced the 5-year sudden death rate in high-risk sustained VT/VF patients to less than 5%.[10–12] This low sudden death rate in ICD-treated patients contrasts to the 50% death rates in historical studies predating the use of ICDs. Even with this remarkable success rate, critics have claimed that previous ICD data were suspect since the data were retrospective and not placebo-controlled. In addition, although sudden deaths were reduced, there was concern that ICDs converted arrhythmic to nonarrhythmic deaths with little impact on long-term survival.[11,13]

Since sotalol, amiodarone, and ICDs have often been used after other antiarrhythmic therapies have failed, little prospective controlled data with these therapies have existed in the past. One small prospective trial[14] demonstrated that early ICD implantation in nondrug-responders resulted in a lower number of outcome events including deaths (0.27 hazard ratio, p=0.02) than the conventional antiarrhythmic drug arm. In patients with previous sustained VT/VF, data from several prospective, randomized, controlled studies to determine the best therapy (antiarrhythmic drugs versus ICD) to prolong survival[15–25] are now available (Table 1).

## Antiarrhythmics Versus Implantable Defibrillators (AVID) Study

The AVID trial[15] studied whether "best" Class III antiarrhythmic therapy (empiric amiodarone or guided sotalol) or ICD therapy were superior in reducing intention-to-treat all-cause mortality in patients with a history of sustained VT/VF. Secondary objectives included quality-of-life assessment and cost effectiveness of the 2 study arms. Inclusion criteria included the fol-

### Table 1

### Sustained VT/VF Trials

|  | AVID | CIDS | CASH |
|---|---|---|---|
| n | 1,016 | 659 | 349 |
| Therapy | ICD vs. empiric amiodarone or guided sotalol | ICD vs. empiric amiodarone | ICD vs. empiric amiodarone metoprolol propafenone |
| Primary End-point | TM | TM | TM |
| Drug Event Rate 2-year ICD | 17.7% | 8.3% | 9.8% |
| Decrease in TM | 27% | 19.6% | 37% |

VT = ventricular tachycardia; VF = ventricular fibrillation; TM = total mortality.

lowing arrhythmia patients: survivors of a VF arrest, sustained VT/syncope, sustained VT/ejection fraction <40%, and sustained VT/near syncope.

One thousand sixteen patients were randomized (509 antiarrhythmic drugs; 507 ICD). Only 2.6% of patients received sotalol long-term and 93% of the ICD group had a nonthoracotomy system implanted. Enrollment was discontinued prematurely because of a significant survival advantage in the ICD group. During an 18.2 ± 12.2-month follow-up period, death rates were 22.0% ± 3.7% in the antiarrhythmic drug versus 15.8 ± 3.2% in the ICD group. One-, 2- and 3-year survival rates were 89.3%, 81.6%, and 75.4% in the ICD group compared to 82.3%, 74.7%, and 64.1% in the drug-treated group (p<0.02), resulting in mortality relative risk reductions of 39%, 27%, and 31% in ICD patients. ICD benefit appeared to be in reducing arrhythmic death since there was no difference between the 2 treatments in nonarrhythmic deaths. The majority of the ICD benefit occurred in the first 9 months. Due to the premature termination of the study, survival in the ICD patients was extended by only 2.7 months. ICD benefit was most prominent in patients with ejection fractions of <35%. ICD therapy was not effective in prolonging survival in patients with ejection fractions >35%. The ICD group had a lower incidence of prior atrial fibrillation/flutter and Class III CHF patients, a higher use of concomitant beta blockers (42%) versus only 17% in the drug-treated group. In an analysis of the AVID study and registry patients, beta-blocker use was independently associated with improved survival in patients with VF or symptomatic VT who were not treated with specific antiarrhythmic therapies.[20] However, beta blockers did not have a protective effect in patients already receiving amiodarone or an ICD.[20] The registry group of patients was clinically similar to the patients randomized into the trial.[16,17] Data from the AVID registry population demonstrated similar high mortality rates in all of the entry subgroups including: cardiac arrest survivors of VF (17%), syncopal VT (21.2%), symptomatic VT (19.7%), stable VT (19.7%), VT/fibrillation with transient/correctable cause (17.8%), and unexplained syncope (12.3%).[18] Thus, front-line use of an ICD is reasonable in all of the above subgroups.

## Cardiac Arrest Study Hamburg (CASH)

The CASH trial[21-23] was initiated to compare the efficacy of empiric antiarrhythmic versus an ICD therapy in survivors of sudden cardiac death unrelated to a myocardial infarction (Table 1). CASH was a prospective, randomized, multicenter open-label trial. The primary end-point was to assess the effects of therapy on total mortality with secondary end-points assessing the recurrence of hemodynamically unstable VT, sudden death, and the incidence of drug withdrawal. In ICD patients, ICD discharges occurring during syncope were counted as VF recurrences, and those occurring during presyncope and/or documented VT were counted as VT recurrences. Baseline studies and pre- and post-therapy programmed electrical stimulation were performed although these studies were not used as part of the clinical decision-making process. Patients were randomized to empiric amiodarone, metoprolol, propafenone or an ICD within 3 months of their cardiac arrest.

An interim report of findings from the first 287 patients was published[22] after the Data and Safety Monitoring Board recommended premature termination of enrollment in the propafenone limb of the study due to a significantly higher mortality (29.5%) and cardiac arrest/sudden death recurrence (23%) occurring in this group compared to a 11.5% total mortality and 0% sudden death rate in patients treated with an ICD. At the time of this analysis, sudden cardiac death was lowest in the ICD arm and total mortality was similar in the ICD, amiodarone, and metoprolol arms of the study.

The study was continued with enrollment to the amiodarone (n=92), metoprolol (n=97), and the ICD (n=99) treatment limbs. The mean age was 58 years with a mean ejection fraction of 44–47%. Over 70% of the patients had coronary artery disease. Preliminary results reported at the 1998 American College of Cardiology meetings[23] noted that the ICD arm decreased total mortality and sudden death by 30% when compared to the combined metoprolol and amiodarone treatment arms of the study (p=0.047). There was no statistical difference in study end-points between the amiodarone and metoprolol treatment arms. Substudy analysis demonstrated that inducibility by programmed electrical stimulation predicted a group of patients with lower 2-year survival rates compared to noninducible patients (p<.001).[24]

## Canadian Implantable Defibrillator Study (CIDS)

The CIDS trial (Table 1)[21,25,26] was a randomized, multicenter trial comparing the efficacy of ICD therapy (n=328) to amiodarone (n=331) in 659 patients with prior cardiac arrest or hemodynamically unstable VT. Enrollment criteria included: documented VF, out-of-hospital cardiac arrest requiring defibrillation, documented sustained VT ≥150 bpm causing presyncope or angina in a patient with an ejection fraction (EF) of ≤35% or syncope with documented spontaneous VT ≥10 seconds or induced sustained VT. The primary end-point compared the above 2 therapies in reducing arrhythmic death. Secondary end-points included quality-of-life assessment and cost-efficacy analyses, all-cause mortality, nonfatal recurrence of VF, sustained VT causing syncope, or cardiac arrest requiring external cardioversion or defibrillation. Patients were followed for 3–5 years.

Results from CIDS were presented by Connolly at the 1998 American College of Cardiology sessions.[26] He reported that all-cause mortality was 25% in the ICD versus 30% in the amiodarone group. Thus, the ICD group tended (p=0.072) toward overall improvement in survival by 19.6% compared to amiodarone after 3 years of follow-up. The results are confounded by the high-crossover rate of this population since many of the ICD patients took concomitant beta blockers (4 times greater than the amiodarone group), sotalol, and amiodarone (30%). In addition, 22% of the amiodarone treatment group later had an ICD implanted. Thus, survival in the amiodarone arm may have been overestimated.

## Clinical Perspective (CASH, AVID, CIDS)

The results of the AVID trial support the use of ICD therapy as a front-line therapy to prolong survival in patients at high risk for sudden death. Since overall survival was improved, the ICD may prolong life further through some undefined nonarrhythmic mechanism. Despite their smaller size and other problems in interpreting these trials, the results of CASH and CIDS support the findings of AVID. The results of all 3 trials, demonstrating ICD superiority in improving survival, are consistent with previous retrospective studies[2] and small prospective trials such as the Dutch Cost-Effectiveness Study.[27] Both CIDS[28] and AVID[29] suggest that patients with sustained VT/VF and depressed ejection fractions less than 35% benefit the most from ICD therapy.

Although the results of these trials are concordant, some differences in the trials exist. AVID and CIDS were powered to determine the overall survival benefit and CASH was not. CIDS had a high treatment crossover rate limiting interpretation of the results. The annual mortality rate was twice as high in the AVID drug-treated group versus CIDS or CASH (Table 1).

Although amiodarone, sotalol, and beta blockers appear to have a beneficial effect on survival in the above patient population, the lack of placebo-controlled studies raises the question of whether these drugs have a beneficial, neutral, or adverse effect on survival. If these drugs had an adverse effect on survival, some of the ICD benefit could be from the lack of any proarrhythmic effect. Based on these 3 trials, estimated 2-year mortality rates of survivors of sustained VT/VF episodes are 40–45% with Class I agents, 20–25% with amiodarone or metoprolol, and 12–20% in ICD patients.[21] Amiodarone discontinuation rates were only about 4% per year, minimizing recurrences secondary to high antiarrhythmic drug withdrawal rates.

The results of all of these studies are confounded by the fact that many of the ICD patients took concomitant beta blockers, sotalol, and amiodarone. Future cost efficacy and quality-of-life analysis will help clinicians in prescribing the most cost-effective therapy.[19]

Myerburg et al.[30] examined the importance of choosing the highest risk yield patient groups for studies and therapies. Although many therapies may be statistically effective, these same therapies may be inefficient and cost ineffective. In AVID, although ICD therapy reduced mortality by 27% (25% in the drug arm versus 18% in the ICD arm), the efficiency of the treatment was only 7%. Preliminary results of cost-effective analyses[19] suggest that even in this high-risk population, an ICD may be 5 times less cost effective than an ICD in the MADIT population[31,32] who had no history of a prior sustained ventricular tachyarrhythmia. The premature termination of AVID underestimates the cost benefit of the ICD arm of the study.

Based on the above studies, the ACC/AHA recently recommended that ICDs should be prescribed with a Class I indication as front-line therapy in patients with hemodynamically destabilizing VT/VF.[33] The above data suggest that ICD therapy is front-line therapy for sustained VT/VF in patients with ejection fractions less than 35% and is a reasonable alternative to sotalol and amiodarone in patients with sustained VT and more preserved ejection fractions. Since 40–70% of ICD patients need the use of a concomitant antiarrhythmic,[34] antiarrhythmic drugs such as beta blockers, sotalol, and amiodarone[35] demonstrated that sotalol decreased the frequency of ICD shocks/sudden death end-point (p<.05) when concomitantly used with an ICD. A CIDS substudy demonstrated that sotalol decreased mortality in the overall patient population when added to either an ICD or amiodarone.[36] The same substudy reported a statistically higher mortality rate when Class I antiarrhythmic agents were added to either amiodarone or an ICD. Data from the CASCADE trial[7] suggested similar benefits when amiodarone was used in ICD patients, since amiodarone therapy statistically ($p=0.32$) reduced syncopal ICD shocks when compared to the use of Class I agents. Depending on baseline structural heart disease (post-MI, congestive heart failure), appropriate nonarrhythmic therapy such as aspirin, statins, and ACE inhibitors[4] should be prescribed. Proper revascularization of patients with high-risk occlusive coronary artery disease should continue to be part of the overall management strategy for preventing sudden cardiac death.[2,37,38] Although ICDs have proven to prolong survival in these secondary prevention trials, the use of ICDs in primary prevention[39] will have the largest future potential impact in the fight against sudden death.

## References

1. Schaffer WA, Cobb LA. Recurrent ventricular fibrillation as mode of death in survivors of out-of-hospital ventricular fibrillation. N Engl J Med 1975; 293:259–262.

2. Gilman JK, Jalal S, Naccarelli GV. Predicting and preventing sudden death from cardiac causes. Circulation 1994; 90:1083–1092.

3. Mason JW, the ESVEM Investigators. A comparison of electrophysiologic testing with Holter monitoring to predict antiarrhythmic drug efficacy for ventricular tachyarrhythmias. N Engl J Med 1993; 329:445–451.

4. Naccarelli GV, Wolbrette DL, Dell'Orfano JT, Patel HM, Luck JC. A decade of clinical trial developments in postmyocardial infarction, congestive heart failure, and sustained ventricular tachyarrhythmia patients: from CAST to AVID and beyond. J Cardiovasc Electrophysiol 1998; 9:864–891.

5. Weinberg BA, Miles WM, Klein LS, Bolander JE, Dusman RE, et al. Five-year follow-up of 589 patients treated with amiodarone. Am Heart J 1993; 125:109–120.

6. Herre J, Sauve M, Malone P, Griffin J, Helmy I, et al. Long-term results of amiodarone therapy with recurrent sustained ventricular tachycardia or ventricular fibrillation. J Am Coll Cardiol 1989; 13:442–449.

7. The CASCADE Investigators. Randomized antiarrhythmic drug therapy in survivors of cardiac arrest (the CASCADE study). Am J Cardiol 1993; 72:280–287.

8. Hallstrom AP, Cobb LA, Yu BH, Weaver WD, Fahrenbruch CE. An antiarrhythmic drug experience in 941 patients resuscitated from an initial cardiac arrest between 1970–1985. Am J Cardiol 1991; 68:1025–1031.

9. Reiffel JA, Hahn E, Hartz, Reiter MJ, for the ESVEM Investigators: Sotalol for ventricular tachyarrhythmias: beta-blocking and Class III contributions, and relative efficacy versus Class I drugs after prior drug failure. Am J Cardiol 1997; 79:1048–1053.

10. Winkle R, Mead H, Ruder M, Gaudiani V, Smith N, et al. Long-term outcome with the automatic implantable cardioverter defibrillator. J Am Coll Cardiol 1989; 13:1353–1361.

11. Newman D, Sauve J, Herre J, Langberg J, Lee M, et al. Survival after implantation of the cardioverter-defibrillator. Am J Cardiol 1992; 69:889–903.

12. Estes M. Clinical strategies for use of the implantable cardioverter-defibrillator: the impact of current trials. PACE 1996; 19:1011–1015.
13. Nisam S. Can Implantable defibrillators reduce non-arrhythmic mortality? J Interventional Cardiac Electrophysiol 1998; 2:371–375.
14. Wever EFD, Hauer RNW, van Capelle FJL, Tijssen JGP, Crijns HJGM, et al. Randomized study of implantable defibrillator as first-choice therapy versus conventional strategy in postinfarct sudden death survivors. Circulation 1995; 91:2195–2203.
15. The Antiarrhythmics versus Implantable Defibrillators (AVID) Investigators. A comparison of antiarrhythmic drug therapy with implantable defibrillators in patients resuscitated from near-fatal ventricular arrhythmias. N Engl J Med 1997; 337:1576–1583.
16. Curtis AB, Hallstrom AF, Klein RC, Nath S, Pinski SL, et al., for the AVID Investigators. Influence of patient characteristics in the selection of patients for defibrillator implantation (the AVID Registry). Am J Cardiol 1997; 79:1185–1189.
17. Kim SG, Hallstrom A, Love JC, Rosenberg Y, Powell J, et al., for the AVID Investigators. Comparison of clinical characteristics and frequency of implantable defibrillator use between randomized patients in the Antiarrhythmics versus Implantable Defibrillators (AVID) trial and nonrandomized registry patients. Am J Cardiol 1997; 80:454–457.
18. Anderson JL, Hallstrom AP, Epstein AE, Pinski SL, Rosenberg Y, et al., and the AVID Investigators. Design and results of the antiarrhythmic versus implantable defibrillators (AVID) registry. Circulation 1999; 99:1692–1699.
19. Larsen GC, McAnulty JH, Hallstrom A, Marchant C, Shein M, et al. Hospitalization charges in the Antiarrhythmics versus Implantable Defibrillators (AVID) Trial: the AVID economic analysis study. Circulation 1997; 96:I-77.
20. Exner DV, Reiffel JA, Epstein AE, et al., and the AVID Investigators. Beta-blocker use and survival in patients with ventricular fibrillation or symptomatic ventricular tachycardia: The Antiarrhythmics versus Implantable Defibrillators (AVID) trial. J Am Coll Cardiol 1999; 334:325–333.
21. Cappato R. Secondary prevention of sudden death: the Dutch study, the Antiarrhythmics versus Implantable Defibrillator Trial, the Cardiac Arrest Study Hamburg, and the Canadian Implantable Defibrillator Study. Am J Cardiol 1999; 83:68D–73D.
22. Siebels J, Cappato R, Ruppel R, Schneider MAE, Kuck KH, and the CASH Investigators. Preliminary results of the Cardiac Arrest Study Hamburg (CASH). Am J Cardiol 1993; 72:109F–113F.
23. Kuck KH, for the CASH Investigators. Cardiac Arrest Study Hamburg (CASH). Presented at the 47th Annual Scientific Sessions of the American College of Cardiology. Late-Breaking Clinical Trials I, 1998.
24. Cappato R, Siebels J, Kuck KH. Value of programmed electrical stimulation to predict clinical outcome in the Cardiac Arrest Study Hamburg (CASH) (abstract). Circulation 1998; 98:I-495.
25. Connolly S, Gent M, Roberts RS, Dorian P, Green MS, et al. Canadian Implantable Defibrillator Study (CIDS): study design and organization. Am J Cardiol 1993; 72:103F–108F.
26. Connolly SJ, for the CIDS Investigators. Canadian Implantable Defibrillator Study. Presented at the 47th Annual Scientific Sessions of the American College of Cardiology. Late-Breaking Clinical Trials I, 1998.
27. Wever EFD, Hauer RNW, van Capelle FJI, Tijssen JGP, Crijns HJGM, et al. Randomized study of implantable defibrillator as first choice therapy versus con-

ventional strategy in postinfarct sudden death survivors. Circulation 1995; 91:2195–2203.

28. Krahn AD, Klein GJ, Yee R, Roberts RS, and the CIDS Investigators. The effect of ejection fraction on the relative benefit of the implantable defibrillator in the Canadian Implantable Defibrillator Study (abstract). Circulation 1998; 98:I-93.

29. Cannom DS, Prystowsky EN. Management of ventricular arrhythmias: detection, drugs, devices. JAMA 1999; 281:172–179.

30. Myerburg RJ, Mitrani R, Interian A, Castellanos A. Interpretation of outcomes of antiarrhythmic clinical trials: design features and population impact. Circulation 1998; 97:1514–1521.

31. Moss AJ, Hall WJ, Cannom DS, Daubert JP, Higgins SL, et al., for the Multicenter Automatic Defibrillator Implantation Trial Investigators. Improved survival with an implanted defibrillator in patients with coronary disease at high risk for ventricular arrhythmia. N Engl J Med 1996; 335:1933–1940.

32. Mushlin AI, Hall WJ, Zwanziger J, Gajary E, Andrews M, et al. Cost-effectiveness of automatic implantable cardiac defibrillators: results from MADIT. Circulation 1998; 97:2129–2135.

33. Gregoratos G, Cheitlin MD, Conill A, Epstein AE, Fellows C, et al. ACC/AHA Guidelines for Implantation of Cardiac Pacemakers and Antiarrhythmia Devices. A report of the American College of Cardiology/American Heart Association Task Force on Practice Guidelines (Committee on Pacemaker Implantation). J Am Coll Cardiol 1998; 31:1117–1209.

34. Naccarelli GV, Dougherty AH, Wolbrette D. Antiarrhythmic drug implantable cardioverter/defibrillator interactions. In: Zipes DP, Jalife J (eds). From Cell to Bedside. W.B. Saunders Co., Philadelphia, 1995, pp 1426–1433.

35. Pacifico A, Hohnsloser SH, Williams JH, Tao B, Saksena S, et al., for the d,l-sotalol Implantable Cardioverter-Defibrillator Study Group. Prevention of implantable-defibrillator shocks by treatment with sotalol. N Engl J Med 1999; 340:1855–1862.

36. Talajic M, Connolly S, Dorian P, Roy D, Mitchell LB, et al. Canadian Implantable Defibrillator Study (CIDS): effects of additional antiarrhythmic drug therapy on survival (abstract). Circulation 1998; 98:I-93.

37. Holmes DR, Davis KB, Mock MB, Fisher LD, Gersch BJ, et al., and the participants in the Coronary Artery Surgery Study. The effect of medical and surgical treatment on subsequent cardiac death in patients with coroanry artery disease: a report from the Coronary Artery Surgical Study. Circulation 1986; 73:1254–1263.

38. Bigger JT, for the CABG Patch Trial Investigators. Prophylactic use of implanted cardiac defibrillators in patients at high risk for ventricular arrhythmias after coronary artery bypass graft surgery. N Engl J Med 1997; 337:1569–1575.

39. Nisam S, Mower M. ICD trials: an extraordinary means of determining patient risk? PACE 1998; 21:1341–1346.

# 47

# Quality of Life in Patients with Implantable Cardioverter-Defibrillators

*Christian Wolpert, MD, Werner Jung, MD, Susanne Herwig, MD, and Berndt Lüderitz, MD*

## Introduction

The implantable cardioverter-defibrillator (ICD) has been proven to reduce the mortality of sudden cardiac death in patients with malignant ventricular tachyarrhythmias since it entered clinical practice. It has become the therapy of choice for patients with aborted sudden cardiac death or hemodynamically unstable ventricular tachycardias and various underlying heart diseases. After transvenous placement of the device, antitachycardia pacing and device miniaturization have been accomplished and safety of the therapy in terms of reliability of hardware and software has been demonstrated, and quality of life in patients with ICDs has gained increasing importance over the years. In the early period of ICD use, painless termination of ventricular tachycardia and the avoidance of inappropriate shocks represented the main clinical points of interest, but today patient acceptance, coping behavior, and psychological integrity are increasingly focused on. Quality-of-life assessment is of great importance in patients with ICDs, because it could be demonstrated that, although ICD therapy improved survival of patients who are at risk of sudden cardiac death, there are also several inherent problems, e.g., inappropriate shocks, fear of shock therapy, and the consciousness of the lifesaving character of the ICD.[1-6] The aim of ICD therapy is only fully achieved if patients regain the maximum possible flexibility, return to their normal activity scale, and reintegrate into family and professional life. A great battery of measuring instruments is in use today to evaluate the quality of life in ICD patients with the intention of obtaining targets and guiding approaches to support this very selective patient population and provide interventional psychological tools.

From: Aliot E, Clementy J, Prystowsky EN (editors). *Fighting Sudden Cardiac Death: A Worldwide Challenge.* ©Futura Publishing Company, Armonk, NY, 2000.

# Definition of Quality of Life

Quality of life has different meanings and contains different items, depending on the perspective of the investigator and the intention for analysis. Although there is no exact definition of quality of life, there is an emerging consensus that quality-of-life assessment can be based on physical condition, psychological well-being, social activity, and everyday activity. These categories can then be further subdivided into a number of aspects such as mobility, self-care, family contact, intimacy, or negativity in terms of depression or anxiety. The approach to quality of life, therefore, must be multidimensional, using a variety of investigatory tools. The limitation of many trials dealing with quality of life is the unidimensional approach, focusing only on restricted issues, e.g., functional status excluding mental or psychological aspects or psychological features, leaving aside functional capacity. Future investigations of quality of life, moreover, will have to address a variety of health-associated sectors including costs, working capacity, or social care in addition to physical and mental integrity, since invasive therapies cause manifold interactions of the individual with the environment and vice versa. The rationale of quality-of-life research should, therefore, use an analytic model and comprehensively include predictors and response variables in a given time frame in which the impact of therapy on quality of life is elicited.

# Design of Quality of Life Measurement Scales

Measurement of quality of life should contain all aspects, subjective and objective, that can be affected by a therapy in each member of a patient population in either a positive or a negative way. This can be achieved only by the use of standardized instruments which have been validated. The primary issue for selection of a specific instrument is the expected performance in a required situation. The choice is guided by the instruments' psychometric properties including validity, reliability, responsiveness, appropriateness to question, use, and practical utility. The common measurement of quality of life is based on complex constructions including items, domains, scales, and instruments. An item is a single question, and a scale contains the available categories or other mechanisms for expressing the response to the question. For instance, a specific question might be answered by filling out an open-ended blank at the discretion of the patient or several categories or a visual analog line, where the patient places a quasidimensional mark. All 3 scales cited here are considered global, since no specific criteria are offered to the patient to demarcate the choice of categories or other expressions. A domain identifies a specific point of interest, such as functional capacity or digestion. This can include a response to single or multiple items.

The instrument itself is a collection of items that is used to gather the required information. An instrument can contain a global question or multiple items that may be categorized into different domains. For the measurement of quality of life, 1 or more instruments may be used. For a single instrument, the output result can be formed in 2 ways: either as a profile, preserving the components and citing individually, or by aggregating the results to a single composite score. Some instruments offer both ways of presentation. The use of instruments and investigatory techniques is influenced by a number of factors: the setting of the evaluation, type of questionnaire used (short form, clinic-based survey, mail-back survey), and others. There are 2 main instruments: (1) *generic instruments* used for surveys in general populations to asses a variety of domains, and (2) *disease-specific instruments* focusing on domains that are most relevant to a certain disease or condition under study. *Disease-specific instruments* are used for clinical trials to assess the influence of specific therapeutic interventions. As an advantage, they are restricted only to relevant dimensions for the specific disease but have a disadvantage concerning comparability with other disease groups. Integration of both generic and disease-specific instruments is possible by using a battery of scales and modular instruments maintaining a core module to address both different disease groups and the therapy under investigation. Finally, studies have demonstrated that the judgment on quality of life is very subject- and observer-dependent. Therefore, a systematic approach to measure quality of life is needed to allow for an improvement of health care professionals' evaluation of quality of life in all fields of medical therapy.

## Quality of Life in Patients with ICDs

Patient acceptance of ICD therapy is influenced by a number of contributing factors, including the preimplant patient history, socialization, environment, and technical aspects such as number of shocks, battery location, device size/ body size, and inappropriate shocks. This means that a patient who easily adapts to the fact of an ICD implant itself may have a very low acceptance of the device during follow-up due to inappropriate or appropriate therapies. A patient may also suffer from the fact that he cannot drive anymore or is not allowed to execute his profession, e.g., mechanical engineer. Many patients do not experience shocks but exhibit a permanent fear of the occurrence of shocks. Therefore, quality-of-life measurements must address not only obvious issues such as device-related, objective data, but also more subjective issues including all of the various perceptions of the individual patient.

In our own patient population, we investigated in a prospective pilot study 57 patients with ICDs, using a variety of quality-of-life issues.[3,6] Eight different questionnaires were used to obtain information on general sociodemographic data and ICD implantation and therapy acceptance, personality (Freiburg Personality Inventory),and quality of life (MOS-SF 36 Inventory). In addition, the patients answered questionnaires concerning fear (State Trait Anxiety Inventory), complaints (Complaint List), depression (Beck Depression Inventory), and coping behavior. The Freiburg Personality Inventory contains 138 questions about a number of expressions of specific behavior, attitudes, and habits. The answer can be given as yes or no. MOS-SF 36 is a generic instrument with good validation and great realibility, and it also offers sufficient sensitivity and specificity. It contains 36 questions about physical, psychological, and social well-being. The State Trait Anxiety Inventory is used for a patient self-evaluation. The test explores 2 different components of fear. Two different scale forms serve to measure the actual fear (State) and general anxiety (Trait). The Complaint List is also a self-evaluation test that detects a broad spectrum of health disturbances such as subjective or negative influence by physical or general complaints. The Beck Depression Inventory deals with different

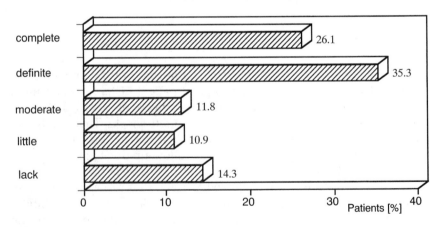

## Quality of Life 12 Months after ICD Implantation

Figure 1. Patient description of quality of life 12 months after ICD implantation. More than half of the patients regain complete quality of life or at least describe a definite positive change. Approximately a quarter of the patients report a lack of or only little loss of quality of life.

dimensions of depression, including dysphoria, hopelessness, fear of failure, guilt feelings, self-hate, suicide tendencies, and others. The Coping Behavior Inventory evaluates the patient's reaction to the fact that he/she has a heart disease and to the changes in behavior during follow-up. In our patient population, 24 of 57 patients answered that they were used to the device after 2 months (Figures 1–3). Thirty-three patients needed a longer period to adapt to the system. The most frequent reply (20 patients) to the question of what causes the greatest fear was fear of ICD discharge, followed by fear of physical discomfort caused by the device, and finally restricted quality of life in profession, sports, and social activities. When asked if they would recommend the device to other patients, a vast majority (56 of 57) answered positively.

In patients ≤40 years of age, Dubin et al. found, using a modified SF-36 health questionnaire, that all patients who answered the questionnaire felt their health to be good to excellent; 38% reported an improvement in health since their ICD implantation.[7] All patients thought they were able to perform activities of daily living and 68% were able to freely manage

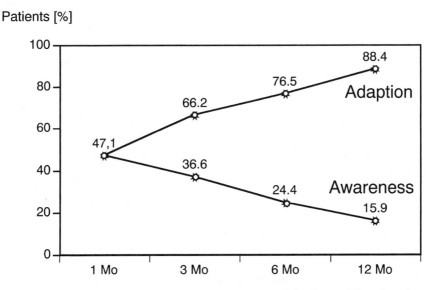

# ICD: Adaption and Awareness

**Figure 2.** Patient adaption to the ICD and awareness of the device. There is a significant increase in adaption over the first 12 months after implant. Awareness continuously decreases over time.

# Symptom Checklist with Respect to Number of Shocks Experienced

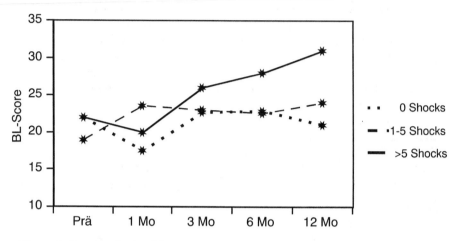

Figure 3. Results obtained from a symptom checklist yield a reduction of quality of life in patients who experience >5 shocks during follow-up indicated by an increase of the complaint list score.

moderate physical activities. In contrast to our own patient population, younger patients, i.e., <50 years of age, had an increased level of anxiety.

Shock incidence was found to be a very important factor that negatively affects quality of life by worsening the degree of depression, complaints, and level of anxiety. In our own study population, more than 5 shocks caused a significantly higher level of anxiety in patients independent of age or sex. These findings are consistent with the data of Dougherty and Hegel, who also assessed a significantly higher level of anxiety and depression in patients with ≤5 discharges compared to patients without any appropriate or inappropriate discharge.[5,8]

The postimplantation period, which is most relevant to the adjustment of the patients to the device and implantation, is described differently in recent studies. Vlay et al. report a 3-month postimplantation period that is necessary for their patients to adapt to the device.[2] Other authors demonstrated that the psychological distress caused by ICD implant and the secondary psychological changes show a decrease over the first 6 months after implant. Heller et al. studied the psychosocial outcome in 58 patients over a mean follow-up of 20 months.[9] In his study there was an increase of positive attitudes toward an ICD from 52% before implant to 76% after implant. The degree of satisfaction showed a strong correlation with less anger and less worry about ICD size. Moreover, an improved attitude was accompanied by less sadness and perceived better health. However, in spite of a successful ICD placement, health concerns increased in 62% of the patients. Furthermore, a support group was attended by 39 patients. Of these, 96% considered the support group to be helpful. Shock incidence $1 shock/patient was associated with various findings. The anxiety about family and reduced activities as well as an increased sadness and more health worries were found in those patients. As a conclusion, the authors state a paradoxical increase in health concerns despite an objective improvement of actual health.

## Future Aspects of Quality of Life in Patients with ICDs

In the very beginning of ICD therapy, the patient population had a significantly longer history of malignant ventricular tachyarrhythmias. The shorter history of patients today is due to better information about the existence of the therapy, earlier detection of patients at risk, and increased survival due to better emergency care networks. Together with expanded indications for implant emerging in the era of primary prevention of sudden death, we will experience even more and younger postmyocardial infarction patients before they are resuscitated and many patients who are completely asymptomatic with respect to arrhythmias.[10] These patients will probably show very different reactions to ICD implant with presumably lower levels of anxiety and fear as well as preserved social activity and psychological flexibility. According to the lack of symptoms attributed to arrhythmias, they may feel implantation to be much more intrusive, since they do not weigh a lifesaving therapy for a potential risk against all restrictions or physical changes, which an ICD system implies. It should not be forgotten that in earlier times, patients usually had gone through serial drug testing, repetitive intensive care stays, and frequently 1 or more episodes of syncope. In these patients, anxiety and fear of a recurrent episode caused by an arrhythmia has a significant impact on overall psychology. To avoid any harmful experience due to arrhythmias, they are more willing and prepared to accept a treatment as long as it helps to reduce in-hospital stay, syncopes with and without injury, and spouses' fears. In the future, an increasing number of patients will enter ICD therapy and follow-up with a prophylactic therapy or will receive shocks for a hemodynamically stable arrhythmia. The perception of the device may thus be inaccurate and lead to a more negative feeling despite a better status of health. Finally, numerous innovations have been implemented into newer ICD devices as better discrimination algorithms for supraventricular and ventricular rhythms or separate atrial therapies and device size will be further decreased. It will be very interesting to see if improvements that will lead to less inappropriate therapies subsequently improve not only device-related and influenced items but also overall quality of life.[11] Similarly, the effect of ICDs with biventricular pacing for treatment of concomitant heart failure on quality of life will be exciting to follow, since the target group makes up a significant number of patients with ICDs. As it has already been shown in several preliminary studies of patients with biventricular pacing without any malignant ventricular tachyarrhythmias, an improvement of the functional status and quality of life can be achieved in a considerable number of patients.[12-14] Resulting from the variety of new developments and the drastic social and economic changes and necessities, quality-of-life assessment will gain increasing importance in the field of ICD therapy since fewer resources and an increasing need for patient mobility, ability to work, and patient independence must be the main goals of the treatment. There is a need for a multidimensional systematic approach using the appropriate instruments to make quality-of-life assessment comparable and a valuable tool for interventional strategies.

## Conclusion

Quality-of-life research has gained increasing importance in patients with ICDs, since not only the electrical efficacy of therapy in terms of a reduction of mortality but also improvement of functional status, patients' well-being, reintegration into their professional environment, and finally, patient mobility and independence are main targets of this lifesaving therapy. To thoroughly assess quality of life with all its subdomains, we are in need of a multidimensional approach, which also yields guidelines for sociopsychological support.

### Reference

1. Sears SF, Todaro JF, Lewis TS, et al. Examining the psychosocial impact of implantable cardioverter defibrillators: a literature review. Clin Cardiol 1999; 22(7):481–489.
2. Vlay SC, Olson LC, Fricchione GL, et al. Anxiety and anger in patients with ventricular tachyarrhythmias: response after automatic internal cardioverter defibrillator implantation. PACE 1989; 12:366–373.
3. Lüderitz B, Jung W, Deister A, et al. Quality of life in multiprogrammable implantable cardioverter-defibrillator recipients. In: Saksena S, Lüderitz B (eds). Interventional Electrophysiology: A Textbook. Futura Publishing Company, Inc., Armonk, NY, 1996, pp 305–313.
4. Kalbfleisch KR, Lehmann MH, Steinmann RT, et al. Reemployment following implantation of the automatic cardioverter defibrillator. Am J Cardiol 1989; 64:199–202.

5. Dougherty CM. Psychological reactions and family adjustment in shock versus no shock groups after implantation of internal cardioverter defibrillator. Heart Lung 1995; 24:281–291.
6. Lüderitz B, Jung W, Deister A, et al: Patient acceptance of implantable cardioverter defibrillator devices: changing attitudes. Am Heart J 1994; 127:1179–1184.
7. Dubin AM, Batsford WP, Lewis RJ, et al. Quality of life in patients receiving implantable cardioverter defibrillators at or before age 40. PACE 1996; 19: 1555–1559.
8. Hegel MT, Griegel LE, Black C, et al. Anxiety and depression in patients receiving implanted cardioverter-defibrillators: a longitudinal investigation. Intl J Psychiatry Med 1997; 27:57–69.
9. Heller S, Ormont M, Lidagoster L, et al. Psychological outcome after ICD implantation: a current perspective. PACE 1998; 21:1207–1215.
10. Moss AJ, Hall WJ, Cannom DS, et al. Improved survival with an implanted defibrillator in patients with coronary disease at high risk for ventricular arrhythmia: Multicenter Automatic Defibrillator Implantation Trial Investigators. N Engl J Med 1996; 335:1933–1940.
11. Jung W, Lüderitz B. Implantation of an arrhythmia management system for patients with ventricular and supraventricular tachyarrhythmias. Lancet 1997; 349:853–854.
12. Holt P, Bucknall C, Chatoor R, et al. Cardiac resynchronization for heart failure: do patients with prior indications for pacing benefit? PACE 1999; 22:A53.
13. Leclerq C, Cazeau S, Alonso C, et al. Long-term results of the French pilot study on multisite biventricular pacing in advanced heart failure. PACE 1999; 22:A65.
14. Sack S, Wolfhard U, Dagres N, et al. Optimized atrioventricular pacing on right, left or biventricular sites impressively improve quality of life. PACE 1999; 22:A52.

# 48

# Economic Aspects of Implantable Cardioverter-Defibrillator Therapy

*Owen A. Obel, MD, and A. John Camm, MD*

## Introduction

Sudden cardiac death (SCD) is a major public health problem accounting for approximately half of all deaths from heart disease,[1] and resulting in approximately 70,000 deaths per year in the United Kingdom alone.[2] Therapy with the implantable cardioverter-defibrillator (ICD) has consistently been shown to provide highly effective treatment for patients with life-threatening ventricular arrhythmias since its inception in 1980,[3,4] and more recently has been shown to confer a survival benefit in a variety of clinical situations. Considerable international variation in ICD implantation rates reflects regional differences in prescribing attitudes among physicians, differences in the amount and method of funding health care that is available, and differences in the number of physicians trained in the field of cardiac electrophysiology. ICD therapy is widely perceived as being expensive. In an age when health services are struggling to keep up with advances in medical diagnostic and therapeutic technology, and the increasing average age of the population, therapeutic effectiveness needs to be balanced against cost. As the potential list of indications for ICD therapy gets broader, and as patients with heart disease survive longer, cost of the ICD needs to be taken into account in order to justify the more widespread use of this form of therapy.

## Efficacy of the ICD Therapy

### Secondary Prevention

It is estimated that fewer than 1 in 3 patients who survive a cardiac arrest are successfully resuscitated and are ultimately discharged from hospital.[5] SCD occurs primarily in patients with established heart disease, par-

From: Aliot E, Clementy J, Prystowsky EN (editors). *Fighting Sudden Cardiac Death: A Worldwide Challenge.* ©Futura Publishing Company, Armonk, NY, 2000.

ticularly those with a history of severe congestive cardiac failure, myocardial infarction (MI), or previous ventricular arrhythmia.[6] Survivors of cardiac arrest in the absence of acute MI are at high risk of future recurrence and have a 1-year mortality of over 30%,[7] and a risk of recurrence of 45% over the subsequent 2 years.[8] In the Antiarrhythmics Versus Implantable Defibrillators (AVID) trial, survivors of cardiac arrest were shown to have a reduced overall mortality when treated with an ICD.[9] The AVID trial recruited a total of 1,016 patients. Inclusion criteria were resuscitation from near-fatal ventricular fibrillation (VF), sustained ventricular tachycardia (VT) with syncope, or sustained VT associated with an ejection fraction (EF) of <0.40 or less, together with symptoms suggesting severe hemodynamic compromise due to the arrhythmia. The majority of patients were male patients with ischemic heart disease, with an average age of approximately 65 years. Patients were randomly assigned to receive either ICD therapy or antiarrhythmic drug therapy that consisted of amiodarone in the majority and sotalol in the remainder. The trial demonstrated a reduction of approximately 30% in death rates as a result of ICD therapy throughout the 3-year follow-up period. The average unadjusted length of additional life associated with ICD implantation was modest, at 2.7 months over the 3 years; however, the outcome curves were continuing to diverge at the end of the follow-up period. The majority of ICD-treated patients received antitachycardia therapy (pacing or shock), and this was more common when the index arrhythmia was VT rather than VF (85% versus 69% at 3 years, respectively). It is noteworthy that more patients in the ICD group received beta blockers compared to the drug therapy group, adjustment for which slightly reduced the estimated survival benefit conferred by ICDs. The results of the CASH and CIDS trials, while not formally published, show a similar survival benefit from ICDs in the secondary prevention of SCD. Together, these trials firmly indicate that the ICD can now be regarded as the treatment of choice in the prevention of SCD in patients who have been resuscitated from cardiac arrest or those with sustained, poorly tolerated ventricular arrhythmia, particularly in the context of a low EF. This high-risk group of patients represents a low proportion of the total group of patients who succumb to SCD. Far more frequent is the situation where SCD is unheralded and occurs as a primary event.

## Primary Prevention

The results of trials of ICD therapy in the primary prevention of SCD have produced divergent results. The Multicentre Automatic Defibrillator Implantation Trial (MADIT) compared ICD (initially transthoracic and then transvenous) therapy with conventional medical therapy in a group of patients at high risk of significant ventricular arrhythmia. Entry criteria included MI (more than 3 weeks) prior to entry, decreased EF (<35%), documented nonsustained VT (NSVT), and inducible VT at electrophysiological study (EPS), which was not suppressed by the administration of procainamide.[10] The trial was stopped prematurely after the recruitment of only 192 patients after a clear mortality benefit in the ICD group was demonstrated. The hazard ratio comparing the risk of death per unit time was 0.46 (95%, confidence interval 0.26 to 0.86) for the ICD versus the conventional group. It is noteworthy that 60% of the patients assigned to an ICD had a shock within 2 years after enrollment; however, the appropriateness of these shocks could not be assessed because the trial began before the time that generators with telemetric capabilities came into routine use. Criticisms of the trial have included the low use of antiarrhythmic drugs (particularly amiodarone) in the conventional arm such that at the time of last follow-up, only 45% of patients were taking the drug, and 23% of patients were not taking any antiarrhythmic drug (including beta blockers) whatsoever. In fact, 11% of patients in the conventional arm were taking Class I antiarrhythmics, which are known to have increased mortality in a very similar group of patients.[11] As in AVID, more patients in the ICD group were on beta-blocker therapy. Since patients had already failed to respond to antiarrhythmic therapy, it might be argued that they were a self-selected group, unlikely to have demonstrated a satisfactory response to conventional therapy.

The recently reported Multicentre Unsustained Tachycardia Trial (MUSTT) examined a similar group of patients.[12] Patients had coronary artery disease (CAD), an EF of less than 40%, asymptomatic, nonsustained VT, and inducible VT at EPS. The trial differed from MADIT mainly in that entry into the trial did not require nonsuppressibility of induced VT, and there was a control group that did not receive any antiarrhythmic therapy (drug or ICD) whatsoever. The treatment arm consisted of 2 subgroups: those prescribed antiarrhythmic drugs, and those implanted with an ICD. Beta-blocker use between the 2 groups was, if anything, higher in the non-therapy group. Median duration of follow-up was more than 3 years; the primary end-point was cardiac arrest or death from arrhythmia. The trial demonstrated a clear mortality benefit in the group treated with antiarrhythmic therapy compared to the group who received no treatment. This reduction appeared to occur purely as a result of ICD therapy and not from antiarrhythmic drugs; however, this was not an observation controlled by prior randomization. The 5-year rate of the primary end-point was 9% in the ICD group compared to 37% in the treatment arm that did not receive ICDs, and there was a more than 50% reduction in overall mortality. The study demonstrated a mortality benefit from ICDs in the primary prevention of SCD in high-risk patients and confirmed the substantial risk to patients who have CAD associated with a reduced EF, nonsustained VT, and inducible VT. The 5-year rate of cardiac arrest or death from arrhythmia was 32% in the group that did not receive antiarrhythmic therapy, and the incidence of spontaneous sustained VT was approximately 20% in both the treated and the nontreated groups.

Although the results of MADIT and MUSTT are encouraging, not all trials of ICD therapy in the primary prevention of ventricular arrhythmias have demonstrated similar effects. The Coronary Artery Bypass (CABG) Patch trial was performed to test the hypothesis that epicardial ICD implantation performed at the time of CABG could further improve the outlook for CAD patients with an EF of less than 36% and abnormalities on the signal-averaged ECG (SAECG).[13] Patients were randomized to ICD implantation or no ICD implantation at the time of surgery. After an average follow-up of 36 ± 12 months, no difference was detected in either cardiac and noncardiac mortality between those who had and those who had not received an ICD. There were, however, significantly more postoperative infections in the ICD group. Fifty-seven percent of the patients with an ICD received a shock within the first 2 years after implantation, although it is noteworthy that the devices used were "committed devices" that deliver shocks even if the index arrhythmia has ceased prior to the end of charging, and could thus deliver inappropriate therapy in cases of nonsustained atrial or ventricular tachyarrhythmia. Furthermore, ICDs at that time were not capable of storing electrograms and thus detailed analysis was impossible.

The reasons for the differences between the CABG Patch trial and trials such as AVID, MADIT, and MUSTT are likely to be several-fold. It is probable that sustained, poorly tolerated ventricular arrhythmia or inducible VTs are more sensitive markers of the future risk of SCD than abnormalities of the SAECG in CAD patients with reduced LV function. The fact that all of the patients in the CABG Patch trial were revascularized may also account for the lack of difference between patient groups since revascularization itself may reduce the incidence of SCD[14] and has a mortality benefit.[15] This is borne out by the lower mortality in the CABG Patch trial than in the other trials.

Overall, ICDs have been shown to offer effective therapy in a variety of contexts, and physicians are reaching consensus regarding the clinical indications for ICD therapy, particularly in the secondary prevention of serious arrhythmic events. The use of ICDs in the primary prevention of arrhythmias is more contentious.

## Cost Effectiveness of ICD Therapy

Several investigators have examined cost effectiveness of the ICD. Until recently, the majority of studies were retrospective and have used secondary cost information or theoretical models to estimate costs. Some studies factored in quality of life, while others used survival data only. Studies have also varied as to whether they have included aspects such as generator replacement costs, and whether the cost of preimplantation screening tests have been included in the analysis.

Using a decision-analytic (Markov) model, Kupperman et al.[16] were the first to report on the cost effectiveness of the ICD. The analysis was retrospective, and charges were obtained from 1984 Medicare databases, the medical literature, individual pharmacies, hospitals, and expert opinion. The authors estimated that the net cost effectiveness of the defibrillator, when used in a group of patients who had suffered at least one cardiac arrest not associated with an MI, was approximately $17,100 per life-year saved. Sensitivity analyses suggested a true value of between $15,000 and $25,000, well within the range of other lifesaving interventions in the United States at the time. The authors also examined a future scenario in which the device would have greater longevity, would be programmable, and would not require thoracotomy. Estimates of the cost effectiveness of the ICD in these circumstances were vastly improved at $7,400 per life-year saved, while sensitivity analyses suggested that the true value lay between a value that is cost saving (less expensive than pharmacological therapy) and $19,600 per life-year saved.

O'Brien[17] performed an observational, descriptive retrospective Markov analysis based on practice in the United Kingdom. The authors studied a hypothetical population of cardiac arrest survivors and used reported treatment information to estimate the incremental cost effectiveness of the ICD compared to amiodarone. Cost effectiveness of ICD treatment was computed over 20 years, and all future costs and effects were discounted at 6% per year. Estimated life expectancy was increased almost 2-fold by ICD therapy (11.1 and 6.7 years over the 20-year period for the ICD and amiodarone, respectively). Discounted 20-year treatment costs were £28,400 for the ICD and £2,300 for amiodarone. Cost effectiveness of ICD treatment was in the range of £8,200 to £15,400 per life-year gained, a figure comparable to interventions such as single-vessel CABG and cholesterol-lowering treatment. A sensitivity analysis in this study showed that cost effectiveness was most sensitive to the magnitude of mortality benefit attributable to ICD therapy.

Kupersmith and colleagues compared the use of the ICD with electrophysiologically guided antiarrhythmic drug therapy in survivors of cardiac arrest.[18] Unlike previous studies, the authors used an empirical clinical dataset for estimation of effectiveness rather than historical controls. Factors such as EP testing, probabilities of repeated hospitalizations, follow-up visits, probability of lead fracture, and generator life were taken into account in the marginal analysis. The authors assumed that the time of first shock in those with an ICD would have been the time of death in those without an ICD, thus patients acted as their own controls. Additional variables such as perioperative mortality, battery life, and discount rate were also incorporated. The study was commenced during the time that transvenous implantation was becoming standard and therefore both epicardial and transvenous ICDs are represented in the analysis. Sensitivity analysis in this study found that a battery life of 4 versus 2 years had a significant effect on cost effectiveness of the ICD, while variations in perioperative mortality rate, discount rate at 0% and 3%, and separate considerations of patients with ICDs who were receiving antiarrhythmics did not. The ICD was more cost effective for patients with an EF <25% than for those with an EF >25%. Performing a preimplant EP study significantly reduced cost effectiveness. Rather surprisingly, the use of the endocardial as opposed to the epicardial ICD had only a modest beneficial effect on cost effectiveness. The study made conservative assumptions such as a 4-year generator life and no periprocedure deaths in the EP-guided antiarrhythmic group. Despite this, the investigators found that ICDs provide cost-effective therapy in relation to other accepted therapies such as hemodialysis and the treatment of hypertension. A limitation of the approach used is the assumption that first shock equilibrates with death in the absence of an ICD since, even today, up to 25% of discharges are inappropriate,[19,20] and even if appropriate, not all ventricular arrhythmias are uniformly fatal, even in survivors of cardiac arrest. Using mortality curves from previously published analysis on EP-guided therapy,[16,20] the authors found a similar cost effectiveness, thus validating their approach of using patients as their own "controls."

Larsen et al.[21] used reports of outcomes of patients treated with ICDs compared to amiodarone for recurrent VT or VF and performed a complex state transition decision model that aims to account for all possible costs (obtained from hospitals' billing records) incurred by the patients in each group. In this study, ICD therapy was found to represent a relatively expensive strategy, costing $29,200 per year per life saved compared to amiodarone. The battery life of the ICD had an important influence in a sensitivity analysis. As with other early studies, the modern applicability of the study is limited by the fact that transthoracic devices were used at the time; furthermore, the authors assumed that no crossover between groups occurred.

In an analysis of ICD therapy, Anderson et al.[2] constructed a simple, reproducible model for cost efficacy by dividing the total cost of ICD therapy by the years of life gained. In addition to survivors of out-of-hospital cardiac arrest, the authors applied the model in a variety of hypothetical clinical settings based on trials of ICD therapy that were in process at that time. Thus, the model was used in patients with nonsustained VT, in patients at high risk after MI, in patients with a low EF and a positive SAECG, and in patients awaiting cardiac transplantation. Finally, the model was used to assess the impact of future technological developments on the cost efficacy of the ICD. By taking this approach, the study was able to provide insight into a variety of clinical scenarios, thus imparting a broader picture of ICD cost efficacy. Uniquely, the costs of screening tests used to identify at-risk patients were included in the analysis that incorporated the cost of the generator, hospitalization costs, and cost of follow-up. The cost of generator replacement, however, was not included in the analysis. In general, use of the ICD in all survivors of SCD was found to be an expensive strategy. However, when a high-risk group of patients was identified by the presence of a low EF (<30%) and inducible ventricular arrhythmia not suppressed by antiarrhythmic drug treatment, cost efficacy improved. The cost efficacy in this group of patients was £22,400 per life-year, whereas in the lowest risk group (ventricular arrhythmia suppressed by drugs; EF>30%) cost rose dramatically to £700,000 per life-year. The authors draw attention to the fact that in the general population, the majority of events occur in the "low-risk" group (although in a low percentage of that group). There is, therefore, a conflict between treating high-risk patient groups with a reasonable cost efficacy and the high costs that would be incurred if ICD therapy were used as a means of reduction in the incidence of SCD in the general population.

In the study by Anderson et al., cost efficacy (based on historical survival data for patients with CAD, reduced EF, and nonsustained VT), in the MADIT study was estimated to be £42,500 per life-year, and £23,500 per life-year for the MUSST study. Post-MI patients were stratified according to the results of noninvasive screening tests. A combination of reduced heart rate variability, >10 ventricular premature contractions/hour, and a positive SAECG identified a high-risk group (SCD rate of 29.9% at 3 years) with a cost efficacy of £36,500 per life-year. An EF of <40% used as a sole criterion in the post-MI group increased cost almost 5-fold to £170,000 per life-year, illustrating again that as the risk profile of the patient group decreases, cost rises. Cost efficacy of the ICD in patients awaiting cardiac transplantation was favorable, particularly when EF was less than 25%. Expected costs for the UK were calculated on the basis of these analyses, and amounted to £22 million per year for survivors of SCD with low EFs. A similar figure was calculated for post-MI patients with inducible, nonsuppressible VT, and £48 million per year was the estimate for post-MI patients with low EFs and inducible arrhythmias. Increasing the life of the generator and reduction in the cost of the generator improved cost efficacy. Interestingly, it was noted that even if the generator was free, cost of ICD therapy remained significant at £19,500 per life-year even in the high-risk postinfarction group. Transvenous implantation had a modest cost benefit over the epicardial method. However, this did not assume a reduced mortality as a result of this method. Screening tests influence total costs, and it was suggested that £250 for the screening test represents the limit beyond which cost efficacy suffered. The combination of the measurement of EF and electrophysiological assessment was better at identifying a cost-effective high-risk subgroup than either of these investigations alone. Furthermore, as the size of the high-risk group became smaller, the cost of the screening test became increasingly important in determining overall cost efficacy of ICD therapy. The authors point out that technological improvements, improved implantation techniques, and competitive prices were all likely to result in an improvement in cost efficacy.

## The Effect of Altering Implant Mortality on the Cost Efficacy of the ICD (Figure 1)

Valenti and colleagues examined the impact of the ICD on hospitalization in patients with drug-refractory VT. Thirty-five such patients were studied with respect to the frequency and duration of hospital stay in the

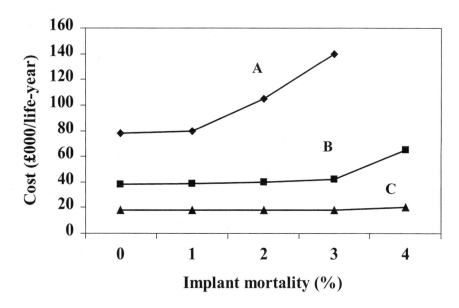

Figure 1. This figure illustrates the effect of altering implant mortality on the cost efficacy of the ICD in 3 populations with differing 3-year sudden death rates: (A) 14%, (B) 28%, (C) 56%. Note that improved implant-related mortality has the greatest effect on cost efficacy where the population group is at a relatively lower risk of sudden death. (Adapted with permission from Anderson MH, et al.[2]

12 months before and after ICD implantation. [22] They found that ICD therapy resulted in a significant decrease in the number of hospitalizations/patient and in the percentage of patients requiring admission to hospital. ICD implantation in this group of patients also resulted in a significant decrease in the duration of hospital stay for all reasons and a decrease of 90% in the total number of hospital days for cardiac reasons. The reason for admission pre-ICD implantation was more likely to be cardiac, while postimplantation admissions were for predominantly noncardiac reasons. Hospital admissions preimplantation were more likely to be to an intensive care unit (30.7% preimplantation versus 3% postimplantation) at a daily cost of nearly 3 times that of admission to general wards. The authors estimated, based on this total reduction of hospital costs, that the initial cost of the ICD would be paid back after a period of 19 months postimplantation. As in other studies, a high rate of actual delivery of ICD therapy was documented. It is noteworthy that in contrast to this study, patients in the ICD group in the AVID trial were in fact hospitalized sooner and more frequently in the first year after enrollment than patients in the antiarrhythmic drug group; however, the respective study groups are not equitable.

The first study to include details of quality of life in the analysis of cost effectiveness of the ICD was performed by Owens et al.[23] This study compared 3 strategies: ICD therapy, amiodarone therapy, and a strategy of amiodarone therapy followed, if necessary, by ICD implantation in a hypothetical group of patients at high/intermediate risk of SCD (57-year-old patients who had suffered a previous cardiac arrest). A Markov analysis was performed, which assigned the patients to particular strategy "trees" (amiodarone, ICD, amiodarone-ICD) and followed patients until they reached a predefined end-point or Markov "node" (e.g., "well" or "neurologic impairment"). The authors assumed a perioperative mortality rate of 1.8% complicated by infection or lead failure rates of 2% and 3%, respectively. The authors assumed a reduction in total mortality of 20–40% at 1 year for the ICD versus amiodarone (with sensitivity analysis performed for each of these levels), and assumed generator replacement every 4 years. In addition to costs of initial hospitalization and costs of ongoing therapy, costs of generator replacement were taken into account, while costs of screening tests were not. The marginal cost effectiveness of treatment with an ICD relative to amiodarone ranged from $37,300 to $74,000 per quality-adjusted life-year (QALY) gained (assuming a reduction in total mortality of 40% and 20%, respectively). The patients in the amiodarone-ICD tree had little benefit compared to the amiodarone only group, and the strategy was expensive relative to the ICD as sole initial therapy. The amiodarone-ICD group was thus excluded from sensitivity analysis, which compared amiodarone with ICD therapy only. Such analysis showed that magnitude of risk reduction as a result of ICD implantation had significant effects on cost effectiveness. As in other studies, an increase in generator longevity had a significant impact such that an increase from 4 to 5 years between generator replacements improved cost effectiveness from $74,400 to $63,800 per QALY. The cost of implantation had only a modest effect on cost effectiveness, while sensitivity analysis accounting for variable values of quality of life had a major impact, a predictable effect given the nature of this particular study.

Wever and colleagues analyzed the economic impact of the ICD while performing an intention-to-treat analysis of the efficacy of ICD therapy as first choice versus a strategy of electrophysiologically guided therapy in postinfarct survivors of out-of-hospital cardiac arrest.[24,25] Unlike previous studies, which were retrospective, this study started accounting medical costs on the day of randomization. Costs were comprehensive and included all medical costs, outpatient visits, investigations, procedures, drug treatment, and domiciliary care. A sensitivity analysis was performed according to variations in cost between 1990 and 1993. A cost-effectiveness ratio (CER) was calculated by dividing the total cost for each patient by the number of days the patient was alive. Quality of life was not taken into account in the primary analysis but was examined separately. Patients allocated to the EP-guided strategy were treated with antiarrhythmic drug therapy first, followed, if necessary, by either catheter ablation or mapguided surgery, and progressing to late ICD implantation if these methods failed to control the arrhythmias. Median follow-up was less for the EP-guided group (676 days) than for the ICD group (871 days) as a result of the higher survival rate in the ICD group. By the end of the study, more than half of the EP-guided patients went on to ICD implantation. Median total costs per patient were higher in the early ICD group during the first 3 months of follow-up; after this point, however, therapy in the EP-guided group was more costly. Patients remaining on antiarrhythmic drugs as sole therapy had the lowest total costs but the highest mortality. The cost of the device, implantation surgery, and hospitalization were the primary contributors to total costs per patient for both strategies. The study found that the early ICD strategy was more cost effective than the EP-guided strategy ($63 versus $94 per patient-day alive). Taking quality-of-life aspects into account enhanced the CER of the ICD even further, while pulse generator replacements and sensitivity analysis for the year of the study did not significantly diminish the CER. The study was performed largely at a time (1990–1993) that transthoracic ICDs were standard. It is likely that improvement in ICD technology such as reduction in generator size, change to transvenous implantation, improved device longevity, and a reduced peri-implantation hospitalization time would result in further improvements in CER. The authors in 1996[26] performed an analysis making the above assumptions, projecting their study to include 1996–2000 as the hypothetical follow-up period. A cost reduction of $11,530 per patient was calculated, and a decrease in the CER to $54 per patient-day alive was estimated. It is noteworthy that both this study and the study by Owen et al. found that when a strategy is used of electrophysiologically guided/antiarrhythmic drug therapy followed later by ICD implantation as necessary, a marked reduction in cost efficacy is the result.

## Costs per Patient for Survivors of Cardiac Arrest Post-MI Managed with Either Early ICD Implantation or EP-Guided Strategy (Figure 2)

The MADIT investigators included a detailed cost-effectiveness analysis as a part of their study, and this represents the first such analysis on the use of the ICD as primary preventive therapy.[27] The data acquisition was prospective and detailed; however, importantly, it did not com-

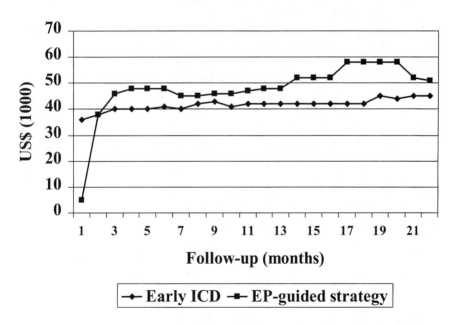

Figure 2. Medians of costs per patient at monthly intervals for survivors of cardiac arrest post-MI managed either with early ICD implantation or an EP-guided strategy. Note that while early ICD implantation was more expensive in the first 3 months, subsequent to this, the EP-guided strategy became the more expensive option. (Adapted with permission from Wever EF, et al.[25])

mence until after patients had been recruited, hence eliminating what must have been substantial costs associated with the lengthy screening process. Initial inpatient costs and subsequent emergency room visits were calculated from patient and physician bills from Medicare rates. Outpatient costs were calculated by adding the cost of reported visits, medication, and services. Costs (within 4 years) assumed a discount rate of 3% per year and the difference between the 2 arms of the trial was calculated. The incremental cost-effectiveness ratio (iCER) was calculated by dividing this value by the discounted years of life saved and represents the extra cost incurred to save 1 year of life within 4 years for the patients randomized to ICD rather than conventional therapy. As expected, the average initial costs were higher in the ICD group. Average monthly costs following this, however, had a tendency to be higher in the conventional treatment arm, and monthly medication costs were significantly higher. The iCER was calculated to be $27,000 per life-year saved, a value that can be seen as representing reasonable cost-effective therapy. Sensitivity analyses taking technological advances into account were also performed. The cost of transvenous ICDs was $6,600 less than transthoracic devices, resulting in a further improvement of the iCER to $22,800 per life-year saved. Eighteen of the 89 patients in the ICD group required a generator change. Assuming an improvement in generator longevity to >4 years improved iCER to $12,500 per life-year. Lowering the cost of the device by 25% and 50% reduced the iCER quite dramatically to $13,100 or $3,300 per life-year, respectively. Patients from both groups who crossed over therapies were also accounted for, resulting in a slight increase in cost. Assuming a reduction in cost of the device along with the exclusive use of transvenous devices, the estimated iCER over a period of 8 years would be approximately $10,000 per life-year. Estimating that 16,000 individuals would meet MADIT criteria annually in the United States, and assuming an average of 2 years of life saved, the authors calculate an annual extra cost of $320 million for 32,000 years of life saved annually.

Cost-effectiveness data from the AVID trial have not been fully published; however, a preliminary analysis has been published in abstract form.[28] Hospital charges for up to 3 years (mean follow-up was 18 months) were collected prospectively on all 1,407 patients and were fully analyzed in 1,230 patients. Average charges at 3 years were $27,580 more for the ICD group than for the antiarrhythmic drug group. Because AVID showed a 2. 9-month survival advantage (0.24 years), cost of the ICD compared to antiarrhythmic drugs was $27,580 X 0.24 and was thus calculated to be $114,917 per year of life saved. The AVID trial was, however, terminated early and the survival curves were continuing to diverge at the time that the trial was terminated, thus survival benefit is likely to be greater and cost effectiveness more favorable than calculated.

Since the patient group in AVID had already suffered life-threatening ventricular arrhythmia, they were probably at similar (if not higher) risk than patients in the MADIT study, which was a primary prevention study. The difference in terms of cost effectiveness between MADIT and AVID ($27,000 vs. $114,917 per life-year saved) may, therefore, at first glance seem to be an inconsistency. There are several differences between both the original trials and the methods of cost-effectiveness analysis that may explain this paradox. Patients receiving antiarrhythmic drugs in AVID had a lower mortality rate (approximately 25%) at 3 years than patients receiving antiarrhythmic drugs in MADIT (approximately 40%), while the mortality rate in both ICD groups was similar. Thus the incremental benefit of the ICD over antiarrhythmic drugs was higher in MADIT than in AVID, and it may therefore be expected that the ICD would prove to be more cost effective. Patients entering MADIT had inducible ventricular arrhythmias that had not been suppressed by antiarrhythmic drugs, and therefore the high mortality in the antiarrhythmic drug group in this trial could be expected. Furthermore, the cost of the extensive screening tests in the MADIT group was not taken into account in the cost analysis, and thus total costs were higher than reported. Finally, due to the fact that the MADIT study was empowered to assess the impact of the ICD on mortality and not cost effectiveness, subsequent numbers were small and confidence intervals were broad.

## Sudden Cardiac Death among Population Subgroups (Figure 3)

In patients who have not experienced a major arrhythmic event, the cost of screening tests is also important in determining the cost effectiveness of therapy. While relatively inexpensive tests such as echocardiography do provide some information, more expensive tests such as EP studies are presently required to define a high-risk group in whom ICD therapy is cost effective. It is noteworthy that in patients who have survived SCD, preimplantation EP studies have been shown to reduce cost effectiveness.[23,25] Noninvasive tests such as heart rate variability (HRV), baroreceptor sensitivity, and SAECG have yet to make their mark as standard clinical screening tools. However, future studies on ICD efficacy will be using novel clinical tests such as HRV as screening tools. Other ongoing primary prevention trials include the SCD-HeFT trial, which is comparing ICD and amiodarone therapy in patients with heart failure. The new trials are likely to have the effect of increasing implantation rates even further, and will raise additional questions regarding cost efficacy, particularly since the magnitude of risk of the study population will tend to fall.

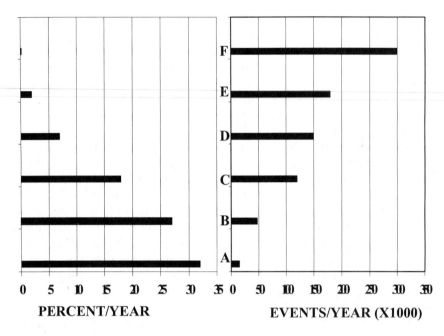

**Figure 3.** Sudden cardiac death among population subgroups. Estimates for incidence (percent per year) and total number of sudden cardiac deaths per year for the United States and for higher risk subgroups: A = patients in the convalescent phase having had VT/VF post-MI; B = survivors of out-of-hospital cardiac arrest; C = patients with heart failure (EF<30%); D = patients who had any prior cardiac event; E = patients at high risk of sustaining a cardiac event; F = overall incidence in the adult population. Note that as risk in a subgroup rises, the total number of SCD cases in the general population that the subgroup represents falls. (Adapted with permission from Myerberg RJ, et al.[29])

Device longevity has been consistently shown to improve cost efficacy of the ICD, and it might be expected that technological advances will result in an improvement in longevity and a decrease in cost. However, coincident with such advances are an increasing number of features being incorporated into modern devices including dual chamber pacing and telemetric facilities, which will have the effect of reducing longevity and increasing costs. The cost of the device itself is a significant determinant of the overall cost effectiveness, and the combined effects of technological improvement and market forces are likely to reduce the overall cost of ICD therapy significantly. Many of the above studies were performed at a time that epicardial ICD implantation was routinely performed, and transvenous implantation was a novel development. Several studies have demonstrated that transvenous ICD implantation is more cost effective than the epicardial method, and as this method has become standard, it will be associated with a more favorable cost efficacy than is quoted.

## Conclusion

The potential for the ICD to effectively reduce mortality in a variety of patient groups has been demonstrated. Most studies suggest that ICD therapy costs from between $17,000 to $40,000 per year of life saved. This is comparable to other therapies such as hemodialysis and some cases of CABG. As discussed, cost effectiveness of the ICD depends to a large extent on the degree of risk of the patients in question. Whereas for the highest risk groups (e.g., survivors of non-MI SCD with a low EF), the ICD appears to be reasonably cost effective, in low-risk groups (e.g., patients with ICD, a normal EF, and noninducible VT), the ICD is unlikely to represent cost-effective therapy at present. Nevertheless, high-risk clinical subgroups do not generate most SCD events within the population. The majority of events in absolute numbers are generated from a relatively lower risk subgroup that is, however, a much larger proportion of the general population.[29] The question as to whether the ICD is cost effective depends on whether the goal is to reduce the incidence of SCD in the population as a whole (in which case the answer is probably no) or whether the goal is to offer a small yet high-risk group of patients effective therapy. One of the dilemmas at this stage is where limits of risk and the limits of expenditure lie. Similar arguments can also be applied to subgroups of patients with a variety of cardiac diseases. For example, patients with cardiomyopathy with relatively preserved functional capacity have lower death rates than those with markedly reduced capacity. However, the fraction of deaths that are sudden in the group with preserved left ventricular function is higher.[29] It should be noted also that the concept of risk is not a static phenomenon since transient and correctable factors such as ischemia, hypoxia, electrolyte disturbances, and drug therapy can play a significant role in the genesis of ventricular arrhythmias in susceptible individuals. Furthermore, survival curves after major cardiac events are nonlinear, with the decrement being steeper in the initial 6–18 months, subsequently leveling out in the ensuing months.[30]

## References

1. Gillum RF. Sudden coronary death in the United States: 1980–1985. Circulation 1989; 79:756–765.
2. Anderson MH, Camm AJ. Implications for present and future applications of the implantable cardioverter-defibrillator resulting from the use of a simple model of cost efficacy. Br Heart J 1993; 69:83–92.
3. Winkle RA, Mead RH, Ruder MA, Gaudiani VA, Smith NA, et al. Long-term

outcome with the automatic implantable cardioverter-defibrillator. J Am Coll Cardiol 1989; 13:1353–1361.

4. Zipes DP, Roberts D, for the Pacemaker-Cardioverter-Defibrillator Trial. Results of the international study of the implantable pacemaker cardioverter-defibrillator: a comparison of epicardial and endocardial lead systems. Circulation 1995; 92:59–65.

5. Weaver WD, Cobb LA, Hallstrom AP, Fahrenbruch C, Copass MK, et al. Factors influencing survival after out-of-hospital cardiac arrest. J Am Coll Cardiol 1986; 7:752–757.

6. Schatzkin A, Cupples LA, Heeren T, Morelock S, Mucatel, et al. The epidemiology of sudden unexpected death: risk factors for men and women in the Framingham Heart Study. Am Heart J 1984; 107:1300–1306.

7. Cobb LA, Baum RS, Alvarez H, Schaffer WA. Resuscitation from out-of-hospital ventricular fibrillation: 4 years follow-up. Circulation 1975; 52:(III)223-(III)235.

8. Liberthson RR, Nagel EL, Hirschman JC, Nussenfeld SR. Prehospital ventricular defibrillation: prognosis and follow-up course. N Engl J Med 1974; 291: 317–321.

9. The Antiarrhythmics Versus Implantable Defibrillators (AVID) Investigators. A comparison of antiarrhythmic drug therapy with implantable defibrillators in patients resuscitated from near-fatal ventricular arrhythmias. N Engl J Med 1997; 337:1576–1583.

10. Moss AJ, Hall WJ, Cannom DS, Daubert JP, Higgins SL, et al. Improved survival with an implanted defibrillator in patients with coronary disease at high risk for ventricular arrhythmia: Multicenter Automatic Defibrillator Implantation Trial Investigators. N Engl J Med 1996; 335:1933–1940.

11. Echt DS, Liebson PR, Mitchell B, Peters RW, Obias-Manno D, et al. , for The Cardiac Arrhythmia Suppression Trial: Mortality and morbidity in patients receiving encainide, flecainide, or placebo. N Engl J Med 1991; 12:781–788.

12. Buxton AE, Lee KL, Fisher JD, Josephson ME, Prystowsky E, et al. A randomized study of the prevention of sudden death in patients with coronary artery disease. N Engl J Med 1999; 341:1882–1890.

13. Bigger JT Jr, for The Coronary Artery Bypass Graft (CABG) Patch Trial Investigators. Prophylactic use of implanted cardiac defibrillators in patients at high risk for ventricular arrhythmias after coronary-artery bypass surgery. N Engl J Med 1997; 337:1569–1575.

14. Every NR, Fahrenbruch CE, Hallstrom AP, Weaver WD, Cobb LA. Influence of coronary bypass surgery on subsequent outcome of patients resuscitated from out of hospital cardiac arrest. J Am Coll Cardiol 1992; 19:1435–1439.

15. Chaitman BR, Fisher LD, Bourassa MG, Davis K, Rogers WJ, et al. Effect of coronary bypass surgery on survival patterns in subsets of patients with left main coronary artery disease: report of the Collaborative Study in Coronary Artery Surgery (CASS). Am J Cardiol 1981; 48:765–777.

16. Kuppermann M, Luce BR, McGovern B, Podrid PJ, Bigger JT Jr, et al. An analysis of the cost effectiveness of the implantable defibrillator. Circulation 1990; 81:91–100.

17. O'Brien M, Buxton, MJ, Rushby JA. Cost effectiveness of the implantable cardioverter-defibrillator: a preliminary analysis. Br Heart J 1992; 68:241–245.

18. Kupersmith J, Hogan A, Guerrero P, Gardiner J, Mellits ED, et al. Evaluating and improving the cost effectiveness of the implantable cardioverter-defibrillator. Am Heart J 1995; 130:507–515.

19. Grimm W, Flores BF, Marchlinski FE. Electrocardiographically documented unnecessary, spontaneous shocks in 241 patients with implantable cardioverter defibrillators. PACE 1992; 15:1667–1673.

20. Neuzner J, Pitschner HF, Konig S, Stohring R, Schlepper M. Stored electrograms in cardioverter/defibrillator therapy: accuracy of rhythm diagnosis in 335 spontaneous arrhythmia episodes. J Ambulatory Monitoring 1995; 1–9.
21. Larsen GC, Manolis AS, Sonnenberg FA, Beshansky JR, Estes N, et al. Cost effectiveness of the implantable cardioverter-defibrillator: effect of improved battery life and comparison with amiodarone therapy. J Am Coll Cardiol 1992; 19:1323–1334.
22. Valenti R, Schlapfer J, Fromer M, Fischer A, Kappenberger L. Impact of the implantable cardioverter-defibrillator on rehospitalizations. Eur Heart J 1996; 17:1565–1571.
23. Owens DK, Sanders GD, Harris RA, McDonald KM, Heidenreich PA, et al. Cost effectiveness of implantable cardioverter defibrillators relative to amiodarone for prevention of sudden cardiac death. Ann Intern Med 1997; 126:1–12.
24. Wever EF, Hauer RN, van Capelle FJ, Tijssen JG, Crijns HJ, et al. Randomized study of implantable defibrillator as first choice therapy versus conventional strategy in postinfarct sudden death survivors. Circulation 1995; 91:2195–2203.
25. Wever EF, Hauer RN, Schrijvers G, van Capelle FJ, Tijssen JG, et al. Cost effectiveness of implantable defibrillator as first-choice therapy versus electrophysiologically guided, tiered strategy in postinfarct sudden death survivors: a randomized study. Circulation 1996; 93:489–496.
26. Hauer RN, Derksen R, Wever EF. Can implantable cardioverter-defibrillator therapy reduce healthcare costs? Am J Cardiol 1996; 78:134–139.
27. Mushlin AI, Hall WJ, Zwanziger J, Gajary E, Andrews M, et al. The cost effectiveness of automatic implantable cardiac defibrillators: results from MADIT: Multicenter Automatic Defibrillator Implantation Trial. Circulation 1998; 97:2129–2135.
28. The Antiarrhythmics Versus Implantable Defibrillators (AVID) Investigators. Hospitalization Charges in the Antiarrhythmics Versus Implantable Defibrillators (AVID) Trial: The AVID Economic Analysis Study. Circulation 1997; 96(Suppl):1–77.
29. Myerburg RJ, Interian A, Mitrani RD, Kessler KM, Castellanos A. Frequency of sudden cardiac death and profiles of risk. Am J Cardiol 1997; 80:(5B),10F-19F.
30. Furukawa T, Rozanski JJ, Nogami A, Moroe K, Gosselin AJ, et al. Time-dependent risk of and predictors for cardiac arrest recurrence in survivors of out-of-hospital cardiac arrest with chronic coronary-artery disease. Circulation 1989; 80:599–608.

# 49

# What Can We Learn From Ongoing Implantable Cardioverter-Defibrillator Trials?

*Martin Fromer, MD*

## Introduction

In the western industrialized world, cardiovascular diseases are the most important causes of death. Congestive heart failure and sudden cardiac death (SCD) are the most frequent manifestations. For several decades, important efforts have been undertaken to reduce cardiovascular death rate, mainly in the form of primary prevention of coronary and hypertensive heart disease or as secondary prevention in patients who were more or less accurately identified to be at high risk.

Beta-blocker trials in postmyocardial infarction (MI) patients and angiotensin converting-enzyme (ACE) inhibitor trials in congestive heart failure patients have shown a beneficial effect on survival of the studied patients. However, antiarrhythmic drug trials using Class Ic drugs or amiodarone or sotalol have shown either a deleterious or at best no effect on total mortality.[1-4] Today, implantable cardioverter-defibrillators (ICDs) can be implanted with almost no perioperative mortality. Observational studies have shown that ICD therapy offers benefit for patients with organic heart disease and a history of sustained ventricular tachycardia (VT) or ventricular fibrillation (VF).[5,6] Since ICD therapy is costly and requires substantial resources in money, time, personnel, specialized knowledge, and infrastructure, the need to base this therapy on rational arguments and scientific evidence has been and is still obvious.[7]

Multicenter ICD trials have been realized to study either the impact of ICD therapy for the prevention of recurrent potentially fatal ventricular tachyarrhythmias (secondary prophylaxis trials) or for prophylaxis of sudden cardiac death in patients screened to be at high risk (primary prophylaxis).

From: Aliot E, Clementy J, Prystowsky EN (editors). *Fighting Sudden Cardiac Death: A Worldwide Challenge.* ©Futura Publishing Company, Armonk, NY, 2000.

# Primary ICD Trials in Postmyocardial Infarction Patients

Patients with old MI and reduced left ventricular ejection fraction (EF) are known to be at high risk for sudden arrhythmic death.[8,9] The trials that studied or are studying patients without a history of sustained VT/VF or cardiac arrest have the following acronyms: MADIT I and II, CABG Patch, MUSTT, DINAMIT, BEST+ICD, IRIS 3, NORDIC 3, SEDET, and for heart failure patients CAT, Pro-ICD, SCD-HeFT, DEFINITE, and PRIDE (Table 1).

## Secondary Prevention Trials

As observational studies have already provided much evidence that ICD therapy is effective in secondary prophylaxis, the design of secondary prevention trials has become more delicate. Already completed studies have the acronyms AVID, CASH, CIDS, and DCS (Table 2).

The AVID trial included patients who had survived VF or had sustained ventricular tachycardia with syncope or sustained VT with EF <40%, or with symptoms of severe hemodynamic compromise.[10,11] The patients were randomized either to ICD or to antiarrhythmic therapy with further randomization to amiodarone versus sotalol. This study was terminated after including 1,016 patients. The ICD group had a 39% reduction in death in the first year, with 27% and 31% reductions in years 2 and 3, respectively. However, subanalysis showed that the benefit was greater

---

### Table 1

### Primary Prevention Trials

| Post-Myocardial Infarction | Cardiomyopathy |
| --- | --- |
| MADIT 1 | Pro-ICD |
| MADIT 2 | SCD-HeFT |
| Best + ICD | PRIDE |
| CABG-Patch | DEFINITE |
| NORDIC | |
| IRIS | |
| SEDET | |
| MUSTT | |
| DINAMIT | |

In PRIDE, patients are also included who presented aborted cardiac arrest or sustained VT, and is in this respect a secondary prevention trial. In MUSTT patients have nonsustained VT.

### Table 2
### Secondary Prevention Trials

AVID
CASH
CIDS

for patients with EF <35% than >35%. The improvement in mortality translates to a mean prolongation in life of only 2.7 months.

Recently, Anderson et al. have published additional data of the AVID registry.[11] This time concerning the patients who were not randomized but who were entered into the register. It shows that patients who did not have severe ventricular dysfunction, but who presented with syncopal VT or unexplained syncope and inducible VT, had a relatively high rate of mortality. Even patients with stable *asymptomatic* VT have a mortality rate similar to patients with symptomatic VT or patients with unexplained syncope. Thus, patients who are considered primarily at low risk had a similar mortality than the high-risk AVID patients.

The Canadian Implantable Defibrillator Study (CIDS) included patients with documented VF or out-of-hospital cardiac arrest, patients with sustained VT and syncope or sustained VT at a rate >150 beats/min, causing presyncope or angina in a patient with EF >35% or unmonitored syncope with subsequent documentation of either spontaneous or induced VT.[12] Patients were randomized either to ICD implantation or to amiodarone. After 3 years of follow-up, patients randomized to the ICD group had a 19.6% relative risk reduction in the primary end-point of all-cause mortality compared to the amiodarone group, a difference that did not reach statistical significance ($p < 0.07$).

The CASH trial was designed as a prospective randomized study comparing ICD therapy with antiarrhythmic drug therapy in patients who have survived a cardiac arrest secondary to a documented sustained ventricular arrhythmia.[13] The primary end-point was total mortality; secondary end-points were SCD and recurrence of cardiac arrest. The antiarrhythmic drugs tested were amiodarone, propafenone, and metoprolol. Propafenone had to be stopped because a significant higher mortality was found in this group compared to the ICD group. The study took almost 10 years to be completed. At the minimum follow-up of 2 years, the all-cause mortality was 19.6% for amiodarone and metoprolol versus 12.1% for the ICD group. This reduction of 37% reached a p value of 0.047. According to an oral communication from Cappato, one of the investigators, there was no difference in the protective effect between amiodarone and metoprolol. Due to the long recruitment time, implantation technique have changed from sternotomy to nonthoracotomy leads and therefore, it is likely that the ICD benefit in the trial was underestimated. Also remarkable is the quite low mortality for the patients treated with amiodarone and metoprolol. The SCD rate in the ICD group was 2% versus 11% in the drug-treated patients (p<0.001).

As neither CASH nor CIDS are published at the time of this review, in-depth analysis of these studies is difficult. In the CIDS trial, the relative risk reduction in the ICD group did not reach statistical significance (25% mortality in the ICD group versus 30% mortality in the amiodarone group; p=0.072). It might be the result of a recruitment of an inhomogeneous patient population with some patients having an unusually good prognosis.

The above-mentioned trials did not investigate ICD therapy in dilated cardiomyopathy patients. The PRIDE trial (Primary Implant of Defibrillators in high risk ventricular arrhythmia) includes patients who suffer from an idiopathic dilated cardiomyopathy with EF <35% and (a) syncope and nonsustained VT or positive signal-averaging electrocardiogram parameters or (b) sustained VT or aborted cardiac arrest. The patients received either immediate ICD therapy or electrophysiologically guided drug therapy. The end-points are all-cause mortality, cost effectiveness, and quality of life. This study is in the enrollment phase. It will give us data on the important patient group with congestive heart failure and it will provide information about the role of electrophysiological (EP) studies in a patient group in which EP studies were considered to give unreliable results, and it will give information as to whether ICD therapy had a beneficial effect on total mortality and not only on arrhythmic mortality in these patients.

The Sudden Cardiac Death in Heart Failure trial (SCD-HeFT) includes patients with a left ventricular EF <35% and ischemic or nonischemic cardiomyopathy, NYHA class II or III (Figure 1). The patients are treated with appropriate ACE inhibitor therapy and have no history of sustained VT or VF.[14] Three treatment arms will be randomized, consisting of placebo and best congestive heart failure therapy, amiodarone and congestive heart failure therapy, and ICD plus congestive heart failure therapy. End-points are all-cause mortality, quality of life, cost effectiveness, morbidity, and incidence of VT or VF. The SCD-HeFT study has a protected sample size of 2,500 patients divided into 3 groups. The study started in 1997. This study looks at SCD and total mortality in symptomatic cardiac dysfunction patients who do not present any specific marker for a high arrhythmogenic risk. It will define whether there is an indication for prophylactic ICD therapy in these patients who do not present an arrhythmogenic profile. This will provide data about the role of amiodarone or ICD in combination with the best anticongestive heart failure therapy and it will give insight into the prognosis of congestive heart failure either based on coronary artery disease or idiopathic disease. MADIT II, discussed later, does not require symptomatic congestive heart failure patients and enrolls only coronary artery disease patients.

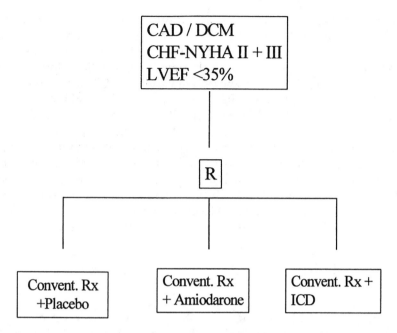

Figure 1. SCD-HeFT patient enrollment.

In the Defibrillator in Non-Ischemic Cardiomyopathy Treatment Evaluation (DEFINITE) trial, the arrhythmogenic risk profile is more evident than in the SCD-HeFT or MADIT II study. Patients with nonischemic cardiomyopathy, EF <35%, and with a history of symptomatic heart failure and nonsustained VT or over 10 premature ventricular contractions/hour are included. The patients are randomized to standard therapy including beta blockers or standard therapy, beta blockers and ICD therapy. All-cause mortality, quality of life, and cost effectiveness are endpoints. The study enrollment might be finished in the year 2000. This study will define the role of beta blockers in congestive heart failure, the contribution of ICD on survival, and the role of premature ventricular contractions in risk stratification.

## Coronary Artery Disease Patients and Primary Prophylaxis

MADIT I trial is followed by the MADIT II study.[14] It includes again coronary artery disease patients with MI and ventricular EF <30%. The arrhythmic risk profile is less evident than in MADIT I. Ventricular arrhythmias on Holter or EP testing for inclusion are not required. The patients do not need clinical symptoms of heart failure. Patients are randomized to ICD versus no ICD therapy. In the no ICD arm, patients are treated with ACE inhibitors and beta blockers. The patients in the ICD arm have programmed ventricular stimulation at the time of implantation. Holter, signal-averaged electrocardiograms, heart rate variability, QT dispersion, and T wave alternans are obtained after randomization. The trial will follow all patients who were eligible but not enrolled. End-points of the study are overall mortality; secondary end-points are the significance of programmed ventricular stimulation and induction of VTs in this type of patient, the role of noninvasive risk assessment, and outcome of screened but not enrolled patients. Inclusion is based solely on cardiac dysfunction post MI, and no symptoms of heart failure are required. It will disclose whether the ICD has any benefit (or harm) in such a patient population that has not been specifically selected with respect to ventricular arrhythmias.

## Best + ICD Trial

The Beta-blocker Strategy + Implantable Cardioverter Defibrillator trial (Figure 2) is a multicenter European study involving mainly centers from Italy and Germany.[15] It tests the hypothesis of whether, in high-risk post-MI patients who are already treated with beta blockers, EP-guided therapy including implantation of ICDs improves survival. Involved are patients who had a recent MI (from 5 to 21 days), left ventricular EF of <35%, and a presence of at least 1 additional risk factor such as premature ventricular contractions >10/hour, abnormal signal-averaging electrocardiogram, or reduced heart rate variability. In addition, patients must tolerate metoprolol to a maximal dose of $2 \times 100$ mg/day. The patients are randomized to either beta blockers and conventional post-MI therapy or to an EP study arm. The patients who are inducible are then randomized to the beta blockers and conventional therapy arm or to ICD therapy plus beta blockers and conventional therapy. Patients who fulfill the MADIT study criteria are excluded from this study. The end-points are all-cause mortality, arrhythmic death, and cost effectiveness. The study also addresses the significance of various noninvasive risk parameters such as heart rate variability, premature ventricular contractions, and late potentials, as well as the role of early ventricular programmed stimulation in these patients. All of the patients who are screened but finally not enrolled in the study are entered into a register for later analysis.

## The DINAMIT Study

The Defibrillator in Acute Myocardial Infarction Trial is looking at a similar patient population. Patients with a recent MI (6 to 31 days) who

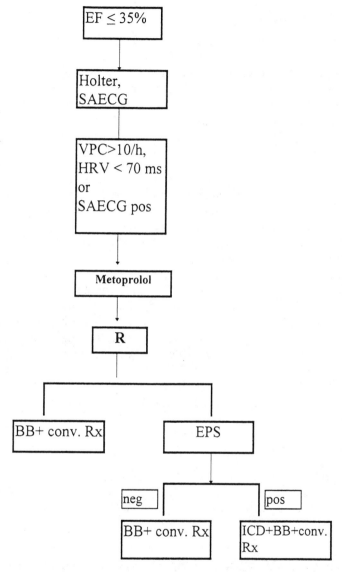

Figure 2. Best + ICD trial patient enrollment.

have a left ventricular EF of <35% and who present either abnormal heart rate variability or a mean heart rate >80 beats/min are randomized to either standard therapy or standard therapy and ICD. This study includes centers from Europe and Canada. The end-points are all-cause mortality, quality of life, and cost effectiveness.

## IRIS

The IRIS study (Immediate Risk Stratification Improves Survival) includes patients with recent MI (5 to 21 days) with short runs of VT or a mean heart rate >100 beats/min and an EF <40% at admission to the hospital. The patients are randomized to conventional therapy or ICD therapy. Conventional therapy includes ACE inhibitors and beta blockers. It has the same end-points as the previously mentioned study.

## The MUSTT Trial

Multicenter Unsustained Tachycardia Trial has included patients from 85 US and Canadian centers. The study investigates whether antiarrhythmic therapy guided by EP study can decrease the risk of arrhythmic death and cardiac arrest in patients with nonsustained VT and EF <40% and coronary artery disease.[16]

If the patients had inducible VT, they were randomized to either ACE inhibitor therapy and beta blockers or EP-guided antiarrhythmic treatment. The patients who have induced sustained VT will be randomized to either serial EP study or to no-antiarrhythmic therapy. Noninduced patients will be followed in a separate database. Serial drug testing includes several antiarrhythmic drugs or combinations. At least 2 drug trials must be performed before amiodarone is started. If no antiarrhythmic drug is found that renders the tachycardia noninducible, the patient will be discharged on the best choice. If no improvement can be found, the patient receives an ICD.

## The SEDET Trial

South European Defibrillator Trial includes patients with a recent MI, not thrombolyzed, with an EF >40%, and nonsustained VT or >10 premature ventricular contractions/hour. They are randomized to ICD or best conventional therapy.

# What Will We Learn From Those Ongoing Studies?

The ongoing trials address new patient groups (Table 3). Cardiomyopathy patients are included in the SCD-HeFT trial and in the DEFINITE trial. The SCD-HeFT will therefore give some information as to whether ICD therapy has to be recommended in NYHA Class II and III patients. On the other hand, the DEFINITE trial excludes ischemic cardiomyopathy but includes patients with a history of symptomatic heart failure and nonsus-

## Table 3

### Patient Characteristics Included in the Various Trials

| Recent Myocardial Infarction | Old Myocardial Infarction | Congestive Heart Failure, Cardiomyopathy |
|---|---|---|
| Best + ICD | MADIT | PRIDE |
| DINAMIT | MUSTT | SCD-HeFT |
| IRIS | | DEFINITE |
| SEDET | | |

tained VTs or >10 premature ventricular contractions/hour and therefore enrolls a group of patients considered to be at high risk for arrhythmogenic death. The treatment arm will define the role of beta blockers as well as the combination of beta blockers with an ICD in this type of patients. However, it cannot answer the contribution of an ICD alone.

Various primary ICD trials will help to define the value of noninvasive risk stratification. Signal-averaging electrocardiograms and heart rate variability are tested in the BEST + ICD trial. Similar, in the DINAMITE study, patients with decreased heart rate variability or increased sinus rate are included. In MADIT II, similar parameters are measured post randomization (Table 4).

Since MADIT I enrolled a highly selected post-MI patient population, MADIT II will enlarge the recruitment, since for enrollment there is no risk stratification by Holter recording and EP studies required. In MADIT II, the single most important enrollment criterion is an EF <30%. It will also allow comparison between programmed ventricular stimulation and noninvasive risk parameters on prediction of device use and mortality.

## Table 4

### Trials that Evaluate Noninvasive Risk Parameters

| Study | Patients | Parameters |
|---|---|---|
| MADIT 2 | old MI | post randomization: SAECG, T wave dispersion HRV |
| PRIDE | CMP | VT, syncope or SAECG |
| Best + ICD | recent MI | HRV, SAECG, PVC |
| DINAMIT | recent MI | HRV, SR>80 b/min |
| NORDIC | acute MI | HRV |

HRV = heart rate variability; SAECG = signal-averaging ECG (late potentials); MI = myocardial infarction; PVC = premature ventricular contraction.

The MUSTT trial studies the role of antiarrhythmic therapy guided by EP studies in patients with coronary artery disease, asymptomatic non-sustained VT and EF <40%. For randomization, the patients had to be inducible. The patients who received no antiarrhythmic therapy received standard therapy. Therefore, the study provides a comparison between ICD therapy and EP-guided antiarrhythmic drug therapy in nonsustained VT patients. According to preliminary results, there is a significant reduction in SCD in the patients treated with an ICD compared to patients treated with EP-guided antiarrhythmic drug therapy.

On the other hand, the SEDET trial looks at high-risk patients who had extended MI and high ventricular instability on Holter. It goes back to the basic question of whether ICDs still improve outcome in such a patient population.

There is a substantial variability in the history of the patients that are included into the various trials. Severe arrhythmias must be present in the the CIDS, CASH, and AVID trials. An intermediate profile is asked in the MUSTT trial with patients showing asymptomatic nonsustained VT. Arrhythmias do not have to be documented in MADIT II. Noninvasive risk parameters are tested in the DINAMIT, CABG Patch, and BEST + ICD trials. Concerning underlying heart disease, the studies will now look at cardiomyopathy patients as in the PRIDE, SCD-HeFT, and DEFINITE trials, or at patients who have a recent MI as in the SEDET, IRIS, DINAMITE, and BEST + ICD trials. In the past, ICD therapy has been compared mainly to amiodarone or sotalol therapy. In IRIS, beta blockers are used in the conventional therapy arm, as well as in BEST + ICD, MADIT II.

In some trials, the included arrhythmia profile is quite varied. In PRIDE, patients have either nonsustained VTs or a history of aborted cardiac arrest, in DEFINITE either nonsustained VTs or premature ventricular contractions. Subgroup analysis will therefore provide further information how to weigh these arrhythmias in these patients. Finally, we hope to tailor the therapy to the individual patient, since we do not treat a group at risk, but an individual person.

## References

1. Ruskin JN. The Cardiac Arrhythmia Suppression Trial (CAST). N Engl J Med 1989; 321:386–388.
2. Julian DG, Camm AJ, Frangin G, Janse MJ, Munoz A, et al, for the European Myocardial Infarct Amiodarone Trial Investigators. Randomised trial of effect of amiodarone on mortality in patients with left-ventricular dysfunction after recent myocardial infarction: EMIAT. Lancet 1997; 349:667–673.
3. Cairns JA, Connolly SJ, Roberts R, Gent M. Randomised trial of outcome after myocardial infarction in patients with frequent or repetitive ventricular premature depolarisations: CAMIAT. The Lancet 1997; 349:675–682.

4. Zipes DP. Atrial fibrillation: a tachycardia-induced atrial cardiomyopathy. Circulation 1997; 95:562–564.
5. Fromer M, Brachmann J, Block M, Siebels J, Hoffman E, et al. Efficacy of automatic multimodal device therapy for ventricular tachyarrhythmias as delivered by a new implantable pacing cardioverter-defibrillator: results of a European multicenter study incorporating 102 implants. Circulation 1992; 86:363–374.
6. Böcker D, Bänsch D, Heinecke A, Weber M, Brunn J, et al. Potential benefit from implantable cardioverter-defibrillator therapy in patients with and without heart failure. Circulation 1998; 98:1636–1643.
7. Kuppermann M, Luce BR, McGovern B, Podrid PJ, Bigger JT Jr, et al. Analysis of the cost effectiveness of the implantable defibrillator. Circulation 1990; 81:91–100.
8. Bigger JT Jr. Identification of patients at high risk of sudden cardiac death. Am J Cardiol 1984; 54:3D–8D.
9. Pierard LA, Chapelle JP, Dubois C, Kulbertus HE. Characteristics associated with early (<3 months) versus late (>3 months to <3 years) mortality after acute myocardial infarction. Am J Cardiol 1989; 64:315–318.
10. Bigger JT Jr. Prophylactic use of implanted cardiac defibrillators in patients at high risk for ventricular arrhythmias after coronary bypass graft surgery. N Engl J Med 1997; 337:1569–1575.
11. Anderson JL, Hallstrom A, Epstein AE, Pinski SL, Rosenberg Y, et al., and AVID Investigators. Design and results of the antiarrhythmics vs implantable defibrillators (AVID) registry. Circulation 1999; 99:1692–1699.
12. Connolly SJ, Gent M, Roberts RS, Dorian P, Green MS, et al. Canadian implantable defibrillator study (CIDS): study design and organisation. Am J Cardiol 1993; 72:103F–108F.
13. Cappato R. Secondary prevention trials of sudden death: the Dutch study, the antiarrythmic versus implantable defibrillator trial, the cardiac arrest study Hamburg, and the Canadian implantable defibrillator study. Am J Cardiol 1999; 83:68D–73D.
14. Klein H, Auricchio A, Reek S, Geller C. New primary prevention trials of sudden cardiac death in patients with left ventricular dysfunction: SCD-HeFT and MADIT-II. Am J Cardiol 1999; 83:91D–97D.
15. Raviele A, Bongiorni MG, Brignole M, Cappato R, Capucci A, et al. Which strategy is "best" after myocardial infarction? The beta blocker strategy plus implantable cardioverter defibrillator trial: rationale and study design. Am J Cardiol 1999; 83:104D–111D.
16. Buxton AE, Lee KL, DiCarlo L, Echt DS, Fisher JD, et al. Nonsustained ventricular tachycardia in coronary artery disease: relation to inducible sustained ventricular tachycardia. Annals Intern Med 1996; 125:35–39.

# 50
# The Future:
# A Hybrid Therapy

### Sanjeev Saksena, MD

## Introduction

The recent publication of a series of clinical trials in patients with symptomatic ventricular arrhythmias has prompted a rush to judgment favoring defibrillator therapy in these populations.[1,2] A more circumspect viewpoint has existed until recently with respect to primary prevention of sudden death with implantable defibrillators. Until the publication of the results of the MUSTT study, the MADIT population was considered as a very small select group in the postmyocardial infarction pool.[3,4] Now, a larger subgroup identified by nonsustained ventricular tachycardia (VT) and varying degrees of ventricular dysfunction is being targeted for device therapy. Many new nuances have emerged in carefully examining trial data. These will be examined in this chapter and the benefits of increasing hybridization of antiarrhythmic therapy will be critically appraised.

## Scrutinizing the Trials

The benefits of the implantable cardioverter-defibrillator (ICD) in the AVID study have been subjected to subgroup analysis.[5] In a recent report, we have noted that the benefits of defibrillator therapy were almost exclusively seen in the patients with a left ventricular ejection fraction <36%. There was no survival advantage in patients with better ejection fractions, and amiodarone remains an option in these patients. Benefit was also diluted in older patients, and in VT patients, but the study was not sufficiently powered to make a definitive statement in this regard. In observational studies, heart failure class has had a significant impact on the benefits of ICD therapy. Bocker and co-workers have reported a decrease in survival benefit with progression from Class I to III heart failure in pa-

From: Aliot E, Clementy J, Prystowsky EN (editors). *Fighting Sudden Cardiac Death: A Worldwide Challenge.* ©Futura Publishing Company, Armonk, NY, 2000.

tients with symptomatic ventricular arrhythmias.[6] It is reasonable to conclude from such analyses that ICDs offer clear survival benefits in certain subgroups of patients with ventricular arrhythmias and remain an important first-line therapeutic option for many others.

Indicators of morbidity such as quality of life are less likely to improve remarkably in these patients. In the AVID study, quality-of-life measures of physical and mental health improved only slightly over the first year with ICDs.[7-9] Antiarrhythmic drugs were often added. Of 470 patients who were discharged with an ICD alone, antiarrhythmic drug therapy was added in 87 patients at an average interval of 162 days. The most common reasons for the crossover included frequent ICD discharges, recurrent VT/ventricular fibrillation, and atrial arrhythmias. There were significant rehospitalization rates in this study. After implantation, the average time to readmission of an ICD patient was approximately 8 months. During a 3-year period of follow-up, these patients accumulated $31,000 in health care charges. Limitations on physical activity imposed by the arrhythmias are not invariably lifted by the implantation of a defibrillator. Most patients are forbidden to drive for 3 to 6 months until the pattern and symptoms associated with arrhythmia recurrence and therapy are defined. In a German study, 20% of patients never returned to driving because of fear or other reasons, 10% experienced device discharges while driving, and 5% had accidents but these were usually unrelated to device therapy.[10]

## A Rationale for Hybrid Therapy

The rationale for hybrid therapy derives from these observations that suggest that ICDs impact survival more than morbidity, combination therapy is often necessary to improve morbidity, and the costs of ICD therapy used nonjudiciously remain daunting even in affluent healthcare systems. There may even be a role for an improved survival hypothesis from existing data with hybrid therapy. In an interesting observation from the AVID registry, patients receiving a combination of antiarrhythmic drug and ICD therapy had survival rates similar to those receiving ICD monotherapy.[11] However, upon adjusting for disease state and arrhythmia variables, the former group would be expected to have inferior outcomes, thus, either hybrid therapy improved survival or monotherapy patients were at increased cardiovascular risk and could have benefited from drug therapy.

Other nonarrhythmic therapies may improve survival. These include angiotensin-converting enzyme (ACE) inhibitors or beta blockers for treatment of concomitant heart failure, HMG coenzyme A reductase inhibitors for coronary patients, antiplatelet agents in patients with prior myocardial infarction, and revascularization in patients with obstructive coronary artery disease. In the carvidelol and CIBIS II studies, these beta blockers reduced all-cause mortality as well as sudden death mortality in patients with heart failure.[12,13] In another subgroup analysis from AVID, Exner et al. showed that beta blocker use was independently associated with improved survival in patients with ventricular fibrillation or symptomatic VT who were not treated with specific antiarrhythmic drug therapy, but a protective effect was not obvious in patients already receiving amiodarone or the ICD.[14] The former was seen in the registry patients who did not receive amiodarone or the ICD.

Morbidity can be reduced with combination therapy. In a prospective randomized clinical trial, *d-l* sotalol in combination with a defibrillator reduced the frequency of defibrillator therapy and increased the time to first therapy significantly.[15] This can translate into fewer mental concerns and physical intolerance for combination antiarrhythmic therapy, perhaps improving quality of life. It may also lift some limitations on resumption of physical activity and driving based on a lesser frequency of need for ICD therapy. Finally, it could reduce rehospitalization rates and follow-up costs associated with recurrent arrhythmias and frequent ICD shocks. In our own experience, the elderly patient is likely to experience earlier defibrillator discharge.[16] These very patients also experience the greatest limitations of physical activity. For them, combination therapy may be especially advantageous. Azimilide may modify certain types of arrhythmic events in defibrillator patients, impacting on the need for antitachycardia pacing but not on overall event rates in early analyses (Procter & Gamble, data on file).

## Future Directions

New avenues in antiarrhythmic and other cardiovascular therapies may offer new directions in hybrid approaches. The extent of efficacy and safety of this evolving approach needs to be critically assessed. Mapping and ablation of ventricular tachycardia is rapidly progressing and could potentially reduce the need for drug and/or device therapy. Schilling et al. utilized noncontact mapping and could delineate the complete circuit in VT in 17 of 24 patients, the exit site in 80 of 81 VTs, and the diastolic limb in 36% of mapping VTs.[17] This improved localization translated into effective radiofrequency ablation of VT in 14 patients. Two target VTs recurred and 5 new VTs emerged during an 18-month follow-up. Nonarrhythmic therapy may have a role in hybrid therapy. Autonomic manipulation, heart failure therapy, and preventive therapy for ventricular dysfunction and coronary disease may also be important partners in an antiarrhythmic regimen.

## References

1. The Antiarrhythmics Versus Implantable Defibrillators (AVID Investigators. A comparison of antiarrhythmic drug therapy with implantable defibrillators in patients resuscitated from near-fatal ventricular arrhythmias. N Engl J Med 1997; 337:1575–1583.
2. Siebels J, Kuck K-H, and the CASH Investigators. Implantable cardioverter defibrillator compared with antiarrhythmic drug treatment in cardiac arrest survivors (the Cardiac Arrest Study Hamburg). Am Heart J 1994; 127(Suppl): 1139–1144.
3. Moss AJ, Hall WJ, Cannom DS, et al. Improved survival with an implanted defibrillator in patients with coronary artery disease at high risk for ventricular arrhythmia. N Eng J Med 1996; 335:1933–1940.
4. Buxton A, for the MUSTT Investigators. Presentation at clinical trial sessions, American College of Cardiology, March 1999.
5. Domanski MJ, Saksena S, Epstein AE, et al. Relative effectiveness of the implantable cardioverter-defibrillator and antiarrhythmic drugs in patients with varying degrees of left ventricular dysfunction who have survived malignant ventricular arrhythmias. J Am Coll Cardiol (in press).
6. Bocker D, Bansch D, Heinecke A, et al. Potential benefit from implantable cardioverter-defibrillator therapy in patients with or without heart failure. Circulation 1998; 98:1636–1643.
7. Steinberg JS, Martins JB, Domanski M, et al. Antiarrhythmic drug use in the implantable defibrillator arm of the Antiarrhythmics vs. Implantable Defibrillators (AVID) study (abstract). J Am Coll Cardiol 1998; 31(Suppl A):514A.
8. Jenkins LS, Steinberg J, Kutalek SP, et al. Quality of life in patients enrolled in the Antiarrhythmics Versus Implantable Defibrillators (AVID) trial (abstract). Circulation 1997; 96(I):I–439.
9. Larsen GC, McAnulty JH, Hallstrom A, et al. Hospitalization charges in the Antiarrhythmics Versus Implantable Defibrillators (AVID) trial: the AVID economic analysis study (abstract). Circulation 1997; 96(I):I–77.
10. Trappe H-J, Wenzlaff P, Grellmann G. Should patients with implantable cardioverter-defibrillators be allowed to drive? Observations in 291 patients from a single center over an 11-year period. J Intervent Cardiac Electrophysiol 1998; 2:193–201.
11. Beckman KJ, Klein RC, Page RL, et al. Effect of antiarrhythmic therapy on survival in patients with ventricular tachycardia or fibrillation in the Antiarrhythmics vs Implantable Defibrillators (AVID) trial registry (abstract). Circulation 1997; 96(I):I–335.
12. Packer M, Bristow MR, Cohn J, et al. The effect of carvedilol on morbidity and mortality in patients with chronic heart failure. N Engl J Med 1996; 334: 1349–1355.
13. The Cardiac Insufficiency Bisoprolol Investigators and Committees. Cardiac Insufficiency Bisoprolol Study (CIBIS II); a randomized trial. Lancet 1999; 353:9–13.
14. Exner DV, Reiffel JA, Epstein AE, et al. Beta blocker use and survival in ventricular fibrillation or symptomatic ventricular tachycardia. The Antiarrhythmics Versus Implantable Defibrillators (AVID) trial. J Am Coll Cardiol 1999; 34:325–333.
15. Pacifico A, Hohnloser SH, Williams JH, et al., for the d,l-Sotalol Implantable Cardioverter-Defibrillator Study Group. Prevention of implantable defibrillator shocks by treatment with sotalol. N Engl J Med 1999; 340:1855–1862.

16. Saksena S, Mathew P, Giorgberidze I, et al. Implantable defibrillator therapy for the elderly. Am J Geriatric Cardiol 1998; 7:11–34.
17. Schilling RJ, Peters NS, Davies DW. Feasibility of a non-contact catheter for endocardial mapping of human ventricular tachycardia. Circulation 1999; 99:2543–2552.

# Index